Aquaphotomics—Exploring Water Molecular Systems in Nature

Aquaphotomics—Exploring Water Molecular Systems in Nature

Editors

Roumiana Tsenkova
Jelena Muncan

MDPI • Basel • Beijing • Wuhan • Barcelona • Belgrade • Manchester • Tokyo • Cluj • Tianjin

Editors

Roumiana Tsenkova
Graduate School of Agriculture Sciences
Kobe University
Japan

Jelena Muncan
Graduate School of Agriculture Sciences
Kobe University
Japan

Editorial Office
MDPI
St. Alban-Anlage 66
4052 Basel, Switzerland

This is a reprint of articles from the Special Issue published online in the open access journal *Molecules* (ISSN 1420-3049) (available at: https://www.mdpi.com/journal/molecules/special_issues/Water_Molecular).

For citation purposes, cite each article independently as indicated on the article page online and as indicated below:

LastName, A.A.; LastName, B.B.; LastName, C.C. Article Title. *Journal Name* **Year**, *Volume Number*, Page Range.

ISBN 978-3-0365-7118-8 (Hbk)
ISBN 978-3-0365-7119-5 (PDF)

Contents

About the Editors ix

Preface to "Aquaphotomics—Exploring Water Molecular Systems in Nature" xi

Jelena Muncan and Roumiana Tsenkova
Aquaphotomics—Exploring Water Molecular Systems in Nature
Reprinted from: *Molecules* **2023**, *28*, 2630, doi:10.3390/molecules28062630 1

Jean-Michel Roger, Alexandre Mallet and Federico Marini
Preprocessing NIR Spectra for Aquaphotomics
Reprinted from: *Molecules* **2022**, *27*, 6795, doi:10.3390/molecules27206795 11

Yan Sun, Wensheng Cai and Xueguang Shao
Chemometrics: An Excavator in Temperature-Dependent Near- Infrared Spectroscopy
Reprinted from: *Molecules* **2022**, *27*, 452, doi:10.3390/molecules27020452 29

Niangen Ye, Sheng Zhong, Zile Fang, Haijun Gao, Zhihua Du, Heng Chen, Lu Yuan and Tao Pan
Performance Improvement of NIR Spectral Pattern Recognition from Three Compensation Models' Voting and Multi-Modal Fusio
Reprinted from: *Molecules* **2022**, *27*, 4485, doi:10.3390/molecules27144485 41

Xiaoyu Cui
Water as a Probe for Standardization of Near-Infrared Spectra by Mutual–Individual Factor Analysis
Reprinted from: *Molecules* **2022**, *27*, 6069, doi:10.3390/molecules27186069 59

Ettore Maggiore, Matteo Tommasini and Paolo Maria Ossi
Raman Spectroscopy- Based Assessment of the Liquid Water Content in Snow
Reprinted from: *Molecules* **2022**, *27*, 626, doi:10.3390/molecules27030626 73

Aleksandar Stoilov, Jelena Muncan, Kiyoko Tsuchimoto, Nakanishi Teruyaki, Shogo Shigeoka and Roumiana Tsenkova
Pilot Aquaphotomic Study of the Effects of Audible Sound on Water Molecular Structure
Reprinted from: *Molecules* **2022**, *27*, 6332, doi:10.3390/molecules27196332 85

Vanessa Moll, Krzysztof B. Beć, Justyna Grabska and Christian W. Huck
Investigation of Water Interaction with Polymer Matrices by Near-Infrared (NIR) Spectroscopy
Reprinted from: *Molecules* **2022**, *27*, 5882, doi:10.3390/molecules27185882 107

Shoichi Maeda, Shunta Chikami, Glenn Villena Latag, Subin Song, Norio Iwakiri and Tomohiro Hayashi
Analysis of Vicinal Water in Soft Contact Lenses Using a Combination of Infrared Absorption Spectroscopy and Multivariate Curve Resolution
Reprinted from: *Molecules* **2022**, *27*, 2130, doi:10.3390/molecules27072130 129

Yasuhiro Miwa, Tomoki Nagahama, Harumi Sato, Atsushi Tani and Kei Takeya
Intermolecular Interaction of Tetrabutylammonium and Tetrabutylphosphonium Salt Hydrates by Low-Frequency Raman Observation
Reprinted from: *Molecules* **2022**, *27*, 4743, doi:10.3390/molecules27154743 139

Jelena Muncan, Satoshi Tamura, Yuri Nakamura, Mizuki Takigawa, Hisao Tsunokake and Roumiana Tsenkova
Aquaphotomic Study of Effects of Different Mixing Waters on the Properties of Cement Mortar
Reprinted from: *Molecules* **2022**, *27*, 7885, doi:10.3390/molecules27227885 . . . . **151**

Harpreet Kaur, Rainer Künnemeyer and Andrew McGlone
Correction of Temperature Variation with Independent Water Samples to Predict Soluble Solids Content of Kiwifruit Juice Using NIR Spectroscopy
Reprinted from: *Molecules* **2022**, *27*, 504, doi:10.3390/molecules27020504 . . . . **187**

Damenraj Rajkumar, Rainer Künnemeyer, Harpreet Kaur, Jevon Longdell and Andrew McGlone
Interactions of Linearly Polarized and Unpolarized Light on Kiwifruit Using Aquaphotomics
Reprinted from: *Molecules* **2022**, *27*, 494, doi:10.3390/molecules27020494 . . . . **203**

Balkis Aouadi, Flora Vitalis, Zsanett Bodor, John-Lewis Zinia Zaukuu, Istvan Kertesz and Zoltan Kovacs
NIRS and Aquaphotomics Trace Robusta-to-Arabica Ratio in Liquid Coffee Blends
Reprinted from: *Molecules* **2022**, *27*, 388, doi:10.3390/molecules27020388 . . . . **215**

Muna E. Raypah, Ahmad Fairuz Omar, Jelena Muncan, Musfirah Zulkurnain and Abdul Rahman Abdul Najib
Identification of Stingless Bee Honey Adulteration Using Visible-Near Infrared Spectroscopy Combined with Aquaphotomics
Reprinted from: *Molecules* **2022**, *27*, 2324, doi:10.3390/molecules27072324 . . . . **229**

Zsanett Bodor, Csilla Benedek, Balkis Aouadi, Viktoria Zsom-Muha and Zoltan Kovacs
Revealing the Effect of Heat Treatment on the Spectral Pattern of Unifloral Honeys Using Aquaphotomics
Reprinted from: *Molecules* **2022**, *27*, 780, doi:10.3390/molecules27030780 . . . . **249**

Laura Marinoni, Marina Buccheri, Giulia Bianchi and Tiziana M. P. Cattaneo
Aquaphotomic, E-Nose and Electrolyte Leakage to Monitor Quality Changes during the Storage of Ready-to-Eat Rocket
Reprinted from: *Molecules* **2022**, *27*, 2252, doi:10.3390/molecules27072252 . . . . **265**

Jelena Muncan, Balasooriya Mudiyanselage Siriwijaya Jinendra, Shinichiro Kuroki and Roumiana Tsenkova
Aquaphotomics Research of Cold Stress in Soybean Cultivars with Different Stress Tolerance Ability: Early Detection of Cold Stress Response
Reprinted from: *Molecules* **2022**, *27*, 744, doi:10.3390/molecules27030744 . . . . **283**

E. Anibal Disalvo, A. Sebastian Rosa, Jimena P. Cejas and María de los A. Frias
Water as a Link between Membrane and Colloidal Theories for Cells
Reprinted from: *Molecules* **2022**, *27*, 4994, doi:10.3390/molecules27154994 . . . . **301**

Keiichiro Shiraga, Yuichi Ogawa, Shojiro Kikuchi, Masayuki Amagai and Takeshi Matsui
Increase in the Intracellular Bulk Water Content in the Early Phase of Cell Death of Keratinocytes, Corneoptosis, as Revealed by 65 GHz Near-Field CMOS Dielectric Sensor
Reprinted from: *Molecules* **2022**, *27*, 2886, doi:10.3390/molecules27092886 . . . . **321**

Mariana Santos-Rivera, Amelia R. Woolums, Merrilee Thoresen, Florencia Meyer and Carrie K. Vance
Bovine Respiratory Syncytial Virus (BRSV) Infection Detected in Exhaled Breath Condensate of Dairy Calves by Near-Infrared Aquaphotomics
Reprinted from: *Molecules* **2022**, *27*, 549, doi:10.3390/molecules27020549 . . . . **335**

About the Editors

Roumiana Tsenkova

Professor Dr. Roumiana Tsenkova holds doctoral degrees in Automation Engineering, from Technical University Rousse, Bulgaria, and in Agriculture, from Hokkaido University, Japan. Her academic career started at the Technical University, Rousse, Bulgaria, in 1978, where she was first introduced to Near-Infrared (NIR) Spectroscopy and started exploring its possibilities for the early diagnosis of mastitis in dairy cows. In 1990, she was awarded a Japanese Monbusho Scholarship for post-doctoral studies at Obihiro University in Japan. In 1992, she moved to Hokkaido University, pursuing the development of NIR technology for the biomonitoring of dairy cows. In 1996, she was offered a tenured position at the Graduate School of Agricultural Science, Kobe University, and she worked there until her retirement in 2021. Following her retirement, she continued scientific and research work. In 2021, she established the Aquaphotomics Research Department at Kobe University, where she is currently working as a specially appointed professor. Since 2015, she has held the position of a visiting professor at the Medical Faculty of Keio University in Tokyo.

Throughout her scientific career, she has been focused on exploring the possibilities of NIR Spectroscopy and ways in which to expand its applications into bio-diagnosis and biomonitoring in life science. She is the first scientist to use NIR Spectroscopy for disease diagnosis and to recognize the untapped well of information that is generated by the interaction of water and light; this has resulted in her theory of Aquaphotomics, a science dedicated to the exploration of this phenomenon. She is the author and co-author of more than 100 peer-reviewed papers and book chapters. Professor Tsenkova is a recipient of many international awards, including the Tomas Hirschfield Award, which is the highest recognition one can receive in the field of near-infrared spectroscopy.

Jelena Muncan

Jelena Muncan obtained her doctoral degree in Biomedical Engineering (2014) at the University of Belgrade, Serbia. She started her career there, first working as a teaching assistant and then as an assistant professor, teaching biostatistics, fractal analysis, spectroscopy methods and techniques, multivariate analysis, and Aquaphotomics. In 2017, she received a post-doctoral research fellowship at Kobe University, Biomeasurement Technology Laboratory, from the Japan Society for the Promotion of Science, ; here, she was researching the possibilities of Aquaphotomics for non-invasive mastitis diagnosis in dairy cows. Since the completion of her postgraduate studies, she has been working as an assistant and associate professor at the newly established Aquaphotomics Research Department at Kobe University. Her research area is very wide and highly multidisciplinary, but is focused on the exploration of water structure and functionality. Her ultimate goal is to translate the research results of Aquaphotomics studies to various technological applications. She is the author and co-author of numerous papers, published in both international journals and books. She is a member of the International Council for Near-Infrared Spectroscopy (ICNIRS) and the International Aquaphotomics Society (IAS), where she also has a role as a board member and secretary. In 2022, she received the prestigious NIR Advance Award from the Japan Council for Near-Infrared Spectroscopy for her contribution to the development of Aquaphotomic near-infrared spectroscopy and research of the functionality of water molecular species in bio-aqueous systems.

Preface to "Aquaphotomics—Exploring Water Molecular Systems in Nature"

Aquaphotomics, as a new "omics" science, was proposed by Roumiana Tsenkova in 2005, and was guided by her vision of exploring the biological world and its aqueous systems in terms of the light–water interaction. In the past, water was seen as a passive element, an inert molecule that hinders useful spectral signals. A radical new approach in spectroscopy—considering the water–light interaction—opened a new door for the world of science. Water, as an active factor, a biomolecule in its own right, and one that builds miscellaneous structures that lead to various functionalities, has been recognized and is slowly becoming a new interdisciplinary scientific platform that connects sciences and technology.

The mission of Aquaphotomics is to understand the role of water, and consider it as a sophisticated molecular network that connects other elements in the system with its rhythm and ability self-organize. All spectroscopy techniques are crucially important for Aquaphotomics, whether they cover visible light, infrared, near-infrared, ultraviolet, Raman, or Terahertz frequencies. The water spectra of the systems under various perturbations create a vast ocean of data. Due to advancements in computer science, data analysis, and new measurement technologies, the spectral studies of water are expanding across disciplines, providing a common platform for diverse technological applications.

This Special Issue of Molecules is devoted to spreading new knowledge regarding the features and functionalities of this most incredibly versatile molecule, and the connections and networks it creates; from these, different functionalities arise. We are immensely pleased to say that interest in this Special Issue has far exceeded our expectations; in this Special Issue, there are 21 scientific papers, reviews and original research works, on a wide variety of topics, which range from basic water structure and science, spectral preprocessing and analysis, to very complex practical applications and their associated problems. We are also excptionally pleased that this first Special Issue collected studies that were performed using different spectroscopy methods, including near–infrared, Raman, infrared and even polarized spectroscopy. It also contains works that are pioneering in nature, that represent emerging areas in the application of Aquaphotomics knowledge, and that propose future directions for its development. This Special Issue is now also available in a book format.

As Guest Editors, we would like to sincerely thank all the authors who contributed to this Special Issue with review and original research articles, and to external editors and reviewers for their efforts in carefully evaluating the received manuscripts. We also would like to sincerely thank the Editorial office of Molecules for its kind assistance in the preparation of this publication. Last, but not least, we would like to express our sincere gratitude to the Tsukino Shizuku Foundation, who kindly supported the article processing charges of several research papers in this publication. Without their support, the range of articles in this first Aquaphotomics Special Issue would have been modest.

Roumiana Tsenkova and Jelena Muncan
Editors

molecules

MDPI

Editorial

Aquaphotomics—Exploring Water Molecular Systems in Nature

Jelena Muncan * and Roumiana Tsenkova *

Aquaphotomics Research Department, Graduate School of Agricultural Science, Kobe University, Kobe 657-8501, Japan
* Correspondence: jmuncan@people.kobe-u.ac.jp (J.M.); rtsen@kobe-u.ac.jp (R.T.)

Since its birth in 2005, when introduced by Prof. Roumiana Tsenkova, and especially in the last five years, the development of aquaphotomics has shown a rising trend. The increasing interest in using aquaphotomics in scientific research can be observed by a rough analysis of the data provided by the Google Scholar search engine (Figure 1). This simple query for the published papers and patents (without citations of those works) on a year-by-year level since the establishment of aquaphotomics in 2005 shows that the slow, steady growth of the first decade is now being replaced with a more rapid trend, with publications doubling in numbers every two years.

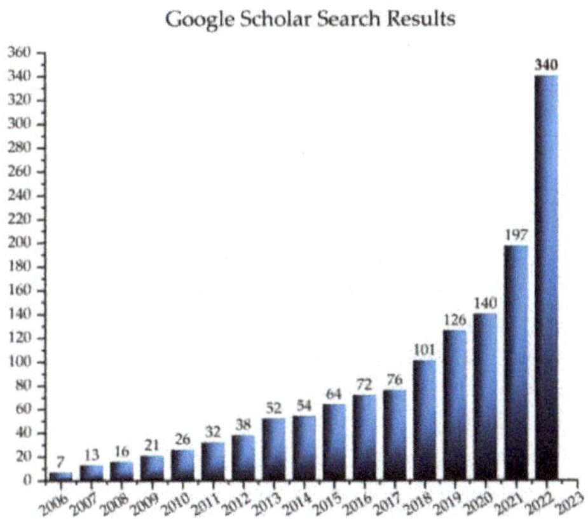

Figure 1. The results of analysis using Google Scholar search tool for articles and patents (excluding citations) mentioning word "aquaphotomics" since its establishment until 2022.

A similar query performed using Web of Science provided more information about the categories of published scientific articles which featuring the word "aquaphotomics" [1]; there were 25 (Figure 2). The two categories to which the majority of the published works belong to are multidisciplinary chemistry (23.81%) and analytical chemistry (20.00%), which together comprise almost half of all the results, followed by biochemistry/molecular biology (19.05%) and spectroscopy (18.10%). Out of the 25 found categories, 4 contain the words "multidisciplinary", 2 "inter-disciplinary", and 3 "applied" or "applications".

This "character" of aquaphotomics as an inter-disciplinary field with lots of applications across many disciplines is well-reflected in this book, which in one place collected high-quality, original research articles and reviews that were originally published as open access articles in a Special Issue of Molecules titled "Aquaphotomics—Exploring Water Molecular Systems in Nature".

Citation: Muncan, J.; Tsenkova, R. Aquaphotomics—Exploring Water Molecular Systems in Nature. *Molecules* **2023**, *28*, 2630. https://doi.org/10.3390/molecules28062630

Received: 2 March 2023
Accepted: 5 March 2023
Published: 14 March 2023

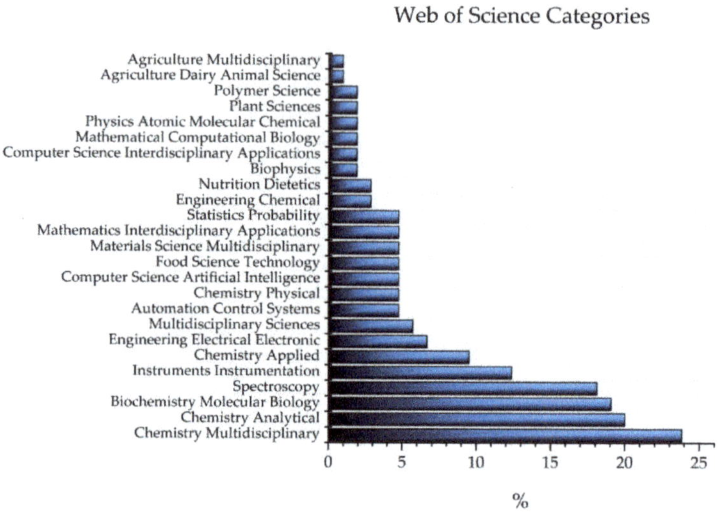

Figure 2. The results of Web of Science search for documents containing word "aquaphotomics" sorted according to categories defined by Web of Science. The majority of results (almost 50%) can belong to the categories of multidisciplinary chemistry and analytical chemistry.

Out of the 21 published articles, 3 were reviews [2–4] and 18 were original research papers [5–22], that can be roughly separated into 6 categories (Figure 3).

The majority of the articles, approximately one third, belongs to the field of applications in agriculture and food science [8,9,12–14,21,22], a field from which aquaphotomics originated, and probably the reason why this category is still at the forefront of aquaphotomics development. Following this category are the preprocessing and chemometrics [2,4,15,18] and fundamental studies [5,6,10,17]. The former category reflects an important issue that aquaphotomics is trying to resolve, namely, the necessity of developing appropriate tools for dealing with the spectra of highly aqueous samples, and that significant efforts are being invested in resolving the issues of extracting the information from very subtle spectral signals. The papers that can be classified as belonging to the Fundamental studies show a recognition of aquaphotomics as a novel tool that can provide new insights into many puzzling phenomena in nature where water plays the role. They also show the possibility of opening new research directions and novel fields of applications.

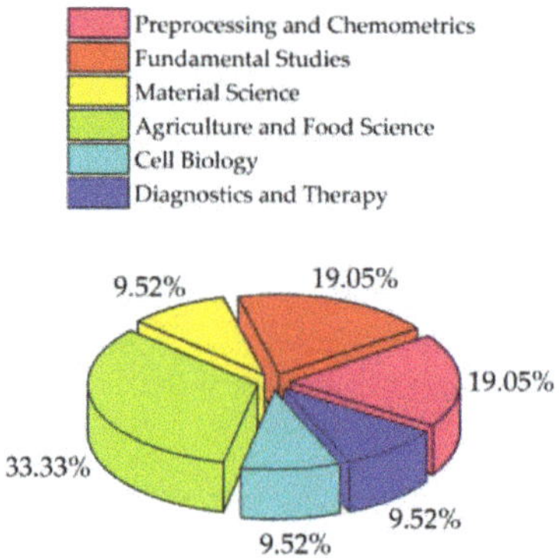

Figure 3. The main categories of scientific articles published in the Special Issue "Aquaphotomics—Exploring Water Molecular Systems in Nature".

This is exactly something that can be said about the category of material science [7,16], a relatively new area where aquaphotomics is slowly starting to make progress. The last two categories, cell biology [3,20] and diagnostics and therapy [11,19], do not feature many research papers because of the difficulty of conducting research with living systems. However, these two categories, and perhaps life science in general, still represent an important direction of growth that holds the strongest potential for making an impact and lasting change in our world, by transforming the current practices and offering non-destructive, real-time monitoring and early diagnostics that hopefully one day will be replaced with prevention.

Another interesting aspect of the original research articles is the measurement methods the researchers employed (Figure 4). Contrary to expectations that this would be the major portion, only four of the original research papers reported results obtained by using near-infrared (NIR) spectroscopy in the area of the first overtone of water (1300–1600 nm) [5,6,19,22].

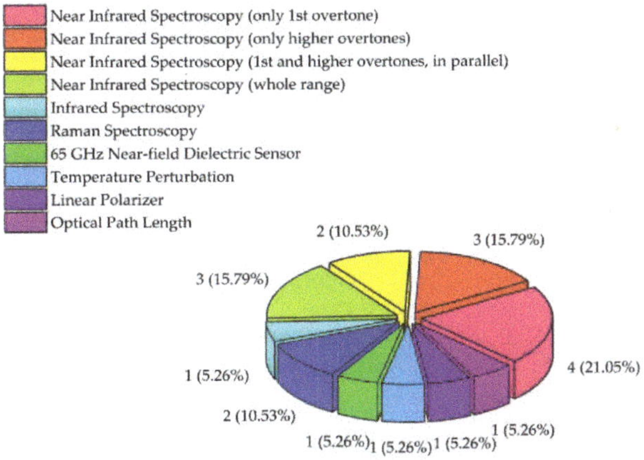

Figure 4. The types of measurement methods and perturbation techniques used by researchers in original research articles of the Special Issue "Aquaphotomics—Exploring Water Molecular Systems in Nature". The numbers beside each category indicate the total number of papers that used a specific measurement method, while the numbers in parentheses represent the percentage of the total number of publications in the Special Issue.

The use of only the first overtone of water in analysis has been the dominant choice in aquaphotomics publications for a long time. This is because aquaphotomics relies on specific water bands as water matrix coordinates (WAMACs), which have been well-defined through studies in this region. As a result, there is now a clear understanding of the assignments of these water absorbance bands and their relation to water functionality. Nevertheless, it is very encouraging to notice that the use of short wavelength NIR spectroscopy is gaining popularity. In this Issue, three papers reported the use of short wavelength NIR spectroscopy, in the approximate range of 750–1000 nm, where the 2nd and 3rd overtone of water are located [9,13,21]. Furthermore, two research groups presented the results, in parallel, for both the first overtone of water region and higher overtones, demonstrating increased efforts in gaining more clarity in the nature of information that can be gained from each of the regions, and attempts at defining WAMACs similar to the existing ones in the first overtone [23]. Additionally, three studies were performed over the entire (~750–2500 nm) [16,18], or nearly the entire range, of the NIR spectrum (1100–2500 nm) [15]. This testifies to increased interest in the water spectral features over the entire range, which may result in many benefits for both scientific and practical aspects.

It is especially encouraging to witness that the light–water interaction over the whole electromagnetic spectrum is a source of valuable information, as stated in aquaphotomics.

One paper reported the results in the mid-infrared region [7], and two used Raman spectroscopy [10,17]. There were also two papers reporting on the exploration of a newly developed measurement technique that employs GHz sensors [20], and also perturbation by polarization filters [13], for the first time in aquaphotomics. Studies such as those challenge the current understanding of what exactly is the nature of light–water interaction and bring attention to the importance of the design of instruments and the choice of light, which is a measurement and a perturbation tool in aquaphotomics.

In this book, all the papers from the Special Issue are organized to follow the trend from fundamentally important topics from which all the readers can benefit, through the rising complexity of the aqueous and biological systems that were investigated. That is why the beginning of the book presents papers dealing with the topics of preprocessing, chemometrics, and the related tools that should lead to improved ways of extracting the relevant information from the spectra. In the first review of this Issue, Roger, Mallet, and Marini [2] provided a comprehensive overview of the most useful preprocessing and chemometrics techniques that are particularly relevant for the nature of signals aquaphotomics is dealing with. If one should choose just one, the most important message of this review should be as follows: "It is important to look at the "raw" spectra before deciding which preprocessing to use!". This is something that cannot be emphasized enough. It is a common mistake in novices to rush and apply chemometrics or create aquagrams according to the explanations provided in the literature [24,25] and jump to interpretations based on the aquagram only. However, this review, through three examples of data, show how inadequate preprocessing, and overlooking the critical step in seeing the spectra before creating aquagrams, can result in a distorted view and misinterpretations. It is our expectation that this review and the techniques proposed are going to be of major significance for future aquaphotomics studies, and readers and researchers are strongly encouraged to start exploring and using the proposed preprocessing techniques. The review paper by Sun, Cai, and Shao [4] summarized novel findings regarding the extraction of structural and quantitative information from the temperature-dependent NIR spectra using chemometrics methods. Shao and his team are leaders in the development of temperature-dependent spectroscopy [26–32], where they utilize the phenomena of using the water spectral changes with temperature when the system undergoes changes in composition. In these applications, water plays the role of a "scanner", acquiring information through the changes in its structure caused by the changes in concentration. The current paper, in addition to providing an overview of chemometrics techniques that can be used in temperature-dependent NIR spectroscopy, highlighted also some of the associated challenges, such as the need for a large number of reference samples and difficulties in finding the most appropriate chemometrics method.

In her work, Cui tackled one of the major issues that can happen in both research and industrial settings: the need to correct the spectral variations caused by the different instruments, measurements, and sample conditions [15]. This problem is of particular importance for all aquaphotomics studies because it uses the high variability of aqueous samples due the very nature of hydrogen bonding in the water molecular network and the water response to even subtle changes either in its own composition or in the environment, and the accuracy and uniformity of the instruments are very important. Cui proposed a newly developed algorithm, called mutual-individual factor analysis (MIFA), which takes advantage of the sensitivity of water to perturbations, to divide the water spectral region into mutual and individual parts, which derive from the spectral features among instruments (mutual) and differences in the sample and measurement conditions (individual). The effectiveness of the newly developed MIFA algorithm for the calibration transfer was successfully demonstrated on two datasets of corn and wheat, showing a novel solution for the standardization of spectra derived from different instruments when measurements are affected by multiple factors.

In one of the very innovative and creative works, Ye et al. developed a new discriminating analysis for the purpose of application in problems of the classification and identification of water samples with small differences in the component content; this is a very hot topic, especially in the quality control of drinking water [18]. The work is rich in novelty in many aspects: they utilized the optical path length of cuvette as a perturbation factor, performed fusion modeling on multi-optical path measurements, and developed a new pattern recognition method that effectively discriminated between three types of drinking water with a very similar content. The novel approach could widely be applied to other types of samples or in other fields.

When it comes to studies that reveal some fundamental new insights, the work by Stoilov et al. [6] stands out, reporting for the first time that the frequency of applied sound perturbation results in distinctive changes in water's molecular structure, that was captured in a water absorbance spectral pattern. The team which investigated two types of water concluded that perturbation by sound produces a measurable impact on water's molecular structure which depends on the nature of the water samples used, as well as the frequency at which at the sound is tuned to. Similarly, very novel results are reported by Muncan et al. [5], who investigated how the water used in mixing for cement production influences the mechanical properties of the final products. The study showed that differences in water defined the properties of cement mortar very early, within the first 24 h. All the waters used in the study satisfy all the conditions as defined by current standards, but contrary to the expectations, they result in very different properties of the final products, showing the need for the recognition of water's molecular structure as one of the aspects that needs to be taken into consideration and incorporated into future practices. Another study showing the importance of the knowledge of water's molecular structure in order to predict the material properties is a study conducted by Maggiore, Tommasini, and Ossi [10]. The study was focused on using Raman spectroscopy to measure the amount of liquid water in snow. In snow, the water can exist in three phases simultaneously, solid, liquid, and vapor, but the content of liquid water is important to estimate snowmelt runoff and wet avalanche risk. This paper is another fascinating example of how the structure of water defines the mechanical properties of the material which, in this case, is snow. By reproducing the water percolation in snow in laboratory settings and monitoring the presence of liquid water using the Raman spectral features of ice and liquid water, the researchers were able to detect the presence of liquid water in a snow volume and to follow the evolution of the progressive filling of snow with the liquid phase in a non-destructive and minimally invasive optical approach. They also proposed the measures needed to upgrade the measurements from laboratory to on-field applications.

The study by Miwa et al. [17] used a similar technique: low-frequency Raman spectroscopy (which is a type of Terahertz spectroscopy) to study the phenomena of semi-clathrate hydrates, which are very popular materials with a wide range of applications due to their ability to store heat. The temperature at which they can store heat can be changed depending on the selection of certain guest-ions, and it is influenced by their size, hydrophilicity, crystal structure, and other properties. Employing low-frequency Raman spectroscopy, the team were able to observe interactions between the ions in semi-clathrate hydrates and found that the temperature at which they stored heat was related to the interactions between the ions, as shown by the position of peaks in the low-frequency Raman spectra.

Interesting and very novel papers are emerging from the area of material science, where for a long time, mid-infrared spectroscopy and Raman spectroscopy were dominant. Moll et al. [16], in contrast, focused on the near-infrared spectroscopic exploration of water in polymers with varying hydrophobicity. One of the most interesting findings of this study is that the changes in the NIR spectrum of water can be observed even in the interaction with highly hydrophobic polymers, leading the authors to conclude that hydrophilicity is not an exhaustive enough parameter to fully account for the interaction of a polymer with water. This also confirms one of the aquaphotomics postulates regarding the sensitivity of water towards its chemical environment and that it is so clearly manifested in the NIR spectra.

Meada et al. [7] employed mid-infrared spectroscopy to study polymers, but their study was performed from an unusual angle: they investigated vicinal water in soft contact lenses. The water in the vicinity of material surfaces has a significant impact on a variety of phenomena stemming from the interfaces, such as chemical reactions, adsorption, friction, adhesion, and biocompatibility. In the paper, the authors devised and proposed a new method to study the behavior of water near polymer materials using conventional ATR infrared spectroscopy. The method involves the application of pressure to a hydrated contact lens, which results in a deformation and change in the ratio of bulk and vicinal water. The spectral signature of vicinal water was then extracted using multivariate curve resolution–alternating least squares (MCR-ALS) analysis. The results showed that the shape of the OH-stretching band in the infrared region, which reflects the hydrogen bonding state of vicinal water, is different depending on the chemical structure of the polymers constituting the contact lenses. This method is also proposed to probe the hydration states of other materials whose function requires water, such as porous materials, hollow fibers, and other soft materials.

In the agricultural sector, aquaphotomics development in the area of food adulteration seem to be increasingly popular. Three papers in the Special Issue tackled challenges in food adulteration, specifically honey [8,21] and coffee [14]. While honey adulteration was a subject of investigations in several previous publications [33–35], the current ones contain two novelties. First, a study by Bodor et al. [14] for the first time reports the aquaphotomics results in the detection of honey adulteration by heat processing. Their results prove that even at a low temperature treatment (40 °C), measurable changes occur in the spectra of the honey, as demonstrated in aquagrams of three types of honey (sunflower, bastard indigo, and acacia), and that these spectral changes are mainly related to the transformation of the highly bonded water to less-bonded water or free water. Raypah et al. [21] investigated the potential of aquaphotomics for honey adulteration, but for the first time in a stingless bee honey, which is made of the nectar of trees, not flowers, and typically has a higher moisture content. Another novelty is the employment, for the first time, of short NIR spectroscopy and the detection of three types of adulterants: water, apple cider, and fructose syrup. This team presented a simple aquagram-based method for the detection of adulteration in the region 800–1100 nm, a very convenient region, where the majority of the most common photodetectors available on the market offer the best sensitivity. Another important contribution of this paper is in the assignments and interpretation of the absorbance bands found to be important for honey adulteration, and their importance from the standpoint of honey functionality. The coffee adulteration work by Balkis et al. [14] is another achievement in food adulteration detection, a particular research topic for which the group of Prof. Kovacs from Hungary is becoming increasingly recognized for. The coffee adulteration work was able to accurately determine the ratio of coffees Robusta (less expensive and easier to cultivate; therefore, commonly used as adulterant in higher-price coffee blends [36,37]) to Arabica in both ground and liquid forms. A classification accuracy of 100% was achieved for pure Arabica and Robusta, and the prediction of the Robusta to Arabica ratio occurred with an error of 2.4%. The aquaphotomics approach provided typical spectral fingerprints for each coffee blend and was able to accurately discriminate and estimate the Robusta content of marketed blends.

Marinoni et al.'s study [22], which focused on utilizing the potential of aquaphotomics to assess the freshness of ready-to-eat rocket salad, may mark the initiation of a promising new realm of applications. The work employed several techniques, including a portable E-nose, the electrolyte leakage test, NIR spectroscopy, and aquaphotomics to evaluate and monitor changes during storage of salad in three types of modified atmosphere at 4 °C. Although preliminary, the results suggest the potential of NIR spectroscopy to provide the modeling of the shelf-life of stored products, the identification of the most suitable atmosphere for maintaining freshness, and increasing insights into the role of water in the preservation/deterioration of fresh vegetables. In this study, in particular, the author found importance of water solvation shells for the description of time-related changes during storage.

Kaur et al. [12] performed an aquaphotomics study aimed at understanding the changes in the water structure of kiwifruit juice with changes in temperature. This study was performed in a style typical for Kaur, where she was focused on one very practical application point of aquaphotomics, the identification of problems and overcoming them by developing new tools and solutions, and, additionally, the study provided new information regarding the water spectral features and assignments, adding to the increasing aquaphotome database. This particular work identified that the influence of an increasing temperature on the peak absorbance of kiwifruit juice spectra manifests as a lateral (wavelength) shift in the first overtone and a vertical shift in the second overtone region of water. Further, experimenting with different preprocessing techniques (orthogonalization and extended multiplicative scatter correction), a temperature-independent partial least square regression model for predicting the soluble solids concentration (SSC) of kiwifruit juice were built for both overtones of water, significantly reducing the prediction bias. Additionally, most importantly, the approach employed in this work, may be applied to other problems such as the prediction of various properties of other fruit juices, intact fruit, or other types of samples, whenever robustness against temperature changes is desirable.

One highly novel work came from Rajkumar et al. [13], who used NIR spectroscopy and aquaphotomics to assess the spectral changes between linearly polarized and unpolarized light in commercially grown yellow-fleshed kiwifruit. Measurements were taken on both unpeeled and peeled kiwifruit using a handheld NIR instrument. The results showed that linearly polarized light activated more free water states, while unpolarized light activated more bound water states. These differences were attributed to the surface layers of the fruit. The soluble solid content (SSC) in the fruit was not a factor in these results as the aquagrams generated for SSC were similar for all configurations. However, within the aquaphotomics framework, it is a significant finding that bound water absorbed more unpolarized light than polarized light, which calls into question the nature of the light–water interaction and how the light properties or the way light is administrated to the sample actually influences the results of the measurements and modeling of the properties of interest. The authors provided a plausible possible explanation that differences are due to polarization sensitive structures, particularly in the near surface layers, but further work is needed and encouraged in this direction.

Only one of the papers in this Special Issue was devoted to plant physiology, using aquaphotomics to explore the cold stress response in five different cultivars of soybean that were engineered to encompass varying levels of tolerance to cold stress [9]. The study showed that all soybean cultivars have a different water molecular structure in the leaves when the plants are exposed to even mild stress conditions, which is very easy to detect very early. Specific water molecular structures in the leaves of soybean cultivars were found to be highly sensitive to the temperature, showing their crucial role in the cold stress response. Further, the study revealed differences among genetically modified cultivars, suggesting that the genetic modification is actually aimed at the end at achieving a specific water molecular structure in the leaves which is more stable in the conditions of temperature change.

Two more papers of this Special Issue report interesting new theories and findings in cell biology. First, the review paper by Disalvo et al. [3] focused on the role of water in biomembranes, the structures commonly thought as surrounding and protecting the cells. In this review, the authors strongly and persuasively present evidence that water should be considered a structural and thermodynamic component of membranes and suggests incorporating this into current theories about the role of membranes in cells. The idea is that membranes should be seen as open and responsive systems that are affected by metabolic events and changes in water. The authors also suggest that the relationship between water and the membranes should be considered in terms of free energy and other thermodynamic properties, which play a role in the behavior of these crowded systems.

Shiraga et al. [20], in their original research paper, further experimentally confirmed some of these aspects. They employed a newly developed measurement system based on a near-field CMOS dielectric sensor operating at 65 GHz, that enabled measurements of the bulk water content in cells with a high precision and single cell resolution. The system was used to evaluate the changes in the bulk water content during the process of cell death in keratinocytes. The results showed that there was a significant increase in the bulk water content approximately 1 h before the membrane disruption, suggesting that the calcium flux may play a role in triggering the increase in water content.

Santos-Rivera et al. [11] conducted a pioneering work, using aquaphotomics for the rapid detection of bovine respiratory syncytial virus (BRSV) infection in cattle, based on the spectra of exhaled breath condensate. This is the first report on utilizing this type of sample to perform diagnosis that holds immense promise, especially for screening purposes in human population. It is worth noting that BRSV is a very contagious viral disease spread by aerosols and via contact between animals. The results showed that changes in the composition of the exhaled breath condensate during infection could be accurately differentiated from the pre-infection stage with an accuracy of over 93%. These findings suggest that NIR aquaphotomics could be used to develop a non-invasive, in-field diagnostic tool for detecting not only BRSV infection in cattle, but similar infections in the human population.

In a very interesting case study, Scholkmann and Tsenkova [19] used aquaphotomics NIR spectroscopy as a tool to monitor the effects of a blood cleaning treatment called double-filtration plasmapheresis (DFPP). The analysis of the spectra acquired from a hand of one subject subjected to DFFP treatment showed that the water properties in the tissue changed after the treatment, characterized by an increase in small water clusters, free water molecules, and a decrease in hydroxylated water and superoxides. The changes in tissue water suggest that the positive effects of DFPP may be linked to improvements in the water quality in blood and tissues, related to the respective water molecular structures. This study is the first to document these changes after DFPP treatment in human tissue, and it is worth noting the existence of similarities between this study and some preliminary findings reported about the hemodialysis and the blood filtration treatment, namely, a marked increase in free water molecules after the filtration [38].

The works performed by the researchers who authored the articles in the Special Issue are all at the cutting-edge of aquaphotomics. Many of the works are the first of their kind, pioneering in nature and showcasing the new phenomena explored through the prism of water–light interaction. However, when one finishes the reading, it becomes apparent that some questions are still left without certain answers, and, furthermore, that new questions have emerged. It is now down to us to encourage others to be stimulated by these new questions, take this challenge, and have courage to create new paths into as of yet unexplored lands.

Acknowledgments: All the authors who kindly contributed to this Special Issue are gratefully acknowledged. The editors are especially grateful to Tsuki no Shizuku Foundation who provided financial support for article processing charges to several contributors.

Conflicts of Interest: The authors declare no conflict of interest.

References

1. Web of Science, Copyright Clarivate 2023. Web of Science Search Results for "aquaphotomics". Available online: https://www.webofscience.com/wos/woscc/analyze-results/1af7d1e6-a927-4f1d-9599-89baa6d264d7-6d791c7c (accessed on 2 February 2023).
2. Roger, J.; Mallet, A.; Marini, F. Preprocessing NIR Spectra for Aquaphotomics. *Molecules* **2022**, *27*, 6795. [CrossRef]
3. Disalvo, E.A.; Rosa, A.S.; Cejas, J.P.; Frias, M.d.l.A. Water as a Link between Membrane and Colloidal Theories for Cells. *Molecules* **2022**, *27*, 4994. [CrossRef]
4. Sun, Y.; Cai, W.; Shao, X. Chemometrics: An Excavator in Temperature-Dependent Near-Infrared Spectroscopy. *Molecules* **2022**, *27*, 452. [CrossRef] [PubMed]
5. Muncan, J.; Tamura, S.; Nakamura, Y.; Takigawa, M.; Tsunokake, H.; Tsenkova, R. Aquaphotomic Study of Effects of Different Mixing Waters on the Properties of Cement Mortar. *Molecules* **2022**, *27*, 7885. [CrossRef]

6. Stoilov, A.; Muncan, J.; Tsuchimoto, K.; Teruyaki, N.; Shigeoka, S.; Tsenkova, R. Pilot Aquaphotomic Study of the Effects of Audible Sound on Water Molecular Structure. *Molecules* **2022**, *27*, 6332. [CrossRef] [PubMed]
7. Maeda, S.; Chikami, S.; Latag, G.V.; Song, S.; Iwakiri, N.; Hayashi, T. Analysis of Vicinal Water in Soft Contact Lenses Using a Combination of Infrared Absorption Spectroscopy and Multivariate Curve Resolution. *Molecules* **2022**, *27*, 2130. [CrossRef]
8. Bodor, Z.; Benedek, C.; Aouadi, B.; Zsom-Muha, V.; Kovacs, Z. Revealing the Effect of Heat Treatment on the Spectral Pattern of Unifloral Honeys Using Aquaphotomics. *Molecules* **2022**, *27*, 780. [CrossRef]
9. Muncan, J.; Jinendra, B.M.S.; Kuroki, S.; Tsenkova, R. Aquaphotomics Research of Cold Stress in Soybean Cultivars with Different Stress Tolerance Ability: Early Detection of Cold Stress Response. *Molecules* **2022**, *27*, 744. [CrossRef] [PubMed]
10. Maggiore, E.; Tommasini, M.; Ossi, P.M. Raman Spectroscopy-Based Assessment of the Liquid Water Content in Snow. *Molecules* **2022**, *27*, 626. [CrossRef]
11. Santos-Rivera, M.; Woolums, A.R.; Thoresen, M.; Meyer, F.; Vance, C.K. Bovine Respiratory Syncytial Virus (BRSV) Infection Detected in Exhaled Breath Condensate of Dairy Calves by Near-Infrared Aquaphotomics. *Molecules* **2022**, *27*, 549. [CrossRef]
12. Kaur, H.; Künnemeyer, R.; McGlone, A. Correction of temperature variation with independent water samples to predict soluble solids content of kiwifruit juice using nir spectroscopy. *Molecules* **2022**, *27*, 504. [CrossRef] [PubMed]
13. Rajkumar, D.; Künnemeyer, R.; Kaur, H.; Longdell, J.; McGlone, A. Interactions of Linearly Polarized and Unpolarized Light on Kiwifruit Using Aquaphotomics. *Molecules* **2022**, *27*, 494. [CrossRef] [PubMed]
14. Aouadi, B.; Vitalis, F.; Bodor, Z.; Zaukuu, J.L.Z.; Kertesz, I.; Kovacs, Z. NIRS and Aquaphotomics Trace Robusta-to-Arabica Ratio in Liquid Coffee Blends. *Molecules* **2022**, *27*, 388. [CrossRef] [PubMed]
15. Cui, X. Water as a Probe for Standardization of Near-Infrared Spectra by Mutual–Individual Factor Analysis. *Molecules* **2022**, *27*, 6069. [CrossRef]
16. Moll, V.; Beć, K.B.; Grabska, J.; Huck, C.W. Investigation of Water Interaction with Polymer Matrices by Near-Infrared (NIR) Spectroscopy. *Molecules* **2022**, *27*, 5882. [CrossRef]
17. Miwa, Y.; Nagahama, T.; Sato, H.; Tani, A.; Takeya, K. Intermolecular Interaction of Tetrabutylammonium and Tetrabutylphosphonium Salt Hydrates by Low-Frequency Raman Observation. *Molecules* **2022**, *27*, 4743. [CrossRef]
18. Ye, N.; Zhong, S.; Fang, Z.; Gao, H.; Du, Z.; Chen, H.; Yuan, L.; Pan, T. Performance Improvement of NIR Spectral Pattern Recognition from Three Compensation Models' Voting and Multi-Modal Fusion. *Molecules* **2022**, *27*, 4485. [CrossRef]
19. Scholkmann, F.; Tsenkova, R. Changes in Water Properties in Human Tissue after Double Filtration Plasmapheresis—A Case Study. *Molecules* **2022**, *27*, 3947. [CrossRef]
20. Shiraga, K.; Ogawa, Y.; Kikuchi, S.; Amagai, M.; Matsui, T. Increase in the Intracellular Bulk Water Content in the Early Phase of Cell Death of Keratinocytes, Corneoptosis, as Revealed by 65 GHz Near-Field CMOS Dielectric Sensor. *Molecules* **2022**, *27*, 2886. [CrossRef]
21. Raypah, M.E.; Omar, A.F.; Muncan, J.; Zulkurnain, M.; Abdul Najib, A.R. Identification of Stingless Bee Honey Adulteration Using Visible-Near Infrared Spectroscopy Combined with Aquaphotomics. *Molecules* **2022**, *27*, 2324. [CrossRef]
22. Marinoni, L.; Buccheri, M.; Bianchi, G.; Cattaneo, T.M.P.P. Aquaphotomic, E-Nose and Electrolyte Leakage to Monitor Quality Changes during the Storage of Ready-to-Eat Rocket. *Molecules* **2022**, *27*, 2252. [CrossRef]
23. Tsenkova, R. Aquaphotomics: Dynamic spectroscopy of aqueous and biological systems describes peculiarities of water. *J. Near Infrared Spectrosc.* **2009**, *17*, 303–313. [CrossRef]
24. Tsenkova, R. Aquaphotomics: Water in the biological and aqueous world scrutinised with invisible light. *Spectrosc. Eur.* **2010**, *22*, 6–10.
25. Tsenkova, R.; Munćan, J.; Pollner, B.; Kovacs, Z. Essentials of Aquaphotomics and Its Chemometrics Approaches. *Front. Chem.* **2018**, *6*, 363. [CrossRef] [PubMed]
26. Cui, X.; Zhang, J.; Cai, W.; Shao, X. Chemometric algorithms for analyzing high dimensional temperature dependent near infrared spectra. *Chemom. Intell. Lab. Syst.* **2017**, *170*, 109–117. [CrossRef]
27. Han, L.; Cui, X.; Cai, W.; Shao, X. Three–level simultaneous component analysis for analyzing the near–infrared spectra of aqueous solutions under multiple perturbations. *Talanta* **2020**, *217*, 121036. [CrossRef]
28. Tan, J.; Sun, Y.; Ma, L.; Feng, H.; Guo, Y.; Cai, W.; Shao, X. Knowledge-based genetic algorithm for resolving the near-infrared spectrum and understanding the water structures in aqueous solution. *Chemom. Intell. Lab. Syst.* **2020**, *206*, 104150. [CrossRef]
29. Shao, X.; Cui, X.; Yu, X.; Cai, W. Mutual factor analysis for quantitative analysis by temperature dependent near infrared spectra. *Talanta* **2018**, *183*, 142–148. [CrossRef]
30. Cui, X.; Sun, Y.; Cai, W.; Shao, X. Chemometric methods for extracting information from temperature-dependent near-infrared spectra. *Sci. China Chem.* **2019**, *62*, 583–591. [CrossRef]
31. Shan, R.; Zhao, Y.; Fan, M.; Liu, X.; Cai, W.; Shao, X. Multilevel analysis of temperature dependent near-infrared spectra. *Talanta* **2015**, *131*, 170–174. [CrossRef]
32. Cui, X.; Liu, X.; Yu, X.; Cai, W.; Shao, X. Water can be a probe for sensing glucose in aqueous solutions by temperature dependent near infrared spectra. *Anal. Chim. Acta* **2017**, *957*, 47–54. [CrossRef] [PubMed]
33. Bázár, G.; Romvári, R.; Szabó, A.; Somogyi, T.; Éles, V.; Tsenkova, R. NIR detection of honey adulteration reveals differences in water spectral pattern. *Food Chem.* **2016**, *194*, 873–880. [CrossRef]
34. Yang, X.; Guang, P.; Xu, G.; Zhu, S.; Chen, Z.; Huang, F. Manuka honey adulteration detection based on near-infrared spectroscopy combined with aquaphotomics. *LWT* **2020**, *132*, 109837. [CrossRef]

35. Omar, A.F.; Mardziah Yahaya, O.K.; Tan, K.C.; Mail, M.H.; Seeni, A. The influence of additional water content towards the spectroscopy and physicochemical properties of genus Apis and stingless bee honey. *Opt. Sens. Detect. IV* **2016**, *9899*, 98990Y. [CrossRef]
36. Wang, X.; Lim, L.T.; Fu, Y. Review of Analytical Methods to Detect Adulteration in Coffee. *J. AOAC Int.* **2020**, *103*, 295–305. [CrossRef] [PubMed]
37. Combes, M.C.; Joët, T.; Lashermes, P. Development of a rapid and efficient DNA-based method to detect and quantify adulterations in coffee (Arabica versus Robusta). *Food Control* **2018**, *88*, 198–206. [CrossRef]
38. Muncan, J.; Tsenkova, R. Aquaphotomics-From Innovative Knowledge to Integrative Platform in Science and Technology. *Molecules* **2019**, *24*, 2742. [CrossRef]

molecules

Review

Preprocessing NIR Spectra for Aquaphotomics

Jean-Michel Roger [1,2,*], Alexandre Mallet [3] and Federico Marini [4]

1 ITAP, INRAE Montpellier Institut Agro, University Montpellier, 34196 Montpellier, France
2 ChemHouse Research Group, 34196 Montpellier, France
3 BioEnTech, 74 Av. Paul Sabatier, 11100 Narbonne, France
4 Department of Chemistry, University of Rome "La Sapienza", Piazzale Aldo Moro 5, 00185 Rome, Italy
* Correspondence: jean-michel.roger@inrae.fr

Abstract: Even though NIR spectroscopy is based on the Beer–Lambert law, which clearly relates the concentration of the absorbing elements with the absorbance, the measured spectra are subject to spurious signals, such as additive and multiplicative effects. The use of NIR spectra, therefore, requires a preprocessing step. This article reviews the main preprocessing methods in the light of aquaphotomics. Simple methods for visualizing the spectra are proposed in order to guide the user in the choice of the best preprocessing. The most common chemometrics preprocessing are presented and illustrated by three real datasets. Some preprocessing aims to produce a spectrum as close as possible to the absorbance that would have been measured under ideal conditions and is very useful for the establishment of an aquagram. Others, dedicated to the improvement of the resolution of the spectra, are very useful for the identification of the peaks. Finally, special attention is given to the problem of reducing multiplicative effects and to the potential pitfalls of some very popular methods in chemometrics. Alternatives proposed in recent papers are presented.

Keywords: near infrared spectroscopy; preprocessing; aquaphotomics; chemometrics

Citation: Roger, J.-M.; Mallet, A.; Marini, F. Preprocessing NIR Spectra for Aquaphotomics. *Molecules* **2022**, 27, 6795. https://doi.org/10.3390/molecules27206795

Academic Editor: Jaan Laane

Received: 31 July 2022
Accepted: 8 October 2022
Published: 11 October 2022

1. Introduction

Infrared spectroscopy is based on the phenomenon of absorption of photons by molecular bonds. The phenomenon of absorption obeys the Beer–Lambert law, which relates linearly the absorbance to the concentration (see Section 2). Each vibration of the molecular bonds, such as elongations or deformations, is responsible for a fundamental absorption [1]. These absorption bands are observed in the mid-infrared range (MIR, from 2.5 μm to 25 μm, corresponding to 4000–400 cm^{-1}). However, near infrared spectroscopy (NIR, from 0.8 μm to 2.5 μm, i.e., 800 nm to 2500 nm, corresponding to 12,500–4000 cm^{-1}), which contains the harmonics and combinations of the MIR bands, is by far the most used technique. One reason for this success is that the interaction between matter and NIR radiation is both weak and real [2]. Because it is weak, the photons can pass through a large amount of matter, typically several millimeters or even centimeters. Because it is effective, it results in an informative spectrum. However, the absorption peaks are weak and intricated. Moreover, measurements can be distorted by equipment drift, temperature/humidity changes, or sample presentation. The NIR spectra must, therefore, be processed by multivariate dedicated techniques, which constitute the toolbox of chemometrics. Among them, pretreatments are used to get closer to the Beer–Lambert theory and, thus, be able to apply linear calibration models.

Aquaphotomics is a new discipline [3,4], which appeared in the early 2000s. It studies water as a multiple-element medium, thus gaining the advantage of being described in a multi-dimensional space, such as that offered by NIR spectroscopy. NIR is typically used to estimate concentrations of chemical compounds, or to determine the membership of a sample in a group. In contrast to this use, aquaphotomics aims to use NIR spectroscopy to better understand the state of water and its interactions with other compounds and complex systems. For this purpose, the concept of aquaphotome is defined [3]. It is based on a set of absorbance values at different wavelengths, defining a water absorbance spectral pattern (WASP), usually presented by an aquagram [4]. The aquagram is a kind of radar graph representing the absorbance intensities at a set of wavelengths. As a consequence, aquaphotomics requires efficient tools to retrieve, on the one hand, the wavelength position of peaks and, on the other hand, relative absorbance intensities at several wavelengths. Preprocessing must, therefore, preserve the extraction of these two pieces of information, or even improve it.

This article proposes a critical review of the preprocessing methods classically used in chemometrics for NIR spectra, putting them in perspective of their use in the context of aquaphotomics studies.

2. Why to Preprocess NIR Spectra?

When electromagnetic radiation passes through a material medium, it undergoes several phenomena, including absorption. When the radiation is in the NIR range, this absorption is caused mainly by the bonds of nonsymmetrical molecules, including carbon, oxygen, hydrogen and nitrogen. This is why NIR spectroscopy is used in analytical chemistry of biological compounds. When a sample is measured under ideal conditions, i.e., in transmission, at low concentration of the analyte(s) of interest and without light scattering, Beer–Lambert law applies (see Figure 1 and Equation (1)).

$$A_0(\lambda) = -log\left(\frac{I(\lambda)}{I_0(\lambda)}\right) = \varepsilon(\lambda)LC \quad (1)$$

where $A_0(\lambda)$ is the absorbance of the analyte at wavelength λ, $I(\lambda)$ and $I_0(\lambda)$ represent the intensity of the transmitted and incident light at the same wavelength, $\varepsilon(\lambda)$ is the molar absorptivity (molar extinction coefficient) of the chromophore, whose concentration is C, and L is the optical pathlength.

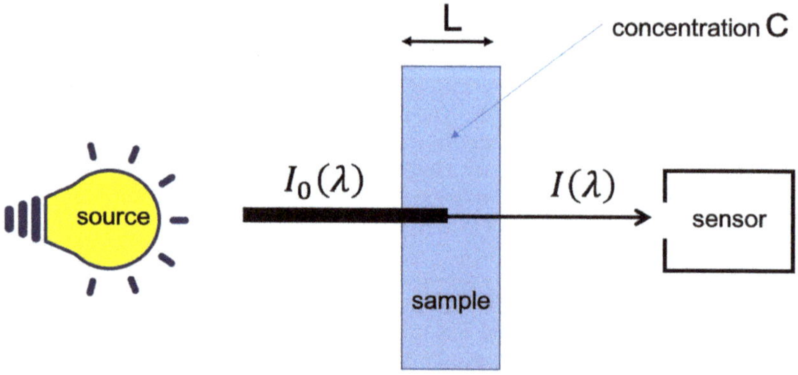

Figure 1. Ideal measurement of the absorption.

However, under current measurement conditions, a number of phenomena are added to the molecular absorption and Beer–Lambert's law no longer applies. Thus, the interaction of radiation with particles and changes in optical index have the effect of modifying the path of photons. This results in a light scattering. This scattering has two consequences, illustrated by Figure 2. The first is a lengthening of the optical path, which introduces a multiplicative term. The second is a loss of photons, which will be falsely counted as an absorption and, thus, introduces an additive term. Some specific optical assemblies, using integrating spheres, allow getting rid of these phenomena. However, these systems require measurements in contact with the product (which may not always be possible), so that acquiring the signal simply in reflection mode is the option often preferred.

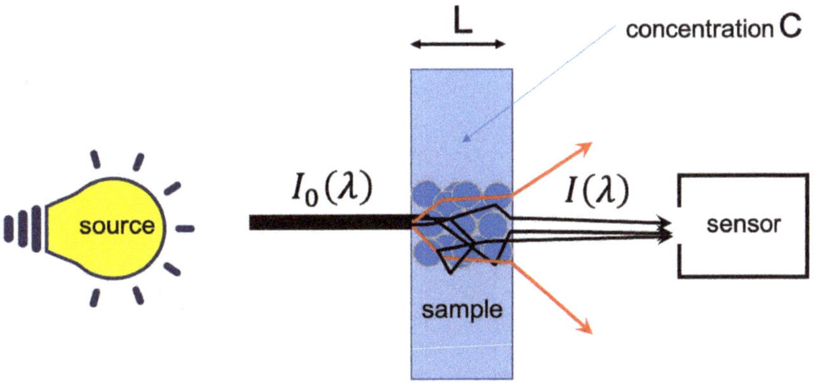

Figure 2. Real measurement of the absorption.

It is usually admitted that the multiplicative term does not depend on the wavelength and that the additive term does. This dependency can be modeled as a polynomial of λ of low degree (up to 2 or 3), and this additive term is, thus, called the baseline [5]. In turn, extra random and stochastic noise is added to the absorbance measurement, which finally results in Equation (2).

$$A(\lambda) = \varepsilon(\lambda)kLC + A_b(\lambda) + A_n(\lambda) = kA_0(\lambda) + A_b(\lambda) + A_n(\lambda) \quad (2)$$

where k, $A_b(\lambda)$ and $A_n(\lambda)$ are a multiplicative factor, a baseline and a random noise, respectively.

When the measured spectra are used to estimate the concentration of a compound, by means of a calibration, or to explain variations related to this concentration, by means of an unsupervised analysis, the additive and multiplicative effects can be detrimental. Thus, in chemometrics, preprocessing aims to correct the experimentally measured absorbance, as expressed in Equation (2), so as to make the relation between the spectra and the concentration C more adherent to the postulated linear model [6,7]. Thus, preprocessing methods are dedicated to reduce or linearize the multiplicative and additive effects. In aquaphotomics, preprocessing aims to reveal a signal as close as possible to the real absorbance, as expressed in Equation (1). For this purpose, pretreatments that reveal hidden peaks and those that restore absorbance intensities are relevant.

3. Data

To illustrate the different preprocessing methods, three sets of data will be used along this paper:

- The first one contains 187 NIR spectra of virgin olive oils from Southern France measured in transmission [8]. The spectra were recorded at 612 wavelengths regularly spaced every 2 nm over the range 1000–2222 nm. The spectra were converted in absorbance.
- The second one contains 150 Vis-NIR spectra of grapes measured in transmission [9]. The spectra were recorded at 256 wavelengths regularly spaced every 3.30 nm over the range 303–1146 nm. No transformation was conducted on the spectra which are, thus, raw intensity spectra.
- The third one contains 126 NIR spectra of flour measured in reflectance mode [10]. The spectra were recorded at 209 wavelengths regularly spaced every 6.28 nm over the range 1118–2425 nm. A log transformation was conducted on the spectra which are, thus, expressed as pseudo absorbances (log(1/R)).

The oil spectra (Figure 3a) are affected by a small additive effect. The grape spectra (Figure 3b) are affected by a huge multiplicative effect, due to the size of the measured berries. The flour spectra (Figure 3c) are affected by noise of two kinds: positive and negative spikes, between 2000 and 2200 nm, and uniform noise after 2200 nm. They also are affected by additive and/or multiplicative effects due to the scattering of the light into the flour.

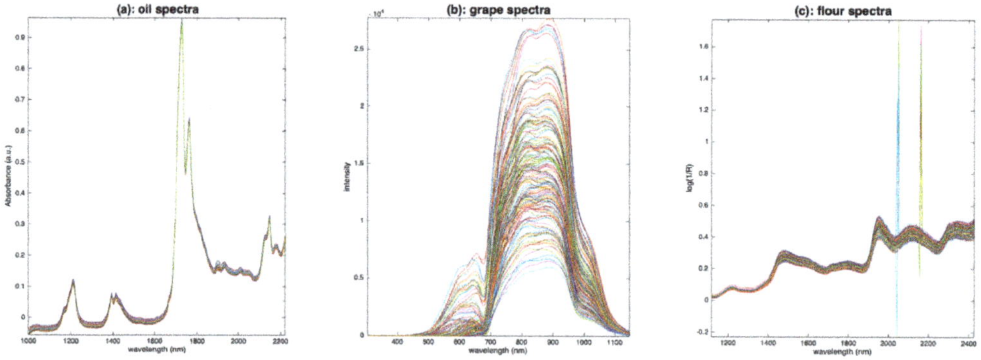

Figure 3. Spectra of olive oil (**a**), grapes (**b**) and flour (**c**).

4. Looking at the Data

It is important to look at the spectra before deciding which preprocessing to use. Several tools are available for this purpose.

4.1. Spectra Plot

One of the simplest visualization tools is to plot all the spectra, as a function of the average spectrum, using a scatter plot. Figure 4 shows the result of this visualization tool for the three datasets. Figure 4a clearly shows that the oil spectra are much more similar to one another than those of grapes (Figure 4b) or flour (Figure 4c). They differ by a small translation, corresponding to an additive effect not depending on the absorbance level. Figure 4b shows a very large variability between the spectra of grapes. All spectra are contained within a cone with the vertex at (0,0). This is characteristic of a pure multiplicative effect, due here to differences in the size of the measured berries. Figure 4c shows that the flour spectra are affected by isolated erroneous measurements, which dilate the vertical scale (spikes). Apart from these outliers, the flour spectra are organized in a cone but also appear to be affected by an additive effect. It is difficult to say whether these spectra contain a multiplicative effect or an additive effect increasing with wavelength.

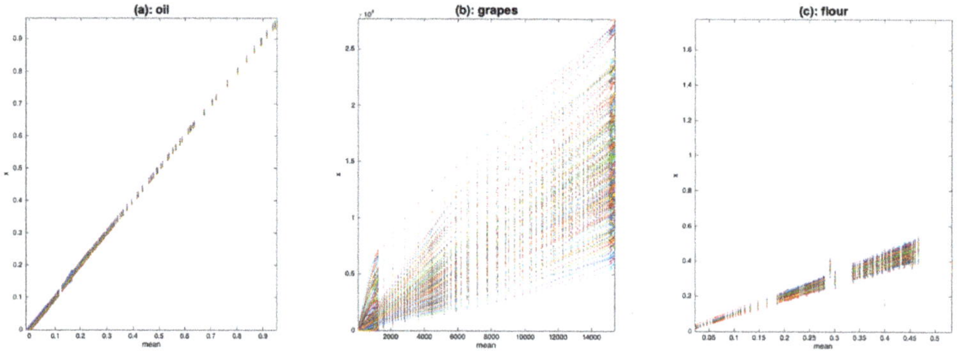

Figure 4. Scatter plot of the spectra as a function of the mean spectrum for (**a**): oil data, (**b**): grape data, (**c**): flour data.

4.2. PCA

Another visualization tool is principal component analysis (PCA). It allows, by examining the scores, observation of the variability between the spectra. Examining the loadings also allows us to understand the source of the observed variability and to infer hypotheses about the presence of multiplicative or additive effects, and, thus, to guide the preprocessing step. Figure 5 shows the scores along the first two components of a PCA performed on the three sets of spectra. Figure 6 shows the corresponding loadings resulting from these PCA, together with the mean spectra of the three datasets. The scores of the grapes spectra (Figure 5b) show, from another point of view, the cone structure already observed in Figure 4b. In addition, the loadings on the PC1 axis (Figure 6b) are very similar to the mean spectrum (Figure 6e). Both observations are characteristic of a multiplicative effect. The reason for this is illustrated in Figure 7. It represents the spectra in the multi-dimensional wavelength space. When the spectra are impacted by a dominant multiplicative effect, they are organized in a very fine conical structure, passing through the origin of the space. When the data are centered, the canonical co-ordinate system is moved to the center of mass, at the end of the mean spectrum ($\overline{\mathbf{x}}$). Then, the axis of greatest inertia (PC1) is calculated and, due to the shape of the spectra set, this axis is aligned with the mean spectrum. The score plot and the loadings of the flour spectra (Figure 6c,f) reveal that the presence of the spikes dominates. As a consequence, this dataset must be cleaned from these spikes before any other processing. The score plot and the loadings of the oil spectra (Figure 6a,d) do not reveal any particular structure.

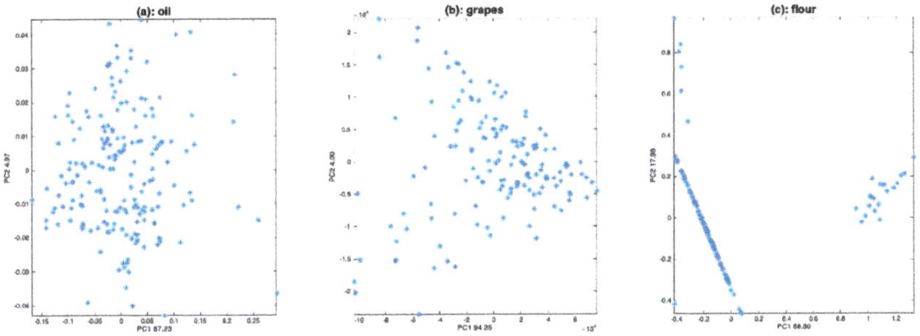

Figure 5. Scatter plot of the two first scores of a PCA calculated on (**a**): oil spectra, (**b**): grape spectra, (**c**): flour spectra.

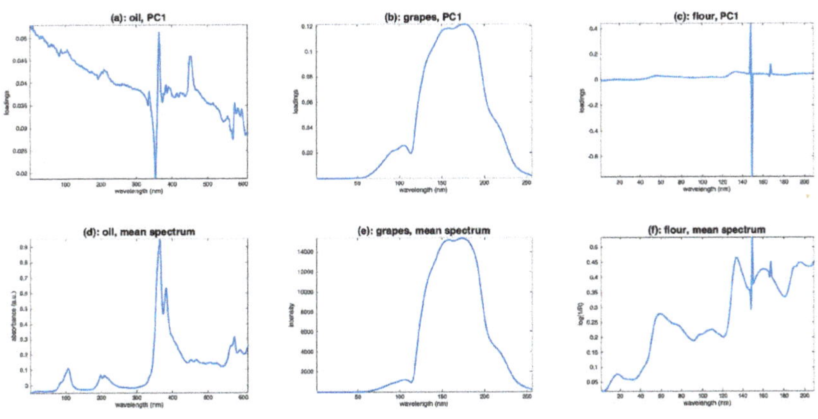

Figure 6. Loadings of a PCA calculated on (**a**): oil spectra, (**b**): grape spectra, (**c**): flour spectra, and mean spectra of (**d**): oil, (**e**): grape and (**f**): flour.

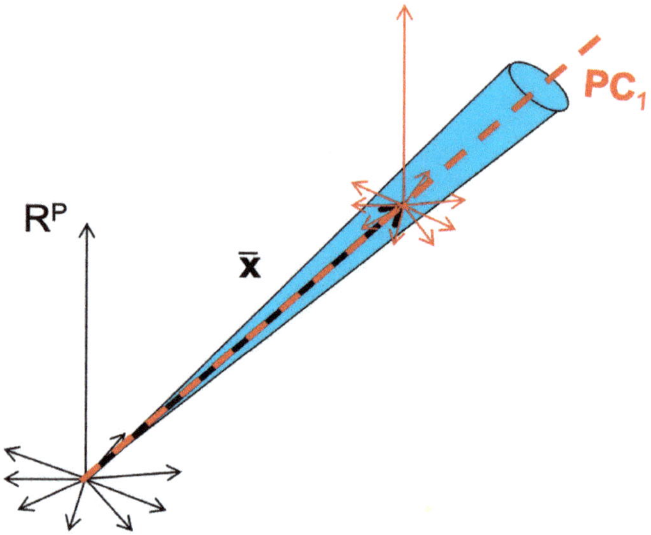

Figure 7. Illustration of the phenomenon of alignment between the mean spectrum and the first axis of the PCA in the case of the presence of multiplicative effects.

5. Most Usual Preprocessing

5.1. Noise Removal

Noise corresponds to random variations in amplitude from one point to another in the spectrum. It is represented by the term $A_n(\lambda)$ of Equation (2). From a signal processing point of view, noise is considered as a high-frequency component. All NIR pre-processing dedicated to noise suppression is, therefore, based on low-pass filters, also called smoothing. In this section, the most commonly used smoothing methods are presented.

5.1.1. Moving Averaging

A simple smoothing method is to replace the value of each point i in the spectrum by the average of the point values over a window of width w, centered on point i. The window is moved along the spectrum, hence the name moving average window or boxcar filter. This calculation cannot be applied to the first and last points of the spectrum. To overcome this problem, one can either extend the spectrum to the left and right before smoothing or keep the nonsmoothed points at both ends.

Figure 8a shows the right-hand side of eight flour spectra for wavelengths above 2245 nm. We can notice the presence of noise, certainly due to the low sensitivity of the sensor often observed at the ends of the spectral range. Despite this noise, we can observe that the spectra show an increasing slope, from 2260 to 2320 nm, followed by a plateau until 2368 nm. This plateau is marked by a slight dip around 2315 nm and a decreasing slope from 2340 to 2368 nm. Figure 8b,c show the same spectra, once smoothed by a moving average of width 5 and 11, respectively. With a window of 5, the noise is not completely removed. The general shape of the spectra has been preserved, but the dip at 2315 nm has disappeared. The decreasing slope after 2340 nm has been preserved. With a window of 11, the noise is completely corrected, but the shape of the spectra has been dramatically altered. The increasing slope now ends at 2320 nm instead of 2300 nm; the dip at 2315 nm, as well as the decreasing slope after 2340 nm, have disappeared. We see on this example a limitation of the moving average smoothing method. When noise removal requires a window that is too wide, some low-frequency features may disappear, such as the dip at 2315 nm in our example. This limitation can be extremely problematic for aquaphotomics, which is based on the observation and measurement of such features.

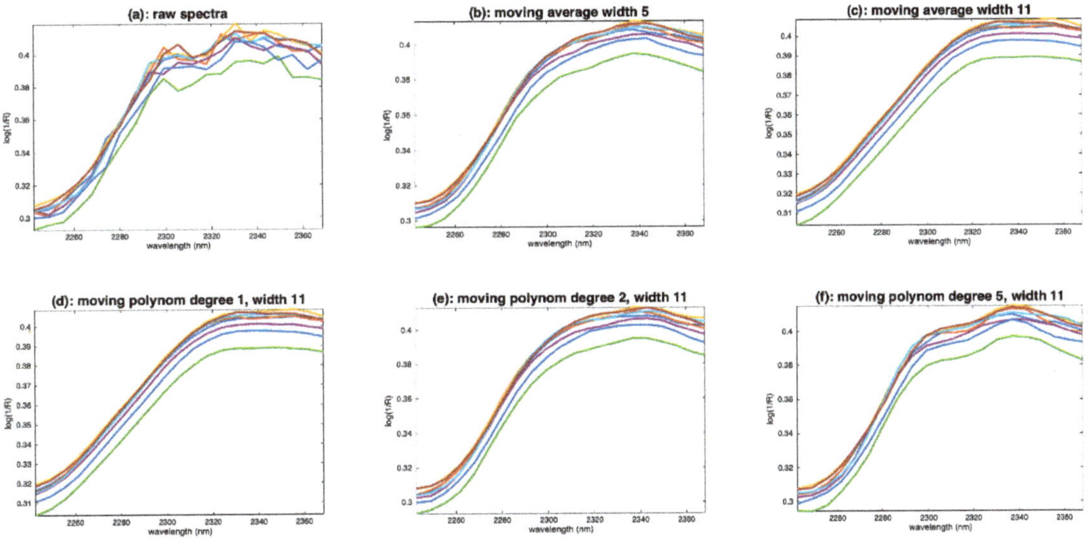

Figure 8. Examples of flour spectra in the wavelength range 2245–2368 nm. (**a**): Raw spectra, (**b**): spectra smoothed by a moving window average, width 5, (**c**): spectra smoothed by a moving window average, width 11, (**d**): spectra smoothed by a moving polynomial fitting, degree 1, width 11, (**d**): spectra smoothed by a moving polynomial fitting, degree 1, width 11, (**e**): spectra smoothed by a moving polynomial fitting, degree 2, width 11, (**f**): spectra smoothed by a moving polynomial fitting, degree 5, width 11.

5.1.2. Moving Polynomial Fitting

To overcome this problem, it is possible to use a mobile polynomial smoothing. Mobile polynomial smoothing consists of identifying a polynomial of degree d in a window of width w centered on point i. The value of the point i is replaced by the value taken by the polynomial. The window is then moved by one point and the calculation is repeated. The same computational problem as for the moving average method arises at the ends of the spectra, and the same trick can be used to solve it. This method preserves the medium-frequency features modeled by the polynomial.

Figure 8d shows the result of smoothing using a window of width 11 and a polynomial of degree 1. We see the same problem as in Figure 8c. Figure 8e shows the result of smoothing with the same window width but using a polynomial of degree 2. We find a correct shape, with the main slope stopping at 2300 nm and the presence of the small decreasing slope after 2340 nm. On the other hand, the dip at 2315 nm is still absent. It is partially recovered by using a polynomial of degree 5, as shown in Figure 8f.

Moving window smoothing, irrespectively of whether it uses the average or the polynomial, is in fact a special case of the general filtering method of Savitsky and Golay, which will be detailed further.

5.1.3. Frequency Filtering

By assimilating the wavelength scale to a time scale, another category of methods consists of decomposing the spectra on a frequency basis. These methods are based on transformations, such as Fourier or wavelet transforms. The signal is projected into a basis of signals of different frequencies. The higher-frequency components are eliminated, and the smoothed spectrum is obtained by the inverse transform. While the most common method to perform such a filtering is the Fourier transform, the wavelet transform is sometimes preferred for its ability to model complex shapes. These methods will not be further discussed here. The interested reader could find more details in [11].

5.1.4. Median Filter

A special case of noise is in the form of peaks affecting a single wavelength, as in the example of flour spectra (Figure 3c). These peaks can originate from dead pixels in hyperspectral cameras. The elimination of such noise cannot be conducted using classical methods, such as moving averages. Instead, a median filter is used, which simply consists of replacing the value of the point i of the spectrum by the median of its neighbors. Figure 9a shows one spectrum of the flour database. We notice an intense spike around 2050 nm. Figure 9b shows the result of a moving average filtering on a window of five points. We can see that the filtering did not work because the noise is not zero mean. Figure 9c shows the result with a moving median filtering. The result is much better.

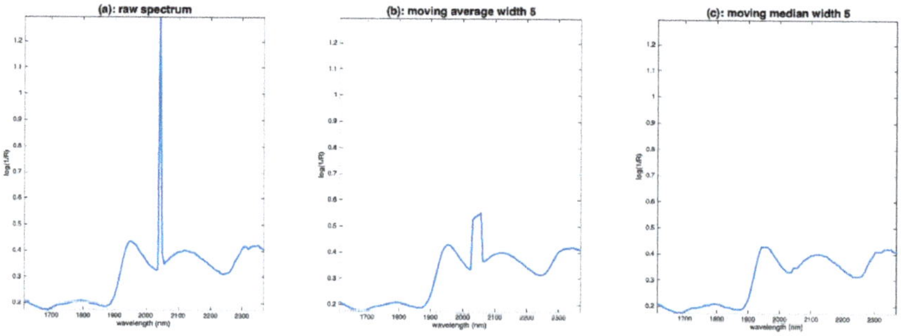

Figure 9. Illustration of the median filter on the first spectrum of the flour dataset. (**a**): Raw spectrum, (**b**): spectrum filtered by moving average, (**c**): spectrum filtered by moving median.

5.2. *Baseline Removal*

Baselines are low-frequency features added to the spectrum. They can be of different shapes. In NIR spectroscopy, baselines are due to light scattering, which causes a loss of photons arriving at the detector. They correspond to the term $A_b(\lambda)$ in Equation (2). They are almost always considered as polynomial functions of the wavelength. Thus, most of the preprocessing techniques dedicated to baseline removal use this model.

5.2.1. Detrending

Since baselines are assumed to be low-order polynomial functions, a simple method of removing them is to fit the spectrum to a polynomial of a chosen degree and replace the spectrum with the residuals of the fit. This method, usually called "detrending", is mathematically defined as follows [7]:

Let $\mathbf{v}$ be a column vector containing the wavelength values or even $[1, 2, \cdots, p]^T$, if the wavelengths are equally spaced. Let $\mathbf{V}_k$ be the $(p, k+1)$ matrix defined as follows:

$$\mathbf{V}_k = \left[\mathbf{v}^0\mathbf{v}^1\mathbf{v}^2\cdots\mathbf{v}^k\right] = \begin{bmatrix} 1 & \lambda_1 & \lambda_1^2 & \cdots & \lambda_1^k \\ 1 & \lambda_2 & \lambda_2^2 & \cdots & \lambda_2^k \\ \vdots & \vdots & \vdots & & \vdots \\ 1 & \lambda_p & \lambda_p^2 & \cdots & \lambda_p^k \end{bmatrix}$$

If $\mathbf{X}$ contains the spectra to be detrended, the baselines contained in the rows of $\mathbf{X}$ are calculated by $\mathbf{V}_k$:

$$\mathbf{L}_k = \mathbf{X}\,\mathbf{V}_k\left(\mathbf{V}_k^T\mathbf{V}_k\right)^{-1}\mathbf{V}_k^T$$

and then removed from $\mathbf{X}$:

$$\mathbf{X}_{det} = \mathbf{X} - \mathbf{L}_k = \mathbf{X} - \mathbf{X}\,\mathbf{V}_k\left(\mathbf{V}_k^T\mathbf{V}_k\right)^{-1}\mathbf{V}_k^T \quad (3)$$

Figure 10 shows the result of applying detrending with polynomial order 0, 1 and 2 on the oil, grapes and flour spectra. Compared with the raw oil spectra (Figure 3a), the detrended oil spectra have been cleaned from their inter-sample baseline variability. Already, by fitting a 0-order baseline (Figure 10a), we see that the spectra match perfectly, except after 1900 nm. This region, attributed to combinations of fundamental vibrations of C-H bonds, was identified by the authors of [7] as one of the most discriminating in the dataset. It can be seen that, with higher polynomial orders (Figure 10d,g), the parts without absorptions, before 1200 nm and between 1300 and 1400 nm, are no longer horizontal. In conclusion, for the oil spectra, a detrend of order 0 allows a very satisfactory shape to be obtained for the spectra. The application of detrending to the grape spectra (Figure 10b,e,h) does not give a good result. Indeed, the left and right parts of the spectra, which were naturally close to 0, are now completely shifted. In fact, regardless of the order of the polynomial used, detrending has added baselines to the spectra that originally contained none. This example illustrates how the application of preprocessing dedicated to additive effects is counterproductive when applied to spectra containing only multiplicative effects. Figure 10c,f,i show the application of detrending to the flour spectra. With a polynomial of degree 0 (Figure 10c), the baselines are corrected only in the center of the wavelength range. With a degree 1 (Figure 10f), the correction is better. The peaks at 1210 nm (fat), 1490 nm (starch), 1940 (water) and 2100 nm (proteins) are clearly exalted. It can be noticed that the use of a degree 2 (Figure 10i) does not bring anything better, which indicates that the baselines of the flour spectra are straight lines.

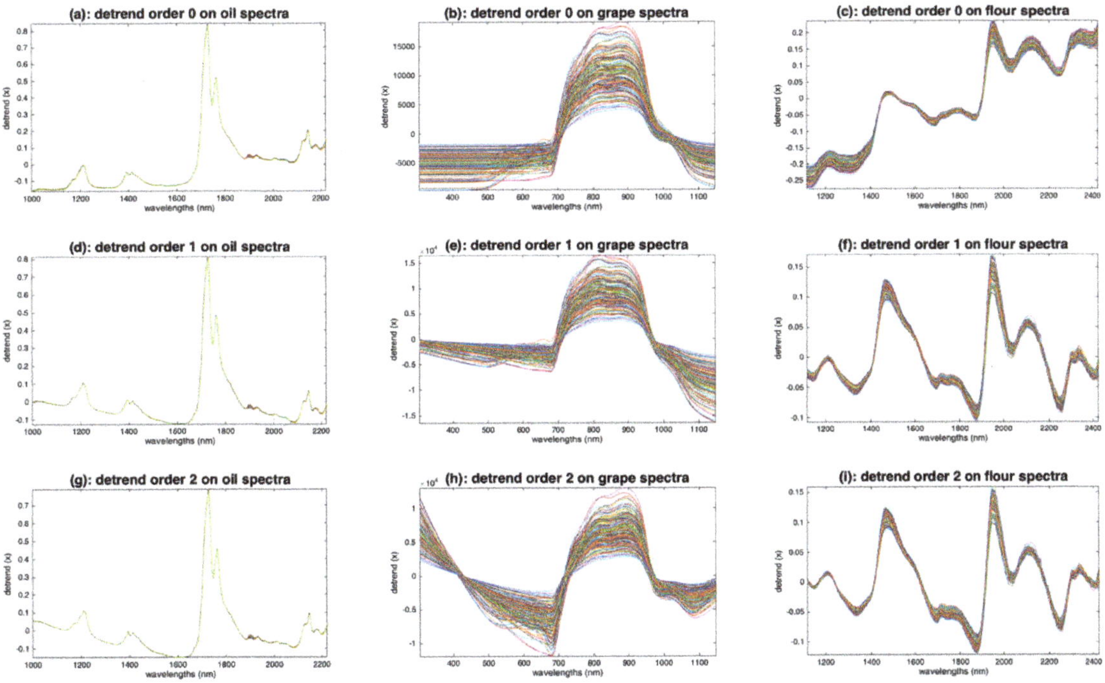

Figure 10. Illustration of the detrending preprocessing. (**a**,**d**,**g**): Oil spectra, (**b**,**e**,**h**): grape spectra, (**c**,**f**,**i**): flour spectra after median filtering (w = 3). (**a**–**c**): Order 0, (**d**–**f**): order 1 and (**g**–**i**): order 2.

In chemometrics, detrending is often used because it removes sources of high variance, allowing the model to focus on useful information. In aquaphotomics, it allows the peaks to be highlighted, as can be seen on the example of the flour spectra, and it can also correct distortions that are detrimental to the construction of aquagrams.

5.2.2. Derivatives

If the baselines are polynomials added to the spectra, a derivative of sufficient order will eliminate them. Thus, a baseline of degree 1 will be eliminated with a derivative of order 2. If $A(\lambda) = \varepsilon(\lambda)LC + A_b(\lambda)$ and if $A_b(\lambda)$ is a polynomial of degree d, then:

$$\frac{\partial^{d+1}(A(\lambda))}{\partial\lambda^{d+1}} = \frac{\partial^{d+1}(\varepsilon(\lambda))}{\partial\lambda^{d+1}}LC$$

To avoid increasing the noise of the spectra, the derivation operation must be performed with a particular algorithm. One of the most used algorithms in NIR spectroscopy is that of Savitzky and Golay [12]. To calculate the derivative at a point i, a polynomial of degree d is fitted to the points of a window centered on i and of width w; then, the polynomial is derived analytically and the value of the derivative at point i is adopted. Figure 11 shows the application of this algorithm to the three spectra sets, with a window of width 11, a polynomial of degree 3 and a derivative of order 2. One can see that all the base lines have disappeared and that a lot of peaks now appear.

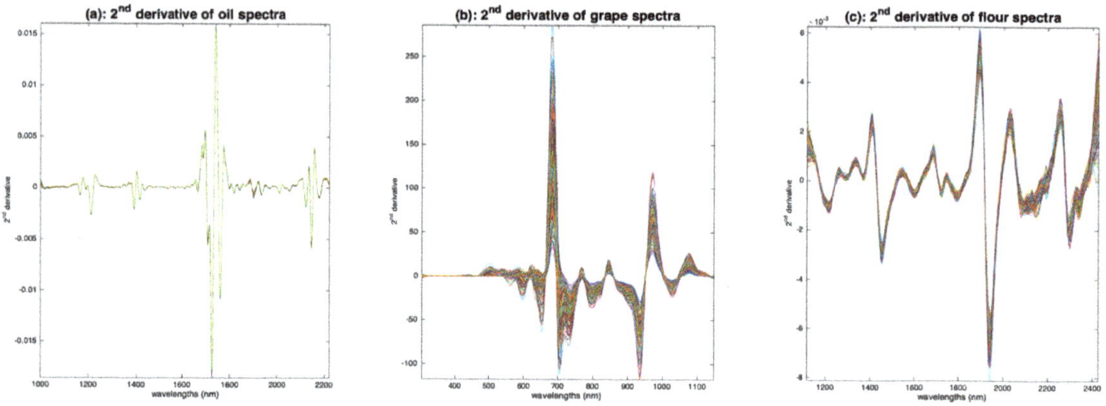

Figure 11. Illustration of the calculation of 2nd order derivatives by the Savitzky and Golay Algorithm. (**a**): Oil, (**b**): grapes, (**c**): flour. All the derivatives have been calculated using an 11 point window and a degree 2 polynomial.

The advantage of the derivatives is that the proportionality with the concentration is recovered. Moreover, this way of removing baselines acts locally, unlike detrending. Thus, if the baseline equation changes with wavelength, the derivation remains effective. The major disadvantage is that the spectrum shape is completely changed, because what appears in the derived spectrum is not the extinction spectrum $\varepsilon(\lambda)$ but its derivative.

However, this feature can be very advantageous for peak identification, and thus for aquaphotomics. For example, in [13], the second derivative of the water spectrum, calculated by the algorithm of Savitzky and Golay, allowed the identification of five species of water, differentiated by the H-bonding of their molecules. This method of pretreatment also allowed the authors to explore the behavior of these species when the temperature of the water changes. In [14], thanks to the peak deconvolution offered by second derivatives, the authors have put forward the existence of two peaks at 1412 nm and at 1462 nm corresponding to two OH-bond vibrational states. These spectacular results were obtained on very pure water. From our experience, second derivative can also reveal hidden peaks on more complex media where OH bond peaks are numerous and intricated, such as wet cellulosic products.

5.2.3. Asymmetric Least Squares

Asymmetric least squares (ALS) allows complex baselines to be eliminated, while preserving the shape of the spectra [15]. It is a technique often used in Raman spectrometry to eliminate the fluorescence background. This method is actually a Whittaker filter, a standard signal processing tool. This method is based on the estimation of a spectrum **z**, approximating as well as possible the spectrum **x**, while having a smooth aspect. This is conducted by minimizing the expression:

$$\sum_i \alpha_i (x_i - z_i)^2 + \beta \sum_i (z_i - 2z_i + z_{i+1})^2$$

where α_i is a weight assigned to each wavelength and β is a penalty term. Minimizing the first term of this sum tends to fit **z** to **x** and minimizing the second one tends to smooth **z**. In order to obtain positive smoothed spectra, the ALS idea is to calculate the weights as follows: $\alpha_i = q$ if $x_i > z_i$ and $\alpha_i = 1 - q$ otherwise. The two parameters β *and* q are user-defined and regulate the degree of smoothness of the estimated baseline and to what extent it is allowed to pass through the peaks.

Figure 12 shows the results of applying ALS on the three sets of spectra. On the oil spectra (Figure 12a), the result is spectacular. The baselines have completely disappeared. All spectra are now based on a zero baseline and are positive, resembling pure absorbance spectra. The peaks appear clearly and so do the inter-sample variations. For the grape spectra (Figure 12b), the result is less convincing, certainly because this set of spectra is mainly affected by multiplicative effects. Nevertheless, the result is much better than the one obtained with detrending (Figure 10). The result on the flour spectra (Figure 12c) is very interesting. The baselines have disappeared, and the peaks and variations appear as clearly as with detrending (Figure 10). The advantage, compared to detrend, is that the spectra are positive.

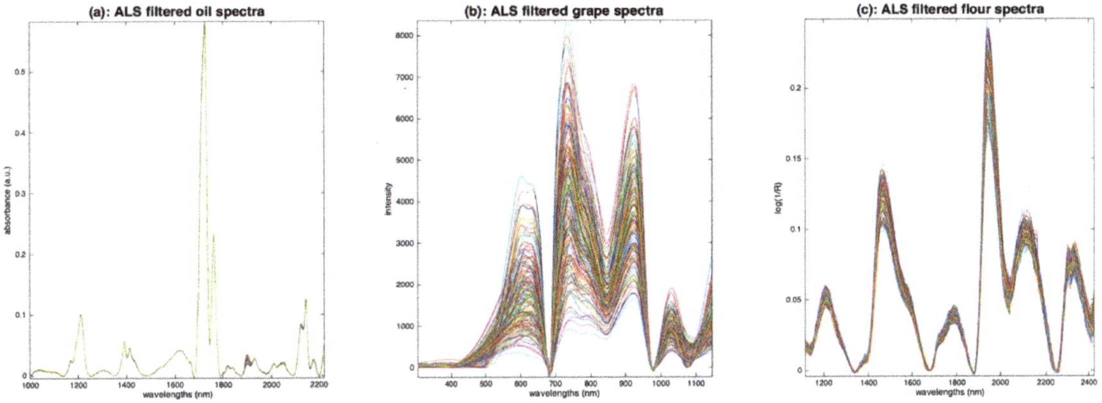

Figure 12. Illustration of asymmetric least squares filtering. (**a**): Oil, (**b**): grapes, (**c**): flour.

The ALS pretreatment appears to be very relevant for aquaphotomics. Indeed, it produces positive spectra, with baselines at zero and clear peaks, which, in some cases, seem quite close to the ideal spectra.

5.3. Multiplicative Effect Removal

As expressed in Equation (2), a multiplicative effect is related to the factor k, which is assumed to multiply the measured values equally for all the wavelengths. This effect is very detrimental in chemometrics because it cannot be compensated by the linear models, contrarily to the additive effect. For this reason, preprocessing of multiplicative effects is often performed before calibration modeling of NIR spectra [16].

5.3.1. Normalization

The basic idea of normalizing a spectrum, as explained in detail in [17], is to divide each of its variables by a quantity calculated from the spectrum and, if possible, affected only by the multiplicative effect. Formally, if $f(.)$ is this quantity, and using the expression in Equation (2) (omitting the additive terms), the normalization preprocessing can be written:

$$A^*(\lambda) = \frac{kA_0(\lambda)}{f(kA_0(\lambda))} = \frac{k\,A_0(\lambda)}{k\,f(A_0(\lambda))} = \frac{1}{f(A_0(\lambda))}A_0(\lambda) \quad (4)$$

We can notice in Equation (4) that the factor k has disappeared and that it has been replaced by a factor depending only on $A_0(\lambda)$. A side effect of this transformation can be to radically change the shape and physical meaning of the spectrum. Caution should, therefore, be paid when choosing the function f. A simple and intuitive choice for f consists of choosing a particular value of the spectrum, which is affected by k. Thus, the maximum of the spectrum is sometimes chosen. However, there are two problems with this choice: the first is that this point may be located on an absorption peak and, in this case, the normalization will remove some useful information. The second is that the wavelength of this point may change from one spectrum to another, which makes the normalization unstable. It is, therefore, preferable to choose, if it exists, a point in the spectrum with a large enough value but independent of the compound of interest. However, the value of a single point in the spectrum has some measurement noise. Dividing the spectrum by this value has the effect of increasing the overall noise of the spectrum. In order to avoid this phenomenon, it is preferable to use a function f calculated on the entire spectrum, such as the area, the mean, the sum, the norm or the standard deviation. When the spectrum contains only positive values, all these functions are almost equivalent. However, if the spectrum contains negative values, as, for example, if the spectrum has been differentiated before, the area, the sum or the mean can be close to zero and, thus, pose stability problems. For this reason, the most used function is the norm or the standard deviation.

Figure 13a–c show the results of normalization by the norm for the three sets of spectra. The effect on the oil spectra (Figure 13a) is almost nonexistent, because these spectra contain no multiplicative effects. The application on the grape spectra is spectacular. The visible part of the spectrum, from 400 to 700 nm, shows several groups of different colors (with peaks at 550 nm or 600 nm), which corresponds well to the ground truth (i.e., different grape varieties). The VNIR part, from 700 to 1150 nm, is much less impacted by the multiplicative effect, although there is still some left. The peak at 960 nm, due to water, now appears more clearly. The flour spectra (Figure 13c) have also benefited from this normalization. The spectra are now much more clustered.

The explanations given, especially by Equation (4), assume that the spectra are free of additive effects. Figure 13d–f show the results of the normalization on the three sets of spectra after application of the ALS filter. It can be seen in Figure 13d that normalization did not alter the oil spectra, which were already near perfect after ALS filtering. On the other hand, the grape spectra, which were highly altered by ALS filtering (Figure 12b), do not give a good result after normalization. Finally, the application of normalization on the ALS-filtered flour spectra (Figure 13f) shows interesting results. The intensity variations that remained on the ALS-filtered spectra (Figure 12c) were significantly reduced. However, it can be seen that variations remain in areas where no chemical absorption takes place, such as between 1300 and 1400 nm. This can be explained by the fact that the spectrum norm, which is used in the normalization procedure, contains chemical information and is, therefore, not the best candidate for the function f. To avoid this problem, several methods have been proposed [17–19]. They all consist of estimating a function f related as much as possible to the multiplicative effect, and as little as possible to the chemistry of the sample.

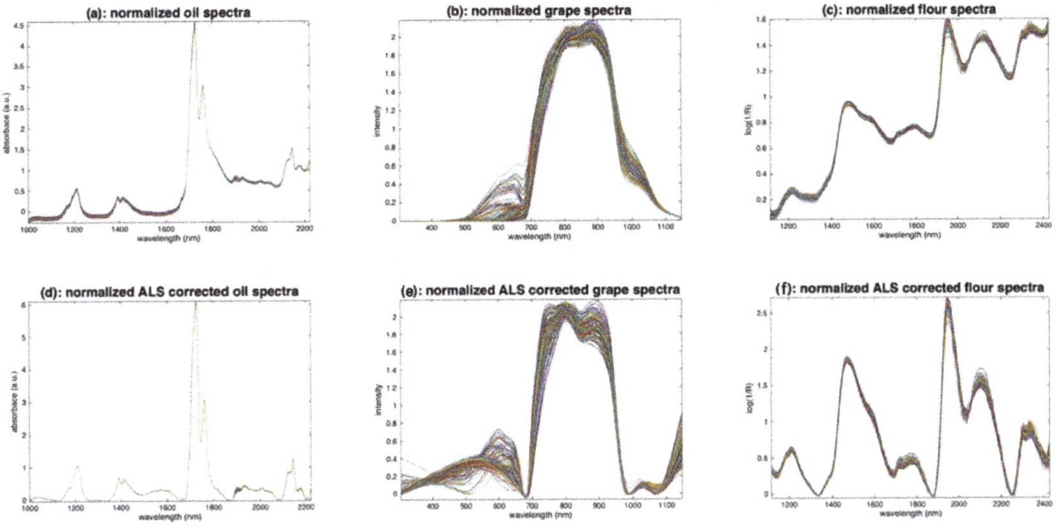

Figure 13. Illustration of normalization. (**a**,**d**): Oil, (**b**,**e**): grapes, (**c**,**f**): flour. (**a**–**c**): Raw spectra are divided by their norm. (**d**–**f**): Raw spectra are first corrected by ALS and then divided by their norm.

5.3.2. Probabilistic Quotient Normalization (PQN)

PQN proposes to estimate $f(\mathbf{x})$ on only a part of the wavelengths in order to avoid the problem mentioned above. It calculates the quotients of the values of all the variables of the spectrum $\mathbf{x}$ over those of the corresponding wavelengths in a reference signal $\mathbf{x}_{\text{ref}}$, thus producing as many divisors as wavelengths. Then, $f(\mathbf{x})$ is calculated as the most probable of these values, i.e., the mode of the divisor distribution. In practice, since it is often impossible to find the mode of a real distribution, the median is taken as an estimate of the most probable value. This method assumes that the variables affected only by the multiplicative effect are more numerous than those also affected by the compound of interest. This condition is rarely met in NIR spectroscopy applied to complex products but it could be met in some aquaphotomics applications.

Figure 14a–c show the results of PQN for the three sets of spectra. Globally, as expected, the results are very similar to those of classical normalization (Figure 13).

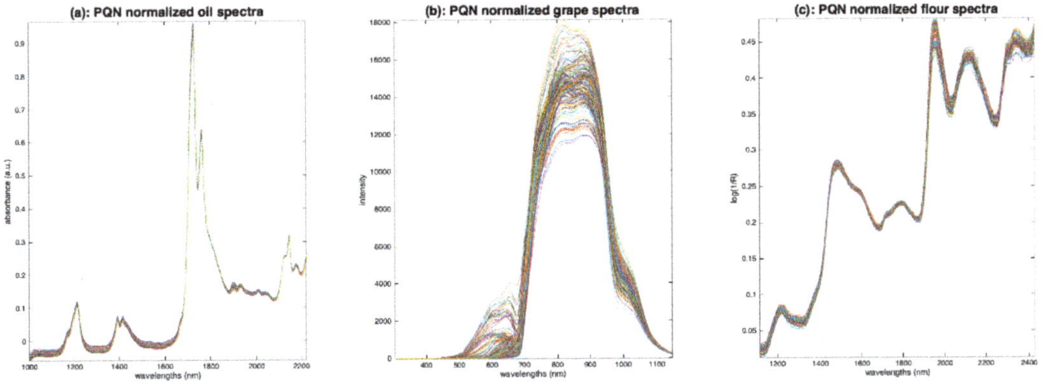

Figure 14. Illustration of probabilistic quotient normalization. (**a**): Oil, (**b**): grapes, (**c**): flour.

5.4. Combined Methods

Methods have been developed to correct for additive and multiplicative effects simultaneously. This is the case of standard normal variate [20], which applies a detrend of order 0 and then a normalization by the standard deviation of the spectrum. This is a very popular method in the NIR community. SNV will be discussed in depth later, in Section 7.

Multiplicative scatter correction (MSC) [21] proposes explicitly correcting each spectrum $\mathbf{x}$ of a set of spectra $\mathbf{X}$ with respect to a reference spectrum $\mathbf{x}_{ref}$. The idea is to remove from each spectrum the additive and multiplicative effects that distinguish it from $\mathbf{x}_{ref}$ and, thus, to align all the spectra on a common global direction. In practice, as $\mathbf{x}_{ref}$ is often unknown, it is usually replaced by the average of $\mathbf{X}$. Concretely, using the point of view of Figure 4, the following model is written:

$$\mathbf{x} = a\mathbf{x}_{ref} + b + \mathbf{r} \tag{5}$$

Then, for each spectrum, a and b are derived by means of a linear regression, and $\mathbf{x}$ is corrected by:

$$\mathbf{x}_{msc} = \frac{\mathbf{x} - b}{a} = \mathbf{x}_{ref} + \frac{1}{a}\mathbf{r} \tag{6}$$

In other words, each spectrum is modified so that it is as close as possible to the reference spectrum. Using the formalism of Equation (2), the idea is that all preprocessed spectra share the same k and $A_b(\lambda)$ as the reference spectrum.

MSC is theoretically closely related to SNV [22]. It, therefore, suffers from the same problems as SNV (see Section 7). However, extended multiplicative scatter correction (EMSC) [5] differs from it by proposing more complex models. EMSC extends the MSC model by modeling the spectrum as a mixture of the reference spectrum and other spectral contributions, such as chemical interferents, temperature effects [23], optical scattering laws, etc. In this sense, EMSC is really a spectroscopic modeling method, as shown by the first sentence of [5]: "Knowledge-driven versus data driven modelling". EMSC is, therefore, a tool of choice for aquaphotomics [24].

6. A Focus on Log Transform

While, in most cases, the additive and multiplicative effects are randomly distributed amongst the spectra, it was recently shown that these effects could be, in fact, directly related to the moisture content of the measured scattering media [25]. By using the EMSC framework to get rid of the additive effects, it could be shown that the path-length modifications (responsible of a multiplicative effect) can be directly related to moisture content by a simple power law. Coming back to Equation (2), this results in the following new equation:

$$A(\lambda) = \varepsilon(\lambda)kLC + \varepsilon_w(\lambda)k_wL_wC_w^p + A_b(\lambda) + A_n(\lambda) \tag{7}$$

where all the variables subscripted by w relate to water, and p is the power coefficient.

In the specific case when moisture content is predicted, applying a log transformation of both the signal (after getting rid of the additive terms) and the predicted variable yields better models, as the log transform linearizes the relationship.

For a broader use, in aquaphotomics, when running multivariate curve resolution experiments, for example, the water effects on scattering could be included as a component, where a hard-modeling constraint could be applied on the shape of the component's score/concentration (i.e., force the shape to be a power law type). Such information added as a constraint could help obtain a better resolution of the mixing problem.

7. A Focus on SNV

SNV is a very popular method in the NIR community; the paper describing this method has been cited more than 3400 times in about 30 years. The reason for such success is that the method is simple and effective in removing most of the variability due to scattering, which is unavoidable in case of backscatter measurements. It is widely used as a preprocessing for linear model calibrations, such as PLS regression. However, when the goal is to recover fundamental spectral components, such as pure spectra, as with $\varepsilon(\lambda)$ in Equation (1), or to recover an accurate level of absorbance, this preprocessing can be detrimental, as shown in the following example.

Figure 15a represents a set of simulated spectra, where four peaks are present, with only the two left hand ones, related to the compounds of interest, varying. In Figure 15b, the same spectra have been assigned a baseline and a multiplicative effect, both independent of wavelength. Figure 15c shows the result of applying SNV on these spectra. The result is far from the pure spectra. For example, the variations at the two right peaks, which should be weak, are comparable to the ones of the peaks of interest. The problem is that SNV estimates the additive and multiplicative effects by the mean and standard deviation of the whole spectrum, respectively. However, these quantities, in our example (spectra in Figure 15b), are very largely influenced by the variations of the compound of interest. Thus, after applying the correction, the variations due to the compound of interest are distributed over the whole spectrum.

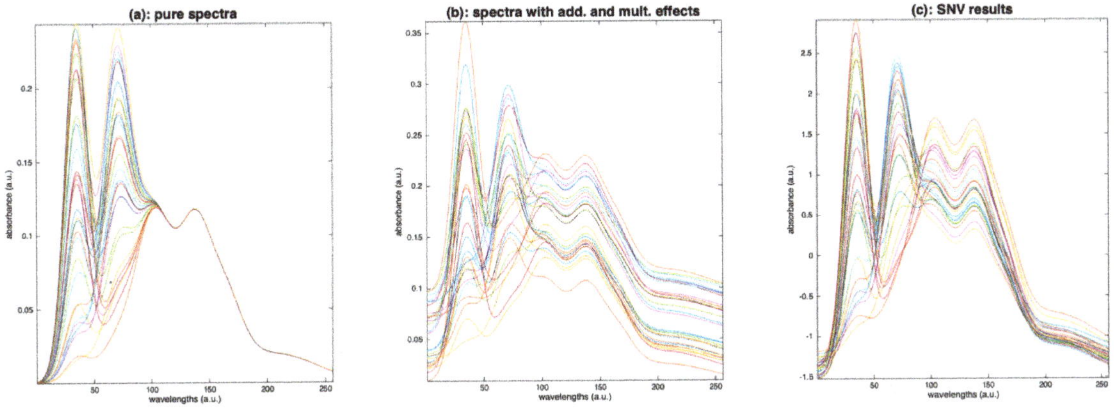

Figure 15. Illustration of the detrimental effect of SNV. (**a**) Simulated pure spectra, (**b**): simulated spectra after addition of baselines and multiplicative factors, (**c**): result of SNV performed on the spectra in (**b**).

A solution consists of performing the estimation of the baseline and the multiplicative effect, preferentially using the wavelengths that are mainly related to the additive and multiplicative effects. This can be conducted using a diagonal matrix $\mathbf{W}$ of weights, between 0 and 1, which is then used in SNV and detrending:

- Compute the standard deviation of $\mathbf{xW}$ in place of $\mathbf{x}$;
- Replace Equation (3) of detrending by: $\mathbf{x}_{det} = \mathbf{x}(\mathbf{I} - \mathbf{W}\,\mathbf{L}\,(\mathbf{L}'\,\mathbf{W}\,\mathbf{L})^{-1}\mathbf{L}')$.

As an example, Figure 16c shows the result of a weighted SNV, using the weights plotted in Figure 16b. The result is perfect, because the additive and multiplicative effects have been estimated using the part of the spectra affected only by these effects.

The variable sorting for normalization (VSN) method [17] automatically calculates these weights $\mathbf{W}$ from the experimental data matrix $\mathbf{X}$. It uses an RANSAC-type algorithm [26] to classify the points of each spectrum into two classes: the inliers are the wavelengths that all share the same additive and multiplicative effect pattern; the outliers are the wavelengths related to nonsystematic variations, thus related to the compounds of interest. The final weight is determined as the probability that each wavelength belongs to the inlier class. VSN also determines the best-suited degree of the polynomial for the baseline.

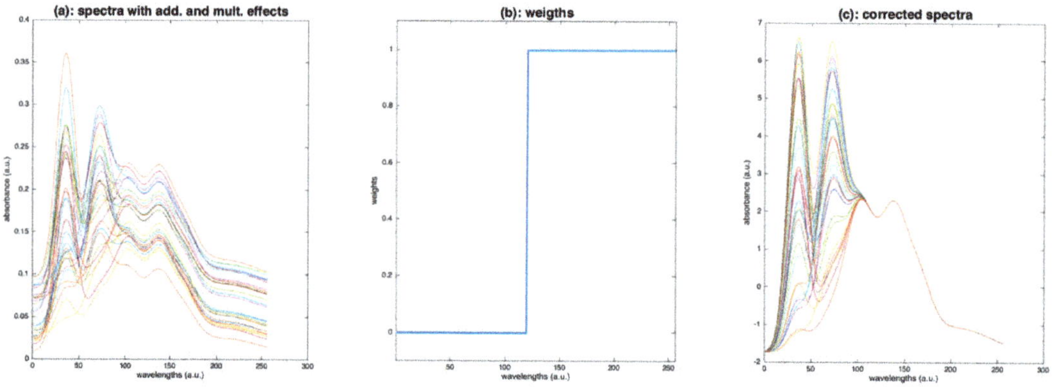

Figure 16. Illustration of the weighted SNV. (**a**): Spectra to be processed, (**b**): weights, (**c**): spectra after preprocessing by weighted SNV.

Figure 17 illustrates the application of VSN to the three sets of oil, grape and flour spectra. Figure 17a–c show the corrected spectra; Figure 17d–f show the weights found by the algorithm. For the oil spectra, VSN retained baselines of degree 1 and calculated the weights plotted in Figure 17d. These weights are overall low, indicating that all wavelengths are mostly related to chemistry. The two least informative areas, and, therefore, the most efficient for calculating additive and multiplicative effects, are the two dips around 1300 and 1500 nm. The resulting spectra reported in Figure 17a are very similar to those yielded by a detrending of order 1 (Figure 10d). For the grape spectra, VSN has identified that only multiplicative effects exist. The weights (Figure 17e) are very contrasting. They are very close to 1 at both ends of the spectral range, i.e., before 500 nm and after 1100 nm, and close to 0 in the 550–1000 nm region, which corresponds well to the region of pigments and metabolic compounds. The resulting spectra (Figure 17b) are quite similar to those obtained with PQN (Figure 14b). This illustrates that, when the spectra are only impacted by multiplicative effects, VSN and PQN are, in fact, two very close solutions to achieve a robust normalization. For the flour spectra, VSN found a model with baselines of degree 1, which corresponds to the result found after applying detrending (Figure 10). The weights (Figure 17f) show that the areas around 1400 nm and above 2000 nm should not be used for the calculation of multiplicative and additive effects. This result is consistent with the absorption areas of O-H bonds (water, cellulose) and proteins. The preprocessed spectra (Figure 17c) globally resemble those obtained with detrending (Figure 10). However, in detail, it can be seen that the area from 1900 nm to 2500 nm was less shrunk by the preprocessing than the rest of the spectrum, suggesting that variations due to chemistry are visible in this area.

It is clear that weighted versions of EMSC or SNV (thanks to PQN or VSN) appear most suitable for aquaphotomics studies. Indeed, while aquaphotomics focuses on the first O-H overtone region (1300–1600 nm), the preprocessing of physical effects should be conducted based on regions where absorbance bonds related to chemical phenomena are absent (in water spectra, this usually corresponds to the following spectral ranges: 1000–1300 nm, 1600–1800 nm, and 2000–2400 nm).

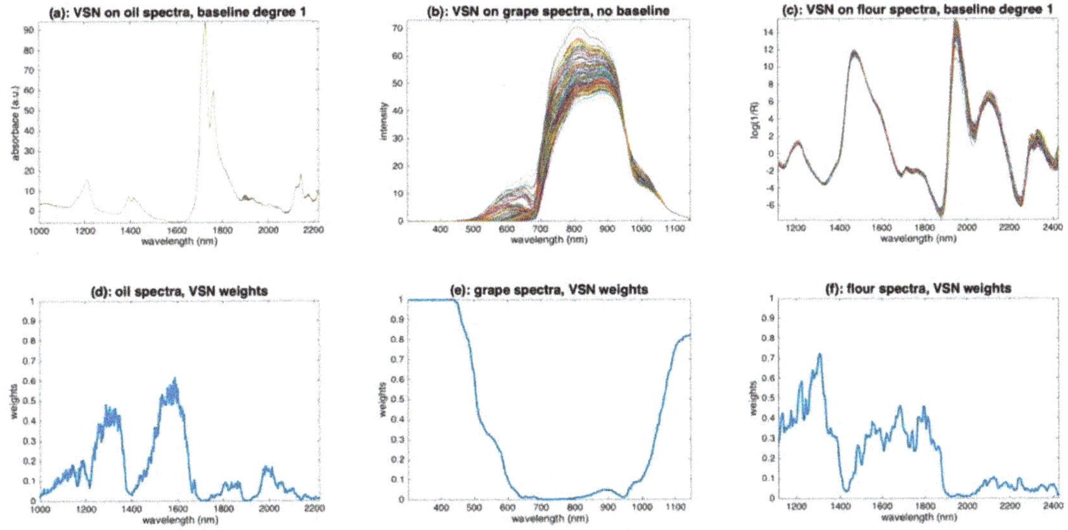

Figure 17. Illustration of the application of VSN. (**a**): VSN corrected oil spectra, (**b**): VSN corrected grape spectra, (**c**): VSN corrected flour spectra, (**d**): VSN weights for the oil spectra, (**e**): VSN weights for the grape spectra, (**f**): VSN weights for the flour spectra.

8. Conclusions

This paper has reviewed the main preprocessing of NIR spectra, with a view to their use in aquaphotomics. Simple visualization methods have been proposed in order to identify the nature of undesirable effects, even before the application of a preprocessing. The most commonly used preprocessing in chemometrics has been presented and illustrated by three sets of spectra, each showing the advantages and disadvantages of each method. Some preprocessing aims to produce a spectrum as close as possible to the absorbance that would have been measured under ideal conditions and can, therefore, be very useful for the establishment of an aquagram. Others, dedicated to the improvement of the resolution of the peaks, prove to be very useful for the identification of hidden peaks. A special focus on the correction of multiplicative effects has shown the interest of logarithmic transformation and weighted normalization methods. This highlights the fact that much preprocessing that has been designed in chemometrics to improve the performance of calibration models should be used with care in aquaphotomics.

Author Contributions: Conceptualization, J.-M.R. and F.M.; methodology, J.-M.R., A.M. and F.M.; software, J.-M.R., A.M. and F.M.; data curation, J.-M.R.; writing—original draft preparation, J.-M.R.; writing—review and editing, J.-M.R., A.M. and F.M. All authors have read and agreed to the published version of the manuscript.

Funding: This research received no external funding.

Institutional Review Board Statement: Not applicable.

Informed Consent Statement: Not applicable.

Conflicts of Interest: The authors declare no conflict of interest.

References

1. Siesler, H.W.; Kawata, S.; Heise, H.M.; Ozaki, Y. (Eds.) *Near-Infrared Spectroscopy: Principles, Instruments, Applications*; John Wiley & Sons: Hoboken, NJ, USA, 2008.
2. Pasquini, C. Near infrared spectroscopy: A mature analytical technique with new perspectives–A review. *Anal. Chim. Acta* **2018**, *1026*, 8–36. [CrossRef]

3. Tsenkova, R. Visible-near infrared perturbation spectroscopy: Water in action seen as a source of information. In Proceedings of the 12th International Conference on Near-Infrared Spectroscopy, Auckland, New Zealand, 1 September 2005; pp. 607–612.
4. Muncan, J.; Tsenkova, R. Aquaphotomics—From innovative knowledge to integrative platform in science and technology. *Molecules* **2019**, *24*, 2742. [CrossRef]
5. Martens, H.; Stark, E. Extended multiplicative signal correction and spectral interference subtraction: New preprocessing methods for near infrared spectroscopy. *J. Pharm. Biomed. Anal.* **1991**, *9*, 625–635. [CrossRef]
6. Rinnan, Å. Pre-processing in vibrational spectroscopy–when, why and how. *Anal. Methods* **2014**, *6*, 7124–7129. [CrossRef]
7. Roger, J.-M.; Boulet, J.-C.; Zeaiter, M.; Rutledge, D.N. Pre-processing Methods*. In *Reference Module in Chemistry, Molecular Sciences and Chemical Engineering*; Elsevier: Amsterdam, The Netherlands, 2020.
8. Dupuy, N.; Galtier, O.; Ollivier, D.; Vanloot, P.; Artaud, J. Comparison between NIR, MIR, concatenated NIR and MIR analysis and hierarchical PLS model. Application to virgin olive oil analysis. *Anal. Chim. Acta* **2010**, *666*, 23–31. [CrossRef]
9. Chauchard, F.; Cogdill, R.; Roussel, S.; Roger, J.M.; Bellon-Maurel, V. Application of LS-SVM to non-linear phenomena in NIR spectroscopy: Development of a robust and portable sensor for acidity prediction in grapes. *Chemom. Intell. Lab. Syst.* **2004**, *71*, 141–150. [CrossRef]
10. Data of a Challenge Proposed at 2022 Chimiométrie Conference, 7–8 June 2022, Brest, France. Available online: https://chimiobrest2022.sciencesconf.org/resource/page/id/5 (accessed on 15 December 2021).
11. Mobley, P.R.; Kowalski, B.R.; Workman, J.J., Jr.; Bro, R. Review of chemometrics applied to spectroscopy: 1985-95, part 2. *Appl. Spectrosc. Rev.* **1996**, *31*, 347–368. [CrossRef]
12. Savitzky, A.; Golay, M.J. Smoothing and differentiation of data by simplified least squares procedures. *Anal. Chem.* **1964**, *36*, 1627–1639. [CrossRef]
13. Maeda, H.; Ozaki, Y.; Tanaka, M.; Hayashi, N.; Kojima, T. Near infrared spectroscopy and chemometrics studies of temperature-dependent spectral variations of water: Relationship between spectral changes and hydrogen bonds. *J. Near Infrared Spectrosc.* **1995**, *3*, 191–201. [CrossRef]
14. Renati, P.; Kovacs, Z.; De Ninno, A.; Tsenkova, R. Temperature dependence analysis of the NIR spectra of liquid water confirms the existence of two phases, one of which is in a coherent state. *J. Mol. Liq.* **2019**, *292*, 111449. [CrossRef]
15. Eilers, P.H.; Boelens, H.F. Baseline correction with asymmetric least squares smoothing. *Leiden Univ. Med. Cent. Rep.* **2005**, *1*, 5.
16. Rinnan, Å.; Van Den Berg, F.; Engelsen, S.B. Review of the most common pre-processing techniques for near-infrared spectra. *TrAC Trends Anal. Chem.* **2009**, *28*, 1201–1222. [CrossRef]
17. Rabatel, G.; Marini, F.; Walczak, B.; Roger, J.M. VSN: Variable sorting for normalization. *J. Chemom.* **2020**, *34*, e3164. [CrossRef]
18. Dieterle, F.; Ross, A.; Schlotterbeck, G.; Senn, H. Probabilistic quotient normalization as robust method to account for dilution of complex biological mixtures. Application in 1H NMR metabonomics. *Anal. Chem.* **2006**, *78*, 4281–4290. [CrossRef] [PubMed]
19. Guo, Q.; Wu, W.; Massart, D.L. The robust normal variate transform for pattern recognition with near-infrared data Anal. *Chim. Acta.* **1999**, *382*, 87–103. [CrossRef]
20. Barnes, R.J.; Dhanoa, M.S.; Lister, S.J. Standard normal variate transformation and de-trending of near-infrared diffuse reflectance spectra. *Appl. Spectrosc.* **1989**, *43*, 772–777. [CrossRef]
21. Isaksson, T.; Næs, T. The effect of multiplicative scatter correction (MSC) and linearity improvement in NIR spectroscopy. *Appl. Spectrosc.* **1988**, *42*, 1273–1284. [CrossRef]
22. Dhanoa, M.S.; Lister, S.J.; Sanderson, R.; Barnes, R.J. The link between multiplicative scatter correction (MSC) and standard normal variate (SNV) transformations of NIR spectra. *J. Near Infrared Spectrosc.* **1994**, *2*, 43–47. [CrossRef]
23. Gowen, A.A.; Marini, F.; Tsuchisaka, Y.; De Luca, S.; Bevilacqua, M.; Donnell, C.O.; Downey, G.; Tsenkova, R. On the feasibility of near infrared spectroscopy to detect contaminants in water using single salt solutions as model systems. *Talanta* **2015**, *131*, 609–618. [CrossRef]
24. Gowen, A.A.; Stark, E.W.; Tsuchisaka, Y.; Tsenkova, R. Extended multiplicative signal correction as a tool for aquaphotomics. *NIR News* **2011**, *22*, 9–13. [CrossRef]
25. Mallet, A.; Tsenkova, R.; Muncan, J.; Charnier, C.; Latrille, é.; Bendoula, R.; Steyer, J.P.; Roger, J.M. Relating Near-Infrared Light Path-Length Modifications to the Water Content of Scattering Media in Near-Infrared Spectroscopy: Toward a New Bouguer-Beer-Lambert Law. *Anal. Chem.* **2021**, *93*, 6817–6823. [CrossRef] [PubMed]
26. Fischler, M.A.; Bolles, R.C. Random sample consensus: A paradigm for model fitting with applications to image analysis and automated cartography. *Commun. ACM* **1981**, *24*, 381–395. [CrossRef]

molecules

MDPI

Review

Chemometrics: An Excavator in Temperature-Dependent Near-Infrared Spectroscopy

Yan Sun, Wensheng Cai and Xueguang Shao *

Research Center for Analytical Sciences, Frontiers Science Center for New Organic Matter, College of Chemistry, Nankai University, Tianjin Key Laboratory of Biosensing and Molecular Recognition, State Key Laboratory of Medicinal Chemical Biology, Tianjin 300071, China; sunyan@mail.nankai.edu.cn (Y.S.); wscai@nankai.edu.cn (W.C.)

* Correspondence: xshao@nankai.edu.cn; Tel.: +86-22-2350-3430

Abstract: Temperature-dependent near-infrared (NIR) spectroscopy has been developed and taken as a powerful technique for analyzing the structure of water and the interactions in aqueous systems. Due to the overlapping of the peaks in NIR spectra, it is difficult to obtain the spectral features showing the structures and interactions. Chemometrics, therefore, is adopted to improve the spectral resolution and extract spectral information from the temperature-dependent NIR spectra for structural and quantitative analysis. In this review, works on chemometric studies for analyzing temperature-dependent NIR spectra were summarized. The temperature-induced spectral features of water structures can be extracted from the spectra with the help of chemometrics. Using the spectral variation of water with the temperature, the structural changes of small molecules, proteins, thermo-responsive polymers, and their interactions with water in aqueous solutions can be demonstrated. Furthermore, quantitative models between the spectra and the temperature or concentration can be established using the spectral variations of water and applied to determine the compositions in aqueous mixtures.

Keywords: temperature-dependent near-infrared spectroscopy; chemometrics; water structure; structural analysis; quantitative analysis

Citation: Sun, Y.; Cai, W.; Shao, X. Chemometrics: An Excavator in Temperature-Dependent Near-Infrared Spectroscopy. *Molecules* **2022**, 27, 452. https://doi.org/10.3390/molecules27020452

Academic Editors: Roumiana Tsenkova and Jelena Muncan

Received: 13 December 2021
Accepted: 10 January 2022
Published: 11 January 2022

1. Introduction

Near-infrared (NIR) spectroscopy has been recognized as a powerful technique to study the structure of water [1]. Due to the strong absorption, the spectral information of the water structures with different hydrogen bonds can be measured, and the structures can be distinguished by analyzing the spectrum [1,2]. Aquaphotomics proposed by Tsenkova provides a framework for understanding the structural change of water caused by various perturbations such as temperature and solutes in aqueous and biological systems [3,4]. The spectral change of water can be used not only as a mirror to reflect the properties of the solutes in aqueous systems, but also as a probe to diagnose diseases or abnormalities non-invasively [5–7]. The spectral pattern describing the structures of water is used to measure the quality of water under different filtration treatments [8], to monitor the lactic acid bacteria fermentation in yogurt production [9], and to understand the physiological strategies of the resurrection plant during desiccation and rehydration procedure [10].

Temperature-dependent NIR spectroscopy is developed based on the temperature effect on the spectrum [11–13]. In 2010, the temperature dependency of NIR spectra on the temperature was studied, and a quantitative spectra–temperature relationship (QSTR) model between the NIR spectra of water and the temperature was established using partial least squares (PLS) regression [11,12]. Then, methods for analyzing the high-dimensional data matrices, including N-way principal component analysis (NPCA), parallel factor analysis (PARAFAC), and alternating trilinear decomposition (ATLD) were employed to analyze high-dimensional temperature-dependent NIR spectra [14]. The spectral variations induced by both the temperature and the concentration were obtained. The former can be used for structural analysis, and the latter can be used for building a calibration model for quantitative analysis. To simplify the calculation, low-dimensional algorithms were also proposed for analyzing high-dimensional temperature-dependent NIR spectral data. Mutual factor analysis (MFA) was proposed, and multilevel simultaneous component analysis (MSCA) was applied for the quantitative analysis of glucose solutions and serum samples [15–17]. A quantitative model was established for predicting the glucose content in aqueous and serum samples. Furthermore, the spectral variation of water induced by the temperature reflects the structural changes and interactions of water and solutes in aqueous solutions. Chemometric methods to improve the spectral resolution and extract temperature-induced spectral variations were studied for structural analysis, including continuous wavelet transform (CWT), independent component analysis (ICA), and Gaussian fitting.

In 2019, a review was published, in which chemometric methods and the applications in the resolution, quantitative, and structural analysis of temperature-dependent NIR spectra were summarized [13]. In this review, further works on extracting structural and quantitative information from temperature-dependent NIR spectra by chemometric methods were summarized. In temperature-dependent NIR spectroscopy, the perturbation of the temperature is taken as a source of spectral information reflecting the variation of systems. When the composition or concentration in the system changes, the temperature dependency of the spectra changes accordingly. Therefore, the temperature-induced spectral features can be used to reflect the properties of the systems. To capture the temperature-induced spectral information of water, chemometric algorithms were proposed for improving the resolution of NIR spectra. The spectral features of water reflecting the structural changes and interactions were obtained. Through the temperature-induced spectral variation, the interactions of water with small molecules, proteins, and polymers were investigated, and the role of water in the chemical and biological processes was revealed. Furthermore, quantitative determination can also be achieved using the spectral variation of water with the temperature or concentration and successfully applied to the quantification of the compositions in aqueous mixtures.

2. Structural Information of Water

The structure of water has been an interesting subject in chemistry and biology for decades due to the complex and flexible patterns of hydrogen bonding [18–21]. The effect of the temperature on the NIR spectrum of liquid water was studied as early as in 1925 [22], and over the past few decades, a number of works reported the temperature dependency of the NIR spectra of water [23–28]. Most of the researches focused on the absorption band around 6900 cm^{-1} measured at different temperatures, where an isosbestic point can be observed, implying the variation of the overlapped spectral components with the change of the temperature. With the help of chemometric methods, the spectral features of water structures with different hydrogen bonds were obtained, and the relative abundances of different water structures that change with the temperature were found [27,28]. Thus, the temperature-dependent NIR spectroscopy combined with chemometrics provides an efficient way to explore the structure of water in aqueous systems.

To investigate the effect of the temperature on the NIR spectra of water, a method for selecting the temperature-dependent variables from the temperature-dependent NIR spectra was developed. Figure 1A shows the temperature-dependent NIR spectra of water measured from 30 to 60 °C in the spectral range of 6000–10,000 cm^{-1}. It can be seen that with the increase of the temperature, a shift of the peak around 6900 cm^{-1} to a higher wavenumber was observed, which is caused by the change of the overlapped spectral components corresponding to different water structures. To obtain the temperature-dependent information from the spectra, a method combined CWT and Monte-Carlo uninformative variable elimination (MC-UVE) was proposed for the selection of the temperature-dependent variables (wavenumbers) from the NIR spectra measured at different temperatures [29]. CWT was used to decompose the spectra into the spectral components with different frequencies, and then MC-UVE was employed to evaluate the importance of the variables in the quantitative model of the spectra and temperature. Figure 1B shows the stability of the transformed water spectra obtained by MC-UVE, which is named as "fountain graph". In the fountain for the peak around 6900 cm^{-1}, seven variables with a significant temperature dependency can be found. This indicates the complexity of water structures and suggests that there are different water species of which the spectral features change differently with the temperature. Furthermore, the temperature-dependent NIR spectra of the aqueous solutions containing NaCl, glucose, and human serum albumin (HSA) were investigated. Figure 1C shows the transformed spectra of water and solutions by CWT and the locations of the selected variables. It can be seen that the selected variables are located at similar but not identical wavenumbers for different solutions, indicating that the variables can be used for the discrimination of different solutions. Furthermore, using the selected variables, quantification can also be achieved. The results indicate that temperature-dependent NIR spectra can be severed as a mirror to reflect the complexity of water structures and identify the aqueous solutions of different compositions.

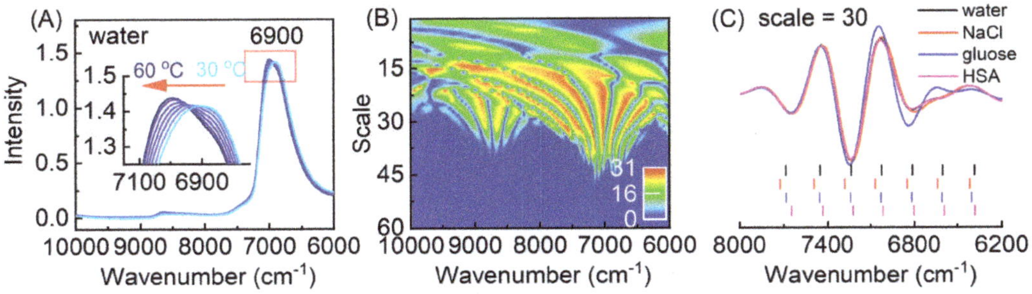

Figure 1. Temperature-independent near-infrared (NIR) spectra of water in the range of 6000–10,000 cm^{-1} measured from 30 to 60 °C (**A**), the fountain graph (**B**), and the selected variables for the samples of water, NaCl (5.8 g L^{-1}), glucose (20 g L^{-1}), and HSA (5.0 g L^{-1}) solutions (**C**).

To understand water structures in liquid water and aqueous solutions, Gaussian fitting was adopted to analyze the temperature-dependent NIR spectra of water. Six spectral components were used to fitting the spectra, corresponding to different water species with no (S_0), one (S_1), two (S_2), three (S_3), and four (S_4) hydrogen bonds, as well as the rotation vibration (S_r) of the water molecule [30]. To describe the complex water structures more exactly, a model was proposed by denoting the proton acceptor (oxygen) with A and the proton donor (hydrogen) with D. The water molecule with *m* hydrogen bonds on oxygen atom and *n* hydrogen bonds on hydrogen atom is represented by A*m*D*n*, where *m* and *n* equal to 0, 1, or 2. Therefore, nine water structures can be defined, i.e., A0D0, A0D1, A1D0, A0D2, A1D1, A2D0, A1D2, A2D1, and A2D2. Ten spectral components corresponding to the nine water structures and S_r were obtained from the temperature-dependent spectra of water and glucose solutions by Gaussian fitting with a knowledge-based genetic algorithm [31]. Figure 2 is one of the results obtained by the fitting. It can be seen that the fitted spectrum coincides well with the measured one. The integral intensity of the 10 peaks was investigated using the NIR spectra measured at different temperatures. With the increase of the temperature, the content of A0D0 increases, while that of A2D2 decreases, indicating the weakening of the hydrogen bonds and the dissociation of the water structures with more hydrogen bonds into that with less hydrogen bonds. Furthermore, through the variation of the spectral components of these water structures with the glucose concentration, the enhancement of the ordered (tetrahedral) hydrogen-bonded water structures induced by the interaction of water and glucose were found, providing a proof for the explanation of the protective effect of glucose on the bio-molecules in aqueous solutions.

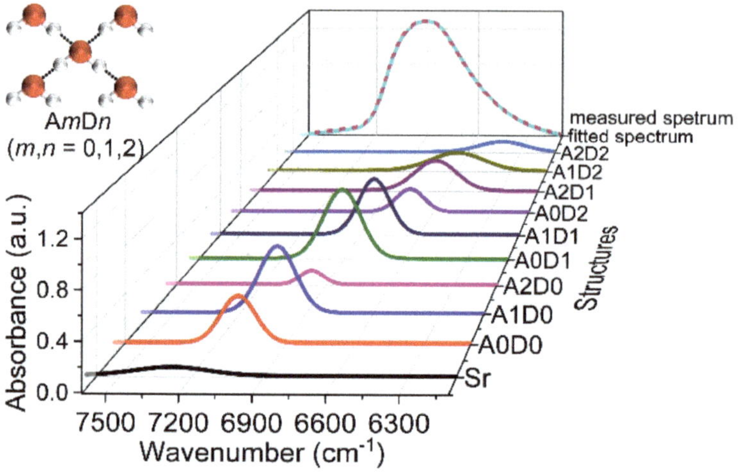

Figure 2. Result of Gaussian fitting for the NIR spectra of water measured at 30 °C.

CWT has been proven to be a powerful tool for the resolution enhancement in the spectral analysis [32–35]. To analyze the spectral features of water in mixtures of water and ethanol, the fourth-order derivative of the temperature-dependent NIR spectra of the mixtures was calculated by CWT [36]. The overlapped peaks were separated, and the spectral features of OH and CH with various intermolecular interactions were identified in the fourth derivative spectra. By fitting the derivative spectra of the mixtures by those of pure water and ethanol, the obtained coefficients for ethanol show a linear relation with the content, but those for water exhibit a non-linear relation, which provides clear evidence for the interactions of ethanol and water in the mixtures. Furthermore, from the residual spectra after the fitting, the structures of water species, aggregations of ethanol, hetero clusters of ethanol–water, and their variation with the content were analyzed. The residual spectra calculated by high-order derivatives provide a very good way to uncover the spectral information about the interactions. These results indicate that the spectral information of water structures with different hydrogen bonds can be extracted from the temperature-dependent NIR spectra, and the temperature-induced spectral features can be a probe to reveal the structural changes and interactions in aqueous solutions.

3. Interaction of Water and Solutes

Water plays an important role in chemical and biological processes. The interaction of water and solutes is of great significance for understanding the properties of aqueous solutions or bio-systems [37]. Due to the sensitivity of NIR spectra to water structures, the spectral changes of water under different perturbations can be a probe to reveal the interactions in aqueous solutions. The interaction of water and bio-organisms including carbohydrate molecules and oligopeptide was investigated using the NIR spectra of aqueous solutions measured at different concentrations and temperatures [30,31,38–41]. The spectral components related to different water structures were obtained from the NIR spectra. Through the variation of these structures with the temperature and the solute concentration, an increase of the tetrahedrally hydrogen-bonded water structure induced by bio-molecules was observed, showing that the thermal stability of water structures may be enhanced in bio-systems.

The interaction of water and ethanol was studied using the temperature-dependent NIR spectroscopy with high-order chemometric algorithms, including NPCA, PARAFAC, and ATLD [14]. The spectral features of water and ethanol in the mixtures were obtained by the three methods. Through the variation of the spectra with the concentration, it was revealed that ethanol promotes the formation of water clusters. To obtain more spectral information of the interactions of water and ethanol, a new method was proposed based on the rotation of the loadings in principal component analysis (PCA) [42]. The calculated spectra were found to be more reliable to reflect the structures in the mixture, from which the spectral features of different water species (S_0–S_4), ethanol clusters, and the interaction of OH and CH groups were observed. Through the difference between the calculated and experimental spectra, it was found that, when ethanol is added into water, the contents of large water clusters with two, three, and four hydrogen bonds increase, and the interaction of water and ethanol varies nonlinearly with the concentration.

The structure of water at low temperatures is related to many special phenomena. For example, the freezing point of water reduces when an antifreeze is added, and water in polar fish does not freeze below the freezing point. The structure of water at low temperatures and the mechanism of the cryoprotectant dimethyl sulfoxide (DMSO) in reducing the freezing point of water were investigated using the NIR spectra measured at low temperatures [43]. CWT was adopted to enhance the resolution of the NIR spectra. The spectral features reflecting the interaction of DMSO and water were found from the resolution-enhanced spectra, and two hydrogen-bonded DMSO–water structures (DW2 and D2W) were identified in the mixtures with different DMSO/water ratios. Through the variation of the spectral features, it was found that DW2 structure inhibits the formation of tetrahedral water structures at low temperatures, which may be the reason for DMSO reducing the freezing point of the mixture. To further understand the effect of protein on the antifreezing performance of the DMSO–water system, the effect of formamide (FA) on the hydrogen bonding of DMSO and water was studied [44]. From the resolution-enhanced spectra by CWT, the spectral feature of the interaction of DMSO and water (S=O . . . H–O) was observed. When FA exists in the mixture, the intensity of the peak decreases with the increase of FA content, indicating that FA may replace the water molecules to form the hydrogen bond of S=O and H–N. Furthermore, the spectra of the three-component mixtures were analyzed by ATLD. Two varying spectral features due to water and DMSO were obtained, but the spectral feature variation with the content of FA was not found. This result implies that, although FA may reduce slightly the antifreezing effect, DMSO is still the key component to prevent water from icing.

4. Structural Change of Water in the Aggregation of Proteins and Polymers

Compared with that of small molecules and water, the interaction of macromolecule and water is more complex, and the interactions are easier to be affected by temperature. For understanding the phase transition mechanism and the role of water in the aggregation of proteins and polymers, the variation of water structures in the aggregation process was studied by using temperature-dependent NIR spectroscopy and chemometrics. The structural change of water in the thermal denaturation of proteins was investigated by analyzing the temperature-dependent NIR spectra of HSA and ovalbumin (OVA) solutions [45–47]. From the resolution-enhanced spectra by CWT, the spectral features of the protein (α-helix and β-sheet) and different water species (S_0–S_4) were observed. Through the variation of the peak intensities related to water species with temperatures, the structural change of the proteins was revealed, indicating that water can be a probe for investigating the structural variation of the proteins in aqueous solutions.

Tau is a class of intrinsically disordered proteins, of which the mistaken aggregation leads to neurodegenerative diseases, typically Alzheimer's disease (AD). Investigating the interaction between tau protein and water during the aggregation is helpful to understand the pathogenesis of the disease. The variation of hydration water during the aggregation of the core fragment of tau, R2/wt, induced by heparin, was investigated using NIR spectroscopy combined with PCA and two-dimensional (2D) correlation spectroscopy [48]. The spectral information due to the structural change of R2/wt was observed from the resolution-enhanced NIR spectra, showing a two-stage variation during the aggregation. Furthermore, the spectral features of water species with one and two hydrogen bonds around NH and CH groups were found in the loadings of PCA, and the variation of the water species during the aggregation was analyzed by 2D correlation spectroscopy. Water species with one hydrogen bond change before the water molecules with free OH and with two hydrogen bonds. The result demonstrates that the hydrogen-bonded water with the NH groups disassociates at first, leading to the formation of the β-sheet structure, and then the hydration water around CH groups releases. This result shows the mechanism for the aggregation of tau protein, i.e., the dehydration of NH groups changes the hydrogen bonding network of the hydration water, and then, the water molecules near the hydrophobic side chains release from the R2/wt, resulting in the formation of the ordered amyloid fibers.

Biological processes such as protein folding mostly occur in cells. Water in a cell has different structures from that in bulk water because of the crowding and confined environment, of which the effect on the structure of biomolecules is considered to be the main reason for explaining the stability and activity of biomolecules [37]. To understand the function of water on the thermal stability of the proteins in a confined environment, the water structures in reverse micelles (RMs) were studied by temperature-dependent NIR spectroscopy [49]. The NIR spectra of aqueous solutions and RMs containing bovine serum albumin (BSA), HSA, and OVA were measured at different temperatures. After enhancing the resolution of the spectra, the spectral features of α-helix in proteins and water species with non-hydrogen bond (NHB), weak hydrogen bonds (WHB), and strong hydrogen bonds (SHB) were observed. The intensity change of the α-helix with the temperature shows a clear denaturation of the protein in aqueous solutions, but not in RMs, indicating the effect of the confined environment on the stability of the proteins. To further understand the water structures in RMs, PCA was performed on the transformed spectra. From the result, the spectral feature of a specific water structure in RMs was found, i.e., the bridging water connecting NH in the protein and S=O in the inner surface of RMs, which only exists in RMs with the protein. This water structure may be the reason for enhancing the thermal stability of the protein in RMs.

Temperature-sensitive polymers exhibit phase separation in aqueous solutions above the lower critical solution temperature (LCST). The interaction of water and the polymer is supposed to be the key factor in driving the aggregation. The temperature-dependent NIR spectra of poly(N,N-dimethylaminoethyl methacrylate) (PDMAEMA) in aqueous solutions were measured for investigating their interactions during the aggregation [50]. The spectral changes of the polymer and water during the aggregation with the temperature were analyzed by NPCA. In a low-concentration solution, a two-stage conformational change was observed in the phase transition, i.e., the hydrated chains tend to form an intermediate state of the loose hydrophobic structure and then aggregate into a micelle at the LCST. In the aggregation process, the S_2 water species increases gradually and then a sudden decrease occurs after the LCST, indicating that S_2 plays an important role in the formation of the intermediate. S_2 water species acts as a bridge to connect the polymer chains in the loose hydrophobic structure, and the dissociation of the S_2 at high temperatures leads to the formation of the micelle. Furthermore, the effect of urea on the interaction of water and the polymer poly(N-isopropyl acrylamide) (PNIPAM) was studied by NPCA for understanding the denaturation in aqueous environments [51]. The results indicate that the water species with three hydrogen bonds (S_3) plays an important role in the stabilization of PNIPAM, which may connect the NH and CO groups in the polymer. The S_3 water species stabilizes the coil state of the polymer, and the release of the species leads to the phase transition. When urea is added, urea may reduce the S_3 content by the hydrogen bonding with the hydrophilic groups in the polymer, thus leading to a phase transition at a lower temperature.

5. Quantitative Analysis of Aqueous Solutions

NIR spectroscopy and chemomtric methods have been extensively used for quantitative determination in various fields [52,53], in which multivariate analysis is generally employed. In the analysis of aqueous solutions, the NIR spectrum contains the spectral information of structures and interactions. Both the information is related to the quantity of the composition. Therefore, quantitative determination can be achieved, with the aid of chemometrics, by analyzing the temperature-induced spectral changes in temperature-dependent NIR spectroscopy. A QSTR model between NIR spectra and the temperature was established based on PLS regression and applied to the quantitative determination of the compositions in aqueous solutions of methanol, ethanol, n-hexane, and their mixtures [11,12]. The results show that both the temperature and the quantity of the composition in mixture solutions can be predicted using the models.

The temperature-dependent NIR spectra measured at different conditions are generally composed of high-dimensional data. For example, the spectral data of a group of samples with different concentrations measured at different temperatures are a three-way matrix with the dimension of wavenumber, concentration, and temperature. Thus, high-order chemometric algorithms have been employed to deal with high-dimensional data. NPCA, PARAFAC, and ATLD were adopted to explore the spectral information from the temperature-dependent NIR spectra of a binary water–ethanol and a ternary water–ethanol–isopropanol mixture solutions [14]. The temperature- and concentration-induced spectral variations were obtained by these algorithms, and the quantitative model was successfully built. For the four-way data array of the ternary mixtures, the algorithms were also proven to be a powerful tool for extracting the quantitative information from the spectral data. The result indicates that high-order chemometric algorithm may be a powerful tool for resolving the temperature-dependent NIR spectra to obtain the quantitative information of aqueous solutions.

In order to simplify the calculation, two-dimensional algorithms were also proposed for analyzing high-dimensional data. MFA was developed for the analysis of temperature-dependent NIR spectra [15,16]. The method unfolds a high-dimensional data array into a combined data matrix and then extracts the common spectral feature contained in the spectra of different temperatures or different concentrations by PCA. The relative quantity of the extracted spectral feature can be used to build the calibration model for quantitative analysis. The method of MFA was employed for the quantitative determination of both low- and high-concentration glucose solutions. The result shows that MFA can achieve the accurate quantification of the glucose content even in low-concentration solutions. Besides, the feasibility of the method was also validated using human serum samples. A calibration model with a good correlation coefficient was obtained for the measurement of the glucose content. More importantly, the calculations were based on the spectral information of water, demonstrating that MFA provides a potential way for detecting the components in complex bio-systems.

High-dimensional data can also be analyzed by MSCA through unfolding a data array into a two-dimensional matrix. A two-level MSCA model was employed to capture the temperature- and concentration-induced spectral variations in the spectra of water–ethanol–isopropanol mixtures [54]. The MSCA contains a between-temperature (QSTR) model describing the effect of the temperature and a within-temperature (QSCR) model describing the concentration variation. In the within-temperature model, the temperature-induced spectral changes are minimized, and the concentration-induced changes can be reflected. Therefore, quantitative analysis can be achieved by the coefficients in the model. The two-level MSCA was also used to detect glucose in aqueous glucose solutions and human serum samples [17]. Using the spectral changes of water, the relationship between the temperature or concentration and NIR spectra can be effectively described by the QSTR model from the first level and the QSCR model from the second level model.

Furthermore, the NIR spectra changing with more factors were analyzed by MSCA. The NIR spectra of proline aqueous solutions in different pH and concentrations were measured at different temperatures [55]. A three-level MSCA (3-MSCA) model was established to investigate the pH-, concentration-, and temperature-induced spectral variations. Figure 3 shows the loadings and scores of the three-level models by the method. The first loading of the first-level model describes mainly the spectral information of the CH_2 groups in proline. The corresponding score goes down first and then up at the isoelectric point, which is due to the structural changes of the proline. The second loading from the first-level model is mainly composed of the spectral information of water, and the corresponding score has the same inflection, which is related to the structural change of water with pH. The first-level model gives a good description of the effect of pH on the spectra, and the spectral changes can be used to analyze the structural change of proline and water. Figure 3(B1,B2) show the first loading and score of the second-level model. The former shows the spectral information of water, and the latter shows the variation of the spectral component with the concentration. The perfect quantitative relationship was obtained, which is a good proof that the interaction between water and proline can be used to describe the change of the composition quantitatively. After the pH- and concentration-induced spectral changes are minimized, the temperature-induced change of water is reflected in the loading and score of the third-level model, as shown in Figure 3(C1,C2), respectively. The relationship is a good QSTR model to quantitatively describe the change of the spectra with the temperature and to predict the temperature of the solution. Therefore, by extracting the information about the structural change of water with three factors in proline solutions, the quantitative models for the determination of pH, concentration, and temperature were obtained. The results further demonstrated that water can be a good probe for sensing quantitative information.

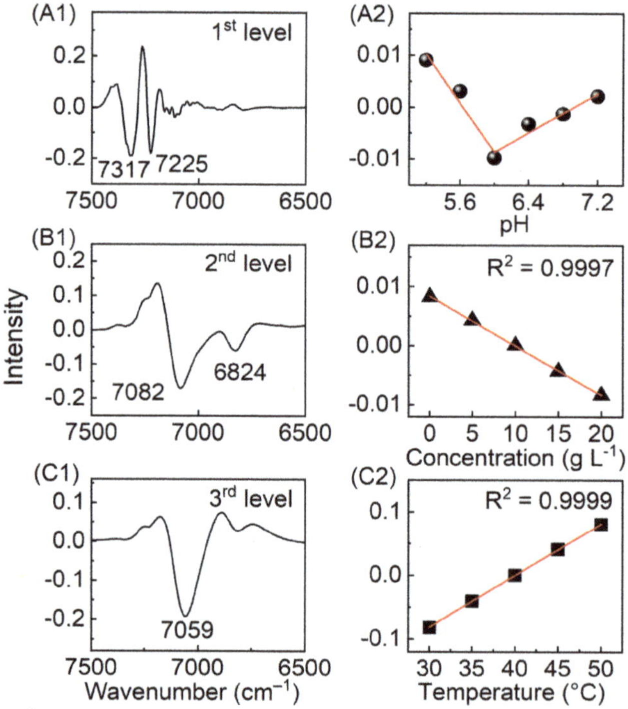

Figure 3. The loadings (**A1–C1**) and scores (**A2–C2**) of the three-level models obtained by three-level multilevel simultaneous component analysis (3-MSCA).

6. Conclusions

Temperature-dependent NIR spectroscopy provides a powerful tool for aquaphotomic studies in both the structural analysis and quantitative determination of aqueous systems. Chemometric methods can be a powerful excavator to mine the temperature-induced information from the overlapping NIR spectra. The spectral features of water structures with different hydrogen bonds can be captured. Through the spectral variation of the water, the structural changes and interactions of water and small molecules, proteins and thermo-responsive polymers can be obtained. Furthermore, quantitative determination can also be achieved using the spectral variation of water with the temperature, concentration, and pH. With the advance of chemometrics, temperature-dependent NIR spectroscopy may be a promising technique for quantitative determination and understanding the properties or functions of analytes in aqueous solutions and biological systems.

Author Contributions: Conceptualization, Y.S. and X.S.; writing of the original draft preparation, Y.S.; writing of review and editing, X.S.; funding acquisition, X.S. and W.C. All authors have read and agreed to the published version of the manuscript.

Funding: This research was funded by the National Natural Science Foundation of China (No. 22174075), the Natural Science Foundation of Tianjin, China (20JCYBJC01480), the Frontiers Science Center for New Organic Matter, Nankai University (No. 63181206), and the Fundamental Research Funds for the Central Universities, Nankai University (No. 63211019).

Institutional Review Board Statement: Not applicable.

Informed Consent Statement: Not applicable.

Data Availability Statement: Not applicable.

Conflicts of Interest: The authors declare no conflict of interest.

References

1. Czarnecki, M.A.; Morisawa, Y.; Futami, Y.; Ozaki, Y. Advances in molecular structure and interaction studies using near-infrared spectroscopy. *Chem. Rev.* **2015**, *115*, 9707–9744. [CrossRef]
2. Ishigaki, M.; Yasui, Y.; Kajita, M.; Ozaki, Y. Assessment of embryonic bioactivity through changes in the water structure using near-infrared spectroscopy and imaging. *Anal. Chem.* **2020**, *92*, 8133–8141. [CrossRef]
3. Tsenkova, R. Aquaphotomics: Water absorbance pattern as a biological marker for disease diagnosis and disease understanding. *NIR News* **2007**, *18*, 14–16. [CrossRef]
4. Tsenkova, R. Aquaphotomics: Dynamic spectroscopy of aqueous and biological systems describes peculiarities of water. *J. Near Infrared Spectrosc.* **2009**, *17*, 303–313. [CrossRef]
5. Sae, T.; Tsenkova, R.; Masato, Y. Details of glucose solution near-infrared band assignment revealed the anomer difference in the structure and the interaction with water molecules. *J. Mol. Liq.* **2021**, *324*, 114764.
6. Goto, N.; Bázár, G.; Kovacs, Z.; Kunisada, M.; Morita, H.; Kizaki, S.; Sugiyama, H.; Tsenkova, R.; Nishigori, C. Detection of UV-induced cyclobutane pyrimidine dimers by near-infrared spectroscopy and aquaphotomics. *Sci. Rep.* **2015**, *5*, srep11808. [CrossRef] [PubMed]
7. Takemura, G.; Bázár, G.; Ikuta, K.; Yamaguchi, E.; Ishikawa, S.; Furukawa, A.; Kubota, Y.; Kovacs, Z.; Tsenkova, R. Aquagrams of raw milk for oestrus detection in dairy cows. *Reprod. Domest. Anim.* **2015**, *50*, 522–525. [CrossRef]
8. Muncan, J.; Matovic, V.; Nikolic, S.; Askovic, J.; Tsenkova, R. Aquaphotomics approach for monitoring different steps of purification process in water treatment systems. *Talanta* **2020**, *206*, 120253. [CrossRef] [PubMed]
9. Muncan, J.; Tei, K.; Tsenkova, R. Real-time monitoring of yogurt fermentation process by aquaphotomics near-infrared spectroscopy. *Sensors* **2020**, *21*, 177. [CrossRef]
10. Kuroki, S.; Tsenkova, R.; Moyankova, D.; Muncan, J.; Morita, H.; Atanassova, S.; Djilianov, D. Water molecular structure underpins extreme desiccation tolerance of the resurrection plant Haberlea rhodopensis. *Sci. Rep.* **2019**, *9*, 3049. [CrossRef] [PubMed]
11. Shao, X.; Kang, J.; Cai, W. Quantitative determination by temperature dependent near-infrared spectra. *Talanta* **2010**, *82*, 1017–1021. [CrossRef] [PubMed]
12. Kang, J.; Cai, W.; Shao, X. Quantitative determination by temperature dependent near-infrared spectra: A further study. *Talanta* **2011**, *85*, 420–424. [CrossRef]
13. Cui, X.; Sun, Y.; Cai, W.; Shao, X. Chemometric methods for extracting information from temperature-dependent near-infrared spectra. *Sci. China Chem.* **2019**, *62*, 583–591. [CrossRef]
14. Cui, X.; Zhang, J.; Cai, W.; Shao, X. Chemometric algorithms for analyzing high dimensional temperature dependent near infrared spectra. *Chemom. Intell. Lab. Syst.* **2017**, *170*, 109–117. [CrossRef]

15. Shao, X.; Cui, X.; Yu, X.; Cai, W. Mutual factor analysis for quantitative analysis by temperature dependent near infrared spectra. *Talanta* **2018**, *183*, 142–148. [CrossRef]
16. Wang, M.; Cui, X.; Cai, W.; Shao, X. Temperature-Dependent Near-Infrared Spectroscopy for Sensitive Detection of Glucose. *Acta Chim. Sin.* **2020**, *78*, 125–129. [CrossRef]
17. Cui, X.; Liu, X.; Yu, X.; Cai, W.; Shao, X. Water can be a probe for sensing glucose in aqueous solutions by temperature dependent near infrared spectra. *Anal. Chim. Acta* **2017**, *957*, 47–54. [CrossRef] [PubMed]
18. Ball, P. Water-an enduring mystery. *Nature* **2008**, *452*, 291–292. [CrossRef]
19. Naserifar, S.; Goddard, W.A. Liquid water is a dynamic polydisperse branched polymer. *Proc. Natl. Acad. Sci. USA* **2019**, *116*, 1998–2003. [CrossRef] [PubMed]
20. Perakis, F.; De Marco, L.; Shalit, A.; Tang, F.; Kann, Z.R.; Kühne, T.D.; Torre, R.; Bonn, M.; Nagata, Y. Vibrational spectroscopy and dynamics of water. *Chem. Rev.* **2016**, *116*, 7590–7607. [CrossRef]
21. Loerting, T.; Fuentes-Landete, V.; Tonauer, C.M.; Gasser, T.M. Open questions on the structures of crystalline water ices. *Commun. Chem.* **2020**, *3*, 109. [CrossRef]
22. Collins, J.R. Change in the infra-red absorption spectrum of water with temperature. *Phys. Rev.* **1925**, *26*, 771–779. [CrossRef]
23. Waggener, W.C. Absorbance of liquid water and deuterium oxide between 0.6 and 1.8 microns. comparison of absorbance and effect of temperature. *Anal. Chem.* **1958**, *30*, 1569–1570. [CrossRef]
24. Segtnan, V.H.; Sasic, S.; Isaksson, T.; Ozaki, Y. Studies on the structure of water using two-dimensional near-infrared correlation spectroscopy and principal component analysis. *Anal. Chem.* **2001**, *73*, 3153–3161. [CrossRef] [PubMed]
25. Sasic, S.; Segtnan, V.H.; Ozaki, Y. Self-modeling curve resolution study of temperature-dependent near-infrared spectra of water and the investigation of water structure. *J. Phys. Chem. A* **2002**, *106*, 760–766. [CrossRef]
26. Czarnik-Matusewicz, B.; Pilorz, S. Study of the temperature-dependent near-infrared spectra of water by two-dimensional correlation spectroscopy and principal components analysis. *Vib. Spectrosc.* **2006**, *40*, 235–245. [CrossRef]
27. Renati, P.; Kovacs, Z.; De Ninno, A.; Tsenkova, R. Temperature dependence analysis of the NIR spectra of liquid water confirms the existence of two phases, one of which is in a coherent state. *J. Mol. Liq.* **2019**, *292*, 111449. [CrossRef]
28. Xu, J.; Dorrepaal, R.M.; Martinez-Gonzalez, J.A.; Tsenkova, R.; Gowen, A.A. Near-infrared multivariate model transfer for quantification of different hydrogen bonding species in aqueous systems. *J. Chemom.* **2020**, *34*, 3274. [CrossRef]
29. Cui, X.; Zhang, J.; Cai, W.; Shao, X. Selecting temperature-dependent variables in near-infrared spectra for aquaphotomics. *Chemom. Intell. Lab. Syst.* **2018**, *183*, 23–28. [CrossRef]
30. Cui, X.; Cai, W.; Shao, X. Glucose induced variation of water structure from temperature dependent near infrared spectra. *RSC Adv.* **2016**, *6*, 105729–105736. [CrossRef]
31. Tan, J.; Sun, Y.; Ma, L.; Feng, H.; Guo, Y.; Cai, W.; Shao, X. Knowledge-based genetic algorithm for resolving the near-infrared spectrum and understanding the water structures in aqueous solution. *Chemom. Intell. Lab. Syst.* **2020**, *206*, 104150. [CrossRef]
32. Leung, A.K.-M.; Chau, F.-T.; Gao, J.-B. Wavelet transform: A method for derivative calculation in analytical chemistry. *Anal. Chem.* **1998**, *70*, 5222–5229. [CrossRef]
33. Shao, X.; Cai, W. Wavelet analysis in analytical chemistry. *Rev. Anal. Chem.* **1998**, *17*, 235–283. [CrossRef]
34. Shao, X.; Leung, A.K.M.; Chau, F.-T. Wavelet: A new trend in chemistry. *Accounts Chem. Res.* **2003**, *36*, 276–283. [CrossRef] [PubMed]
35. Sun, Y.; Cui, X.; Cai, W.; Shao, X. Understanding the complexity of the structures in alcohol solutions by temperature–dependent near–infrared spectroscopy. *Spectrochim. Acta Part A Mol. Biomol. Spectrosc.* **2020**, *229*, 117864. [CrossRef] [PubMed]
36. Shao, X.; Cui, X.; Wang, M.; Cai, W. High order derivative to investigate the complexity of the near infrared spectra of aqueous solutions. *Spectrochim. Acta Part A Mol. Biomol. Spectrosc.* **2019**, *213*, 83–89. [CrossRef]
37. Ball, P. Water as an active constituent in cell biology. *Chem. Rev.* **2008**, *108*, 74–108. [CrossRef]
38. Beganović, A.; Moll, V.; Huck, C.W. Comparison of multivariate regression models based on water-and carbohydrate-related spectral regions in the near-infrared for aqueous solutions of glucose. *Molecules* **2019**, *24*, 3696. [CrossRef]
39. Beganović, A.; Beć, K.B.; Grabska, J.; Stanzl, M.T.; Brunner, M.E.; Huck, C.W. Vibrational coupling to hydration shell–Mechanism to performance enhancement of qualitative analysis in NIR spectroscopy of carbohydrates in aqueous environment. *Spectrochim. Acta Part A Mol. Biomol. Spectrosc.* **2020**, *237*, 118359. [CrossRef]
40. Dong, Q.; Guo, X.; Li, L.; Yu, C.; Nie, L.; Tian, W.; Zhang, H.; Huang, S.; Zang, H. Understanding hyaluronic acid induced variation of water structure by near-infrared spectroscopy. *Sci. Rep.* **2020**, *10*, 1387. [CrossRef]
41. Cheng, D.; Cai, W.; Shao, X. Understanding the interaction between oligopeptide and water in aqueous solution using temperature-dependent near-infrared spectroscopy. *Appl. Spectrosc.* **2018**, *72*, 1354–1361. [CrossRef]
42. Shao, X.; Cui, X.; Liu, Y.; Xia, Z.; Cai, W. Understanding the molecular interaction in solutions by chemometric resolution of near−infrared spectra. *ChemistrySelect* **2017**, *2*, 10027–10032. [CrossRef]
43. Zhao, H.T.; Sun, Y.; Guo, Y.C.; Cai, W.S.; Shao, X.G. Near infrared spectroscopy for low-temperature water structure analysis. *Chem. J. Chin. Univ.* **2020**, *41*, 1968–1974.
44. Su, T.; Sun, Y.; Han, L.; Cai, W.S.; Shao, X.G. Revealing the interactions of water with cryoprotectant and protein by near-infrared spectroscopy. *Spectrochim. Acta Part A Mol. Biomol. Spectrosc.* **2022**, *266*, 120417. [CrossRef]
45. Fan, M.; Cai, W.; Shao, X. Investigating the structural change in protein aqueous solution using temperature-dependent near-infrared spectroscopy and continuous wavelet transform. *Appl. Spectrosc.* **2017**, *71*, 472–479. [CrossRef]

46. Liu, X.-W.; Cui, X.-Y.; Yu, X.-M.; Cai, W.-S.; Shao, X. Understanding the thermal stability of human serum proteins with the related near-infrared spectral variables selected by Monte Carlo-uninformative variable elimination. *Chin. Chem. Lett.* **2017**, *28*, 1447–1452. [CrossRef]
47. Ma, L.; Cui, X.; Cai, W.; Shao, X. Understanding the function of water during the gelation of globular proteins by temperature-dependent near infrared spectroscopy. *Phys. Chem. Chem. Phys.* **2018**, *20*, 20132–20140. [CrossRef] [PubMed]
48. Sun, Y.; Ma, L.; Cai, W.; Shao, X. Interaction between tau and water during the induced aggregation revealed by near-infrared spectroscopy. *Spectrochim. Acta Part A Mol. Biomol. Spectrosc.* **2020**, *230*, 118046. [CrossRef]
49. Wang, S.; Wang, M.; Han, L.; Sun, Y.; Cai, W.; Shao, X. Insight into the stability of protein in confined environment through analyzing the structure of water by temperature-dependent near-infrared spectroscopy. *Spectrochim. Acta Part A Mol. Biomol. Spectrosc.* **2021**, *267*, 120581. [CrossRef]
50. Wang, L.; Zhu, X.; Cai, W.; Shao, X. Understanding the role of water in the aggregation of poly(N,N-dimethylaminoethyl methacrylate) in aqueous solution using temperature-dependent near-infrared spectroscopy. *Phys. Chem. Chem. Phys.* **2019**, *21*, 5780–5789. [CrossRef]
51. Ma, B.; Wang, L.; Han, L.; Cai, W.; Shao, X. Understanding the effect of urea on the phase transition of poly(N-isopropylacrylamide) in aqueous solution by temperature-dependent near-infrared spectroscopy. *Spectrochim. Acta Part A Mol. Biomol. Spectrosc.* **2021**, *253*, 119573. [CrossRef] [PubMed]
52. Moros, J.; Garrigures, S.; Guardia, M. Vibrational spectroscopy provides a green tool for multi-component analysis. *TrAC Trends Anal. Chem.* **2010**, *29*, 578–591. [CrossRef]
53. Pasquini, C. Near infrared spectroscopy: A mature analytical technique with new perspectives—A review. *Anal. Chim. Acta* **2018**, *1026*, 8–36. [CrossRef]
54. Shan, R.; Zhao, Y.; Fan, M.; Liu, X.; Cai, W.; Shao, X. Multilevel analysis of temperature dependent near-infrared spectra. *Talanta* **2015**, *131*, 170–174. [CrossRef] [PubMed]
55. Han, L.; Cui, X.; Cai, W.; Shao, X. Three–level simultaneous component analysis for analyzing the near–infrared spectra of aqueous solutions under multiple perturbations. *Talanta* **2020**, *217*, 121036. [CrossRef] [PubMed]

molecules

MDPI

Article

Performance Improvement of NIR Spectral Pattern Recognition from Three Compensation Models' Voting and Multi-Modal Fusion

Niangen Ye †, Sheng Zhong †, Zile Fang, Haijun Gao, Zhihua Du, Heng Chen, Lu Yuan and Tao Pan *,†

Department of Optoelectronic Engineering, Jinan University, Guangzhou 510632, China; yng2020@stu2019.jnu.edu.cn (N.Y.); zhongsheng@stu2019.jnu.edu.cn (S.Z.); fangzile@stu2019.jnu.edu.cn (Z.F.); haijungao@stu2019.jnu.edu.cn (H.G.); dzh0905@stu2019.jnu.edu.cn (Z.D.); hengchen@stu2019.jnu.edu.cn (H.C.); yuanlu9835@stu2020.jnu.edu.cn (L.Y.)
* Correspondence: tpan@jnu.edu.cn
† These authors have contributed equally to this work.

Citation: Ye, N.; Zhong, S.; Fang, Z.; Gao, H.; Du, Z.; Chen, H.; Yuan, L.; Pan, T. Performance Improvement of NIR Spectral Pattern Recognition from Three Compensation Models' Voting and Multi-Modal Fusion. *Molecules* **2022**, *27*, 4485. https://doi.org/10.3390/molecules27144485

Academic Editors: Roumiana Tsenkova and Jelena Muncan

Received: 5 June 2022
Accepted: 11 July 2022
Published: 13 July 2022

Abstract: Inspired by aquaphotomics, the optical path length of measurement was regarded as a perturbation factor. Near-infrared (NIR) spectroscopy with multi-measurement modals was applied to the discriminant analysis of three categories of drinking water. Moving window-*k* nearest neighbor (MW-kNN) and Norris derivative filter were used for modeling and optimization. Drawing on the idea of game theory, the strategy for two-category priority compensation and three-model voting with multi-modal fusion was proposed. Moving window correlation coefficient (MWCC), inter-category and intra-category MWCC spectra, and *k*-shortest distances plotting with MW-kNN were proposed to evaluate weak differences between two spectral populations. For three measurement modals (1 mm, 4 mm, and 10 mm), the optimal MW-kNN models, and two-category priority compensation models were determined. The joint models for three compensation models' voting were established. Comprehensive discrimination effects of joint models were better than their sub-models; multi-modal fusion was better than single-modal fusion. The best joint model was the dual-modal fusion of compensation models of one- and two-category priority (1 mm), one- and three-category priority (10 mm), and two- and three-category priority (1 mm), validation's total recognition accuracy rate reached 95.5%. It fused long-wave models (1 mm, containing 1450 nm) and short-wave models (10 mm, containing 974 nm). The results showed that compensation models' voting and multi-modal fusion can effectively improve the performance of NIR spectral pattern recognition.

Keywords: near-infrared spectroscopic pattern recognition; multi-optical-path; two-category priority's compensation models; three-model voting fusion; moving-window-*k*-nearest neighbor; Norris derivative filter

1. Introduction

The water system samples, (e.g., drinking water, dairy product, and blood) are important analysis objects in the fields of food, environment, and biomedicine. Water can be used not only as a direct analysis object, (e.g., the safety detection and classification identification of drinking water) but can also be used as the most common background solvent of liquid samples, which is a very important analyte. Qualified drinking water has undergone strict safety testing before it can enter the market for social use. Due to the huge market demand for drinking water, some brands of high-end bottled drinking water are expensive and increasingly popular, and they can be easily counterfeited. Using water that has not undergone safety testing to counterfeit high-end drinking water will not only damage the rights and interests of producers and consumers but may also cause large-scale safety problems of drinking water. The authenticity identification of drinking water brands on the market is an important problem that needs to be solved urgently. The current water quality testing methods mainly include quantitative analysis of water quality safety indexes (multiple trace components), which are complex and expensive. Due to the very similar component structures, the above quantitative methods are still difficult to achieve accurate identification of different drinking water brands, and there have been no related results reported so far. Therefore, a fast and easy detection method that can be used in the field is urgently needed.

Near-infrared (NIR) spectra mainly reflect the vibrational absorption of the overtones and combined frequencies of the hydrogen-containing groups X-H. This measurement method usually does not require reagents to measure samples directly, which has the advantage of being quick and easy. Water system samples have significant NIR absorption, and NIR spectroscopy has been applied to a variety of water-based analysis samples in agriculture and food [1–5], environment [6,7], and biomedicine [8–12].

The qualitative discriminant analysis of NIR spectroscopy is one of the hot research directions in recent years. For the classification and identification of samples with small differences in component content, the discriminant analysis is more effective and simpler than quantitative analysis. This discriminant analysis involves pattern recognition technology of multiple spectral populations, which needs to make full use of the spectral similarities of the same population, and spectral differences of different populations. It has been applied to sample identification in many fields in recent years, such as melon genotype [13], edible oil type [14], transgenic sugarcane leaf [15,16], milk powder adulteration identification [17], wine identification [18], rice seed authenticity identification [19] and thalassemia screening [16,20]. However, the application of NIR spectral discriminant analysis to the identification of water samples has not been reported yet. Efficient discriminant analysis methods for spectral populations with small differences are also rare.

Water sample identification involves multi-category discriminant analysis of spectral populations, which is more challenging than the two-category discriminant analysis problems. Partial least squares discriminant analysis (PLS-DA) is a well-performed method of two-category discriminant analysis. When using PLS-DA for multi-category discriminant analysis, it is necessary to perform multiple two-category analysis and their comprehensive evaluation. This process is complicated and difficult to popularize. Principal component analysis–linear discriminant analysis (PCA–LDA) is another effective two-category discriminant analysis method. When using PCA–LDA to process n-category discriminant analysis, it is necessary to determine the optimal classification surface of n-1 dimensions in n-dimensional space, which is mathematically complicated and difficult. Therefore, PLS-DA and PCA–LDA methods are not suitable to deal with the multi-classification problem.

The k-nearest neighbor (kNN) [21–25] is one of the most commonly used multi-classification algorithms. When it was applied to a supervised multi-category problem, the idea was as follows: based on the spectra of calibration samples containing multiple categories, the Euclidean (or Mahalanobis) distances between the unknown sample and all calibration samples were calculated; the k nearest calibration samples were determined; finally, the unknown sample was categorized as the category with the largest number among the k nearest samples.

The kNN uses two cyclic parameters of sample number and k value, and determines the optimal k based on discriminant effect, which has better robustness and applicability than the ordinary Euclidean distance classification method. It is not limited by the number of categories and is especially suitable for multi-category spectral discriminant analysis. The kNN has been applied to multi-category discriminant analysis based on various spectral techniques, such as, NIR [21], mid-infrared [22], Raman [23,24], and laser-induced breakdown spectroscopies [25].

On the other hand, the wavelength model optimization can enhance the characteristic attributes of the spectral category, reduce the interference of redundant data and model complexity, and provide valuable reference for the design of a dedicated spectrometer. Since further wavelength optimization requires higher-dimensional algorithm integration, there are few works on kNN-based wavelength model optimization.

The moving-window waveband screening combined with PLS regression [2,3,9,10] is a well-executed method in the quantitative analysis of NIR spectroscopy. However, its combination with qualitative discriminant analysis algorithms, (e.g., kNN) is still rare. In the current study, "tap water" and two kinds of drinking water brands (C'estbon and Nongfu Spring), a total of three categories of water samples, were used as identification samples. NIR spectroscopy combined with kNN were used to establish the discriminant analysis models for three categories of drinking water. An ensemble algorithm based on kNN and moving-window waveband screening was established, denoted as MW-kNN, and applied to the wavelength optimization of the three-category discrimination model for drinking water. Among them, the initial wavelength and the number of wavelengths were used as the cyclic parameters of MW-kNN to realize the modeling and optimization of all sub-wavebands.

Considering the small spectral differences of different categories of water, new in-depth research on population differences in water spectra is required. The recently emerging aquaphotomics method [26–28] uses specific disturbance factors, (e.g., temperature, pH) and makes changes to the dynamic measurement of water-system samples to obtain a "curved surface" spectrum of water absorption peak disturbances, that is, the spectral disturbance set of a sample, and further use omics method to achieve quantitative and qualitative analysis of weak features. The curved surface spectrum has rich information features with higher dimensions than the line spectrum, which can enhance the information capacity or population difference of the samples, thereby improving the accuracy of quantitative and qualitative analysis of weak analytes. The water spectrum has one strong absorption peak near 1940 nm in the NIR combination frequency region (1900–2500 nm), twelve slightly weaker absorption peaks in NIR double overtones frequency region (1300–1600 nm), and two weaker absorption peaks in the NIR high-overtone frequency region (900–1300 nm) [26–28].

As we know, using a transmission measurement accessory with a longer optical path (>1 mm) can increase the significance of the water absorption peaks in the short-wave NIR region, while using a transmission measurement accessory with a shorter optical path (<1 mm) can avoid saturated absorption of water in long-wave NIR region. Therefore, using long and short optical path transmission accessories to extract the spectral information in the short- and long-wave NIR regions, respectively, and perform model fusion, is expected to comprehensively improve the differences of water spectral populations and improve the accuracy of spectral identification. Inspired by aquaphotomics, the optical path length of the transmission measurement accessory was used as a perturbation factor, and a novel method for multi-modal spectra fusion modeling based on multi-optical-path measurement was proposed. The multi-modal NIR spectra based on the short, medium, and long optical paths (1 mm, 4 mm, and 10 mm) were used to establish the discriminant analysis models for three categories of drinking water.

A comprehensive judgment method based on the three models' voting was also proposed for the model fusion. Each sample was judged three times, and the sample category of comprehensive judgment was obtained according to the principle of "two wins in three games", and thereby a joint model of three-model voting was established. On the other hand, drawing on the idea of game theory, for the 3-category discriminant analysis problem, a strategy of two-category priority compensation was proposed and used for three-model voting fusion. Its goal was that the comprehensive discrimination effect of the fusion model was better than its three sub-judgments. Moreover, in the process of two-category priority compensation and three-model voting fusion, all joint models based on the same and different measurement modals were used. The joint voting of the multi-modal compensation models can highlight the spectral differences from two dimensions, which is expected to improve the discrimination accuracy of the spectral population with small differences.

The strategy of three compensation models' voting and multi-modal fusion was applied for performance improvement of NIR spectral pattern recognition of three categories of drinking water. Furthermore, the spectra of the moving-window correlation coefficient, intra-class correlation coefficient, and inter-class correlation coefficient were also proposed to evaluate weak differences between two spectral populations.

2. Results and Discussion

2.1. Spectra of Three Groups of Water Samples Based on Three Measurement Modals

Using the transmission accessories of 1, 4, and 10 mm cuvettes, the Vis–NIR spectra of three categories of water samples (one-, two-, three-category) in the desaturated wavebands are shown in Figure 1. In the case of the long optical path measurement, the spectra of the water samples exhibited saturated absorption, so the spectra of 4 and 10 mm cuvettes showed only the unsaturated region. In order to facilitate viewing in the same figure, the absorbance values of samples of two-, and three-category were increased by 1.5 and 3, respectively. Seeing Figure 1, the spectra in desaturated wavebands of three groups of water samples based on three measurement modals, no significant difference was observed.

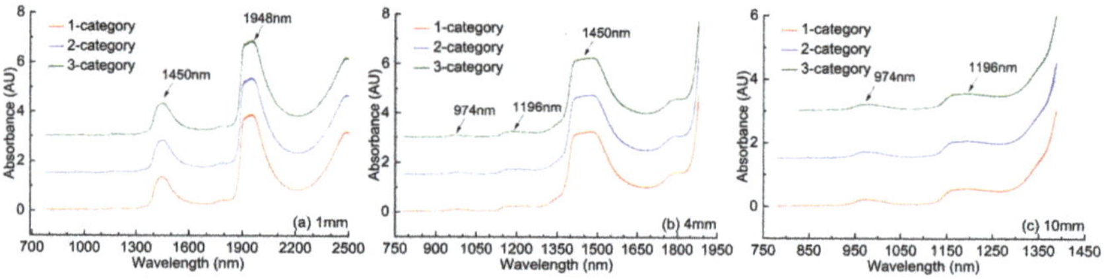

Figure 1. Spectra in desaturated wavebands of three groups of water samples based on three measurement modals: (**a**) 1 mm, (**b**) 4 mm, (**c**) 10 mm.

Note that, in the spectra of the 1 mm measurement modal, one strong absorption peak near 1948 nm in the NIR combination frequency region, and one slightly weaker absorption peak near 1450 nm in the NIR double-overtone frequency region were observed; in the spectra of the 10 mm measurement modal, two weaker absorption peaks (974 nm, 1196 nm) in NIR high-overtones frequency region were observed, while in the spectra of the 4 mm measurement modal, the absorption peak near 1450 nm began to appear saturable absorption, the two weaker absorption peaks (974 nm, 1196 nm) were less obvious.

2.2. Intra-Category and Inter-Category Correlation Coefficient Spectra

In order to evaluate the weak difference between two spectral populations, the moving-window correlation coefficient (MWCC) spectrum between any two spectra was first proposed. In the symmetrical wavelength window (number of wavelengths: $m = p + 1 + p$), the correlation coefficient between the two spectra was calculated as the local correlation coefficient of the center wavelength. Through the moving window, the local correlation coefficients of each central wavelength were calculated, and thereby the MWCC spectrum corresponded to m was obtained, as follows:

$$R_{i,m}=\frac{\sum_{k=-(m-1)/2}^{(m-1)/2}\left(x_{i+k}-\overline{x}_{i,m}\right)\left(y_{i+k}-\overline{y}_{i,m}\right)}{\sqrt{\sum_{k=-(m-1)/2}^{(m-1)/2}\left(x_{i+k}-\overline{x}_{i,m}\right)^2\sum_{k=-(m-1)/2}^{(m-1)/2}\left(y_{i+k}-\overline{y}_{i,m}\right)^2}} \quad (1)$$

where i was the serial No. of central wavelength.

Next, for the two spectral populations, their respective average spectrum was calculated separately. Within each spectral population, the MWCC spectrum between each spectrum and the average spectrum was calculated, and then the average spectrum of all MWCC spectra was further calculated, called the intra-category MWCC spectrum. For two spectral populations, the MWCC spectrum between each spectrum in a spectral population and the average spectrum of another spectral population was calculated, and then the average spectrum of all MWCC spectra was further calculated, called inter-category MWCC spectrum.

Here, the MWCC spectrum, intra- and inter-category MWCC spectra of spectral populations of any two categories of samples were calculated to evaluate the weak differences between the two categories of water spectra. Since the numerical difference was small, the different spectrum of the intra- and inter-category MWCC spectra were further calculated to observe their differences.

For the spectral datasets of 1, 4, and 10 mm, the intra-category and inter-category MWCC spectra were calculated for the 1–3 category, 2–3 category and 1–2 category spectral groups, respectively. Additionally, the different spectra between two intra-category MWCC spectra and one inter-category MWCC spectrum were further calculated, see Figure 2. As can be seen from Figure 2a, for the dataset of the 1 mm measurement modal, the differences between the two categories of water spectra were mainly at 1072 nm, 1106 nm, 1198 nm, 1258 nm, 1448 nm, 1682 nm, 1806 nm, 1944 nm, 1948 nm, 2212 nm. Among them, 1448 nm was in the wavelength range of 1448–1454 nm (OH-$(H_2O)_{4,5}$, one of the twelve characteristic water wavelengths) [28], and 1944 nm, 1948 nm located near the strong absorption peak of water at 1948 nm (see Figure 1). As can be seen from Figure 2b, for the dataset of the 4 mm measurement modal, the differences between the two categories of water spectra were mainly at 798 nm, 858 nm, 980 nm, 1078 nm, 1104 nm, 1198 nm, 1258 nm, 1440 nm, 1454 nm. Among them, 1440 nm and 1454 nm were in the wavelength ranges of 1432–1444 nm and 1448–1454 nm, respectively (S_1 and OH-$(H_2O)_{4,5}$, two of the twelve characteristic water wavelengths) [28], and they were also located near the absorption peak of water at 1450 nm (see Figure 1). As can be seen from Figure 2c, for the dataset of the 10 mm measurement modal, the differences between the two categories of water spectra were mainly at 794 nm, 980 nm, 1078 nm, 1196 nm, and 1260 nm. Among them, 980 nm and 1196 nm were located near the weaker absorption peaks of water at 974 nm and 1196 nm, respectively (see Figure 1). In the six difference spectra, positive values were almost all observed, indicating that the intra-category correlations were significantly better than inter-category correlations, thus indicating the existence of weak differences between the two categories of spectral populations.

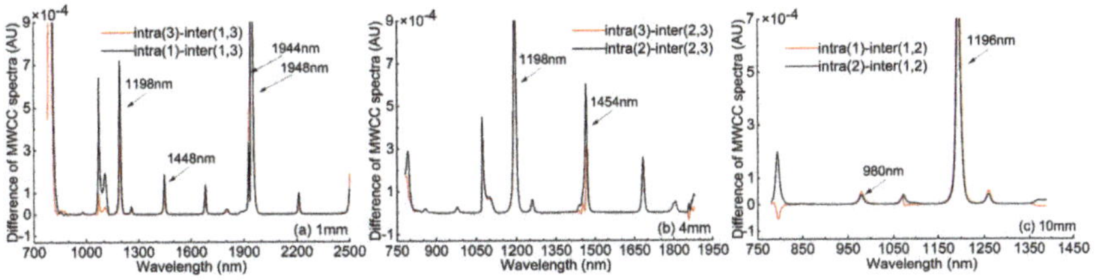

Figure 2. Difference spectra between intra-category and inter-category MWCC spectra: (**a**) 1 mm, 1–3 category, (**b**) 4 mm, 2–3 category, (**c**) 10 mm, 1–2 category.

2.3. MW-kNN Models

First, for the three modal spectral datasets, using direct kNN method, the three-category discriminant analysis models based on desaturated wavebands were established, respectively. See Table 1 for their optimal k values and modeling discriminant effects. The results showed that the case of 10 mm achieved a better discrimination effect (RAR_{Total} = 82.9%).

Table 1. Modeling discrimination effects of kNN models of three measurement modals based on desaturated wavebands.

Modal	Waveband (nm)	*N*	*k*	RAR_{Total}
1 mm	780–2498	860	4	64.4%
4 mm	780–1880	551	1	44.9%
10 mm	780–1388	305	3	82.9%

Then, the MW-kNN models were built for each modal dataset. For the two-dimensional parameter combination (*I*, *N*) of the initial wavelength (*I*) and the number of wavelengths (*N*), the 3D effect diagrams of the modeling discriminant effect (RAR_{Total}) of kNN models of three measurement modals are shown in Figure 3. Among them, the indicated points of the arrow were the optimal parameter combinations (*I*, *N*). Additionally, the corresponding optimal wavebands of the three measurement modals (1 mm, 4 mm, 10 mm) were 966–1894, 938–1402, and 964–1378 nm, respectively.

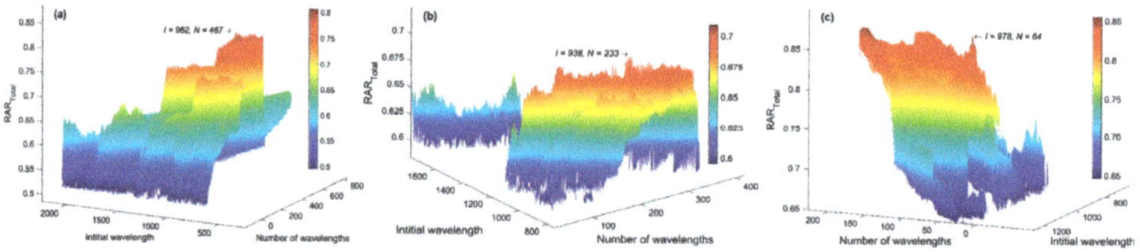

Figure 3. The 3D effect diagrams of the modeling discrimination effect of MW-kNN models of three measurement modals for the initial wavelength (*I*) and the number of wavelengths (*N*): (**a**) 1 mm, (**b**) 4 mm, (**c**) 10 mm.

The modeling discrimination effects of the optimal MW-kNN models of three measurement modals are summarized in Table 2. The results show that the modeling effect of the optimal MW-kNN models of the three modals were significantly better than the previous direct kNN models (Table 1), and the number of wavelengths used were also significantly reduced, so the models were simpler.

Table 2. Modeling discrimination effects of the optimal MW-kNN models of three measurement modals.

Modal	*I*	*N*	*k*	RAR_{Total}
1 mm	966	465	3	80.7%
4 mm	938	233	3	70.9%
10 mm	964	208	3	85.3%

As described above, the optimal MW-kNN models reached the better modeling discrimination effects for three categories of water samples. As described in Figure 1, the spectral shapes of the three categories of water samples were very similar and no significant differences were observed. Therefore, it is necessary to reanalyze the differences of the three spectral populations based on the principle of the kNN method.

Note that the optimal *k* value for all three optimal MW-kNN models was 3 (Table 2). According to the principle of kNN, each prediction sample was determined as the category with the most occurrence among the categories of the three calibration samples that had the minimum distance from it. In view of this, based on the Euclidean distance of the spectra, a visualization method described the differences of spectral populations was proposed: for a specific spectral range, the distances of the spectrum of each prediction sample from the spectra of all calibration samples were calculated, and the first three shortest distances were selected and plotted corresponding to the serial number of the sample. Among them, if the selected distance was the distance between samples of the same category, its value was displayed in a green hollow circle, and if the selected distance was the distance between different samples, its value was displayed in a red hollow circle. Among the first three shortest distances of each prediction sample, if the number of green hollow circles was greater than or equal to 2, it indicated that the sample was correctly identified; otherwise, the sample was incorrectly identified.

The effect of the above visualization of spectral population differences was directly related to the selection of spectral waveband. Using the MW-kNN method for waveband selection can highlight the differences in spectral populations. Here, based on the optimal MW-kNN wavebands for three measurement modals, the visualization of spectral population differences for three categories of water samples was presented. To avoid crowding of data points, the first 60 prediction samples of each spectral population were used for display; the three points on the same horizontal coordinate represented the first three shortest distances of the same sample, which were connected by vertical lines for easy observation; in addition, a pentagram (red or green) was added at the bottom of the same horizontal coordinate to show whether the judgment was correct or not: green meant correct judgment, red meant wrong judgment. In the case of 1 mm, based on the optimal waveband (966–1894 nm), the first three shortest distances between the first 60 one-category prediction samples and all calibration samples are shown in Figure 4a. In the case of 4 mm, based on the optimal waveband (938–1402 nm), the first three shortest distances between the first 60 two-category prediction samples and all calibration samples are shown in Figure 4b. In the case of 10 mm, based on the optimal waveband (964–1378 nm), the first three shortest distances between the first 60 three-category prediction samples and all calibration samples are shown in Figure 4c. As can be seen from the figures, for those prediction samples, the first three shortest distances were mostly green, a small part was red, and the green pentagrams were much more than the red pentagrams, indicating that most samples were correctly identified. In particular, in the case of 10 mm, in almost all the three-category prediction samples, the corresponding first three shortest distances were green (green pentagrams), indicating that the three-category samples (10 mm) were precisely recognized (RAR_3 = 99.3%).

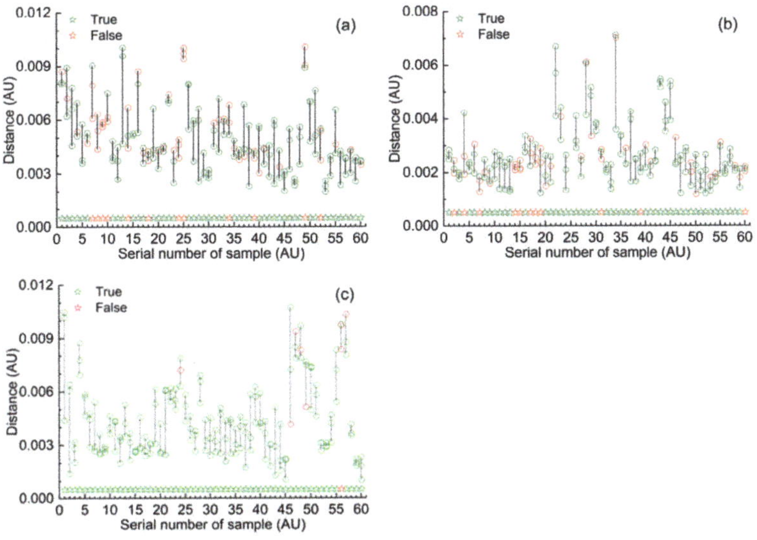

Figure 4. First three shortest distances between each prediction sample and all the calibration samples based on the optimal MW-kNN waveband in the three measurement modals: (**a**) 1-category, 1 mm, 966–1894 nm; (**b**) 2-category, 4 mm, 938–1402 nm; (**c**) 3-category, 10 mm, 964–1378 nm.

In fact, based on the principle of kNN and the wavelength model optimization, a plotting approach of the first k-shortest distances was proposed here. It can describe the differences of spectral populations, and it is also expected to be applied to other analytic objects.

2.4. Two Categories Priority's Compensation Models

Using the method of priority compensation model described later in Section 3.5, the two-category priority compensation models $\Phi_{1,2}$, $\Phi_{1,3}$, $\Phi_{2,3}$ of three modals were determined, respectively. The selected corresponding wavebands were 1704–1868, 858–1896, and 844–1890 nm for 1 mm, 798–1412, 986–1402, and 1080–1332 nm for 4 mm, and 970–1378, 960–1140, and 924–1384 nm for 10 mm. The modeling discrimination effects of the two-category priority compensation models of three measurement modals are summarized in Table 3.

Table 3. Modeling discrimination effects of the 2-category priority's compensation models of three measurement modals.

Modal	Submodel	I	N	k	$RAR_{1,2}$	$RAR_{1,3}$	$RAR_{2,3}$	RAR_{Total}
1 mm	$\Phi_{1,2}$	1704	83	2	81.0%			68.0%
	$\Phi_{1,3}$	858	520	3		84.7%		78.9%
	$\Phi_{2,3}$	844	524	1			80.7%	76.9%
4 mm	$\Phi_{1,2}$	798	308	4	85.3%			69.6%
	$\Phi_{1,3}$	986	209	3		66.0%		70.0%
	$\Phi_{2,3}$	1080	127	1			72.3%	70.0%
10 mm	$\Phi_{1,2}$	970	205	4	78.3%			85.1%
	$\Phi_{1,3}$	960	88	4		95.3%		82.2%
	$\Phi_{2,3}$	924	231	3			90.3%	85.1%

2.5. Optimal Norris Parameters

Using the Norris derivative filter algorithm, based on each modal, the parameter optimization of spectral preprocessing for the optimal MW-kNN model and the two-category priority compensation models was performed.

Take the optimal MW-kNN model (waveband) of 1 mm modal as an example, for the two-dimensional parameter combination (S, G) of the number of smoothing points (S) and the number of differential gaps (G), the 3D-effect diagram (RAR_{Total}) of all kNN models processed by NDF (D = 1) is shown in Figure 5. Additionally, the indicated point of the arrow was the optimal parameter combination (S, G).

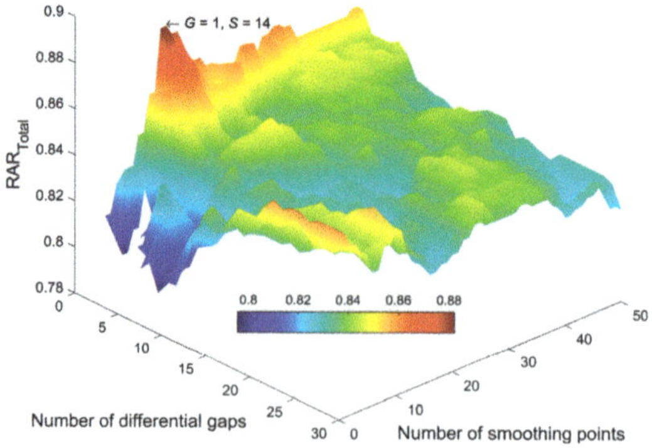

Figure 5. The 3D effect diagram of the modeling discrimination effect of kNN models processed by NDF for the number of smoothing points (S) and the number of differential gaps (G).

The modeling discrimination effects of the optimal MW-kNN models processed by optimal NDF parameters are summarized in Table 4. Comparing Tables 2 and 4, after using NDF preprocessing, the effect of each model had been significantly improved.

Table 4. Modeling discrimination effects of the optimal MW-kNN models processed by optimal NDF parameters.

Modal	*I*	*N*	*k*	*D*	*S*	*G*	RAR_{Total}
1 mm	966	465	3	1	14	1	88.2%
4 mm	938	233	3	2	2	1	73.8%
10 mm	964	208	3	2	1	1	85.6%

The modeling discrimination effect of the two-category priority compensation models of three measurement modals processed by optimal NDF parameters are summarized in Table 5. Comparing Tables 3 and 5, after using NDF preprocessing, the performance of almost every model also had been significantly improved.

Table 5. Modeling discrimination effect of the 2-category priority's compensation models of three measurement modals processed by optimal NDF parameters.

Modal	Submodel	*D*	*S*	*G*	*k*	$RAR_{1,2}$	$RAR_{1,3}$	$RAR_{2,3}$	RAR_{Total}
1 mm	$\Phi_{1,2}$	2	26	5	2	98.3%			88.2%
	$\Phi_{1,3}$	1	18	2	3		88.3%		85.6%
	$\Phi_{2,3}$	1	12	1	1			90.0%	88.9%
4 mm	$\Phi_{1,2}$	0	4	–	4	86.0%			69.8%
	$\Phi_{1,3}$	2	6	2	3		71.3%		73.3%
	$\Phi_{2,3}$	1	36	6	1			77.3%	73.6%
10 mm	$\Phi_{1,2}$	2	1	1	3	78.7%			85.6%
	$\Phi_{1,3}$	2	20	5	2		95.7%		77.8%
	$\Phi_{2,3}$	0	3	–	3			90.0%	85.1%

2.6. *Joint Models Based on Three-Model Voting Fusion*

2.6.1. Fusion Based on Single-Modal Models

After processing by the optimal NDF parameters, using the method described later in Section 3.5, based on the three two-category priority compensation models of each single-modal, the joint model based on three-model voting was established. The modeling discrimination effect of the three joint models are summarized in Table 6. Comparing Tables 4 and 6, for each measurement modal, the comprehensive effect of the joint model was better than that of the corresponding optimal MW-kNN model. Among them, the joint model of the 1 mm's modal was the best.

Table 6. Modeling discrimination effect of the joint models for three compensation models' voting based on single-modal.

Modal	Submodel			RAR_1	RAR_2	RAR_3	RAR_{Total}	RAR_{SD}
1 mm	$\Phi_{1,2}$	$\Phi_{1,3}$	$\Phi_{2,3}$	96.0%	94.0%	90.0%	93.3%	3.1%
4 mm	$\Phi_{1,2}$	$\Phi_{1,3}$	$\Phi_{2,3}$	76.0%	94.7%	68.7%	79.8%	13.4%
10 mm	$\Phi_{1,2}$	$\Phi_{1,3}$	$\Phi_{2,3}$	85.3%	75.3%	100.0%	86.9%	12.4%

2.6.2. Fusion Based on Multi-Modal Models

The experimental design of three-model voting fusion based on multi-modal spectra was considered using the method described later in Section 3.5.

Firstly, various cases of the joint voting of three models based on two modals were considered: the three sub-models of priority compensation were first sorted as the basic order of $\Phi_{1,2}$, $\Phi_{1,3}$, $\Phi_{2,3}$, and then all possible structures and arrangements of two modals were filled in, such as 1 mm-$\Phi_{1,2}$,10 mm-$\Phi_{1,3}$, 1 mm-$\Phi_{2,3}$. They were divided into three groups (structures): 1 mm and 4 mm, 1 mm and 10 mm, 4 mm and 10 mm; each group (take 1 mm and 10 mm as an example) was further divided into two sub-groups, (e.g., two 1 mm and one 10 mm or two 10 mm and one 1 mm); according to the order of collocation, each sub-group had three cases in total, (e.g., the first sub-group included three cases of 1 mm-$\Phi_{1,2}$, 1 mm-$\Phi_{1,3}$, 10 mm-$\Phi_{2,3}$; 1 mm-$\Phi_{1,2}$, 10 mm-$\Phi_{1,3}$, 1 mm-$\Phi_{2,3}$, and 10 mm-$\Phi_{1,2}$, 1 mm-$\Phi_{1,3}$, 1 mm-$\Phi_{2,3}$). In summary, there were eighteen dual-modal fusion cases. Modeling had been completed for each case, and the optimal case is summarized in Table 7.

Table 7. Modeling discrimination effects of the optimal joint models for three-model voting fusion based on multi-modal.

Modal	Modal (mm)-Submodel			RAR_1	RAR_2	RAR_3	RAR_{Total}	RAR_{SD}
Dual modal	1-$\Phi_{1,2}$	10-$\Phi_{1,3}$	1-$\Phi_{2,3}$	98.7%	95.3%	94.0%	96.0%	2.4%
Triple-modal (global)	1-Φ_{global}	4-Φ_{global}	10-Φ_{global}	89.3%	92.0%	98.7%	93.3%	4.8%
Triple-modal (compensatory)	1-$\Phi_{1,2}$	10-$\Phi_{1,3}$	4-$\Phi_{2,3}$	97.3%	96.7%	92.7%	95.6%	2.5%

Secondly, various cases of the joint voting of three models based on three modals were considered: the three sub-models of priority compensation were still sorted as the basic order of $\Phi_{1,2}$, $\Phi_{1,3}$, $\Phi_{2,3}$, and then all possible structures and arrangements of three modals were filled in; that is, the three sub-models used for joint voting belong to three different modals (1mm, 4mm, 10mm), and belong to three different priority compensation types ($\Phi_{1,2}$, $\Phi_{1,3}$, $\Phi_{2,3}$), respectively, such as 1 mm-$\Phi_{1,2}$, 10 mm-$\Phi_{1,3}$, 4 mm-$\Phi_{2,3}$; the three modals were arranged sequentially, and there were six cases as follows: (1) 1 mm-$\Phi_{1,2}$, 4 mm-$\Phi_{1,3}$, 10 mm-$\Phi_{2,3}$; (2) 1 mm-$\Phi_{1,2}$, 10 mm-$\Phi_{1,3}$, 4 mm-$\Phi_{2,3}$; (3) 4 mm-$\Phi_{1,2}$, 1 mm-$\Phi_{1,3}$, 10 mm-$\Phi_{2,3}$; (4) 4 mm-$\Phi_{1,2}$, 10 mm-$\Phi_{1,3}$, 1 mm-$\Phi_{2,3}$; (5) 10 mm-$\Phi_{1,2}$, 1 mm-$\Phi_{1,3}$, 4 mm-$\Phi_{2,3}$; (6) 10 mm-$\Phi_{1,2}$, 4 mm-$\Phi_{1,3}$, 1 mm-$\Phi_{2,3}$. In addition, the global optimal MW-kNN models of the three modals were also used as sub-models for joint voting, that was, the fusion of 1 mm-Φ_{global}, 4 mm-Φ_{global} and 10 mm-Φ_{global}. In summary, there were seven different triple-modal fusion cases. Modeling had been completed for each case. The modeling discrimination effect of the optimal model of six joint models based on compensation models' fusion is summarized in Table 7. The modeling discrimination effect of the joint model based on the global optimal MW-kNN models' fusion is also summarized in Table 7.

Seeing Table 7, the three selected fusion models all reached high discrimination accuracy and good category balance, the optimal RAR_{Total} and RAR_{SD} are 96.0% and 2.4%.

2.6.3. Comparison before and after Model Fusion

Table 8 showed the comparison of the modeling discrimination effects for the optimal joint models of the three-model voting fusion and their sub-models. It showed that the effect of each joint model was better than its sub-models. Among them, the highest increasement of discrimination accuracy rate was 22.0%.

2.7. Independent Validation

The validation samples that were not involved in modeling were used to validate the four optimal joint models of three-model voting fusion. Table 9 showed the validation discrimination effect of the four optimal joint models based on the fusion of single-modal or multi-modal models. The four joint models had reached high validation discrimination accuracy and good balance, the best of which was the dual-modal fusion of 1 mm-$\Phi_{1,2}$, 10 mm-$\Phi_{1,3}$, 1 mm-$\Phi_{2,3}$, the RAR_{Total} was 95.5%, and the corresponding waveband combination (nm) was 1704–1868 (1 mm), 960–1140 (10 mm) and 844–1890 (1 mm). Among them, two models in the NIR overtones frequency region of the 1 mm modal (containing the absorption peak at 1450 nm) and one model in the NIR high-overtone frequency region of the 10 mm modal (containing the absorption peak at 974 nm) were jointly used.

Table 8. Comparison of the modeling discrimination effects for the optimal joint models of the three-model voting fusion and their sub-models.

Modal	Modal (mm)-Submodel			Joint Model RAR_{Total}	Increase Rate of RAR_{Total}		
	Model 1	Model 2	Model 3		Model 1	Model 2	Model 3
Single modal	1-$\Phi_{1,2}$	1-$\Phi_{1,3}$	1-$\Phi_{2,3}$	93.3%	5.1%	7.7%	4.4%
Dual modal	1-$\Phi_{1,2}$	10-$\Phi_{1,3}$	1-$\Phi_{2,3}$	96.0%	18.2%	7.8%	7.1%
Triple-modal (global)	1-Φ_{global}	4-Φ_{global}	10-Φ_{global}	93.3%	5.1%	19.5%	7.7%
Triple-modal (compensatory)	1-$\Phi_{1,2}$	10-$\Phi_{1,3}$	4-$\Phi_{2,3}$	95.6%	7.4%	22.0%	17.8%

Table 9. Validation discrimination effect of the four optimal joint models based on the fusion of single-modal or multi-modal models.

Modal	RAR_1	RAR_2	RAR_3	RAR_{Total}	RAR_{SD}
Single modal	95.5%	94.2%	84.0%	91.2%	6.3%
Dual modal	97.4%	98.1%	91.0%	95.5%	3.9%
Triple-modal (global)	88.5%	91.7%	98.1%	92.7%	4.9%
Triple-modal (compensatory)	95.5%	99.4%	90.4%	95.1%	4.5%

In fact, if the optical-path length of the transmission measurement accessory is regarded as a perturbation factor, the three-model voting fusion modeling approach based on multi-measurement modals is similar to the idea of aquaphotomics. The comprehensive use of the multi-modal spectral features of samples can improve the accuracy of discrimination.

Figure 6 showed the schematic diagrams of the recognition effect of the optimal joint model (dual-modal) based on a three-model voting fusion for the validation samples. Among them, the true value of the category value of the *i*-th sample was set to i, i = 1, 2, 3; its predicted value was set to δ_i, $\delta_i \in \{1,2,3\}$; when $\delta_i = i$, the recognition was correct, otherwise was wrong. The second category of drinking water samples reached the highest validation discrimination accuracy rate (RAR_2 = 98.1%).

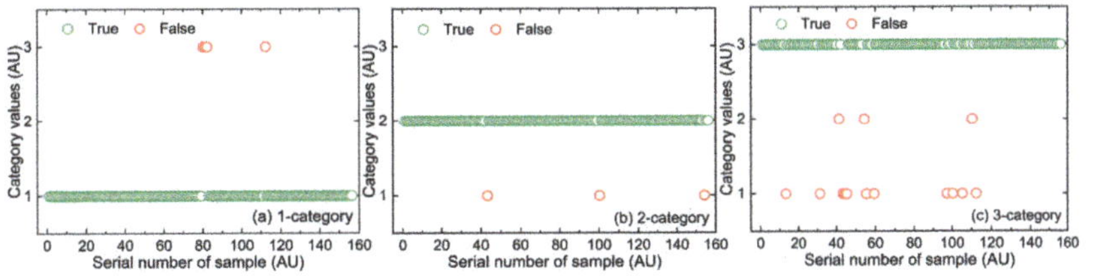

Figure 6. Schematic diagrams of the recognition effect of the optimal joint model based on three-model voting fusion for three categories of validation samples: (**a**) 1-category, (**b**) 2-category, (**c**) 3-category.

3. Materials and Methods

3.1. Experimental Materials, Instruments, and Measurement Methods

Two kinds of drinking water brands (C'estbon and Nongfu Spring) and "tap water" for users after municipal treatment, a total of three categories of water samples were collected as identification samples (not in order, denoted as 1-category, 2-category, 3-category). Among them, 162 tap water samples were collected successively from multiple tap water supply points on the university campus where the experiment was located; C'estbon and Nongfu Spring were purchased from regular commercial channels, 162 bottles of each category, one sample was taken from each bottle; in total, 486 samples were obtained. Two drinking water brand samples were purchased through formal channels, so the authenticity of their brands can be guaranteed, and their sample categories can serve as a reference for spectral pattern recognition.

The XDS Rapid Content^{TM} Liquid Grating Spectrometer (FOSS, Denmark) and a transmission accessory with multiple cuvettes were used for spectral measurement. Spectral scope ranged from 780–2498 nm with a 2 nm wavelength interval. Wavebands of 780–1100 nm and 1100–2498 nm were used for Si and PbS detection, respectively. Using the cuvettes of three optical paths of short, medium, and long (1 mm, 4 mm, 10 mm), each sample was measured three times. The obtained NIR spectra of multiple measurement modals were used for modeling and validation. The experimental temperature and humidity were 25 ± 1 °C and $45 \pm 1\%$, respectively.

3.2. Calibration-Prediction-Validation Framework and Evaluation Indicators

A sample-independent experimental design in calibration–prediction–validation was adopted. The spectral data of the calibration and prediction sets were used for modeling and parameter optimization; the spectral data of the validation set that does not participate in the modeling was used to validate the established models. For each measurement modal, each category of water samples (162) was randomly divided into the calibration (60), prediction (50), and validation (52) sets. In total, for the numbers of the samples and spectra, the division was calibration (180 samples, 540 spectra), prediction (150 samples, 450 spectra), and validation sets (156 samples, 468 spectra).

The evaluation indicators were set as the recognition accuracy rate (RAR_i, $i = 1, 2, 3$) of each category sample and their standard deviation (RAR_{SD}), as well as the total recognition accuracy rate (RAR_{Total}) of all samples, as follows:

$$RAR_i = \frac{\widetilde{M_i}}{M_i},\ i = 1,2,3 \tag{2}$$

$$RAR_{Total} = \frac{\sum_{i=1}^{3} \widetilde{M_i}}{\sum_{i=1}^{3} M_i} \tag{3}$$

where $M_i (i = 1,2,3)$ was the number of samples of i-th category of the prediction (or validation) set, and $\widetilde{M_i}$ was the number of accurately identified samples in i-th category samples of the prediction (or validation) set. In the modeling process, the global optimal model was preferred according to the indicator RAR_{Total}. In order to consider balance, RAR_{SD} was used as the second optimization indicator.

3.3. Norris Derivative Filter Algorithm

In spectral preprocessing, appropriate smoothing and derivatives can effectively eliminate noises and improve spectral information quality. The famous Norris derivative filter (NDF) is an effective spectral pretreatment method, which is an algorithm group with various parameters [29,30]. NDF includes two steps: the moving average smoothing and differential derivation and uses three parameters: the derivative order (D), the number of smoothing points (S, odd), and the number of differential gaps (G) [12,31,32]. Here, the loop parameters were set to $D = 0, 1, 2$; $S = 1, 3 \ldots, 49$; $G = 1, 2 \ldots, 30$. Any combination of parameters (D, S, G) corresponding to the Norris derivative mode, a total of $25 + 2 \times 25 \times 30 = 1525$ modes were obtained. Based on variation of multiple parameters, the Norris derivative spectra were more diverse and applicable than the raw spectra. Norris parameters combination (D, S, G) should not be specified artificially but should be reasonably optimized according to the analysis object and modeling discrimination effect. Next, an algorithm platform for Norris parameter optimization based on kNN modeling was constructed by using MATLAB version 7.6 software.

For all Norris derivative modes, using the kNN algorithm, the calibration–prediction models were established corresponding to the Norris derivative spectra, which were called the Norris-kNN models. The recognition accuracy rate (RAR_i, i = 1, 2, 3) of each category of prediction samples and the total recognition accuracy rate (RAR_{Total}) of all prediction samples were calculated. Additionally, based on the total prediction effect (RAR_{Total}), the optimal Norris parameters combination (D^*, S^*, G^*) was preferred, as follows:

$$\text{RAR}_{\text{Total}}\left(D^*,S^*,G^*\right) = \max_{\substack{D \in \{0,1,2\} \\ S \in \{1,3,\cdots,49\} \\ G \in \{1,2,\cdots,30\}}} \text{RAR}_{\text{Total}}\left(D,S,G\right). \tag{4}$$

3.4. MW-kNN Algorithm

Moving-window waveband screening and kNN were combined. The total indicator RAR_{Total} was adopted as the optimization goal and taken into account the balance indicator RAR_{SD}, and a wavelength optimization platform (MW-kNN) of qualitative discriminant analysis was established by using MATLAB version 7.6 software. The parameters of MW-kNN were set as: (a) the initial wavelength I, (b) the number of wavelengths N. By looping these two parameters, all sub-wavebands were traversed to establish all kNN models, and the optimal model was determined based on the total prediction effect (RAR_{Total}).

Corresponding to the spectral unsaturated absorption regions of the three measurement models, the parameters of moving-window waveband screening were set as the follows: for the dataset of 1 mm, $I \in \{780, 782, \cdots, 2498\}$, $N \in \{2, 3, \cdots, 859, 860\}$; for the dataset of 4 mm, $I \in \{780, 782, \cdots, 1880\}$, $N \in \{2, 3, \cdots, 550, 551\}$; for the dataset of 10 mm, $I \in \{780, 782, \cdots, 1388\}$, $N \in \{2, 3, \cdots, 304, 305\}$. The parameter k of kNN was set as $k \in \{1, 2, \cdots, 5\}$. For the three datasets of 1 mm, 4 mm and 10 mm, based on the total prediction effect (RAR_{Total}), the optimal parameters combinations (I^*, N^*, k^*) were preferred, respectively, as follows:

$$\text{RAR}_{\text{Total}}\left(I^*,N^*,k^*\right) = \max_{\substack{I \in \{780,782,\cdots,2498\} \\ N \in \{2,3,\cdots,859,860\} \\ k \in \{1,2,\cdots,5\}}} \text{RAR}_{\text{Total}}\left(I,N,k\right), \tag{5}$$

$$\text{RAR}_{\text{Total}}\left(I^*,N^*,k^*\right) = \max_{\substack{I \in \{780,782,\cdots,1882\} \\ N \in \{2,3,\cdots,550,551\} \\ k \in \{1,2,\cdots,5\}}} \text{RAR}_{\text{Total}}\left(I,N,k\right), \tag{6}$$

$$\text{RAR}_{\text{Total}}\left(I^*,N^*,k^*\right) = \max_{\substack{I \in \{780,782,\cdots,1388\} \\ N \in \{2,3,\cdots,304,305\} \\ k \in \{1,2,\cdots,5\}}} \text{RAR}_{\text{Total}}\left(I,N,k\right). \tag{7}$$

3.5. Strategy for 2-Category Priority's Compensation and Three-Model Voting Fusion

Drawing on the idea of game theory, the strategy for 2-category priority's compensation and three-model voting fusion was proposed.

The two-category priority compensation models were proposed first. For any two categories of samples of i, j ($i, j = 1, 2, 3$, $i < j$), the total recognition accuracy rate ($RAR_{i,j}$), as follows:

$$\text{RAR}_{i,j} = \frac{\widetilde{M_i} + \widetilde{M_j}}{M_i + M_j}, \tag{8}$$

where M_i, M_j were the number of samples of i-th category and j-th category of the prediction (or validation) set, respectively, and $\widetilde{M_i}$, $\widetilde{M_j}$ were the number of accurately identified samples in i-th category and j-th category samples of the prediction (or validation) set, respectively. For the three categories of samples of 1, 2, and 3, there were three compensation models for the two categories of priority: $\Phi_{1,2}$, $\Phi_{1,3}$, $\Phi_{2,3}$. Among them, according to the optimal total recognition accuracy rate ($RAR_{i,j}$) of i, j-category samples, the corresponding compensation model ($\Phi_{i,j}$) was selected, $i, j = 1, 2, 3, i < j$. For the three datasets of 1 mm, 4 mm and 10 mm, based on the $RAR_{i,j}$, the optimal parameter combinations (I^*, N^*, k^*) were preferred, respectively, as follows:

$$RAR_{i,j}(I^*,N^*,k^*) = \underset{\substack{I\in\{780,782,\cdots,2498\}\\ N\in\{2,3,\cdots,859,860\}\\ k\in\{1,2,\cdots,5\}}}{\text{Max}} RAR_{i,j}(I,N,k), \quad (9)$$

$$RAR_{i,j}(I^*,N^*,k^*) = \underset{\substack{I\in\{780,782,\cdots,1882\}\\ N\in\{2,3,\cdots,550,551\}\\ k\in\{1,2,\cdots,5\}}}{\text{Max}} RAR_{i,j}(I,N,k), \quad (10)$$

$$RAR_{i,j}(I^*,N^*,k^*) = \underset{\substack{I\in\{780,782,\cdots,1388\}\\ N\in\{2,3,\cdots,304,305\}\\ k\in\{1,2,\cdots,5\}}}{\text{Max}} RAR_{i,j}(I,N,k). \quad (11)$$

The above algorithm was also written in MATLAB version 7.6 software.

Next, the three-model voting fusion was described. Taking $\Phi_{1,2}$, $\Phi_{1,3}$, $\Phi_{2,3}$ as sub-models for three-model voting: each sample was judged three times, then, the sample category of comprehensive judgment was determined according to the principle of "Two wins in three games", so as to establish a joint model (Φ_{Fusion}) of three-model voting.

Assuming that each compensation model ($\Phi_{1,2}$, $\Phi_{1,3}$, $\Phi_{2,3}$) has a high probability of identifying certain two categories of samples, then according to the principle of "two wins in three games" of three models voting, their joint model will likely have a high probability of identifying all three categories sample. Therefore, the total recognition accuracy rate (RAR_{Total}) will likely reach a higher probability recognition effect, which is expected to be better than its three sub-models. See also Table 10.

Table 10. Schematic diagram of voting effect for the three-model fusion's joint model and its sub-models.

Model	1-Category	2-Category	3-Category	All Samples
$\Phi_{1,2}$	High	High		High
$\Phi_{1,3}$	High		High	High
$\Phi_{2,3}$		High	High	High
Φ_{Fusion}	High	High	High	Higher

In fact, the strategy proposed here can be generalized to the n-category discriminant analysis case: the $n-1$ categories priority's compensation models were first determined; the joint model based on n-model voting fusion was further established.

4. Conclusions

Inspired by aquaphotomics, a novel method of multi-modal spectra fusion modeling based on multi-optical path measurement was proposed. The optical path length of the transmission measurement accessory was regarded as a perturbation factor. The three-model voting fusion modeling approach based on multi-measurement modals (1 mm, 4 mm, and 10 mm) was used to establish the NIR spectral discriminant analysis models of three categories of drinking water.

The MW-kNN combined with Norris derivative filter was used to optimize the three-category discriminant analysis models for each spectral modal. Drawing on the idea of game theory, the selection method of the two-category priority compensation models was proposed, and the fusion modeling method of three compensation models' voting was further proposed, aiming to make the joint models achieve a better comprehensive discriminant effect.

Based on the model set of MW-kNN with NDF, the global optimal models and the two-category priority compensation models for each modal were determined, and the joint models based on the fusion of single-modal or multi-modal models were also determined. The comprehensive discrimination effects of all joint models were better than their three sub-models; the effect of multi-modal fusion was better than that of single-modal fusion. The joint voting of the multi-modal compensation models can highlight the spectral differences from two dimensions, thereby improving the discrimination accuracy of the spectral population with small differences. The global optimal joint model was the dual-modal fusion of 1 mm-$\Phi_{1,2}$, 10 mm-$\Phi_{1,3}$, and 1 mm-$\Phi_{2,3}$, and the validation's RAR_{Total} reached 95.5%. Thus, it showed the feasibility of NIR spectroscopy for the multi-classification identification of drinking water.

Furthermore, the MWCC spectrum, inter-category, and intra-category MWCC spectra were also proposed to evaluate small differences between two spectral populations of drinking water samples. Based on the principle of kNN and the wavelength model optimization, the plotting approach of the first *k*-shortest distances was also proposed to describe the differences in spectral populations. Their results showed the spectral differences between the three categories of water sample populations.

In summary, a novel NIR spectral pattern recognition strategy was proposed, which included two aspects: three compensation models' voting and multi-modal fusion, which can significantly improve the discriminant analysis effect of spectral populations with small differences. The idea of this methodology is also expected to be widely applied to spectral discriminant analysis in other fields.

Author Contributions: Conceptualization, T.P.; data curation, N.Y., S.Z., Z.F., H.G., Z.D. and H.C.; formal analysis, T.P.; funding acquisition, T.P.; investigation, N.Y., S.Z., Z.F., H.G., Z.D., H.C. and L.Y.; methodology, N.Y., S.Z. and T.P.; project administration, T.P.; resources, T.P.; software, N.Y., L.Y. and T.P.; visualization, N.Y., S.Z., L.Y. and T.P.; writing—original draft, N.Y., S.Z., Z.F., H.G., Z.D., H.C. and T.P.; writing—review and editing, N.Y., S.Z., L.Y. and T.P. All authors have read and agreed to the published version of the manuscript.

Funding: This research was funded by National Natural Science Foundation of China grant number 61078040 and Science and Technology Project of Guangdong Province of China grant number 2014A020213016, 2014A020212445, and the APC was funded by Jinan University.

Acknowledgments: This work was supported by the National Natural Science Foundation of China (No. 61078040), and the Science and Technology Project of Guangdong Province of China (No.2014A020213016, No.2014A020212445).

Conflicts of Interest: The authors declare no conflict of interest.

Sample Availability: Two categories of drinking water brands (C'estbon and Nongfu Spring) were purchased through formal channels. Another category of samples (Tap water) was collected successively from multiple tap water supply points on the authors' university campus.

References

1. Pudelko, A.; Chodak, M. Estimation of total nitrogen and organic carbon contents in mine soils with NIR reflectance spectroscopy and various chemometric methods. *Geoderma* **2020**, *368*, 114306. [CrossRef]
2. Chen, H.Z.; Pan, T.; Chen, J.M.; Lu, Q.P. Waveband selection for NIR spectroscopy analysis of soil organic matter based on SG smoothing and MWPLS methods. *Chemom. Intell. Lab. Syst.* **2011**, *107*, 139–146. [CrossRef]
3. Pan, T.; Wu, Z.T.; Chen, H.Z. Waveband Optimization for Near-Infrared Spectroscopic Analysis of Total Nitrogen in Soil. *Chin. J. Anal. Chem.* **2012**, *40*, 920–924. [CrossRef]
4. Liu, Z.Y.; Liu, B.; Pan, T.; Yang, J.D. Determination of amino acid nitrogen in tuber mustard using near-infrared spectroscopy with waveband selection stability. *Spectrochim. Acta A* **2013**, *102*, 269–274. [CrossRef] [PubMed]

5. Pan, T.; Han, Y.; Chen, J.M.; Yao, L.J.; Xie, J. Optimal partner wavelength combination method with application to near-infrared spectroscopic analysis. *Chemom. Intell. Lab. Syst.* **2016**, *156*, 217–223. [CrossRef]
6. Sousa, A.C.; Lucio, M.M.L.M.; Bezerra, O.F.; Marcone, G.P.S.; Pereira, A.F.C.; Dantas, E.O.; Fragoso, W.D.; Araujo, M.C.U.; Galvao, R.K.H. A method for determination of COD in a domestic wastewater treatment plant by using near-infrared reflectance spectrometry of seston. *Anal. Chim. Acta* **2007**, *588*, 231–236. [CrossRef]
7. Pan, T.; Chen, Z.H.; Chen, J.M.; Liu, Z.Y. Near-infrared spectroscopy with waveband selection stability for the determination of COD in sugar refinery wastewater. *Anal. Methods* **2012**, *4*, 1046–1052. [CrossRef]
8. Jiang, J.H.; Berry, R.J.; Siesler, H.W.; Ozaki, Y. Wavelength interval selection in multicomponent spectral analysis by moving window partial least-squares regression with applications to mid-infrared and near-infrared spectroscopic data. *Anal. Chem.* **2002**, *74*, 3555–3565. [CrossRef]
9. Pan, T.; Liu, J.M.; Chen, J.M.; Zhang, G.P.; Zhao, Y. Rapid determination of preliminary thalassaemia screening indicators based on near-infrared spectroscopy with wavelength selection stability. *Anal. Methods* **2013**, *5*, 4355–4362. [CrossRef]
10. Chen, J.M.; Yin, Z.W.; Tang, Y.; Pan, T. Vis-NIR spectroscopy with moving-window PLS method applied to rapid analysis of whole blood viscosity. *Anal. Bioanal. Chem.* **2017**, *409*, 2737–2745. [CrossRef]
11. Chen, J.M.; Peng, L.J.; Han, Y.; Zhang, J.; Pan, T. A rapid quantification method for the screening indicator for β-thalassemia with near-infrared spectroscopy. *Spectrochim. Acta A* **2018**, *193*, 499–506. [CrossRef] [PubMed]
12. Tan, H.; Liao, S.X.; Pan, T.; Zhang, J.; Chen, M.J. Rapid and simultaneous analysis of direct and indirect bilirubin indicators in serum through reagent-free visible-near-infrared spectroscopy combined with chemometrics. *Spectrochim. Acta A* **2020**, *233*, 18215. [CrossRef] [PubMed]
13. Seregély, Z.; Deák, T.; Bisztray, G.D. Distinguishing melon genotypes using NIR spectroscopy. *Chemom. Intell. Lab. Syst.* **2004**, *72*, 195–203. [CrossRef]
14. Yang, H.; Irudayaraj, J.; Paradkar, M.M. Discriminant analysis of edible oils and fats by FTIR, FT-NIR and FT-Raman spectroscopy. *Food Chem.* **2005**, *93*, 25–32. [CrossRef]
15. Guo, H.S.; Chen, J.M.; Pan, T.; Wang, J.H.; Cao, G. Vis-NIR wavelength selection for non-destructive discriminant analysis of breed screening of transgenic sugarcane. *Anal. Methods* **2014**, *6*, 8810–8816. [CrossRef]
16. Yao, L.J.; Xu, W.Q.; Pan, T.; Chen, J.M. Moving-window bis-correlation coefficients method for visible and near-infrared spectral discriminant analysis with applications. *J. Innov. Opt. Health Sci.* **2018**, *11*, 1850005. [CrossRef]
17. Capuano, E.; Boerrigter-Eenling, R.; Koot, A.; Ruth, S.M. Targeted and untargeted detection of skim milk powder adulteration by near-infrared spectroscopy. *Food Anal. Method.* **2015**, *8*, 2125–2134. [CrossRef]
18. Santos, C.A.T.d.; Pascoa, R.N.M.J.; Sarraguca, M.C.; Porto, P.A.L.S.; Cerdeira, A.L.; Gonzalez-Saiz, J.M.; Pizarro, C.; Lopes, J.A. Merging vibrational spectroscopic data for wine classification according to the geographic origin. *Food Res. Int.* **2017**, *102*, 504–510. [CrossRef]
19. Chen, J.M.; Li, M.L.; Pan, T.; Pang, L.W.; Yao, L.J.; Zhang, J. Rapid and non-destructive analysis for the identification of multi-grain rice seeds with near-infrared spectroscopy. *Pectrochim. Acta A* **2019**, *219*, 179–185. [CrossRef]
20. Liu, K.Z.; Tsang, K.S.; Li, C.K.; Shaw, R.A.; Mantsch, H.H. Infrared spectroscopic identification of beta-thalassemia. *Clin. Chem.* **2003**, *49*, 1125–1132. [CrossRef]
21. Tsuchikawa, S.; Yamato, K. Discriminant analysis of wood-based materials with weathering damage by near infrared spectroscopy. *J. Near Infrared Spec.* **2003**, *11*, 391–399. [CrossRef]
22. Mabwa, D.; Gajjar, K.; Furniss, D.; Schiemer, R.; Crane, R.; Fallaize, C.; Martin-Hirsch, P.L.; Martin, F.L.; Kypraios, T.; Seddon, A.B.; et al. Mid-infrared spectral classification of endometrial cancer compared to benign controls in serum or plasma samples. *RSC Analyst* **2021**, *146*, 5631–5642. [CrossRef] [PubMed]
23. Stables, R.; Clemens, G.; Butler, H.J.; Ashton, K.M.; Brodbelt, A.; Dawson, T.P.; Fullwood, L.M.; Jenkinson, M.D.; Baker, M.J. Feature driven classification of Raman spectra for real-time spectral brain tumour diagnosis using sound. *RSC Analyst* **2017**, *142*, 98–109. [CrossRef] [PubMed]
24. Ciloglu, F.U.; Saridag, A.M.; Kilic, I.H.; Tokmakci, M.; Kahraman, M.; Aydin, O. Identification of methicillin-resistant Staphylococcus aureus bacteria using surfaceenhanced Raman spectroscopy and machine learning techniques. *RSC Analyst* **2020**, *145*, 7559–7570. [CrossRef]
25. Celani, C.P.; Lancaster, C.A.; Jordan, J.A.; Espinoza, E.O.; Booksh, K.S. Assessing utility of handheld laser induced breakdown spectroscopy as a means of Dalbergia speciation. *RSC Analyst* **2019**, *144*, 5117–5126. [CrossRef]
26. Tsenkova, R. Aquaphotomics: Exploring water–light interactions for a better understanding of the biological world. *NIR News* **2006**, *4*, 10–11. [CrossRef]
27. Tsenkova, R. Aquaphotomics: Acquiring Spectra of Various Biological Fluids of the Same Organism Reveals the Importance of Water Matrix Absorbance Coordinates and the Aquaphotome for Understanding Biological Phenomena. *NIR News* **2008**, *1*, 13–15. [CrossRef]
28. Kinoshita, K.; Miyazaki, M.; Morita, H.; Vassileva, M.; Tang, C.X.; Li, D.S.; Ishikawa, O.; Kusunoki, H.; Tsenkova, R. Spectral pattern of urinary water as a biomarker of estrus in the giant panda. *Sci. Rep.* **2012**, *2*, 856. [CrossRef]
29. Norris, K.H.; Williams, P.C. Optimization of mathematical treatments of raw near-infrared signal in the measurement of protein in hard red spring wheat. I. Influence of particle size. *Cereal. Chem.* **1984**, *61*, 158–165.

30. Norris, K.H. Applying Norris derivatives-understanding and correcting the factors which affect diffuse transmittance spectra. *NIR News* **2001**, *12*, 6–9. [CrossRef]
31. Pan, T.; Zhang, J.; Shi, X.W. Flexible vitality of near-infrared spectroscopy—Talking about Norris derivative filter. *NIR News* **2020**, *31*, 24–27. [CrossRef]
32. Yang, Y.H.; Lei, F.F.; Zhang, J.; Yao, L.J.; Chen, J.M.; Pan, T. Equidistant combination wavelength screening and step-by-step phase-out method applied to near-infrared spectroscopy analysis of serum urea nitrogen. *J. Innov. Opt. Health Sci.* **2019**, *12*, 1950018. [CrossRef]

molecules

MDPI

Article

Water as a Probe for Standardization of Near-Infrared Spectra by Mutual–Individual Factor Analysis

Xiaoyu Cui

BIC-ESAT and SKL-ESPC, College of Environmental Sciences and Engineering, Peking University, Beijing 100871, China; xycui@pku.edu.cn

Abstract: The standardization of near-infrared (NIR) spectra is essential in practical applications, because various instruments are generally employed. However, standardization is challenging due to numerous perturbations, such as the instruments, testing environments, and sample compositions. In order to explain the spectral changes caused by the various perturbations, a two-step standardization technique was presented in this work called mutual–individual factor analysis (MIFA). Taking advantage of the sensitivity of a water probe to perturbations, the spectral information from a water spectral region was gradually divided into mutual and individual parts. With aquaphotomics expertise, it can be found that the mutual part described the overall spectral features among instruments, whereas the individual part depicted the difference of component structural changes in the sample caused by operation and the measurement conditions. Furthermore, the spectral difference was adjusted by the coefficients in both parts. The effectiveness of the method was assessed by using two NIR datasets of corn and wheat, respectively. The results showed that the standardized spectra can be successfully predicted by using the partial least squares (PLS) models developed with the spectra from the reference instrument. Consequently, the MIFA offers a viable solution to standardize the spectra obtained from several instruments when measurements are affected by multiple factors.

Keywords: water probe; mutual–individual factor analysis; calibration transfer; aquaphotomics; near infrared spectroscopy

Citation: Cui, X. Water as a Probe for Standardization of Near-Infrared Spectra by Mutual–Individual Factor Analysis. *Molecules* **2022**, *27*, 6069. https://doi.org/10.3390/molecules27186069

Academic Editors: Roumiana Tsenkova and Jelena Muncan

Received: 6 August 2022
Accepted: 13 September 2022
Published: 17 September 2022

1. Introduction

Water, as one of the most common substances on earth, has numerous functions, including dissolution, stabilization, catalyzation, transportation, etc. [1–3]. However, water is an enduring mystery, due to the intricate and dynamic structures of its intermolecular hydrogen bond network [4]. The molecular interaction is generally affected by perturbations in water's surroundings, such as temperature and additives, resulting in hydrogen bond rearrangement and the alteration of chemical as well as physical performance in the system [5]. Thus, water structure has remained a significant research subject for decades.

Aquaphotomics has been proposed as a new scientific discipline based on innovative knowledge of the water molecular network, which describes the features of water structure from the water spectrum, indirectly reflecting all perturbations, including experimental conditions and sample compositions [6]. The water spectral pattern hence becomes a revelator of the system condition. Several attempts have been made to analyze the experimental conditions by using water spectra. Shao et al. reported that a quantitative spectra–temperature relationship (QSTR) model can be established, and the temperature of a solution can be predicted from the near-infrared (NIR) spectrum with the water region using the model [7,8]. Romanenko et al. developed a new approach, which used three fitted Gaussian features from the water Raman spectra to investigate pressure and solution density [9]. Subsequently, aquaphotomics has gradually broadened as water was applied to be a sensor and an amplifier in the structural and quantitative analysis of aqueous systems [10]. A number of researchers have reported that water was a sensitive probe for analyzing the structural changes and the interactions in aqueous solutions of alcohols [11,12], as well as proteins [13–15], and practical samples [16–18]. On the other hand, the water probe possesses its own advantages when carrying out the component detection [19–21].

Currently, aquaphotomics for experimental conditions and sample compositions in aqueous systems have been investigated simultaneously with chemometric methods [22–24]. The NIR spectra of water in terms of hydrogen bonding were extracted to characterize the perturbations created by the change of temperature and concentration in solutions with the application of multivariate curve resolution–alternating least squares (MCR–ALS) [25], alternating trilinear decomposition (ATLD) [26], and multilevel simultaneous component analysis (MSCA) [27], etc. Furthermore, practical samples were studied [28,29]. The common spectral features that contained the water spectra influenced by temperature were extracted from the spectra of serum samples, and both the temperature and glucose can be successfully measured by using mutual factor analysis (MFA) [29]. Therefore, aquaphotomics provides a common platform for practical applications.

In industrial applications with NIR spectroscopy, standardization or calibration transfer is usually required to correct the spectral variations both caused by the measurement and sample conditions [30]. There are three major pathways for standardizing the NIR spectra measured on different instruments, including the correction of the prediction values [31], alteration of the model coefficients [32,33], and modification of the spectra [34–37]. The last strategy is the most commonly applied. Piecewise direct standardization (PDS) is a very efficient method by which to establish a linear relationship between the spectra measured on different instruments in several small window regions [34]. By using techniques like spectral space transformation (SST) [35], alternating trilinear decomposition (ATLD) [36], and multilevel simultaneous component analysis (MSCA) [37], research was also conducted by determining the relationship between the principal components retrieved from the spectra as an alternative to correcting spectra. However, the majority of standardization methods concentrate on resolving the discrepancy resulting from a straightforward link between the spectra obtained on various instruments and describing the calibration transfer through a mathematical formula. Aquaphotomics may provide a different approach by which to examine spectral differences that are influenced by a variety of circumstances, enhancing interpretability and lowering bias, especially for the spectra of samples containing water, such as agricultural products.

In this work, particular attention is paid to the application of aquaphotomics for calibration transfer to discover more information with physical and chemical meanings. A new algorithm, called mutual–individual factor analysis (MIFA), using water as a probe, was proposed to analyze the water spectra both influenced by different instruments and substances, and the standardization performance of the water probe was validated by two NIR spectral datasets.

2. Theory and Algorithm

2.1. Continuous Wavelet Transform

As an efficient tool for data processing, continuous wavelet transform (CWT) has been generally applied to improve the spectral quality, i.e., resolution enhancement, baseline correction, and smoothing [29,38,39]. In this work, CWT with a Symmlet filter with a vanishing moment 6 (Sym6 filter)) was employed, which is approximately equal to the sixth derivative. With CWT, the resolution improvement and spectrum smoothing can be achieved simultaneously [39]. Due to the property of the sixth derivative, the positive absorption in the raw spectra becomes a negative one. In this study, for the convenience of description, the value of the derivative is reversed.

2.2. Mutual–Individual Factor Analysis

In order to develop the transfer model, the spectra of standard samples collected on different instruments are generally employed for standardization. Following CWT processing, the spectra from three instruments, denoted as $\mathbf{X}_1$, $\mathbf{X}_2$, and $\mathbf{X}_3$ were employed in this investigation. In accordance with MFA [29], the combined spectral matrix, $\mathbf{X}_{comb}$, was first processed to separate the standardized signal (**SS**), which represents the spectral information of samples measured on a reference instrument. The relationship can be presented as

$$\mathbf{X}_{comb} = [\mathbf{X}_1, \mathbf{X}_2, \mathbf{X}_3] = \mathbf{T}\left[\mathbf{P}_1^{\mathrm{T}}, \mathbf{P}_2^{\mathrm{T}}, \mathbf{P}_3^{\mathrm{T}}\right] + \mathbf{E} \tag{1}$$

$$\mathbf{SS} = \mathbf{TP}_{ref}^{\mathrm{T}} = \mathbf{X}_{ref}\left(\mathbf{P}_{ref}^{\mathrm{T}}\right)^{+}\mathbf{P}_{ref}^{\mathrm{T}}, \tag{2}$$

where superscripts T and + denote the mathematical operation of transposition and pseudoinverse of the matrix, respectively, and **E** contains the residuals between the actual spectra and the fitted model. The scores and loadings in a principal component analysis (PCA) model are symbolized as **T** and $\mathbf{P}_i^{\mathrm{T}}$ (i = 1, 2, and 3), respectively. As a result of using the same **T**, $\mathbf{P}_i^{\mathrm{T}}$ represents the variations in the measured conditions or instruments. Then, it is possible to determine how much of the spectral pattern of $\mathbf{X}_i$ is present in $\mathbf{X}_j$ ($i \neq j$) by using the relationship. The relative quantity (z_i) of **SS** contained in each $\mathbf{X}_i$ can be obtained, and score, $\mathbf{t}_i$, in each group of spectra collected on different instruments can be calculated by using the reference loading, $\mathbf{P}_{ref}$. The relationship can be presented as

$$z_i = trace\left(\mathbf{X}_i\mathbf{SS}^{+}\right) \tag{3}$$

$$\mathbf{t}_i = \mathbf{X}_i\left(\mathbf{P}_{ref}^{\mathrm{T}}\right)^{+}. \tag{4}$$

It should be noted that, theoretically, any group of spectra measured on an instrument can be used as the reference; however, generally the spectra collected on the master instrument is applied.

The mutual part between the spectra measured on various instruments can be discovered after MFA processing. However, apart from the spectral alterations driven by the instruments, there are also spectral variations caused by the altered sample structural features as a result of changing measurement conditions. Despite being minor, the spectral variations affect the standardization, especially for the samples containing water, due to the sensitive response of OH in NIR spectra [6]. As a result, the individual factor was introduced to evaluate the variance using PCA model as the following equation,

$$\mathbf{X}_{lef} = \begin{bmatrix} \mathbf{X}_1 - z_1\mathbf{SS}^{+} \\ \mathbf{X}_2 - z_2\mathbf{SS}^{+} \\ \mathbf{X}_3 - z_3\mathbf{SS}^{+} \end{bmatrix} = \begin{bmatrix} \mathbf{T}_{lef,1} \\ \mathbf{T}_{lef,2} \\ \mathbf{T}_{lef,3} \end{bmatrix}\mathbf{P}_{lef}^{\mathrm{T}} + \mathbf{E}_{lef}, \tag{5}$$

where $\mathbf{E}_{lef}$ denotes the remaining data that did not fit into the model, and $\mathbf{T}_{lef,i}$ and $\mathbf{P}_{lef}^{\mathrm{T}}$ reflect the scores and loadings in the PCA model, respectively, after the mutual parts have been removed. As a result, the score of the model merely accounts for the variance affected by the measurement of the sample. Because the essence of the algorithm is to extract the factor mutually and individually contained in the spectral data of different samples, the algorithm is named as mutual–individual factor analysis and abbreviated as MIFA.

By adjusting the coefficients, i.e., z_i and $\mathbf{T}_{lef,i}$, the spectra measured on one instrument can be transferred to another. The details of the standardization can be summarized in two steps, as follows.

(1) Establish MIFA models: The MIFA approach is applied to establish the two models, containing $\mathbf{t}_i$, $\mathbf{P}_i^{\mathrm{T}}$, $\mathbf{T}_{lef,i}$, and $\mathbf{P}_{lef}^{\mathrm{T}}$, from the standard spectra measured on three instruments, $\mathbf{X}_1$, $\mathbf{X}_2$, and $\mathbf{X}_3$. This stage involves determining how many principal components each of the two models has.

(2) Transfer the spectrum: As an illustration, the following computations can be used to transfer the spectrum of instrument 2 ($\mathbf{X}_{2s}$) to instrument 1,

$$\mathbf{t}_s = \mathbf{X}_{2s}\left(\mathbf{P}_1^{\mathrm{T}}\right)^{+} \tag{6}$$

$$\mathbf{T}_{lef,s} = (\mathbf{X}_{2s} - \mathbf{t}_s\mathbf{P}_1^{\mathrm{T}})\left(\mathbf{P}_{lef}^{\mathrm{T}}\right)^{+} \tag{7}$$

$$\mathbf{t}_{Ts} = \mathbf{t}_s(\mathbf{t}_2)^{+}\mathbf{t}_1 \tag{8}$$

$$\mathbf{T}_{lef,Ts} = \mathbf{T}_{lef,s}\left(\mathbf{T}_{lef,1}\right)^{+}\mathbf{T}_{lef,2} \tag{9}$$

$$\mathbf{X}_{T2s} = \mathbf{t}_{Ts}\mathbf{P}_1^{\mathrm{T}} + \mathbf{T}_{lef,Ts}\mathbf{P}_{lef}^{\mathrm{T}}. \tag{10}$$

The scores of $\mathbf{X}_{2s}$ can be calculated by using Equations (6) and (7) through MIFA models, and then transferred from instrument 2 to instrument 1 by using Equations (8) and (9). Finally, Equation (10) can be applied to obtain the transferred spectra by using the loadings ($\mathbf{P}_1{}^{\mathrm{T}}$ and $\mathbf{P}_{lef}{}^{\mathrm{T}}$) and the transferred scores. The spectra from the instrument 3 can be transferred in the same way.

3. Data Description

Two NIR spectral datasets were employed in this investigation. Dataset 1 was downloaded from http://software.eigenvector.com/Data/Corn/index.html (accessed on 25 June 2019), and contains the moisture, oil, protein, and starch contents of 80 corn samples along with the NIR spectra obtained by using three NIR spectrometers (m5, mp5, and mp6). Each spectrum was acquired with 700 data points throughout the wavelength range of 1100–2498 nm with a digitization interval of 2 nm.

Dataset 2 was downloaded from https://www.cnirs.org/content.aspx?page_id=22&club_id=409746&module_id=239453 (accessed on 17 July 2022), and includes 744 NIR spectra analyzed on three instruments (A1, A2, and A3), as well as the protein content of the 248 wheat samples. Each spectrum comprised 741 data points with a digitization interval of 0.5 nm, and was recorded in the wavelength range of 730–1100 nm.

Prior to the calculation, each dataset was divided into a calibration set, a transfer set, and a prediction set using the Kennard-Stone (KS) technique [40]. The calibration set (the spectra of the master) is employed to develop the multivariate calibration model of the master, the transfer set (containing the spectra of all the instruments) is applied to building the transfer model, and the prediction set (the spectra of the salve) is used for validating the effect of the transfer model. For dataset 1, the calibration, transfer, and prediction sets were composed of 30, 30, and 20. For dataset 2, the possible outlier (ID 20140190) was removed, and the remaining 247 samples were divided into a calibration set of 117 samples, a transfer set of 30 samples, and a prediction set of 100 samples.

4. Results and Discussion

4.1. Spectral Analysis and Resolution Enhancement

The spectra of corn samples using three instruments are displayed in Figure 1. Figure 1(a1) shows that there are several broad bands with a ranked background, and the average spectrum intensity from m5 is higher than those from mp5 and mp6. The outcome demonstrates that the background shift appears to be the major source of the overall spectral variance induced by different instruments. To remove the background, CWT with Sym6 was used, which is approximately equal to the sixth derivative [39]. The CWT-processed spectra are shown in Figure 1(b1), illustrating an almost zero baseline. Furthermore, compared with the spectra from the three instruments, the similarity proves that the background shifting among the instruments is the primary cause of the difference. In addition, taking advantage of the high-order derivative, narrower peaks were obtained than the corresponding spectra in Figure 1(a1). It has been reported that compared with the results by the first or second derivatives used in our previous works [11,17,26,28], the CWT-processed spectra from higher-order derivatives illustrate higher resolution, and reveal more information to understand the interactions in aqueous samples [29,41].

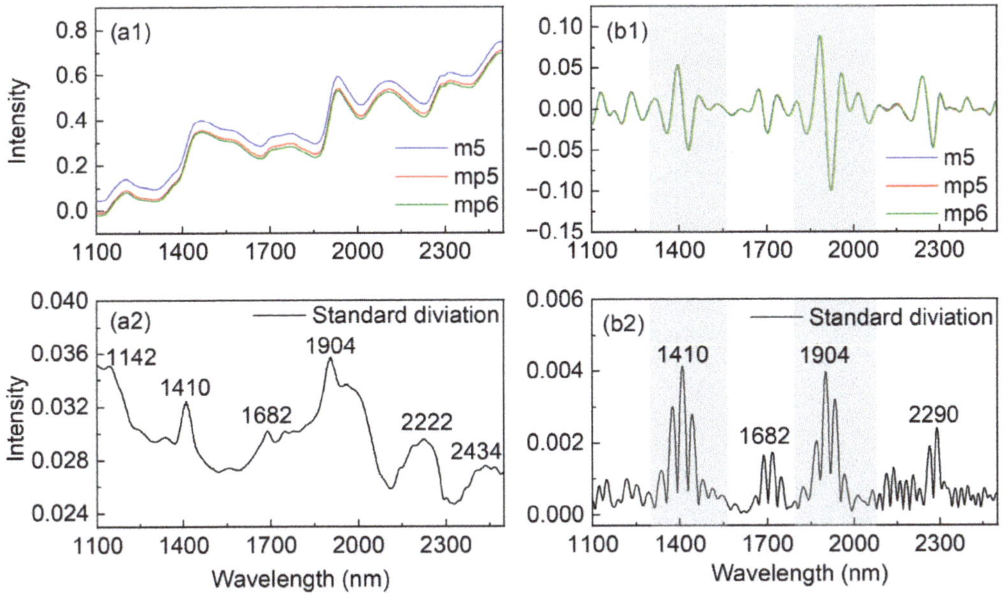

Figure 1. Average NIR spectra of corn samples from instrument m5, mp5, and mp6, respectively (**a1**), standard deviation of the averaged spectra (**a2**), average spectra from each instrument after CWT transformation (**b1**), and standard deviation of the CWT processed spectra (**b2**). The selected ranges were indicated with shadows.

For a further comparison, Figure 1(a2,b2) provides the standard deviation of the sample spectra and the CWT-processed spectra, respectively, where the higher the intensity, the larger the difference. The relatively higher intensity in both subfigures can be seen around 1410 and 1904 nm, which are primarily composed of the overtone and a combination of stretching and bending vibrational modes of OH in water, as well as features of OH, NH, and CH in biological components [6,18]. The others around 1682 and 2200–2300 nm are related to the CH groups in biomolecules and α-helix in protein, respectively, consistent with the assignments of NIR bands from quantum chemical simulations [42,43]. Additionally, the background shift may be the reason of the high intensity around 1142 and 2434 nm in Figure 1(a2), as there are no strong values in these spectral regions of Figure 1(b2). These findings suggest that as detecting conditions change, different instruments alter not just the background but also the spectral intensity of various species in samples, which is consistent with the results of MSCA [37]. Thus, it is necessary to adjust the spectra at both the instrument and sample levels.

Furthermore, the major differences in the shadow reveal that NIR spectra are sensitive to OH, which can easily undergo structural changes due to hydrogen bonding when environmental changes are detected [6,24]. Compared with biomacromolecules, such as oil, protein, and starch in seeds, OH groups in water are relatively more active due to the smaller size and stronger polarity of water, and may cause more spectral changes from different instruments [6,44]. For this reason, by using water as the probe, the spectral ranges (1294–1556 and 1788–2078 nm) associated with water in the shadow in Figure 1(b1) were chosen to build the MIFA model.

4.2. Mutual–Individual Factor Analysis

To investigate the instrument and sample effects on the NIR spectra, MIFA was employed on dataset 1 using water as a probe. First, the numbers of principal components (PC) were required to construct the mutual and individual factor analysis models, respectively.

The commonly used criteria of "explained variance" was utilized in this study to determine the numbers [37]. The number of the PCs that explain 99.9% of the variance was applied. For dataset 1, the parameters for the mutual and individual factor analysis models were 1 and 6, respectively.

Equations (1)–(3) were then applied to calculate the standardized signal (**SS**) and the relative quantity (z_i) using the spectra from m5 as the reference. The **SS** is shown in Figure 2a to estimate instrument-induced variance. As a result, it should be unaffected by instrument changes. The intensity of the signal should be only related to the concentration of the samples. Figure 2b shows the intensity variations at 1882 nm with the mass percentage of moisture to validate the assumption. A linear function can be generated from quantitative analysis of complicated biological samples with a recovery of less than 20%, which is considered a good result when using single-point spectral values for regression. The results suggest that **SS** is related to water in corn, indicating the effectiveness of mutual parts, which are consistent with the MFA conclusion [29].

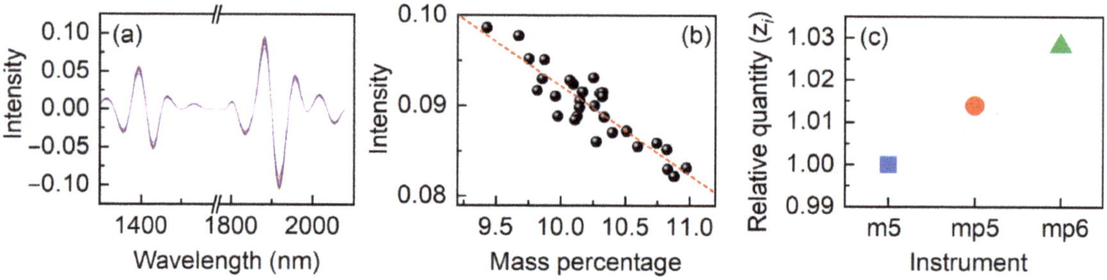

Figure 2. Standardized signal (**SS**) (**a**), the relationship between the intensity at 1882 nm and the mass percentage of moisture (**b**), and the relationship between the relative quantity (z_i) and instruments (**c**). The linear regression appears as the red dash.

Figure 2c depicts z_i in relation to the three instruments. The very small difference in values reflects the minor overall variations between the spectra of three instruments, even if the background was reduced by the CWT. This demonstrates that apart from the background variation, the mutual part contains the sample change with different instruments, indicating the sensitivity of water probe. z_i is a mirror of the spectral variation caused by instruments; hence the relationship between z_i can be utilized to regulate the overall spectral difference caused by the measurement circumstances.

After removing the mutual part from the spectra, PCA was used to evaluate the individual spectral features from the remaining spectra. Figure 3 shows the loadings for each PC, and the spectrum characteristics are related to the hydrated CH, NH, and OH in biomolecules as well as the hydrated OH in water [6,15,16,18,42,43]. The disparities between the PCs may be due to differences in the samples and the measurement of the spectra. In comparison to the other five PCs, the first PC provides additional details concerning the characteristics of the hydrogen-bonded OH at 1444 and 1934 nm, according to aquaphotomics [10]. When samples of corn are measured by using different instruments, the outcomes show that the hydrogen-bonding variance of the chemicals in the corn is what causes the majority of individual differences.

In order to further explore the feasibility of the model transfer, Figure 4 displays the scores of the individual part for the first six PCs. The scores in the models are more essential in this study because the transfer is accomplished by modifying the scores. This implies that measurement-related changes in molecule structures may impact the measured spectra, as not all of the discrepancy can be accounted for by the mutual part or only one model [37]. For adjusting the complicated effects, a multi-step strategy can be a wise solution.

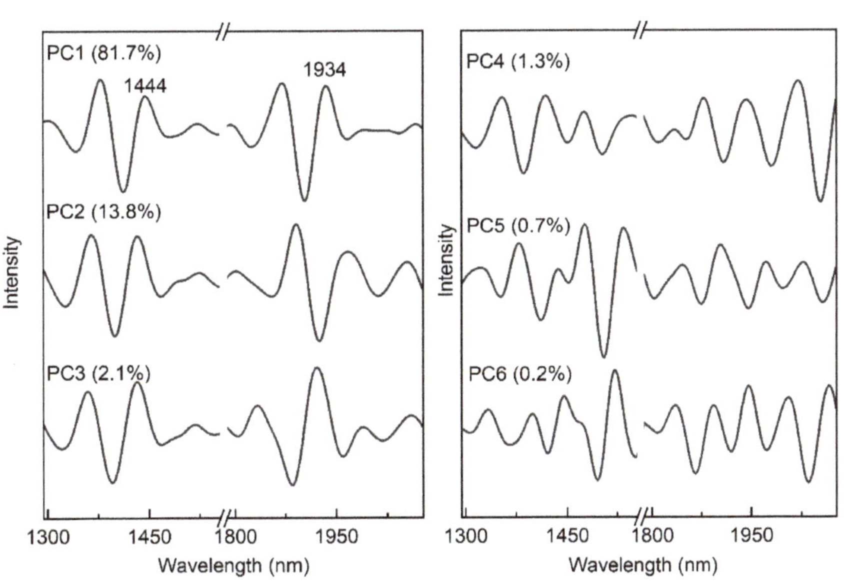

Figure 3. The first through the sixth loadings in the PCA model, after the mutual parts have been removed.

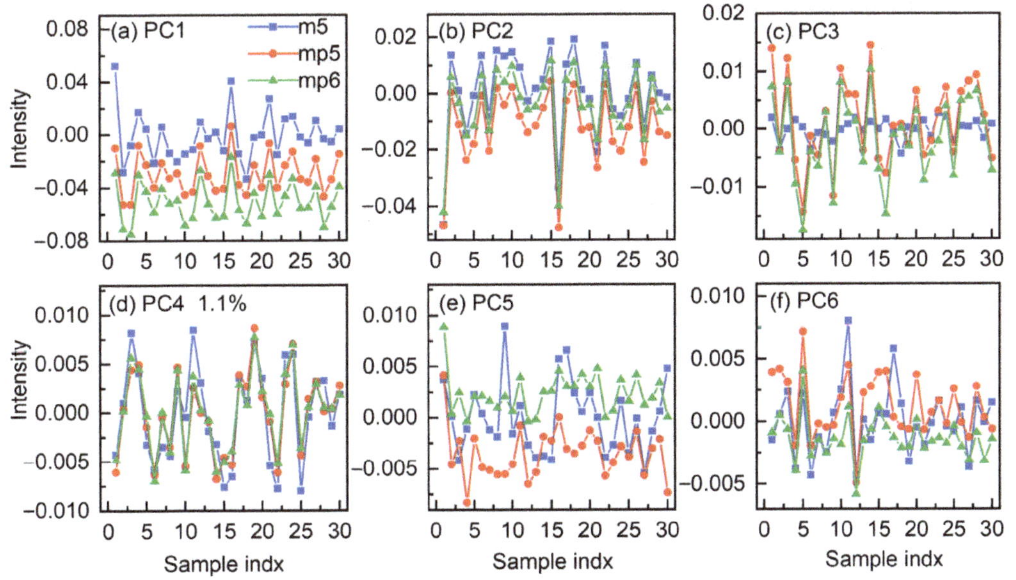

Figure 4. Comparison of the scores in the first through the sixth (**a–f**) PCs in the individual part for the spectra from the instruments m5, mp5, and mp6. The blue square, red circle, and green triangle represent the score for instrument m5, mp5, and mp6, respectively.

In contrast to the scores in PC2–PC6, it is obvious that PC1 shows the largest disparity. In PC1, the scores from mp5 and mp6 show similar changes when compared with that from m5, indicating that structural alterations of hydrogen-bonded water in corn have a regular pattern under different measurement conditions. The findings prove that water probe may be utilized for model transfer and that water spectral features can be used as a comprehensive descriptor to portray the system.

4.3. Standardization of the Spectra

By adjusting the coefficient values in the scores, it is possible to achieve spectral standardization, or the transfer of the spectra from mp5 and mp6 to m5 (mp5–m5 and mp6–m5). Because there is just one value for the mutual part in dataset 1, it is obvious that the transfer may be finished by simply changing the z_i of mp5 and mp6 to m5, respectively. In general, the transfer for the mutual part can be accomplished by Equation (8). Similarly, Equation (9) can be used to determine the transfer of individual part.

Figure 5 displays the spectra measured from m5, mp5, and mp6 for a sample randomly chosen from the prediction set of dataset 1. The transferred spectra by the mutual and mutual–individual parts are also shown in the figure to demonstrate the effects of the standardization by the proposed strategy. Clearly, the spectra from the three instruments differ among one another in the embedded graphs. The spectra of mp5 and mp6 approach closer to the spectrum of m5 once the mutual part has been corrected, although there is still a little divergence. The spectra from m5, mp5–m5, and mp6–m5 are virtually identical after the individual parts have been corrected. The findings unequivocally demonstrate that both mutual and individual parts have an impact on the transfer of the spectra.

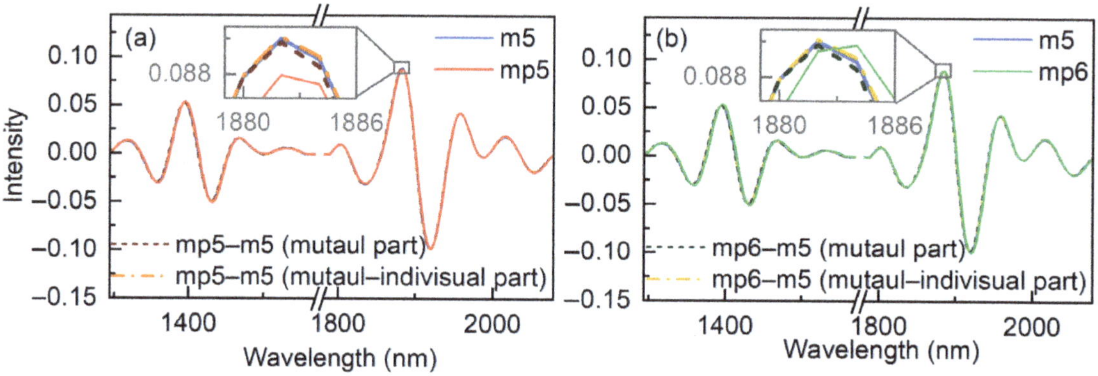

Figure 5. The transfer results for an arbitrarily selected spectrum from mp5 (**a**) and mp6 (**b**) to m5, respectively.

To further assess the transfer effect of the proposed approach, PCA was carried out on the spectra both before and after spectral standardization. Figure 6 displays the transfer outcomes of the spectra from various equipment in the first three PC spaces. The scores from m5 and the other two instruments differ substantially, demonstrating the variation in spectra between them. The disparity between the mp5 and mp6 is not as significant, consistent with the findings in Figure 1. The results show that the score can properly represent the spectral features.

When the scores of the reference and the transferred spectra are compared, it is clear that the ellipsoids with a confidence value of 95% are overlapped, demonstrating that the disparity has been corrected by MIFA. The outcomes unequivocally illustrate that the proposed method is capable of transferring the measured spectra from other instruments to the reference.

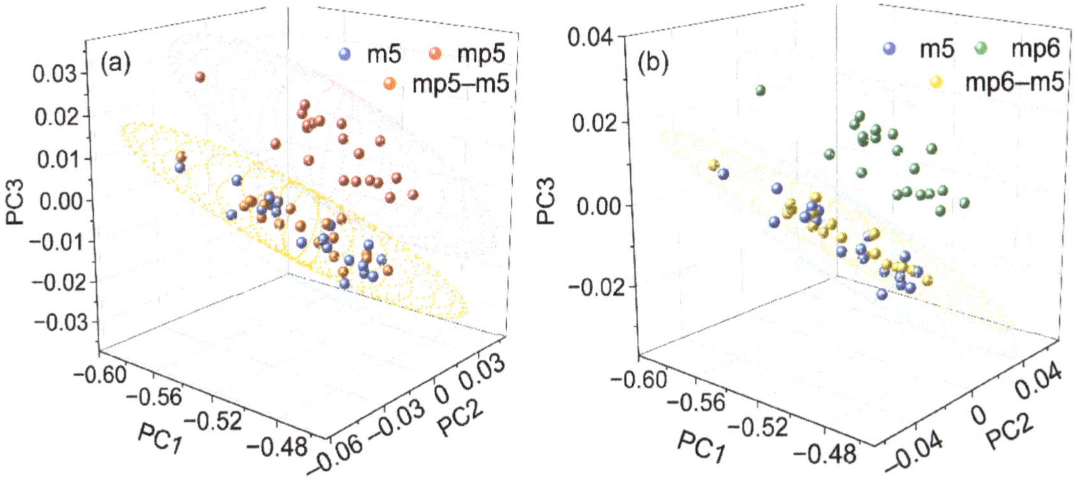

Figure 6. Results of the scores in PC1–PC2–PC3 space for the spectra from m5, mp5, and mp5–m5 (**a**) and spectra from m5, mp6, and mp6–m5 (**b**), respectively. The ellipsoids are determined with the confidence of 95%.

4.4. Validation of the Standardized Spectra

For the final evaluation of the proposed method, a partial least squares (PLS) model was built with the calibration spectra measured on the reference instrument, and then applied to the prediction set from other instruments. Cross-validation is used to establish the optimal number of latent variables (nLV) in the PLS model. For the calibration set of dataset 1, four LVs were employed. Figure 7 depicts the relationship between predicted and original moisture, oil, protein, and starch values based on the spectra from m5 in blue points. The results of the spectra from mp5 and mp6 are displayed in red and green points, and the predicted values of the transferred spectra from mp5 and mp6 are also plotted in orange and yellow for comparison. It is obvious that similar results can be found between the blue and orange or blue and yellow points in the subfigures, respectively. Moreover, the blue and red or blue and green points clearly differ from each other. The results demonstrate that the PLS model from the reference instrument can accurately predict the transferred spectra.

When comparing the correlation coefficient (R^2) of the calibration models, it should be noted that the relationships between the original and predicted values for moisture, protein, and starch are slightly better than that for oil. The moisture quantification result is the best because the water spectral range was chosen. In addition, protein and starch, which interact more strongly with water [2,10], have superior quantification models than oil. Despite the fact that R^2 is slightly lower than others for oil, the quantitative model can be applied for practical samples with the recovery less than 20%.

To further investigate the effectiveness of the proposed approach, Tables 1 and 2 exhibit the predictions made by MIFA for datasets 1 and 2, respectively, compared with the results from PDS and SST. By using one of the instruments as a reference, the values of root mean squared error of prediction (RMSEP) for the oil and protein contents in the validation set are shown in the tables, respectively. Clearly, the direct prediction of spectra from other instruments through the reference model is substantially worse than that of the reference spectra. The RMSEP can be minimized if the transferred spectra are predicted. The results provide a strong validation for the efficiency of the calibration transfer, even though the values are still slightly larger than those of the reference instrument. Additionally, although there is a minor variance, similar results are also obtained for the PDS, SST, and MIFA.

Consequently, the MIFA can be used to successfully transfer the spectra measured by different instruments with the water spectral region. Furthermore, the MIFA approach (using water as a probe) narrows the wavelength range needed by concentrating on the water spectral region, which reflects the major structural changes in the system, providing the opportunity of standardization between miniature instruments.

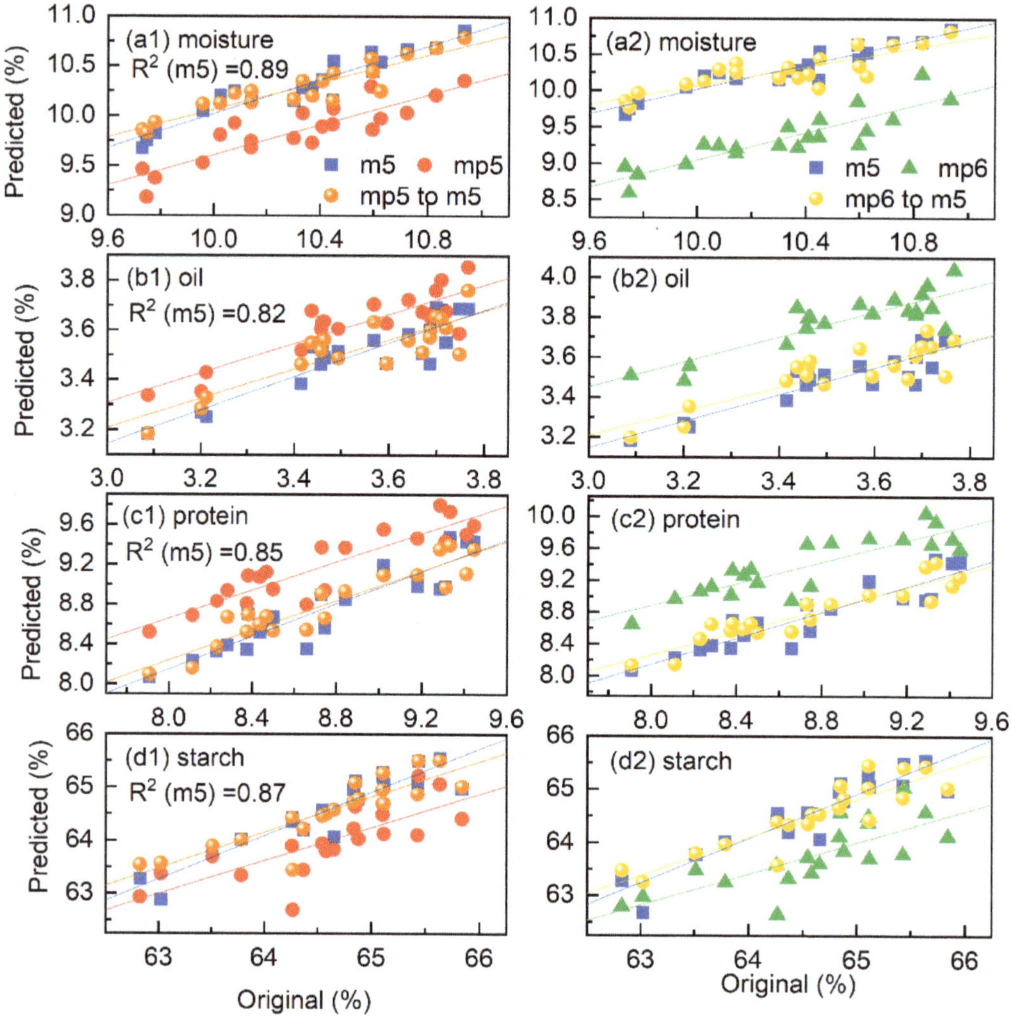

Figure 7. Relationship between the original and the prediction values of moisture (**a**), oil (**b**), protein (**c**), and starch (**d**) obtained from the spectra from m5, mp5, and mp6, as well as the transferred spectra of mp5–m5 and mp6–m5, respectively.

Table 1. Comparison of the results obtained by PDS, SST and MIFA for dataset 1.

Calibration Spectra	Validation Spectra	RMSEP
m5	m5	0.1419
	mp5	0.1667
	mp6	0.2608
	mp5–m5 (MIFA)	0.1435
	mp5–m5 (PDS)	0.1592
	mp5–m5 (SST)	0.1573
	mp6–m5 (MIFA)	0.1424
	mp6–m5 (PDS)	0.1519
	mp6–m5 (SST)	0.1493
mp5	mp5	0.1527
	m5	0.1786
	mp6	0.1669
	m5–mp5 (MIFA)	0.1601
	m5–mp5 (PDS)	0.1642
	m5–mp5 (SST)	0.1639
	mp6–mp5 (MIFA)	0.1546
	mp6–mp5 (PDS)	0.1593
	mp6–mp5 (SST)	0.1572
mp6	mp6	0.1523
	m5	0.1981
	mp5	0.1909
	m5–mp6 (MIFA)	0.1609
	m5–mp6 (PDS)	0.1564
	m5–mp6 (SST)	0.1551
	mp5–mp6 (MIFA)	0.1546
	mp5–mp6 (PDS)	0.1634
	mp5–mp6 (SST)	0.1586

Table 2. Comparison of the results obtained by PDS, SST and MIFA for dataset 2.

Calibration Spectra [1,2]	Validation Spectra	RMSEP
A1	A1	0.6091
	A2	0.8028
	A3	0.9866
	A2–A1 (MIFA)	0.6824
	A2–A1 (PDS)	0.6987
	A2–A1 (SST)	0.6752
	A3–A1 (MIFA)	0.7154
	A3–A1 (PDS)	0.7089
	A3–A1 (SST)	0.7066
A2	A2	0.7475
	A1	0.8538
	A3	0.9274
	A1–A2 (MIFA)	0.8049
	A1–A2 (PDS)	0.8122
	A1–A2 (SST)	0.799
	A3–A2 (MIFA)	0.8106
	A3–A2 (PDS)	0.8324
	A3–A2 (SST)	0.8075

Table 2. *Cont.*

Calibration Spectra [1,2]	Validation Spectra	RMSEP
	A3	0.7044
	A1	0.8316
	A2	1.1068
	A1–A3 (MIFA)	0.7993
A3	A1–A3 (PDS)	0.8237
	A1–A3 (SST)	0.8033
	A2–A3 (MIFA)	0.8196
	A2–A3 (PDS)	0.8169
	A2–A3 (SST)	0.8127

[1] The number of PC for the mutual and individual factor analysis models were 1 and 6 in MIFA, respectively.
[2] PLS model was built with 3 LVs, according to cross-validation.

5. Conclusions

For the purpose of standardizing NIR spectra, a new chemometric technique called mutual–individual factor analysis (MIFA) was developed based on the water spectral region, which used water as a probe. In order to describe the overall differences between the various instruments, the method extracted the spectral feature of the mutual part present in the spectra from different instruments. The difference between the molecular interactions in the samples caused by various measurement conditions was then depicted in each individual part. Furthermore, the spectra measured on one instrument can be effectively transferred to that of another by modifying the coefficients of the mutual and individual parts, respectively. When compared with PDS and SST, MIFA produced a similar result, but provided additional information with physical and chemical meanings by using aquaphotomics. Therefore, in practical applications of NIR spectroscopic analysis, the water probe may offer an effective solution when the spectra are impacted by several complex perturbations, and promote the development of small instruments with limited wavelength ranges.

Funding: This research was funded by the China Postdoctoral Science Foundation, grant number 2020M670048.

Institutional Review Board Statement: Not applicable.

Informed Consent Statement: Not applicable.

Conflicts of Interest: The author declares no conflict of interest.

Sample Availability: Samples of the compounds are not available from the authors.

References

1. Dong, J.; Davis, A.P. Molecular Recognition Mediated by Hydrogen Bonding in Aqueous Media. *Angew. Chem. Int. Ed.* **2021**, *60*, 8035–8048. [CrossRef] [PubMed]
2. Adhikari, A.; Park, W.; Kwon, O. Hydrogen-Bond Dynamics and Energetics of Biological Water. *ChemPlusChem* **2020**, *85*, 2657–2665. [CrossRef] [PubMed]
3. Breynaert, E.; Houlleberghs, M.; Radhakrishnan, S.; Grübel, G.; Taulelle, F.; Martens, J.A. Water as a Tuneable Solvent: A Perspective. *Chem. Soc. Rev.* **2020**, *49*, 2557–2569. [CrossRef]
4. Ball, P. Water—An Enduring Mystery. *Nature* **2008**, *452*, 291–292. [CrossRef] [PubMed]
5. Dereka, B.; Yu, Q.; Lewis, N.H.C.; Carpenter, W.B.; Bowman, J.M.; Tokmakoff, A. Crossover from Hydrogen to Chemical Bonding. *Science* **2021**, *371*, 160–164. [CrossRef]
6. Tsenkova, R. Aquaphotomics: Dynamic Spectroscopy of Aqueous and Biological Systems Describes Peculiarities of Water. *J. Near Infrared Spectrosc.* **2009**, *17*, 303–313. [CrossRef]
7. Shao, X.; Kang, J.; Cai, W. Quantitative Determination by Temperature Dependent Near-Infrared Spectra. *Talanta* **2010**, *82*, 1017–1021. [CrossRef]
8. Kang, J.; Cai, W.; Shao, X. Quantitative Determination by Temperature Dependent Near-Infrared Spectra: A Further Study. *Talanta* **2011**, *85*, 420–424. [CrossRef]
9. Romanenko, A.V.; Rashchenko, S.V.; Goryainov, S.V.; Likhacheva, A.Y.; Korsakov, A.V. In Situ Raman Study of Liquid Water at High Pressure. *Appl. Spectrosc.* **2018**, *72*, 847–852. [CrossRef]

10. Muncan, J.; Tsenkova, R. Aquaphotomics—From Innovative Knowledge to Integrative Platform in Science and Technology. *Molecules* **2019**, *24*, 2742. [CrossRef]
11. Shao, X.; Cui, X.; Liu, Y.; Xia, Z.; Cai, W. Understanding the Molecular Interaction in Solutions by Chemometric Resolution of Near−Infrared Spectra. *ChemistrySelect* **2017**, *2*, 10027–10032. [CrossRef]
12. Dong, Q.; Yu, C.; Li, L.; Nie, L.; Li, D.; Zang, H. Near-Infrared Spectroscopic Study of Molecular Interaction in Ethanol–Water Mixtures. *Spectrochim. Acta Part A Mol. Biomol. Spectrosc.* **2019**, *222*, 117183. [CrossRef] [PubMed]
13. Dong, Q.; Yu, C.; Li, L.; Nie, L.; Zhang, H.; Zang, H. Analysis of Hydration Water around Human Serum Albumin Using Near-Infrared Spectroscopy. *Int. J. Biol. Macromol.* **2019**, *138*, 927–932. [CrossRef] [PubMed]
14. Sun, Y.; Ma, L.; Cai, W.; Shao, X. Interaction between Tau and Water during the Induced Aggregation Revealed by Near-Infrared Spectroscopy. *Spectrochim. Acta Part A Mol. Biomol. Spectrosc.* **2020**, *230*, 118046. [CrossRef]
15. Zhang, M.; Liu, L.; Yang, C.; Sun, Z.; Xu, X.; Li, L.; Zang, H. Research on the Structure of Peanut Allergen Protein Ara H1 Based on Aquaphotomics. *Front. Nutr.* **2021**, *8*, 696355. [CrossRef]
16. Bázár, G.; Romvári, R.; Szabó, A.; Somogyi, T.; Éles, V.; Tsenkova, R. NIR Detection of Honey Adulteration Reveals Differences in Water Spectral Pattern. *Food Chem.* **2016**, *194*, 873–880. [CrossRef]
17. Cui, X.; Yu, X.; Cai, W.; Shao, X. Water as a Probe for Serum–Based Diagnosis by Temperature-Dependent near–Infrared Spectroscopy. *Talanta* **2019**, *204*, 359–366. [CrossRef]
18. Muncan, J.; Tei, K.; Tsenkova, R. Real-Time Monitoring of Yogurt Fermentation Process by Aquaphotomics Near-Infrared Spectroscopy. *Sensors* **2020**, *21*, 177. [CrossRef]
19. Goto, N.; Bazar, G.; Kovacs, Z.; Kunisada, M.; Morita, H.; Kizaki, S.; Sugiyama, H.; Tsenkova, R.; Nishigori, C. Detection of UV-Induced Cyclobutane Pyrimidine Dimers by Near-Infrared Spectroscopy and Aquaphotomics. *Sci. Rep.* **2015**, *5*, 11808. [CrossRef]
20. Mura, S.; Cappai, C.; Greppi, G.F.; Barzaghi, S.; Stellari, A.; Cattaneo, T.M.P. Vibrational Spectroscopy and Aquaphotomics Holistic Approach to Determine Chemical Compounds Related to Sustainability in Soil Profiles. *Comput. Electron. Agric.* **2019**, *159*, 92–96. [CrossRef]
21. Cui, X.; Tang, M.; Wang, M.; Zhu, T. Water as a Probe for PH Measurement in Individual Particles Using Micro-Raman Spectroscopy. *Anal. Chim. Acta* **2021**, *1186*, 339089. [CrossRef] [PubMed]
22. Pasquini, C. Near Infrared Spectroscopy: A Mature Analytical Technique with New Perspectives—A Review. *Anal. Chim. Acta* **2018**, *1026*, 8–36. [CrossRef] [PubMed]
23. Tsenkova, R.; Munćan, J.; Pollner, B.; Kovacs, Z. Essentials of Aquaphotomics and Its Chemometrics Approaches. *Front. Chem.* **2018**, *6*, 363. [CrossRef] [PubMed]
24. Cui, X.; Sun, Y.; Cai, W.; Shao, X. Chemometric Methods for Extracting Information from Temperature-Dependent Near-Infrared Spectra. *Sci. China Chem.* **2019**, *62*, 583–591. [CrossRef]
25. Gowen, A.A.; Amigo, J.M.; Tsenkova, R. Characterisation of Hydrogen Bond Perturbations in Aqueous Systems Using Aquaphotomics and Multivariate Curve Resolution—Alternating Least Squares. *Anal. Chim. Acta* **2013**, *759*, 8–20. [CrossRef]
26. Cui, X.; Zhang, J.; Cai, W.; Shao, X. Chemometric Algorithms for Analyzing High Dimensional Temperature Dependent near Infrared Spectra. *Chemom. Intell. Lab. Syst.* **2017**, *170*, 109–117. [CrossRef]
27. Shan, R.; Zhao, Y.; Fan, M.; Liu, X.; Cai, W.; Shao, X. Multilevel Analysis of Temperature Dependent Near-Infrared Spectra. *Talanta* **2015**, *131*, 170–174. [CrossRef]
28. Cui, X.; Liu, X.; Yu, X.; Cai, W.; Shao, X. Water Can Be a Probe for Sensing Glucose in Aqueous Solutions by Temperature Dependent near Infrared Spectra. *Anal. Chim. Acta* **2017**, *957*, 47–54. [CrossRef]
29. Shao, X.; Cui, X.; Yu, X.; Cai, W. Mutual Factor Analysis for Quantitative Analysis by Temperature Dependent near Infrared Spectra. *Talanta* **2018**, *183*, 142–148. [CrossRef]
30. Feudale, R.N.; Woody, N.A.; Tan, H.; Myles, A.J.; Brown, S.D.; Ferré, J. Transfer of Multivariate Calibration Models: A Review. *Chemom. Intell. Lab. Syst.* **2002**, *64*, 181–192. [CrossRef]
31. Bouveresse, E.; Hartmann, C.; Massart, D.L.; Last, I.R.; Prebble, K.A. Standardization of Near-Infrared Spectrometric Instruments. *Anal. Chem.* **1996**, *68*, 982–990. [CrossRef]
32. Kunz, M.R.; Kalivas, J.H.; Andries, E. Model Updating for Spectral Calibration Maintenance and Transfer Using 1-Norm Variants of Tikhonov Regularization. *Anal. Chem.* **2010**, *82*, 3642–3649. [CrossRef] [PubMed]
33. Nikzad-Langerodi, R.; Zellinger, W.; Lughofer, E.; Saminger-Platz, S. Domain-Invariant Partial-Least-Squares Regression. *Anal. Chem.* **2018**, *90*, 6693–6701. [CrossRef]
34. Wang, Y.; Veltkamp, D.J.; Kowalski, B.R. Multivariate Instrument Standardization. *Anal. Chem.* **1991**, *63*, 2750–2756. [CrossRef]
35. Du, W.; Chen, Z.-P.; Zhong, L.-J.; Wang, S.-X.; Yu, R.-Q.; Nordon, A.; Littlejohn, D.; Holden, M. Maintaining the Predictive Abilities of Multivariate Calibration Models by Spectral Space Transformation. *Anal. Chim. Acta* **2011**, *690*, 64–70. [CrossRef] [PubMed]
36. Liu, Y.; Cai, W.; Shao, X. Standardization of near Infrared Spectra Measured on Multi-Instrument. *Anal. Chim. Acta* **2014**, *836*, 18–23. [CrossRef]
37. Zhang, J.; Guo, C.; Cui, X.; Cai, W.; Shao, X. A Two-Level Strategy for Standardization of near Infrared Spectra by Multi-Level Simultaneous Component Analysis. *Anal. Chim. Acta* **2019**, *1050*, 25–31. [CrossRef]
38. Shao, X.-G.; Leung, A.K.-M.; Chau, F.-T. Wavelet: A New Trend in Chemistry. *Acc. Chem. Res.* **2003**, *36*, 276–283. [CrossRef]

39. Shao, X.; Ma, C. A General Approach to Derivative Calculation Using Wavelet Transform. *Chemom. Intell. Lab. Syst.* **2003**, *69*, 157–165. [CrossRef]
40. Kennard, R.W.; Stone, L.A. Computer Aided Design of Experiments. *Technometrics* **1969**, *11*, 137–148. [CrossRef]
41. Shao, X.; Cui, X.; Wang, M.; Cai, W. High Order Derivative to Investigate the Complexity of the near Infrared Spectra of Aqueous Solutions. *Spectrochim. Acta Part A Mol. Biomol. Spectrosc.* **2019**, *213*, 83–89. [CrossRef] [PubMed]
42. Chu, X.; Guo, L.; Huang, Y.; Yuan, H. (Eds.) *Sense the Real Change: Proceedings of the 20th International Conference on Near Infrared Spectroscopy*; Springer Nature: Singapore, 2022; ISBN 978-981-19488-3-1.
43. Grabska, J.; Beć, K.B.; Ishigaki, M.; Huck, C.W.; Ozaki, Y. NIR Spectra Simulations by Anharmonic DFT-Saturated and Unsaturated Long-Chain Fatty Acids. *J. Phys. Chem. B* **2018**, *122*, 6931–6944. [CrossRef] [PubMed]
44. Zhou, Y.; Dhital, S.; Zhao, C.; Ye, F.; Chen, J.; Zhao, G. Dietary Fiber-Gluten Protein Interaction in Wheat Flour Dough: Analysis, Consequences and Proposed Mechanisms. *Food Hydrocoll.* **2021**, *111*, 106203. [CrossRef]

molecules

MDPI

Article

Raman Spectroscopy-Based Assessment of the Liquid Water Content in Snow

Ettore Maggiore [1], Matteo Tommasini [1] and Paolo Maria Ossi [2,*]

[1] Dipartimento di Chimica, Materiali e Ingegneria Chimica "G. Natta", Politecnico di Milano, 20133 Milano, Italy; ettore.maggiore@polimi.it (E.M.); matteo.tommasini@polimi.it (M.T.)
[2] Dipartimento di Energia, Politecnico di Milano, 20133 Milano, Italy
* Correspondence: paolo.ossi@polimi.it

Abstract: In snow, water coexists in solid, liquid and vapor states. The relative abundance of the three phases drives snow grain metamorphism and affects the physical properties of the snowpack. Knowledge of the content of the liquid phase in snow is critical to estimate the snowmelt runoff and to forecast the release of wet avalanches. Liquid water does not spread homogeneously through a snowpack because different snow layers have different permeabilities; therefore, it is important to track sudden changes in the amount of liquid water within a specific layer. We reproduced water percolation in the laboratory, and used Raman spectroscopy to detect the presence of the liquid phase in controlled snow samples. We performed experiments on both fine- and coarse-grained snow. The obtained snow spectra are well fitted by a linear combination of the spectra typical of liquid water and ice. We progressively charged snow with liquid water from dry snow up to soaked snow. As a result, we exploited continuous, qualitative monitoring of the evolution of the liquid water content as reflected by the fitting coefficient c.

Keywords: snow; water; Raman spectroscopy; OH-stretching band; liquid water content

Citation: Maggiore, E.; Tommasini, M.; Ossi, P.M. Raman Spectroscopy-Based Assessment of the Liquid Water Content in Snow. *Molecules* **2022**, *27*, 626. https://doi.org/10.3390/molecules27030626

Academic Editors: Roumiana Tsenkova and Jelena Muncan

Received: 23 December 2021
Accepted: 17 January 2022
Published: 19 January 2022

1. Introduction

Snow is a granular, porous material made of a mixture of ice crystals with a variety of forms, a fraction of liquid water and water vapor in thermodynamic equilibrium [1]. The initial shape of the crystallites formed in a cloud include plates, needles, hollow columns, dendrites, depending on the combinations of temperature and water vapor supersaturation values they experience along their free fall down to the ground, where they progressively accumulate [2]. After its deposition, natural snow undergoes extensive metamorphism [3] that consists of grain sintering under mechanical compression and thermal gradients through the snowpack thickness due to mass and thermal energy fluxes, driven by the weather conditions it experiences. Sun irradiation, temperature gradients, humidity and wind are the leading factors that concur with the evolution of the layers that progressively accumulate upon successive snowfalls and build up the snowpack. The size and shape of the constituting snow grains concurrently evolve. In the laboratory, strict control of ambient temperature and supersaturation allows us to produce natural-like snow crystals with a degree of perfection higher than that of spontaneously grown crystals [4].

A relevant property of a snowpack is the liquid water content θ_W. This results mostly when melted snow or rainwater infiltrates into the snow, changing its wetness [5]; alternatively, the presence of thermal gradients through the snowpack may drive changes of θ_W in snow layers at specific depths [6]. As such, θ_W in snow is a marker of snowmelt and snow mechanical stability [7]. Accelerated melting under strong Sun irradiation, as well as heavy rain on snow, lead to increased θ_W values and can result in a flood, possibly associated with severe runoff [8] or wet avalanche release. This can be full depth when water reaches the ground behind the snow cover, or, since the shear strength of snow reduces exponentially with increasing the volumetric water content [9], when a wet, buried snow layer becomes the preferential sliding surface of the avalanche. The fate of the snowpack is further affected by the lowered surface albedo of snow progressively impregnated with water [10] since considerable liquid phase amounts favor the formation of ice clusters [11] that act similar to big grains, being more efficient than small crystallites in absorbing light. Indeed, albedo is higher in snow with smaller grains and vice versa [12].

Measuring θ_W is admittedly difficult and demanding [13,14]. To take into account the space–time evolution of meltwater outflow that is correlated with the snowpack stability, continuous recording of θ_W is required. Indeed, associated with θ_W changes are sudden, non-linear alterations of snowpack properties and of the outflow of meltwater. Several in-situ, more or less invasive techniques to measure θ_W were reviewed in the past and include centrifugal, dielectric, calorimetric or dilution approaches [15,16]. The main drawbacks of such techniques are the large amount of snow and the long time necessary to perform a measurement. Thus, no successive tests can be made at a given site since the snowpack is irreversibly altered at every measurement. More gentle, non-destructive methods are based on the changes of spectral reflectance in the NIR region (920–1650 nm) of snow bearing different water contents [17,18] and ground-penetrating radar, by which an electromagnetic signal is generated and the reflected wavefield is measured, from which it is possible to map the values of θ_W in the sampled region. Recent satellite and ground-based remote sensing are based on the analysis of microwave radiation reflected at the Earth's surface in comparison to a signal directly received at an antenna above the ground [19,20]. These methods leave the sampled area intact, but since the satellite repetition time is of the order of days, snow parameters can be checked only intermittently. Mountain areas are challenging for passive microwave systems, mostly due to the coarse spatial resolution, in the range of a few tens of km^2, and to the complicated terrain topography that produces shadowing and foreshortening effects. Thus, presently, satellite-based sensing of snow properties is mostly devoted to flat areas [21].

Here we describe an innovative approach based on Raman spectroscopy for the insitu assessment of the liquid phase content in snow. We conceived this idea from the observations that first, snow consists of frozen water; second, we are concerned with discriminating among snow with different contents of liquid-phase water; and third, in the region of the OH-stretching band, the Raman spectrum (RS) of ice qualitatively differs from that of liquid water. Notably, very recently, we found a single old report (in Russian) where Raman spectroscopy was proposed as a conceptual tool to determine the θ_W of snow [22]. Other optical spectroscopy techniques, such as reflectance spectroscopy, were used to investigate snow metamorphism [23] and to measure snow albedo to derive from it the snow grain size, also taking into account the presence of different concentrations of dust contaminants [24].

In our study, we used two reference types of snow with markedly different average grain sizes (0.2 mm; 1.6 mm). By this choice, we expect that the infiltration strategy of equal, controlled amounts of water, homogeneously deposited on the sample surface, differs in the two snow kinds. We recorded RS from the snow samples at a fixed height below the water-wet surface, at fixed delays with respect to the wetting time. We observed that the RS of snow with different fractional contents of the liquid phase, driven by the degree of water infiltration, can be described well by a weighted linear combination of the spectra of ice and liquid water. For both kinds of tested snow, we plotted vs. time the weighting factor (c) as well as the independently measured liquid phase fraction. We found a smooth behavior of c with two evident thresholds. Each threshold occurs at the same value of liquid phase fraction for both kinds of snow. By our method, we collected RS from specific points in the snow volume. Even though punctual information could be of less interest when the global liquid water content in a snow volume is required, local Raman measurements such as those presented here provide useful insight regarding the progressive accumulation of liquid water at specific locations in the snowpack, e.g., within snow layers that lay on top of a melt-freeze crust. The water content in such layers is critical for a wet avalanche release because the accumulated liquid water reduces the cohesive force among snow grains, thus dramatically decreasing the mechanical stability of the snowpack.

2. Results

In Table 1, we report the measured amounts of water accumulated inside the empty container by spraying water from progressively increasing distances from the top open surface. In our experiments, we sprayed water from a point placed between 3 and 5 cm above the container opening (see Section 4 for details). In such a condition, the average collected water per spray is 0.15 g.

Table 1. Water mass collected in the container after spraying from progressively increased heights above the top open surface.

Height (cm)	Collected Water after 100 Sprays (g)	Average Collected Water per Spray (g)
0	18.3	0.183
5	11.6	0.116
10	3.9	0.039
15	3.3	0.033
20	2.6	0.026

We performed four different experiments in which we added controlled amounts of liquid water to different snow batches, as summarized in Table 2, where the conditions adopted to charge with water the two different kinds of snow, namely natural-like snow (NLS) and natural snow (NS) (see Section 4 for details) are grouped. We remark that the density of NLS (280 kg m^{-3}) differs from that of NS (380 kg m^{-3}). Lower density snow is characterized by a more open microstructure with more pores that result in increased water vapor presence. Around 0 °C enhanced melting is likely to occur. Yet, in our experiments, we discard the role of water vapor due to the dominant weight of the amount of liquid water we deliberately inject in the sample from its top surface.

Table 2. Experimental parameters adopted to add liquid water to the snow samples.

Snow Kind; Injection Method	Initial Snow Mass (g)	Total Mass of Injected Water (g)	Number of Injection Steps	Water Mass per Unit Step (g)
NLS; spray	11.6	4.8	31	0.15
NLS; pipette	3	4.7	100	0.047
NS; pipette 1st	3	4.8	100	0.048
NS; pipette 2nd	3.1	4.2	100	0.042

We collected the reference spectra of bulk ice and liquid water at 0 °C in a mixture of ice/water from a volume of distilled water, focusing the laser spot at the *same* fixed distance for both measurements. We normalized the intensity of both spectra according to the intensity of the most relevant ice peak. The obtained spectra are reported in Figure 1a and clearly show how the different hydrogen-bonding networks that characterize ice and liquid water produce markedly different Raman bandshapes in the OH-stretching region [25]. Such a different spectral profile can be used to *qualitatively* assess, by a least-square fitting procedure, the relative amount of liquid water in snow, as described below.

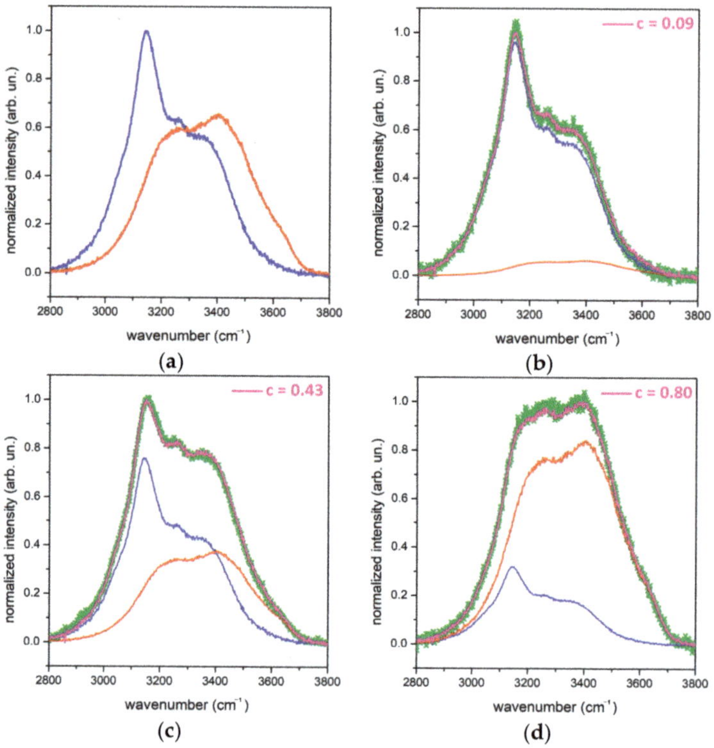

Figure 1. (**a**) RS of ice (blue curve) and liquid water (red curve) at 0 °C normalized to the maximum intensity of the ice spectrum. Panels (**b–d**) are the fits (pink curves) to three representative experimental spectra (green curves), as obtained by Equation (1) with the indicated values of the *c* coefficient. In each panel, we report the different relative intensities of the spectra of ice and water.

After the acquisition of the RS of snow, we first operated spike removal and baseline correction over the range 2800–3800 cm^{-1} (OH-stretching band), and the spectra were normalized. To fit all RS collected from snow samples, we use a linear combination of the ice and water spectra according to:

$$I_{fit}(\omega) = (1 - c) \times I_{ice}(\omega) + c \times I_{water}(\omega), \quad (1)$$

where $I_{ice}(\omega)$ and $I_{water}(\omega)$ are the intensities of the reference spectra of ice (normalized to its maximum) and water (normalized to the maximum of ice spectrum), respectively. c is the fitting coefficient that runs between 0 (pure ice) and 1 (pure liquid water). For a given snow sample, we obtain the value by minimizing the squared sum of the residuals (S^2) computed using the *measured* normalized spectrum of wet snow ($I_{meas}(\omega)$) and the *fitted* spectrum given by Equation (1) in the spectral range of the OH-stretching region (2800 cm^{-1} = $\omega_a < \omega < \omega_b$ = 3800 cm^{-1}), according to:

$$S^2 = \int_{\omega_a}^{\omega_b} \left[I_{meas}(\omega) - I_{fit}(\omega) \right]^2 d\omega \quad (2)$$

In Figure 1 b–d, we show the experimental spectra of wet snow samples containing different amounts of water, fitted with the spectrum associated with the value of the c coefficient (Equations (1) and (2)) that allows the experimental data to match in the best way (i.e., in the least-squares sense).

For this set of experiments (see Section 4 for details), we used the spray bottle, and we collected six RS after each spray in order to establish a stationary distribution of liquid water throughout the snow volume along the time required to take RS. When we used the pipette, we collected a single RS for every addition of water. Since in this experiment the snow volume is smaller, we assumed that water requires less time to obtain a stationary volume distribution with respect to water addition using the spray bottle.

We investigated the percolation of water through the snow by a specific experiment. In Figure 2, we report four representative frames of a video collected during the progressive addition of a diluted (0.03% in volume; see Section 4) water-colored solution to a sample of NS. Moving from plate (a) to plate (d) of the figure, we notice that the fraction of the green-colored area and the intensity of the coloration progressively increase. This coincides with a correspondingly large number of times the fixed liquid water volume (0.04 mL) was uniformly dropped onto the snow surface using the pipette, from 4 (20 s; plate a) to 7 (35 s; plate b) and 14 (70 s; plate c) to 62 (310 s; plate d). We observed that initially (plate a) liquid water was mostly deposited at the top surface of the snow, and it appears as a barely visible green shaded area. The increased intensity of green coloration of plate b coincides with liquid water penetrating down to the bottom of the container through a percolation path. From this point on, water diffusion through snow mostly occurs along the already established path involving progressively larger snow volumes (plate c). After the heaviest water injection, the whole bottom of the container is saturated with liquid water (plate d). The above trend is the same observed in the dye infiltration experiment through snow [26].

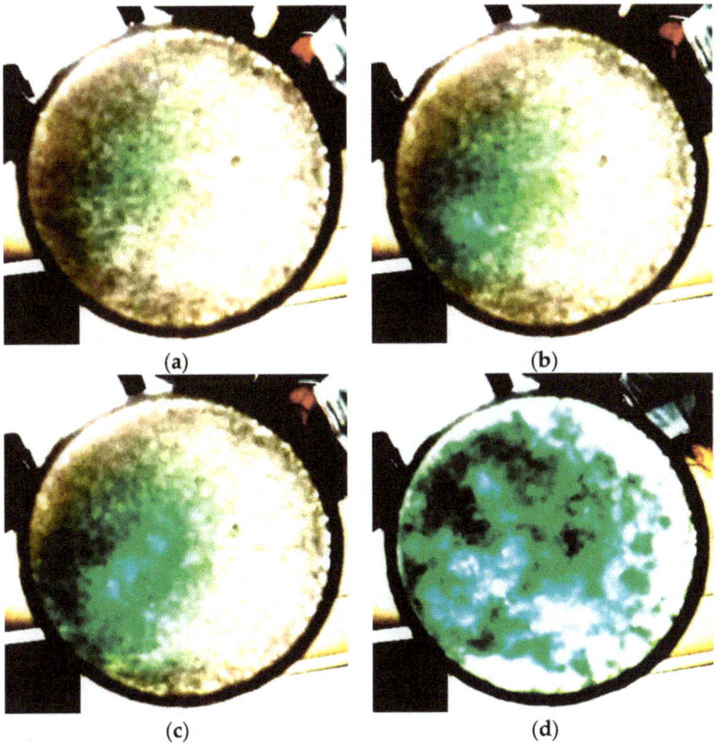

Figure 2. Snow pictures taken from the bottom of the container after uniformly dropping (**a**) 4, (**b**) 7, (**c**) 14, (**d**) 62 pipettes of green-colored water onto the snow top surface. The contrast of the pictures is enhanced to highlight the green-colored areas.

In Figure 3, we show the trend of the *c* coefficient (Equation (1)) vs. time, as represented by the black curves. The red curves provide the liquid water (LW) mass fraction in the samples. Figure 3a refer to NLS that underwent successive water sprayings. After an initial region where *c* values are nearly constant, a sudden vertical discontinuity (disc. 1) at an LW mass fraction value of 0.13 is followed by a region of roughly constant *c* values.

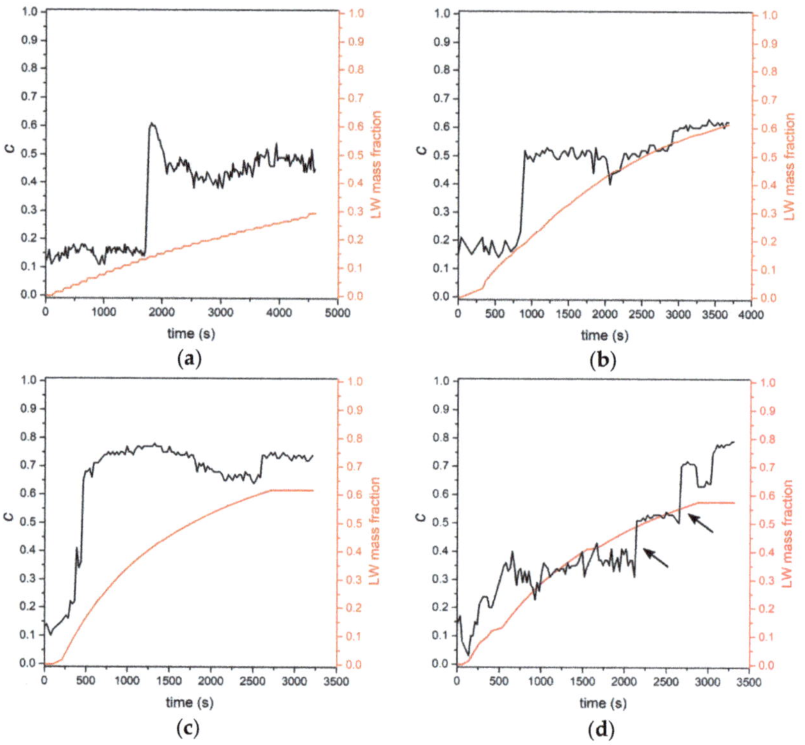

Figure 3. Trend of the *c* coefficient (black curves and ordinate scale) and liquid water mass fraction (red curves and ordinate scale) for selected combinations of snow kind and degree of liquid water injection. (**a**) NLS, spray; (**b**) NLS, pipette; (**c**) NS, pipette 1st; (**d**) NS, pipette 2nd. See text for details.

In Figure 3b, we show the result of an experiment similar to the one discussed in Figure 3a, apart from the more consistent water injection in the snow that was possible when we used a pipette. Indeed, in this case, the mass of the snow sample is about 25% of the sample mass used for spraying measurements (see Table 2). The initial trend of the *c* coefficient is similar to that in Figure 3a: the average *c* value in the initial region is around 0.15. The vertical discontinuity (disc. 1) occurs at the value of LW mass fraction 0.17, and again a nearly flat region of *c* values follows up to a second vertical discontinuity (disc. 2) at the LW mass fraction 0.55. Discontinuity 2 is less marked than discontinuity 1, and it is followed by a region of nearly constant *c* values.

The same kind of measurement just discussed, when performed on a NS sample (Figure 3c), qualitatively mirrors the trend of the *c* coefficient already discussed for Figure 3b. The discontinuities occur at LW mass fraction values of 0.13 and 0.6, respectively. Remarkably, in Figure 3c, the steep increase of the *c* value across the discontinuity region is rather high, around 0.7. We believe that such a large value is due to the combination of the coarse snow grain of this sample (see Figure 4a) and of the focusing conditions. Indeed, since the laser spot diameter is less than the average grain size, it is likely that a small number of snow grains is illuminated, thus magnifying the liquid water contribution in the recorded RS.

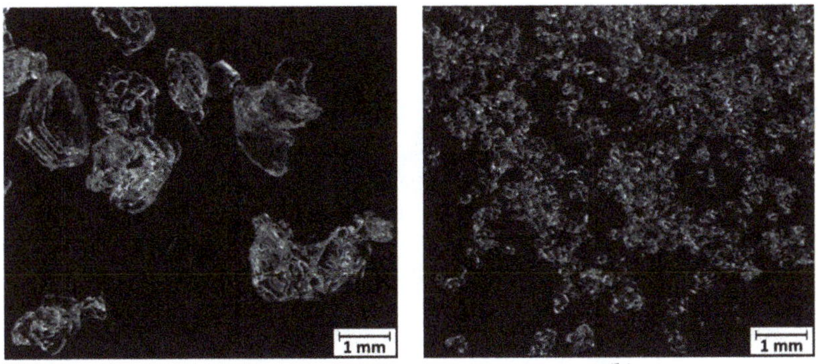

(a) (b)

Figure 4. Stereo-microscopy pictures of (**a**) natural and (**b**) natural-like snow grains.

In Figure 3d, we show the results we obtained when the same measurement as for Figure 3c was performed under defocused laser irradiation. The consequence is a noisier *c* trend. We identify again the two discontinuities placed at LW mass fractions of 0.13 (disc. 1) and 0.55 (disc. 2), respectively. In between the discontinuities, we observe a roughly constant *c* trend centered around 0.3. Notably, disc 1 is less marked than in all other experiments. Our choice for locating the position of such a discontinuity was driven by the observation that there is a jump in *c* values coincident with an LW mass fraction equal to the value evident in Figure 3c. Two discontinuities occur at high LW mass fraction, as indicated by the arrows in Figure 3d: it is, however, irrelevant which one is considered since the LW mass fraction value for both discontinuities is nearly the same (0.48; 0.51).

In Table 3, we display the LW mass fraction values for our samples at discontinuities 1 and 2.

Table 3. LW mass fraction at the *c* discontinuities.

Snow Kind; Injection Methos	LW Mass Fraction at Discontinuity 1	LW Mass Fraction at Discontinuity 2
NLS; spray	0.13	
NLS; pipette	0.17	0.55
NS; pipette 1st	0.13	0.55
NS; pipette 2nd	0.13	0.6

3. Discussion

Some remarks on the results of the evolution of the LW mass fraction in our samples are pertinent. We observe that the initial *c* value differs from 0 in all measurements. This means that even when no liquid water is introduced in the sample, the RS cannot be fitted with the only contribution of bulk ice. We attribute this fact to the role of surfaces in the RS of snow [27] that are covered by a quasi-liquid water layer, the thickness of which becomes relevant over the temperature range −1–0 °C. Such a layer provides liquid water to the RS of snow. Since NLS is made of grains of smaller average size, the contribution of liquid water is larger than in NS. This corresponds to a higher *c* coefficient (about 0.15) for NLS than for NS (on average, 0.1).

Discontinuity 1 observed in Figure 3a–d can be related to the pictures in Figure 2 and to the kinetics of liquid water infiltration through the snow. In the initial stage, the LW content in the volume where the RS is collected is nearly constant. The discontinuity coincides with the time when the liquid waterfront reaches the collection volume of the

RS. Then the water level remains nearly constant until water expands through the entire snow volume. We associate the different values taken by the *c* coefficient along this stage in NLS (about 0.5; see Figure 3b) and in NS (about 0.3; see Figure 3d) to the different average grain sizes of the two kinds of snow that behave in a sponge-like manner. In fact, NLS with smaller grains is a more efficient sponge (larger *c*) able to retain a larger amount of liquid water than NS. The above *c* values are in agreement with the volumetric water content measured with other techniques [28].

Discontinuity 2 is associated with the formation of a layer completely filled with liquid water at the bottom of the sample, as we observed. In this condition, since the laser is focused at a fixed height with respect to the sample bottom, the fractional contribution of liquid water to RS, with respect to that of ice, becomes dominant.

The experiments discussed above appear suitable to detect the presence of liquid water in a snow volume and to follow the evolution of the progressive filling of snow with the liquid phase. This is facilitated by the spectral shape analysis of the RS of the wet snow sample, based on the weighted contributions of the spectral features of ice and water. Indeed, the recorded RS result solely from the vibrational contributions of water and ice. The contributions from other species, such as chemical contaminants and dust, provide additional peaks that can be easily spotted and rejected in the analysis of the RS. Thus, Raman spectroscopy opens the way to the investigation of the spatial-temporal changes in the water content of snow using a non-destructive and minimally invasive optical approach. For on-field applications, a vertical trench across the snowpack thickness is required to take RS at different depths corresponding to progressively accumulated snow layers. For a quantitative estimate of θ_w, we still have to determine the calibration curve of our method against θ_w, as measured by an assessed, independent technique. We plan to exploit this activity in future research.

4. Materials and Methods

We performed our experiments inside a home-built climatic chamber. We recorded the temperature by placing a type K thermocouple at the bottom (immersed in stagnant air) of a commercial freezer. We connected the thermocouple to an Arduino board (model Uno) feedback looped to a relay that acts as a switch and turns on the freezer when the temperature recorded by the thermometer is higher than -1 °C. With this system, we kept the temperature inside the climatic chamber between -2 °C and -0.5 °C. The top opening of the freezer was closed with a 2 cm thick Styrofoam plate; we cut a circular opening at the center of the plate, through which we could inject water on the top surface of the sample. Given the low thermal conductivity of air, we assume that over the temperature range explored during our experiments, neither melting of snow nor freezing of water occurred in association with heat exchanges between the snow samples and the surrounding air.

To reduce, as much as possible, the melting of snow grains during the addition of liquid water, we used distilled water at 0 °C to avoid handling of undercooled water with the associated metastability. We partially frost a volume of water to constantly keep liquid water at 0 °C during the experiments.

We filled a cylindrical Polypropylene container with an external diameter of 39 mm, a height of 6 cm and 2 mm thick lateral surfaces with snow, without compacting it. We removed the bottom of the container, and we closed it with an optically transparent Polyethylene (PE) film (thickness 10 µm) impermeable to liquid water. The film was stretched to obtain folding-free transparent sealing to ensure optimal quality of the recorded RS.

We added liquid water to the snow using a spray bottle and a pipette. Our purpose is to simulate the random fall of raindrops on the snowpack surface.

In the first set of experiments, we used a spray bottle that produced a puff of water droplets of average size between 200 µm and 600 µm. The water mass ejected in each spray was about 0.22 g. The amount of liquid water collected in the container was smaller than the injected water mass because a fraction of the droplets evaporate or fall outside the container. In the second set of experiments, we added liquid water to snow using an adjustable volume pipette (Model: Gilson P1000). The pipette was kept 2 cm above the top open surface of the snow. Under these conditions, the whole ejected water fell onto the snow surface. In all pipette experiments, we set a fixed volume of 0.04 mL per injection.

We used two reference types of snow: natural snow (NS) and natural-like snow (NLS). NS was collected from a field at Gressoney Sant Jean (Aosta Valley, Italy). It was gently collected using a plastic scoop and filled in plastic containers avoiding any compaction. We stored NS inside the closed containers at a temperature of −15 °C for seven months. After this period, the average size (taken out of 20 randomly chosen grains) of NS was 1.6 mm, as shown in Figure 4a, and the density of NS was 380 kg m^{-3}.

We produced NLS using the method described in [29]. NLS was stored under the same temperature conditions as NS for 2 months after synthesis. Due to metamorphism, the average snow grain size increased up to 0.2 mm (taken out of 20 different snow grains), as shown in Figure 4b. The density of NLS was 280 kg m^{-3}.

The pictures of the snow samples were acquired with an Olympus SZX16 stereomicroscope(Tokyo, Japan) connected to an LC30 Olympus digital color camera.

To visually look at the process of water spreading through the two kinds of snow, we colored a sample of liquid water with a diluted solution (0.03% in volume) of a green dye. The color of the solution is transparent greenish. We maintained the solution at 0 °C. We placed 3 g of natural snow inside the cylindrical container, and using the pipette, we carried out successive additions of 0.04 mL each of the colored solution every 5 s. Simultaneously, we acquired a video by using a smartphone to monitor the evolution of the snow-solution mixture at the bottom of the container.

RS were collected with portable Raman equipment BW&TEK (Plainsboro, NJ, USA) Exemplar Plus model (wavelength range 532–680 nm; slit width 10 μm, diffraction grating 1800 lines mm^{-1}, resolution 2 cm^{-1}). All spectra were acquired at the fixed laser wavelength 532 nm and laser power of 50 mW, with an acquisition time of 15 s. We used a BAC102 Raman probe (BW&TEK, Plainsboro, NJ, USA) that operates in backscattering. The focal plane is located at a distance of 5.4 mm from the probe. The diameter of the laser spot at the focal plane is 85 μm.

The Raman probe was placed upward toward the center of the circular bottom side of the container closed with the PE film (Figure 5). We adjusted the probe-container distance in such a way that the focal plane was located within the snow volume far enough from the PE film to facilitate negligible PE contributions to the RS. We estimate that the diameter of the laser spot at the internal surface of PE film was between 0.2 and 0.4 mm.

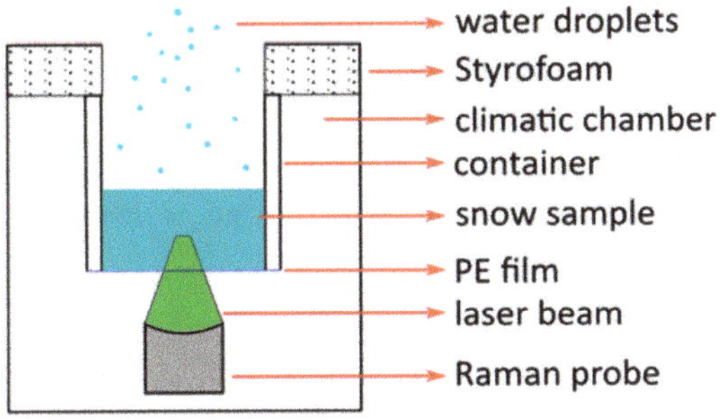

Figure 5. Schematic of the Raman probe disposition with respect to the snow sample. The green triangular area represents the laser focus position within the snow volume.

5. Conclusions

In conclusion, we proved that Raman spectroscopy is a powerful technique to assess the presence of liquid phase in snow. We performed a demonstrative study analyzing in the laboratory qualitatively different kinds of snow, representative of the two extremes of freshly deposited, fine-grained snow characteristic of early winter snowfalls (NLS) and of coarse-grained snow typical of aged layers in a snowpack (NS). We observed two definite discontinuities in the trend of the *c* coefficient vs. time. These are associated with different degrees of snow impregnation with water. The percolation kinetics are different in the two kinds of snow. Raman spectroscopy is appreciable because the instrumentation is light, easy to carry on the field and affordable. The measurements are fast and scarcely invasive. By data analysis procedures, the collected spectra can be processed to easily remove spectral contributions from impurities accidentally present in the snowpack.

Author Contributions: Conceptualization, E.M. and P.M.O.; methodology, E.M.; software, E.M.; validation, E.M.; formal analysis, E.M., M.T. and P.M.O.; investigation, E.M.; resources, P.M.O. and M.T.; data curation, E.M.; writing—original draft preparation, E.M. and P.M.O.; writing—review and editing, M.T. and P.M.O.; visualization, E.M.; supervision, P.M.O. and M.T. All authors have read and agreed to the published version of the manuscript.

Funding: This research received no external funding.

Institutional Review Board Statement: Not applicable.

Informed Consent Statement: Not applicable.

Data Availability Statement: The data presented in this study are available on request from the corresponding author.

Acknowledgments: This research was performed in the frame of the activities of CRYOLAB (Politecnico di Milano).

Conflicts of Interest: The authors declare no conflict of interest.

Sample Availability: Samples of the compounds are not available from the authors.

References

1. Shultz, M.J. Crystal growth in ice and snow. *Phys. Today* **2020**, *71*, 34–39. [CrossRef]
2. Nakaya, U. *Snow Crystals: Natural and Artificial*; Harvard University Press: Cambridge, MA, USA, 1954.
3. Ebner, P.P.; Schneebeli, M.; Steinfeld, A. Metamorphism during temperature gradient with undersaturated advective airflow in a snow sample. *Cryosphere* **2016**, *10*, 791–797. [CrossRef]
4. Libbrecht, K.G. Physical Dynamics of Ice Crystal Growth. *Annu. Rev. Mater. Res.* **2017**, *47*, 271–295. [CrossRef]
5. Ye, H.; Yang, D.; Robinson, D. Winter rain on snow and its association with air temperature in northern Eurasia. *Hydrol. Process.* **2008**, *22*, 2728–2736. [CrossRef]
6. Pfeffer, W.; Humphrey, N. Determination of timing and location of water movement and ice-layer formation by temperature measurements in sub-freezing snow. *J. Glaciol.* **1996**, *42*, 292–304. [CrossRef]
7. Mitterer, C.; Hirashima, H.; Schweizer, J. Wet-snow instabilities: Comparison of measured and modelled liquid water content and snow stratigraphy. *Ann. Glaciol.* **2011**, *52*, 201–208. [CrossRef]
8. De Michele, C.; Avanzi, F.; Ghezzi, A.; Jommi, C. Investigating the dynamics of bulk snow density in dry and wet conditions using a one-dimensional model. *Cryosphere* **2013**, *7*, 433–444. [CrossRef]
9. Yamanoi, K.; Endo, Y. Dependence of shear strength of snow cover on density and water content. *J. Jpn. Soc. Snow Ice* **2002**, *64*, 443–451. [CrossRef]
10. Dietz, A.J.; Kuenzer, C.; Gessner, U.; Dech, S. Remote sensing of snow — a review of available methods. *Int. J. Remote Sens.* **2012**, *33*, 4094–4134. [CrossRef]
11. Colbeck, S. Grain clusters in wet snow. *J. Colloid Interface Sci.* **1979**, *72*, 371–384. [CrossRef]
12. O'Brien, H.W.; Munis, R.H. *Red and Near-Infrared Spectral Reflectance of Snow*; Corps of Engineers, US Army, Cold Regions Research and Engineering Laboratory: Hanover, NH, USA, 1975.
13. Stein, J.; Laberge, G.; Levesque, D. Monitoring the dry density and the liquid water content of snow using time domain reflectometry (TDR). *Cold Reg. Sci. Technol.* **1997**, *25*, 123–136. [CrossRef]
14. Mavrovic, A.; Madore, J.-B.; Langlois, A.; Royer, A.; Roy, A. Snow liquid water content measurement using an open-ended coaxial probe (OECP). *Cold Reg. Sci. Technol.* **2020**, *171*, 102958. [CrossRef]
15. Techel, F.; Pielmeier, C. Point Observations of Liquid Water Content in Wet Snow—Investigating Methodical, Spatial and Temporal Aspects. *Cryosphere* **2011**, *5*, 405–418. [CrossRef]
16. Kinar, N.J.; Pomeroy, J.W. Measurement of the physical properties of the snowpack. *Rev. Geophys.* **2015**, *53*, 481–544. [CrossRef]
17. Pérez Díaz, C.L.; Muñoz, J.; Lakhankar, T.; Khanbilvardi, R.; Romanov, P. Proof of Concept: Development of Snow Liquid Water Content Profiler Using CS650 Reflectometers at Caribou, ME, USA. *Sensors* **2017**, *17*, 647. [CrossRef]
18. Eppanapelli, L.K.; Lintzén, N.; Casselgren, J.; Wåhlin, J. Estimation of Liquid Water Content of Snow Surface by Spectral Reflectance. *J. Cold Reg. Eng.* **2018**, *32*, 05018001. [CrossRef]

19. Schmid, L.; Schweizer, J.; Bradford, J.; Maurer, H. A synthetic study to assess the applicability of full-waveform inversion to infer snow stratigraphy from upward-looking ground-penetrating radar data. *Geophysics* **2016**, *81*, WA213–WA223. [CrossRef]
20. Naderpour, R.; Schwank, M. Snow Wetness Retrieved from L-Band Radiometry. *Remote Sens. Environ.* **2018**, *10*, 359. [CrossRef]
21. Koch, F.; Prasch, M.; Schmid, L.; Schweizer, J.; Mauser, W. Measuring Snow Liquid Water Content with Low-Cost GPS Receivers. *Sensors* **2014**, *14*, 20975–20999. [CrossRef]
22. Bekkiyev, A.Y.; Glushkov, S.M.; Zalikhanov, M.C.; Panchishin, I.M.; Fadeyev, V.V.; Ushakova, L.A.; Klevtsov, A.M. Use of Raman spectroscopy to determine the liquid water content of snow. *Trans. (Dokl.) USSR Acad. Sci. Earth Sci. Sect.* **1988**, *303*, 11–13, (Abstract in English Available).
23. Nakamura, T.; Abe, O.; Hasegawa, T.; Tamura, R.; Ohta, T. Spectral reflectance of snow with a known grain-size distribution in successive metamorphism. *Cold Reg. Sci. Technol.* **2001**, *32*, 13–26. [CrossRef]
24. Kokhanovsky, A.; Lamare, M.; Di Mauro, B.; Picard, G.; Arnaud, L.; Dumont, M.; Tuzet, F.; Brockmann, C.; Box, J.E. On the reflectance spectroscopy of snow. *Cryosphere* **2018**, *12*, 2371–2382. [CrossRef]
25. Duričković, I.; Claverie, R.; Bourson, P.; Marchetti, M.; Chassot, J.M.; Fontana, M.D. Water-ice phase transition probed by Raman spectroscopy. *J. Raman Spectrosc.* **2011**, *42*, 1408–1412. [CrossRef]
26. McGurk, B.; Marsh, P. Flow-finger continuity in serial thick-sections in a melting Sierran snowpack. In *Biogeochemistry of Seasonally Snow-Covered Catchments;* IAHS Publ. No. 228; Tonnessen, K.A., Williams, M.W., Transter, M., Eds.; IAHS Press: Wallingford, UK, 1995; pp. 81–88.
27. Maggiore, E.; Galimberti, D.R.; Tommasini, M.; Gaigeot, M.P.; Ossi, P.M. The contribution of surfaces to the Raman spectrum of snow. *Appl. Surf. Sci.* **2020**, *515*, 146029. [CrossRef]
28. Yamaguchi, S.; Katsushima, T.; Sato, A.; Kumakura, T. Water retention curve of snow with different grain sizes. *Cold Reg. Sci. Technol.* **2010**, *64*, 87–93. [CrossRef]
29. Maggiore, E.; Tommasini, M.; Ossi, P.M. Synthesis of Natural-Like Snow by Ultrasonic Nebulization of Water: Morphology and Raman Characterization Molecules. *Molecules* **2020**, *25*, 4458. [CrossRef]

molecules

MDPI

Article

Pilot Aquaphotomic Study of the Effects of Audible Sound on Water Molecular Structure

Aleksandar Stoilov [1,†], Jelena Muncan [2,†], Kiyoko Tsuchimoto [1], Nakanishi Teruyaki [1], Shogo Shigeoka [1,*] and Roumiana Tsenkova [1,2,*]

1 Yunosato Aquaphotomics Lab, Hashimoto 648-0086, Wakayama, Japan
2 Aquaphotomics Research Department, Graduate School of Agricultural Science, Kobe University, Kobe 657-8501, Hyogo, Japan
* Correspondence: yunosatoaquaphotomicslab@gmail.com (S.S.); rtsen@kobe-u.ac.jp (R.T.); Tel.: +81-73-626-7300 (S.S.); +81-78-803-5911 (R.T.)
† These authors contributed equally to this work.

Abstract: Sound affects the medium it propagates through and studies on biological systems have shown various properties arising from this phenomenon. As a compressible media and a "collective mirror", water is influenced by all internal and external influences, changing its molecular structure accordingly. The water molecular structure and its changes can be observed as a whole by measuring its electromagnetic (EMG) spectrum. Using near-infrared spectroscopy and aquaphotomics, this pilot study aimed to better describe and understand the sound-water interaction. Results on purified and mineral waters reported similar effects from the applied 432 Hz and 440 Hz frequency sound, where significant reduction in spectral variations and increased stability in water were shown after the sound perturbation. In general, the sound rearranged the initial water molecular conformations, changing the samples' properties by increasing strongly bound, ice-like water and decreasing small water clusters and solvation shells. Even though there was only 8 Hz difference in applied sound frequencies, the change of absorbance at water absorbance bands was specific for each frequency and also water-type-dependent. This also means that sound could be effectively used as a perturbation tool together with spectroscopy to identify the type of bio, or aqueous, samples being tested, as well as to identify and even change water functionality.

Keywords: aquaphotomics; near-infrared spectroscopy; water; light; sound; frequency; perturbation; aquagram; molecular dynamics

Citation: Stoilov, A.; Muncan, J.; Tsuchimoto, K.; Teruyaki, N.; Shigeoka, S.; Tsenkova, R. Pilot Aquaphotomic Study of the Effects of Audible Sound on Water Molecular Structure. *Molecules* **2022**, *27*, 6332. https://doi.org/10.3390/molecules27196332

Academic Editor: Stefano Materazzi

Received: 15 August 2022
Accepted: 14 September 2022
Published: 26 September 2022

1. Introduction

Sounds are mechanical waves of pressure that propagate through a transmission medium. Being a wave of pressure, the sound acts as a mechanical stimulus and has an influence on the medium through which it propagates. In physics, sound waves and their properties are widely investigated and generally well-understood, however in life sciences the investigation of sound has not yet received full attention.

There are many records documenting how sound affects biomolecules in water solutions, single-cells and even whole organisms, plants especially [1–7]. One study showed that audible sound in the form of music (38–689 Hz) was able to affect growth, metabolism and antibiotic susceptibility of prokaryotic as well as eukaryotic microbes [8,9]. A study about the influence of sound on chrysanthemum plants, discovered that sound wave accelerated the synthesis of RNA and soluble protein, indicating that some stress-induced genes might be switched on under sound stimulation. Further, another study showed that survival rate in the conditions of water deprivation is significantly higher in sound-treated Arabidopsis adult plants compared to plants kept in silence [2]. This study revealed significant upregulation of 87 genes, the majority of which are responsible for abiotic stress response, pathogen responses and oxidation reduction processes; interestingly, two genes were involved in the responses to mechanical stimulus.

The effects of sound on biological structures was also investigated in vitro, showing, for example, that crystallization of proteins is sensitive to audible sound and is frequency-dependent [6,10]. Sound, however, has not only been seen to induce changes by pure mechanical means, it has also been shown to have an impact on the signal paths of plants and the nervous system of animals. In a study evaluating the effects of different musical frequencies (432 and 440 Hz) on food intake and body weight in rats, it was discovered that different frequencies affect the neuronal expressions of two peptides involved in regulation of food intake in the rat hypothalamus, which stimulated weight increase (higher weight increase was found for 440 Hz) [11]. Listening to low frequency music (432 Hz) was shown to significantly decrease heart rate in high-blood pressure individuals [12].

Recent studies demonstrated clear evidence on sound-induced liquid vibrations that can lead to the formation of chemically (pH or redox) different spatiotemporal domains in solutions. This approach was later used to specifically align nanofibers in solution utilizing fluid flows generated by audible sound vibrations [13,14].

Regardless of the description of sound effects on different organizational levels, from biomolecules to organisms, the specific process of underlying molecular mechanisms, especially in the case of biological systems, is still poorly understood. Up to very recently, scientists were focusing on pinpointing single biomolecules related to sound influence, without considering the contribution of all components, especially without considering water, which is actually a major component of all biological systems. Since biological systems are water systems, the sound-water interaction is of interest and aquaphotomics science and technology [15,16] offer a non-invasive way to investigate this phenomenon. This discipline uses the water molecular network as a mirror [15] or a sensor [16] to characterize the observed system by monitoring the electromagnetic (EMG) spectral pattern of water under various perturbations. With the help of the aquaphotomics method, this pilot study aims to better understand how sound alters the molecular structure and dynamics of water using music tuned at two frequencies—432 Hz and 440 Hz.

The frequency 440 Hz was chosen, as it is the audio frequency which serves as a tuning standard for the musical note A4 above middle C, standardized by the International Organization for Standardization (ISO 16) in 1955 [17]. The 432 Hz was chosen because of the increasing number of claims that this frequency is superior to the standard tuning 440 Hz, affecting the body, emotional response, timbre, sound quality, character and tone; while it is actually unclear if it is humanly possible to discern a difference between the two [18,19]. According to existing scientific studies, music tuned at 432 Hz, compared to 440 Hz, can significantly decrease the heart rate and slightly decrease mean respiratory rate values [19]; it results in better cardiovascular benefits including slowing heart rate and it promotes relaxation [12]. It significantly decreases dental anxiety levels [20,21], significantly improves the sleep scores of patients with spinal cord injuries [22] and leads to increased levels of perceived arousal [23]. On the other hand, there are reports suggesting that listening to 440 Hz music can promote a feeling of anxiety, nervousness or aggression [19]. The research study about the effects of sound of different frequencies found that human DNA is sensitive to music, and that in fact by subjecting stem cells to various frequencies, it is possible to modify their natural organic function [24]. The actual mechanism behind all these phenomena is still unknown. The possibility of influencing the human body on a biomolecular level and stimulating, modifying or repairing the functionality of vital biomolecular structures just by using sound, holds tremendous potential. As a first step towards this goal, it is necessary to understand the role that frequency plays in sound effects and provide the information on which the choice of frequency for sound can be performed.

2. Results

2.1. Reference Measurements

Near-infrared spectroscopy (NIRS) in the range of 900–1700 nm, in parallel with monitoring of several physico–chemical parameters, was used to characterize pure water (hereinafter PW) and a chosen mineral water (hereinafter MW), both measured before and after sound perturbation at the frequencies of 432 Hz and 440 Hz. The mean values and standard deviations of measured electrical conductivity, pH, salinity and temperature of the samples through 10 min of sound are presented in Table 1. pH values were observed to be slightly more resilient to change in samples after the perturbation was applied, where the waters had an average of 0.81% and 0.38% more stable pH, respectively, after being perturbed by the sound with 432 Hz and 440 Hz frequencies. The difference in variance between samples that were perturbed and the control ones was not found to be statically significant (data not shown), however, statistical significance is not the same as practical importance [25]. Increased changes in values were seen for electrical conductivity of more than 18% on average after sound. These parameters are hard to measure precisely for waters, especially for PW. As soon as the vial is opened there is an exchange with the atmosphere of the environment; some evaporation may occur, gases from the atmosphere, such as CO_2 and O_2, may influence the resulting measurements of pH and electroconductivity. The changes in pH are, for example, very small, and due to the inherent probe instability [26] may not reflect accurate values. This all points out the difficulties of reference methods usually used to describe the effects of perturbations that may be very delicate, but nevertheless genuine and consistent, which requires devising other means and more controlled measurements which can completely eliminate possible influences of the environment. There is also a possibility that these physico-chemical parameters may simply be inadequate to capture all of the information relevant for the thorough description of water as a complex system and its dynamics in response to some perturbations [27].

Table 1. Measured water parameters, each presented with its mean and standard deviation (SD), with increase in value stability for the perturbed waters, compared to the control ones in general also having higher standard deviations. A similar trend in changes was seen through all the samples.

	pH	Electrical Conductivity Mean ± SD (μS/cm)	Salinity Mean ± SD (ppb)	Temperature Mean ± SD (°C)
PW-control Before	7.82 ± 0.38	10.25 ± 5.47	0	24.9 ± 0.3
PW-control After	6.95 ± 0.15	37.79 ± 27.7	0	24.6 ± 0.2
MW-control Before	7.09 ± 0.11	302 ± 2	0.15	25 ± 0.1
MW-control After	6.95 ± 0.14	320.5 ± 4.6	0.15	24.6 ± 0.1
PW-432 Hz Before	7.15 ± 0.18	23.7 ± 2.15	0	24.5 ± 0.1
PW-432 Hz After	6.39 ± 0.1	24.4 ± 2.2	0	24 ± 0.1
PW-440 Hz Before	7.49 ± 0.1	19.1 ± 1.19	0	24.3 ± 0.3
PW-440 Hz After	6.81 ± 0.34	64.1 ± 2.17	0	23.7 ± 0.3
MW-432 Hz Before	7.02 ± 0.33	307 ± 2.64	0.15	24.9 ± 0.3
MW-432 Hz After	6.97 ± 0.27	317 ± 2.37	0.15	24.3 ± 0.2
MW-440 Hz Before	7.04 ± 0.18	314 ± 0.6	0.15	24.8 ± 0.1
MW-440 Hz After	6.81 ± 0.27	319 ± 0.8	0.15	24.3 ± 0.1

However, despite this, the current results pointed to some degree of stability of water properties in the presence of sound. One possible way of interpretation this is that sound as a mechanical wave-inducing constant perturbation on the samples, reduces the susceptibility to influences from other factors. This phenomenon is further investigated in the following analyses.

The mean temperature values showed the tendency to decrease after the sound application, irrespective of the water type or the frequency of the applied sound, while the salinity did not change at all, evidencing that sound does not change the chemical components in the water. The change in temperature might be a result of absorbed heat generated by the sound perturbation. Previous works have shown that at least part of the audible sound energy is transformed into heat that can be absorbed by water, and spent on the reorganization of water molecular structure, causing the change in its temperature [6,10].

2.2. *Aquaphotomic Spectral Analysis*

2.2.1. Initial Exploration of Spectra: Raw Spectra of Water, Preprocessed Spectra and Difference Spectra

The raw water absorbance spectra generated during the experiments are presented in Figure 1a. The spectra show absorbance higher than OD = 1 a.u. and are rather flat except for the large, broad peak at lower wavelengths.

However, on closer inspection, several spectral features could be observed: large absorbance band centered around 957–963 nm corresponds to the 2nd overtone of water OH stretching vibrations, smaller band corresponding to the overtone of the combination band of free water molecules can be detected around 1143–1155 nm, and a broad peak corresponding to the 1st water overtone of water stretching vibrations can be seen located in the region 1300–1600 nm. The spectral profiles of PW show a generally higher spectral profile compared to the MW. This baseline shift is generated partially from the unfixed environmental conditions (temperature, humidity, water layer on the surface of the sample's vials, etc.), that may influence scattering of light and lead to differences in the real pathlength of light, but the higher spectral profile of PW can also be due to the higher actual water content since MW contain lots of minerals. When applying SNV preprocessing on the raw data, the baseline effects were removed (Figure 1b). Calculating difference spectra (Figure 1c–f) yielded more information on the effects of sound. This method requires the subtraction of a sample spectrum, usually of the control group (in this case the waters before sound perturbation), from the spectra of the other samples (waters after sound perturbation). The calculated difference spectra presented in Figure 1c,d, respectively, display 432 Hz and 440 Hz datasets with averaged waters' spectra after subtraction of averaged spectrum of the control.

In the subtracted spectra, three groups of common peaks were observed that correspond to well-known water absorbance bands: water confined in a local field of ions or so-called trapped water (1391–1397 nm) [28], water solvation shells and proton hydrates (1347–1385 nm) [15,29–31] and strongly bound water (1515–1590 nm) [15,32].

After averaging the whole spectra of PW and MW (Figure 1e), and subtracting their controls, a common increase in light absorption was observed at 1335–1403 nm and 1515–1600 nm, regions related to free, trapped and strongly-bounded water, respectively, while the absorbance in the in-between region (~1416–1490 nm) showed a decrease after the sound perturbation. The absorbance in the spectral region of absorbance of small water clusters with one hydrogen bond (1440–1444 nm), two hydrogen bonds (1462–1468 nm), three hydrogen bonds (1476–1482 nm) and four hydrogen bonds (1488–1494 nm) [15] showed differences between the two examined waters, but the common feature for both was decreased light absorption in general. The absorbance at absorbance bands corresponding to water solvation shells (1360–1366 nm and 1380–1388 nm) [15], hydronium ions (1434–1438 nm) [15], protonated and hydroxylated water clusters (1564 nm, 1583 nm and 1589 nm) [29–31], as well as water superoxide ions [31], increased after the sound perturbations. Although PW and MW are both waters and exhibited similar spectral curvatures, a contrast emerged describing unique characteristics for each sample type. As a mineral water, having minerals, after sound stimulus, MW was seen with much higher absorption at the bands related to water ions (water solvation shells (1380–1388 nm) [15] and trapped water (1391–1397 nm) [32]).

When calculating average spectra according to the applied sound frequency (Figure 1f), water samples after 432 Hz sound stimulus were characterized by a higher increase in ionic water species, while displaying less free water molecules and small water clusters compared to the molecular structure of water after 440 Hz sound stimulus. This finding suggests that a particular tuning even with only 8 Hz difference could generate different effects, which by themselves are dependent on the type of media/water being perturbed (sample-dependent) and are related to respective changes of water functionalities [15,16,33,34].

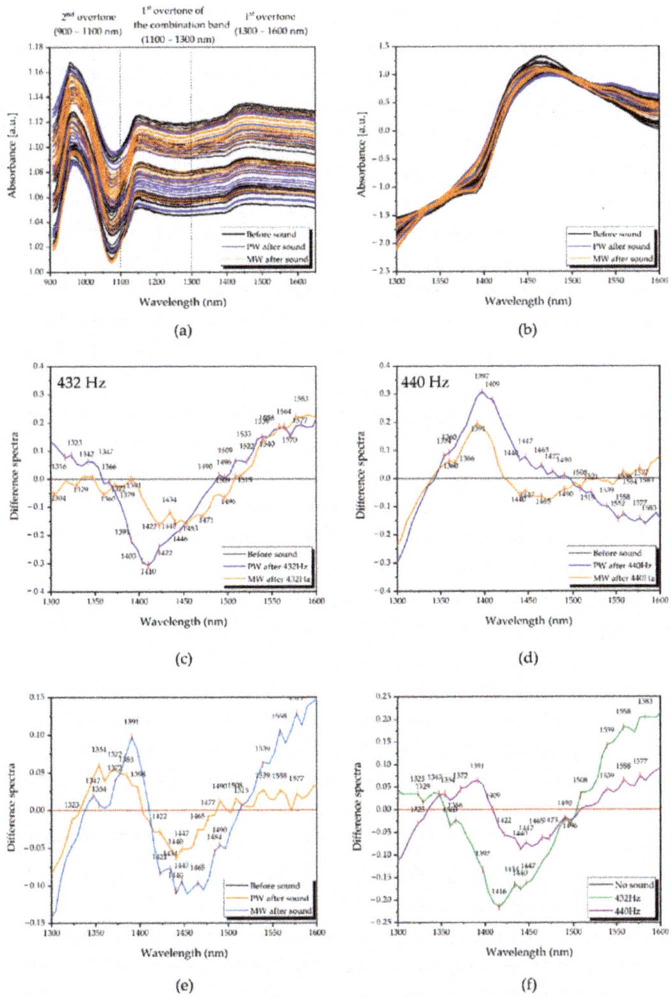

Figure 1. Near-infrared spectra of tested pure and mineral waters and difference spectra analyses (DSA) on defined datasets, preprocessed with SNV: (**a**) Raw spectra, separated into the water overtones; (**b**) raw spectra at the 1st water overtone (1300–1600 nm) transformed with SNV and smoothed with Savitzky–Golay filter using 2nd order polynomial (9 points), showing decreased baseline offset; (**c**) difference spectra analysis of 432 Hz data, with specific spectral patterns for each water; (**d**) difference spectra analysis of 440 Hz data with different spectral patterns than those at 432 Hz; (**e**) difference spectra analysis of averaged water types, displaying similarities in the spectral curves and differences in regions related to small water clusters and water ions; (**f**) difference spectra analysis of averaged frequencies, showing how the gap of 8 Hz can affect water differently.

2.2.2. Exploratory Analysis-Principal Component Analysis (PCA)

In order to better understand the effects of sound and confirm the initial findings, further analysis was performed—PCA (principal component analysis) with mean-centering and SNV preprocessing applied on spectral data. The experimental dataset was split into four datasets, according to the water type and sound frequency (PW–432 Hz, PW–440 Hz, MW–432 Hz, MW–440 Hz) and then PCA was applied to explore if there are any patterns or groupings in the spectra that can be related to the applied sound perturbation (Figure 2). The score plot of PC1 vs. PC2 from each PCA analysis are presented in Figure 2a and show repeatable patterns where generally scores of waters after sound perturbation showed diminished dispersion (inter-class variation) in the PC1–PC2 defined space. This implied that the sound-perturbed waters were more stable, becoming less prone to environmental influences, such as temperature, humidity, light, etc., which is consistent with the previous findings based on water parameters. The separation of the scores before and after sound perturbation was also a common property for all datasets and could be observed in the score space of PC1 vs. PC2. The loadings of PC1 and PC2 are given in Figure 2b and show that the absorbance bands that explain this separation of scores according to the sound perturbation are the same wavelengths already observed in the analysis of the subtracted spectra. The shape of PCA loadings was similar to the spectral profiles of subtracted spectra shown in Figure 1c,d, and again, but here in PC1 loadings, MW showed smaller differences compared to the PW for both 432 Hz and 440 Hz frequencies. On the other hand, PW being more receptive of changes, displayed opposing peaks in the 1366–1490 nm region, with direction shift different for the two frequencies.

Looking at the score plots of PCA analysis of PW (Figure 2a) it can be observed that in both cases, after the sound perturbation, the scores of PW are located in the positive part of PC1. The loading of PC1 for the dataset of sound perturbation by 432 Hz, shows the most prominent spectral feature as a negative peak at 1416 nm, which means that absorbance at this band increases under the sound influence.

For the 440 Hz dataset, the most prominent feature is the peak at 1397 nm, which can be interpreted as an increase in absorbance at this band under the influence of sound. The absorbance band at 1416 nm can be assigned to the free water, but it is more likely that this band can be attributed to so-called hydration water molecules [15], while 1397 nm is assigned to quasi-free water molecules, the single water molecules trapped in the local field of ions [28]. Similarly, for the score plots of PCA analysis of MW, the scores in the case of the 432 Hz dataset are mostly in the negative part of PC1, while in the case of 440 Hz they are in the positive part. In this case, in order to be able to compare the shape and sign of all loadings (Figure 2b), due to the arbitrary assignment of loadings in PCA, the loading vector of PC1 in the case of the MW dataset for 432 Hz frequency had to be multiplied by -1; therefore, the interpretation of the meaning of the scores of the MW dataset for 432 Hz is actually reversed. Having this in mind, it can be observed from the loadings plot (Figure 2b) that most distinctive features are a large negative peak at 1422 nm for the 432 Hz dataset PC1 loading, and a positive peak at 1391 nm in the case of the 440 Hz dataset PC1 loading. In the first case, this result means that sound of 432 Hz leads to an increase of absorbance at 1391 nm (trapped water band), while sound of 440 Hz leads to an increase in absorbance at 1422 nm (hydration band). From this, it can be concluded that the sound of 432 Hz frequency shows common effect for both waters, the increased absorbance of trapped water molecules, while 440 Hz sound increases the absorbance of hydration water. In both cases, this increase comes at the expense of reorganization of hydrogen-bonded water (absorbance bands at wavelengths longer than 1440 nm).

There is also, one more interesting observation. Looking into the percentage of explained variation, it can be seen that PC1 for all datasets explains more than 90% of variation in the spectral data, except in the case of the MW-440 Hz dataset, where PC1 explains only 56.8%, which means that there are additional spectral pattern variations specific for 440 Hz with high variations.

Next, PCA was repeated but this time on two datasets, separated into water type (either only PW or MW) in order to find out what the influence of sound is on waters in general (Figure 3).

In the cases of both waters, the PCA score plots revealed the pattern of separation of scores in groups of "before sound" and "after sound" along the PC2 axis (Figure 3a), whereas the scores corresponding to the "after sound" group were located only on one side of PC2. For the PW dataset, the variance explained by PC2 was 6.8%, while in the case of the MW dataset, a higher percentage of variance (25.2%) was described by the same factor (Figure 3b). Looking at the loadings of PC2 for both PW and MW PCA analysis, familiar absorbance bands similar to the ones from Figure 2b can be seen. This further showed the importance of the already observed bands, as the ones where sound influences the absorbance of water, more precisely, influences particular water molecular structures, especially trapped water (1391–1403 nm) and hydration water (1416–1422 nm). In this analysis, looking at the loadings of PC2, the effects of sound can also be better observed at the region of hydrogen bonded water (1440–1496 nm) where it seems that the small water clusters with 1–4 hydrogen bonds are affected, also, by the sound influence, as well as the strongly bound water (absorbance bands at wavelengths longer than 1508 nm, in particular 1539 nm and 1558 nm).

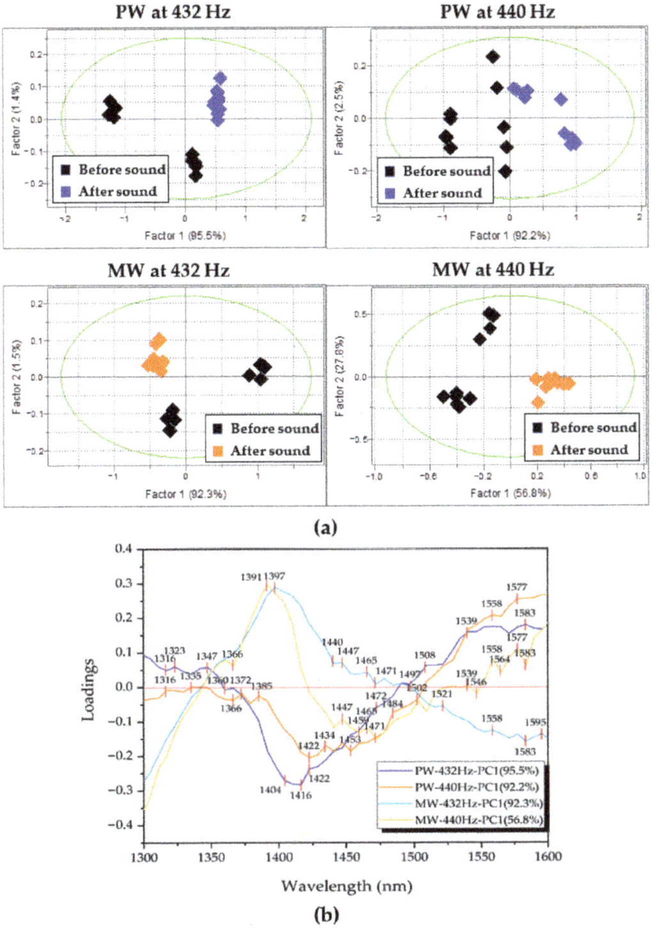

Figure 2. PCA scores and loadings separating samples before and after sound: (**a**) Scores of 1st and 2nd principal components for the 4 datasets; (**b**) loadings of 1st principal components for the 4 datasets, separating before from after samples (it should be noted that the sign of PC loadings is assigned arbitrarily, and due to this, the loading of PC1 for MW at 432 Hz was multiplied by −1).

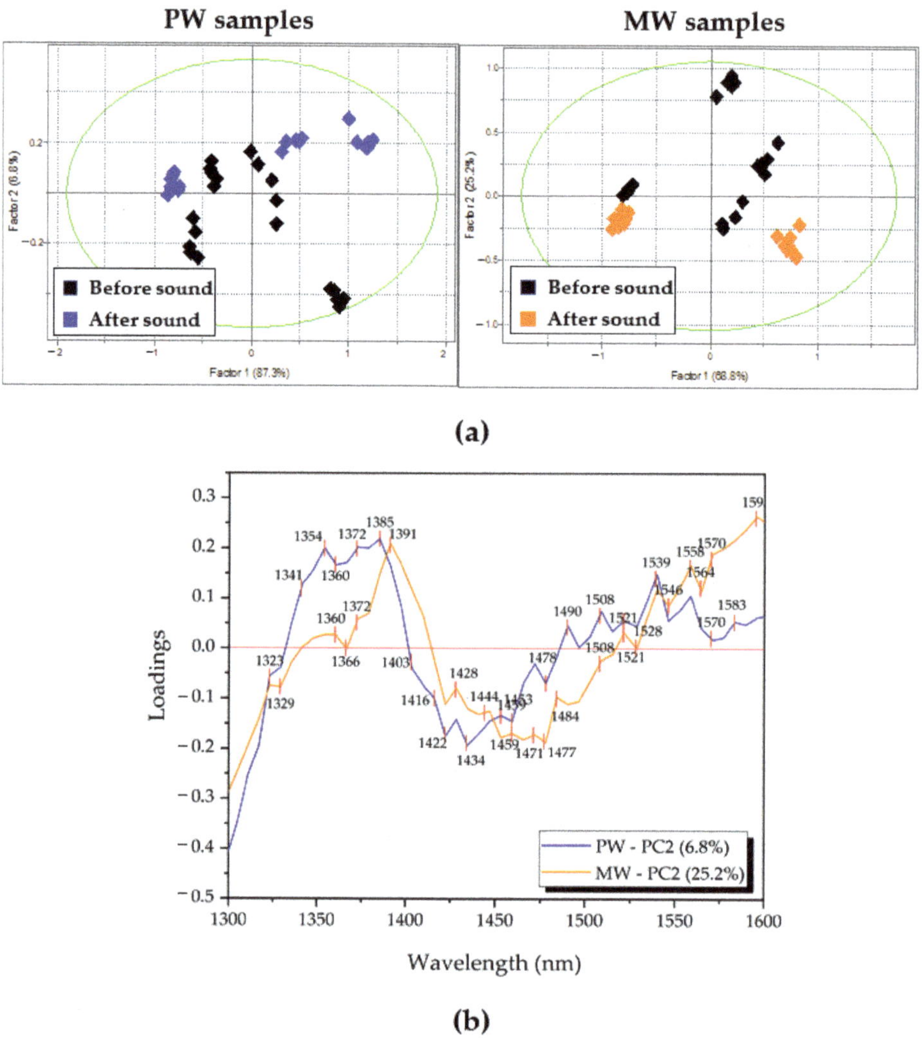

Figure 3. Score plots of PCA analysis of raw spectra preprocessed with SNV for separate PW and MW datasets: (**a**) Score plots for PW data (**left**) and MW (**right**); (**b**) PCA loadings describing influence of sound at PC2 for both waters (positive peaks are related to samples after sound perturbation).

2.2.3. Discriminating Analysis—Soft Independent Modeling of Class Analogies (SIMCA)

Further, classification analysis, SIMCA, was performed on the already SNV-preprocessed data with 5% significance (95% confidence interval). Three different groups of classes were assigned, such as water type (Class1: PW/Class2: MW), frequency (Class1: 432 Hz/Class2: 440 Hz) and sound perturbation (Class1: before sound perturbation/Class2: after sound perturbation) were performed and their distinction from one another was investigated separately.

First, differentiation between PW and MW was performed on four datasets (waters before 432 Hz, after 432 Hz, before 440 Hz and after 440 Hz) with 100% classification accuracy. It was observed that after the sound the Mahalanobis distances (interclass distances) between the waters decreased by 52% for 432 Hz and 46% for 440 Hz. This pointed out the waters displaying similar properties when stimulated by sound, a tendency seen in previous analysis.

Second, the SIMCA analysis performed with the aim of discriminating the samples before and after sound perturbation showed that the classes are different with an interclass distance of 0.76. When the datasets were separated according to the water type, the discrimination accuracy was 98.75% (Figure 4a), but the interclass distances were larger compared to the previous analysis when the waters were put into the same dataset. The values of interclass distances were 1.21 for PW and 1.55 for MW. When the datasets were split into four according to the water type and sound application, and SIMCA analysis was performed once again, the largest value of interclass distance was observed and it was 3.72 between MW before sound and PW after sound. As can be seen from the Cooman's plot in Figure 4a, the spreading of the scores of samples before sound was more pronounced compared to the scores corresponding to samples after sound perturbation. In order to quantify and compare this "spreading", the individual PCA models created by SIMCA for each dataset were examined, and the differences between the scores of the same samples were explained in each case by PC2. The percentage of explained variance by PC2 was 1.45% and 1.28%, respectively for PW and MW before sound, decreasing to 0.72% and 0.55% for the respective waters after sound. This was again consistent with previous analyses and pointed towards the influence of sound that can be described as "equalizing", i.e., reducing the influences of other factors present in the experiment, thus that the measured spectra of the waters showed lower variation among measured replicates.

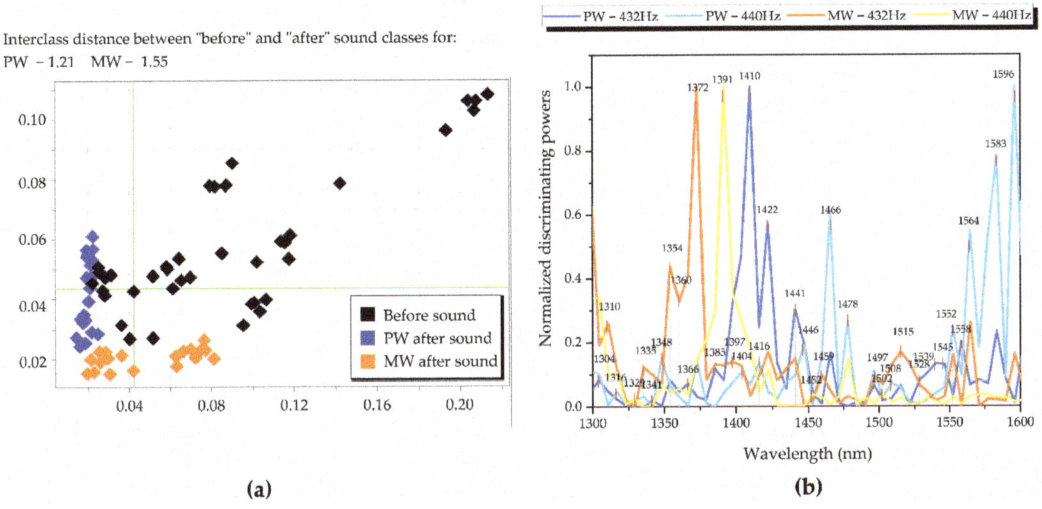

Figure 4. SIMCA classification of waters before and after sound perturbation: (**a**) Cooman's plot with class distances between PW before sound, PW after sound, MW before sound and MW after sound; (**b**) discriminating powers comparison with applied feature scaling (normalized values from 0 to 1) between PW at 432 Hz, PW at 440 Hz, MW at 432 Hz and MW at 440 Hz, displaying prominent bands for distinguishing the sound states.

In the last step, SIMCA was performed on the same four datasets used in PCA analysis (PW at 432 Hz, PW at 440 Hz, MW at 432 Hz and MW at 440 Hz) to explore the differences before and after sound. The generated discriminating powers show the variables with the highest contribution to the separation of the classes (before sound/after sound). Due to these discriminating powers having different magnitudes unique for the analyzed group of spectra, they were adjusted using feature scaling (unity-based normalization that brings all values into the range of 0–1) for easier comparison, where their recalculated normalized values are presented in Figure 4b. Similar to difference spectra and PCA loadings, the water absorbance bands (WABs) important for discrimination between "before sound" and "after sound" groups, were shown to be dependent on the sample type and located in the same wavelength regions. When the discriminating powers' prominent peaks (marked with arrows in Figure 4b) were summarized for comparison (Table 2), there was a repeating pattern of variables that were important for discrimination between before and after sound perturbation, and included the following absorbance bands: asymmetric stretching vibrations (1335–1347 nm) [15], H_2O symmetric stretching proton hydrates $H^+ \cdot (H_2O)_4$ (1372 nm) [29,30], trapped and free water molecules (1391–1409 nm), water molecules with four hydrogen bonds (1490–1496 nm) [15] and protonated water pentamer (1552–1564 nm) [35]. These water bands were consistent through the four datasets, pointing to a similar effect generated from the perturbation by sound. Small water clusters with three and less hydrogen bonds were also repeatedly seen to be prominent (1440–1477 nm), together with several other wavelength coordinates related to water solvation shells and hydroxylated water clusters (1360–1366 nm) [36,37], hydration band (1422 nm), proton hydrates at 1329–1335 nm [29,35] and at 1583–1589 nm [29].

Table 2. Water absorbance bands (WABs) prominent for distinguishing samples perturbed by sound from the ones used as a control (before sound perturbation). From yellow to red, repeatability of the same band activation increases in the 4 displayed datasets, where most consistent and notable water matrix coordinates (WAMACS) were shown in darker color.

PW-432 Hz	1304			1347	1354	1372	1385	1398	1409	1422	1440	1447	1465		1496		1515	1528		1546	1564		1583
PW-440 Hz	1304	1316	1335	1347		1372		1398	1416		1434	1447	1465	1477	1496	1508				1552	1564		1583
MW-432 Hz	1310		1335	1354	1366	1372	1385	1398	1403	1422	1440		1459	1477	1496		1515			1552	1564		
MW-440 Hz	1304	1316	1329	1347	1360	1372		1391	1409	1422		1453		1477	1490	1502	1515		1533	1552	1564	1577	1589

2.2.4. Aquagrams

As an important visualization tool of aquaphotomics, aquagrams [15,34,38]—radial graphs presenting the WASP (water spectral pattern) of samples at chosen WABs (water absorbance bands)—were prepared in several ways to emphasize different aspects of the investigation (Figures 5 and 6).

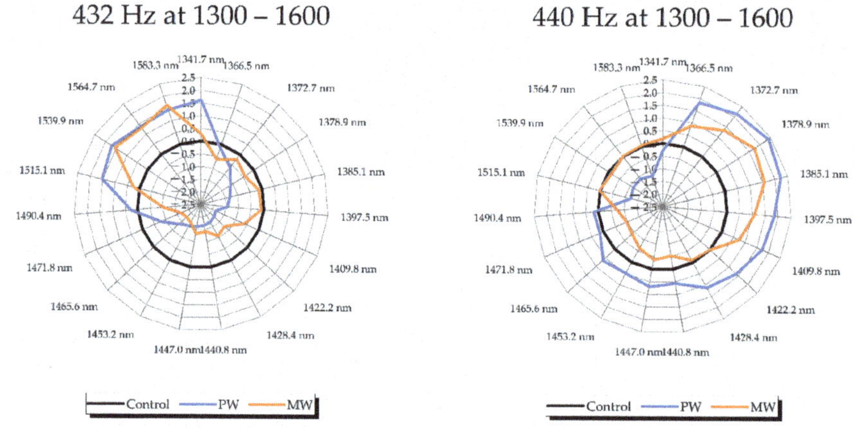

(a) (b)

Figure 5. Aquagrams on waters, using prominent WABs from previous analyses, illustrating consistent WASPs at: (**a**) 432 Hz PW and MW at 1300–1600 nm with consistent WASP illustrated as increase in absorbance bands related to aqueous protons and strongly-bounded water; (**b**) 440 Hz PW and MW at 1300–1600 nm with a differently-consistent WASP characterized by higher concentration of water solvation shells, trapped and free water molecules.

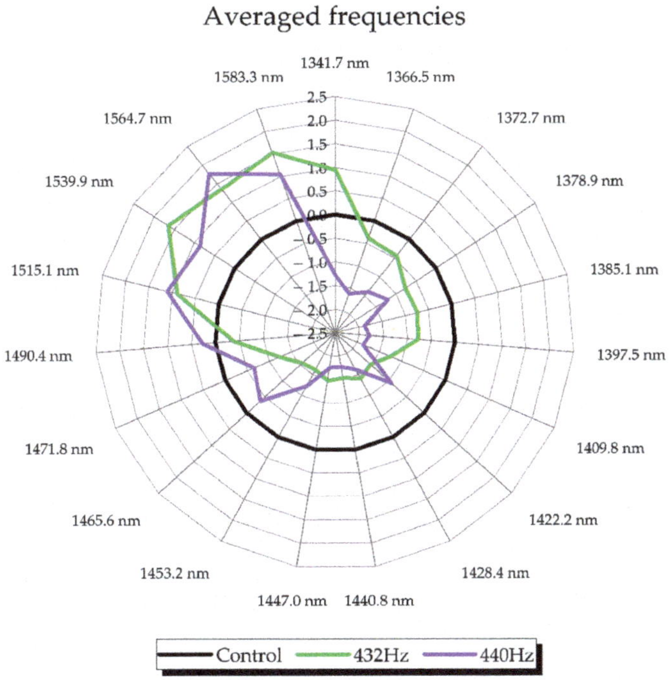

Figure 6. Aquagrams showing average WASPs of water perturbed by sound with 432 Hz and 440 Hz frequencies.

In the first step, spectral absorbance values were standardized using the mean and standard deviation for each wavelength, followed by averaging of PW and MW separately for samples corresponding to before and after sound perturbation. This process was performed for datasets obtained using different sound frequencies, 432 Hz and 440 Hz, in order to present in the aquagram, what the difference in effects of sound is depending on the applied frequency. This result is presented in Figure 5 and distinction between the frequencies was observed at regions related to "ice-like" (strongly-bonded) and "vapor-like" (less bonded) water, respectively [33].

Even though the absorbance in the region of small water clusters (1434–1492 nm) decreased after sound perturbation, some specific bands corresponding to the absorbance of water dimer (1440 nm), trimer (1465 nm), tetramer (1472 nm) and pentamer (1490 nm), were still prominent in the case of 440 Hz, but only for the PW. In this case, absorbance was also high at the hydration water band (1422–1428 nm). One more difference between frequencies was observed at the band of proton hydrates (1342 nm), where in the case of 432 Hz, the absorbance was very high, in contrast to the 440 Hz spectral pattern. For 432 Hz samples (Figure 5a), both PW and MW waters shared similar spectral patterns in the 1546–1563 nm region, where the absorbance of hydrogen bonded water and protonated water clusters was increased, while intermediate water species, such as water trimer (1464 nm) and water tetramer (1474 nm) [15], showed tendency of decreased absorbance. Water solvation shells (1364 nm, 1387 nm) and trapped water molecules (1398 nm) did not show changes in MW at that frequency, possibly due to the presence of minerals resulting in the stability of these water species. For PW, proton hydrates (1344 nm) and strongly bound water (1518–1563 nm) were seen to drastically increase, suggesting stronger rearrangements in response to sound. These characteristics, however, were unique for the 432 Hz frequency. At 440 Hz, PW displayed contrasting properties, with a decrease in strongly bound water, while increasing all small water clusters and "vapor-like" water structures (1344–1410 nm). MW, with slightly different pattern, was seen to preserve strongly bound water, while increasing the absorbance of proton hydrates and solvation shells (1364–1387 nm) which may indicate an increase in solvation ability. There was also an increase in the absorbance of water molecules confined between ions (1398 nm).

In the next step, the aquagrams were calculated with both waters' spectra taken together to try to obtain more general water spectral patterns, irrespective of the water type, and to see what the difference between water spectral patterns is depending on the frequency of the applied sound, and what exactly sound does to water molecular structure independent of sound frequency (Figure 6). The specific WASPs for 432 Hz and 440 Hz were generated when the averaged spectra of controls were subtracted from their corresponding datasets and averaging according to the frequency was performed.

Even though there were differences at specific water absorbance bands depending on the sound frequency, in general it can be concluded that the effect of sound on water resulted in increased absorbance of strongly bound, ice-like water. In another words, if the differences between the waters are not considered, on average, sounds at 432 Hz and 440 Hz frequency promoted crystallization of water. However, the aquagrams in Figure 6 can be somewhat misleading as they are calculated using averaged spectra of both waters together and may look contradictory to the previously presented aquagrams, especially the ones given in Figure 5b, which display WASPs of waters perturbed by 440 Hz sound. This apparent contradiction is exactly the result of averaging, where the much stronger influence of sound of 432 Hz masked the less influential effects of 440 Hz. This just emphasizes the importance of the finding that the effects of the sound on water molecular network are sample- and frequency-dependent.

3. Discussion

In this study, aquaphotomics methodology was applied to investigate the influence of sound effects on water samples monitored using near infrared spectroscopy. Using the water matrix coordinates (WAMACS) [15,38], as is usual in aquaphotomics, the changes in the molecular network of water samples as a result of sound perturbation were described. The most important, prominent WABs in characterizing the sound effects are summarized in Table 3, where those that appeared consistently during different spectral analyses are marked with darker color and could be considered as WAMACs—absorbance bands of water at which the effect of the sound can be measured.

Table 3. WABs seen activated through analyses in the region 1300–1600 nm. From lighter to darker (yellow to red) color, repeatability of the same band increases in the displayed 4 datasets. Consistent common bands were found at 1335–1347 nm, 1391–1403 nm, 1409–1416 nm, 1422–1427 nm, 1447 nm, 1484–1496 nm and 1552–1558 nm for sound perturbation, while specific bands were distinguished according to the frequencies and water types.

PW at 432 Hz																							
DSA		1316		1347		1372		1391	1403	1422					1496		1515		1539		1564		1583
PCA			1323	1347	1366		1385			1422		1453		1471	1490	1508			1539	1558	1564		1583
SIMCA	1304			1347	1354	1372	1385	1398	1409	1422	1440	1447	1465		1496		1515	1528		1546	1564		1583
PLS-DA	1310	1323	1335	1354	1360	1378		1398	1416	1428	1434	1447	1459	1477	1490	1502	1515	1521	1533	1552	1564	1577	1595
PW at 440 Hz																							
DSA			1329	1354				1398	1409	1428		1447	1465	1477	1490			1521	1539	1558		1577	
PCA			1335	1354	1360			1398	1409	1428		1447	1465	1477	1490			1521		1558		1577	
SIMCA	1304	1316	1335	1347		1372		1398	1416		1434	1447	1465	1477	1496	1508				1552	1564		1583
PLS-DA	1304	1323	1335	1354		1372	1385	1398	1416	1422	1447	1453		1471	1490	1508	1521	1539	1546	1558		1570	1595
MW at 432 Hz																							
DSA			1323	1347		1378		1391			1434	1447	1459		1496		1515			1558		1577	
PCA		1316	1335	1347		1372	1385		1409		1434	1447	1459		1484	1508			1539	1558		1577	
SIMCA	1310		1335	1354	1366	1372	1385	1398	1403	1422	1440		1459	1477	1496		1515			1552	1564		
PLS-DA	1310	1323	1335	1347	1366	1378		1398	1416		1434	1447	1465	1477	1490	1508		1533	1546	1558	1564	1577	1583
MW at 440 Hz																							
DSA			1329		1360			1391	1403	1428		1447	1465		1490	1502	1515	1527	1539	1558		1577	
PCA				1347	1360			1391	1403	1428		1447	1465		1484	1502	1521	1527	1539	1558		1577	
SIMCA	1304	1316	1329	1347	1360	1372		1391	1409	1422		1453		1477	1490	1502	1515		1533	1552	1564	1577	1589
PLS-DA	1304	1323	1341	1347	1360	1378		1398	1416	1428	1440	1447		1471	1484	1502		1528	1539	1552	1564	1570	1583

Repeatedly-present water species in all the conducted analyses for "after sound" samples were indicative of sound perturbation, most consistent of which at the 1300–1600 nm region was the water pentamer (1484–1496 nm), or water molecules bound by four hydrogen bonds [15]. This water molecular species is well-known as temperature-sensitive, where the absorbance at this band increases with the decrease in temperature [39]. The importance of this band for description of the influence of sound agrees with what was observed in measurements of temperature of the samples after the sound perturbation, where the common change for all samples was a decrease in temperature. This is further evidence of the stimulating effect of sound on hydrogen bond making.

Our results showed that despite the small difference of only 8 Hz, perturbation by sound using frequencies of 432 Hz and 440 Hz produced large and consistent differences in water samples as multiple analyses confirmed and established that they are water-dependent. In other words, it was determined that sound affected pure and mineral water in a different way. This has two implications. First, it provides basis for the future use of sound in perturbation spectroscopy to differentiate between the samples, and second, it implies that other water-based systems may be affected in different ways by the sound of the same frequency. When it comes to the effect of sound on water, in general, it was observed that, on average it led to the reduction in the samples' variability during the measurements and the samples became more stable against environmental influences. This was observed not only in the spectral analysis, but also in the measurements of physico-chemical parameters. This stability can be explained, as it was succinctly presented in aquagrams, by the effect of sound on the molecular network of water which promotes crystallization. In simpler words, the water which is strongly hydrogen bonded is not easily changed, and therefore it is more stable against influences from the environment. The temperature measurements also support this explanation, as the temperature of all the samples was shown to decrease after sound perturbation. However, if the effects of sounds of different frequencies are considered separately, which was shown to be the most correct, the effect of sound with 432 Hz frequency promotes crystallization, and the effects are much stronger compared to the effects of 440 Hz sound, which are actually opposite and could be said to enhance evaporation and solubilization.

Our findings, even though based on investigation of sound effects on the simplest aqueous systems and only two frequencies, may prove to have wider implications, especially considering the major role water plays as a matrix for biological systems. Recent scientific reports showed that audible sound promotes crystallization of proteins, which is frequency-dependent, and shows some variation based on protein type; this was found to be connected with the change of temperature and evaporation of protein solution [6,10]. Although the mentioned studies were performed using different frequencies and even variable-frequency sound perturbation, there is a common link with our study—sound affects water-based systems and changes their molecular structure in a frequency- and sample-type-dependent manner.

In conclusion, this study successfully applied NIR spectroscopy for rapid and non-invasive characterization of sound effects on water, and aquaphotomics inquiry allowed for the interpretation of the molecular dynamics after the applied perturbation, giving a better understanding of the sound-water interaction. Future research efforts will be directed towards exploration of the effects of additional frequencies on specific water systems, including biological.

4. Materials and Methods

4.1. Experimental Setup

As water samples, purified water (PW) (Organo, Purelite-α, Tokyo, Japan) and Yunosato Gold mineral water (MW) (Yunosato Onsen, Hashimoto, Japan) were used. The content of the mineral water is described in the following table (Table 4):

Both waters were kept in similar containers (plastic bottles and glass vials, depending on the experiment) and conditions (at room temperature). Music tuned separately at 432 Hz and 440 Hz was played by the Japanese pianist and composer Acoon Hibino on a YAMAHA MOTIF XF8 synthesizer, sounded by a pair of BOSE L1 Compact stereo speakers.

The PW and MW samples were placed a meter away from the sound source inside glass vials, specifically made for measurements with a MicroNIR spectrophotometer by VIAVI Solutions (Scottsdale, AZ, USA). Each water type was prepared with 2 replicates in a total of 4 vials per frequency, each measured 5 consecutive times. Sample replicates at every frequency were measured in random order, first spectra were taken at 432 Hz, then at 440 Hz, for a total of 80 spectra.

Table 4. Mineral content for Yunosato Gold mineral water (MW) as described on the bottle's label.

Nutritional Information Per 1000 mL	
Calories from proteins, fats, carbohydrates	0 mg
Na	40 mg
Ca	23 mg
Mg	8.7 mg
K	2.2 mg

Several sample parameters were measured before and after sound by LAQUA Horiba F-74BW meter, such as pH, electrical conductivity, electrical resistivity, salinity and sample temperature (Figure 7).

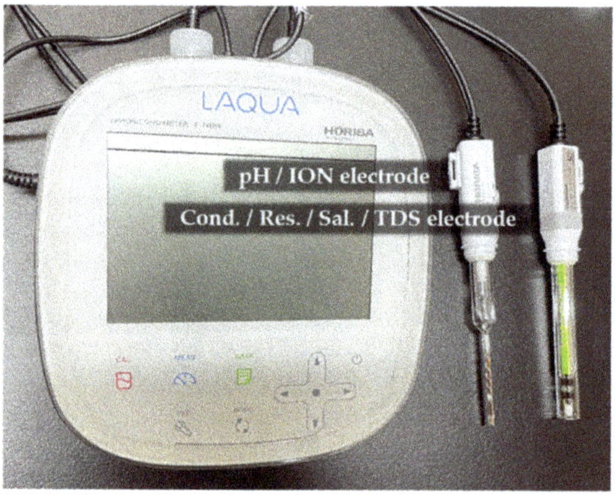

Figure 7. LAQUA Horiba F-74BW meter with pH electrode (left) and electrical conductivity/resistivity/salinity electrode (right).

4.2. *Near-Infrared Spectroscopy*

Near-infrared spectroscopy was selected as it is a rapid, non-destructive and non-invasive measurement technique, that requires very little or no sample preparation at all, and it can also be used for real-time monitoring. In the near-infrared spectral region (780–2500 nm) there are four main water absorbance maxima located at around 970 nm, 1190 nm, 1450 nm and 1940 nm, due to the 2nd overtone of the OH stretching band, the combination of the first overtone of the OH stretching and OH bending band, 1st overtone of the OH stretching bands and combination of the OH stretching band and OH bending band, respectively [40]. Following the aquaphotomics findings and systematization of the knowledge about water, these main bands are even further resolved and currently there are more than 500 known absorbance bands in this region [41], which is why this technique is specifically chosen to investigate the molecular structure of water under influence of sound perturbation.

The spectrophotometer used for this study was a MicroNIR 1700-ES (Viavi Solutions, Scottsdale, AZ, USA), capable of acquiring spectra in the wavelength range of 908.1–1676.2 nm, with a wavelength step of approximately 6 nm. The device was set on reflectance mode and used with its vial-holder attachment and a 3D-printed light-shutter cap (Figure 8a). During the experiments, samples were measured before and after the played sounds, where each vial had its spectra taken 5 times consecutively and represented as 1 sample.

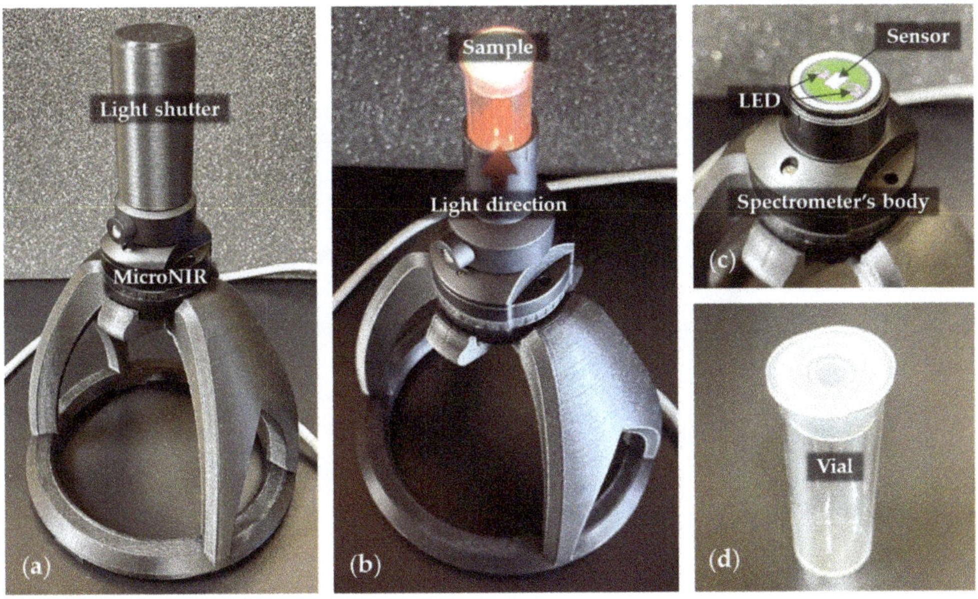

Figure 8. Near-infrared spectroscopy setup: (**a**) MicroNIR 1700-ES mounted on a 3D-printed stand and with a 3D-printed light shutter cap; (**b**) setup without light shutter, showing the sample's position and measurement; (**c**) MicroNIR 1700-ES device; (**d**) empty glass vial as a sample container, with 2 replicates per water at specific frequency, in a total of 40 spectra acquired (2 waters at 2 frequencies with 2 replicates, each measured 5 consecutive times).

The entire experimental flow is given schematically in Figure 9. Steps 1–3 were first performed for the sound perturbation using 432 Hz music, then the entire experiment was repeated, using the 440 Hz frequency.

4.3. Aquaphotomics Spectral Analysis

In this study, the main focus of the analysis was placed on the 1st water overtone (1300–1600 nm), where several analytical methods were applied to the acquired spectral data, such as calculation of difference spectra and MVA (multi-variate analysis), including PCA (principal component analysis) [42] and SIMCA (soft independent modeling by class analogy) [43]. This particular wavelength region was chosen since it is by far the best studied in aquaphotomics; there is almost no overlap with the absorbance of other functional groups and it provides the most information about the molecular structure of water [15].

Difference spectra were calculated by subtracting the values of a control's selected wavelength $\lambda_{control}$ (subtrahend) from the same wavelength of the sample in focus λ (minuend), where the difference is represented as λ_{DSA}:

$$\lambda_{DSA} = \lambda - \lambda_{control} \quad (1)$$

With this calculation applied to all spectra, fundamental and environmental effects are reduced, being left only with other perturbations that have occurred and are not present equally in all samples (such as sound).

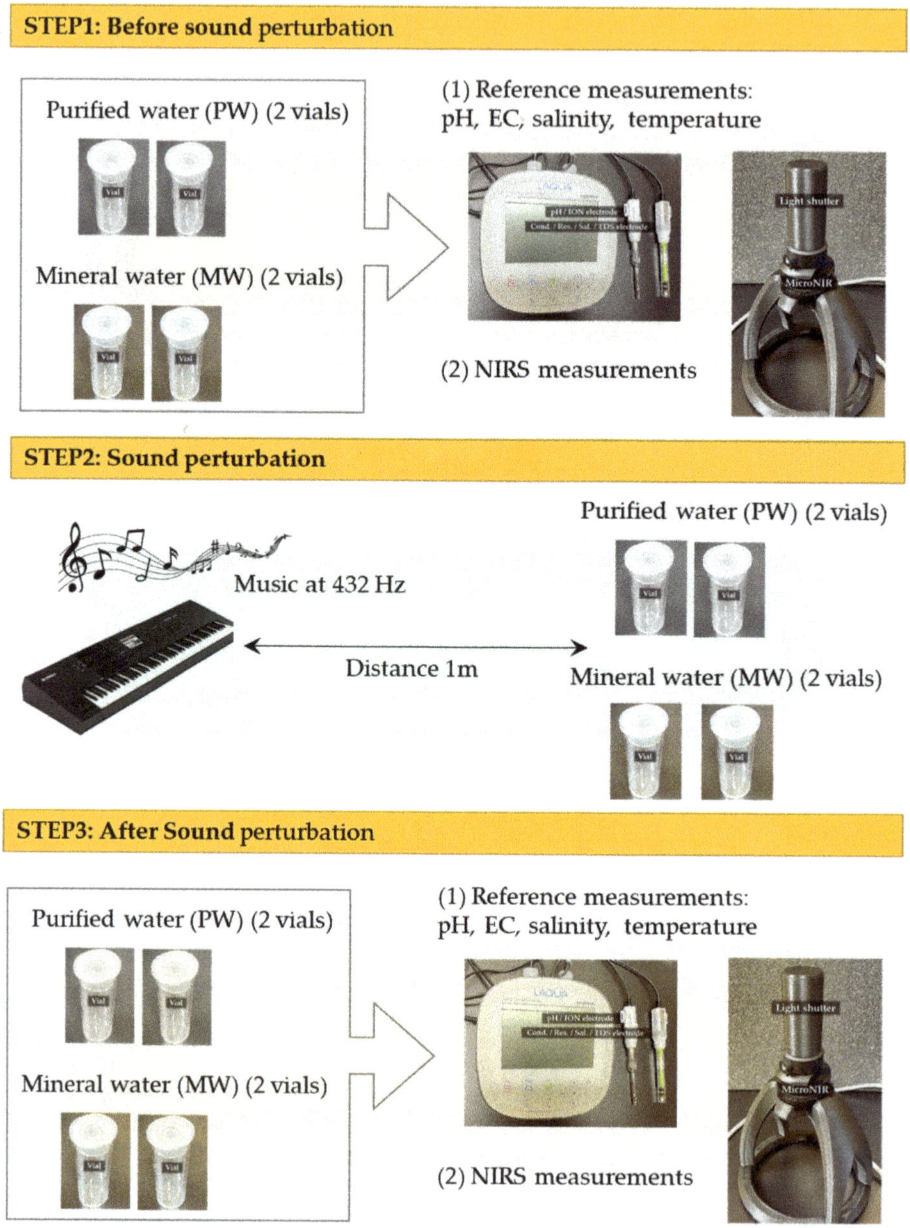

Figure 9. Schematic representation of the experimental flow. The experiment was first performed in steps 1–3 with the frequency of music set to 432 Hz, and then the entire procedure was repeated with the only difference being setting of the frequency to 440 Hz.

As preprocessing, SNV (standard normal variate) [44] was performed in this and all other analyses to reduce spectral baseline offset. In addition to SNV, the spectral data were smoothed using the Savitzky–Golay 2nd order polynomial filter (9 points) [45].

As an exploratory analysis, PCA (principal component analysis) was used, a statistical procedure that forms the basis of all used MVA (multi-variate analysis). It allows summarizing of information content in large data tables by means of a smaller set of "summary indices" that can be more easily visualized and analyzed; in the form of scores and loading plots in this study. Scores are projections of original spectra in the pattern spaces defined by principal components, while loadings show the weight coefficients of original variables. Mean-centering was applied only in PCA calculations as an additive transformation, after which each sample became relative to the global mean and analyses were of the variance around the global mean. Another statistical method used in this study is SIMCA (soft independent modeling by class analogy), applied for supervised classification of data, with confidence interval at 95%. Classification of spectra is based on a comparison of Mahalanobis distance, which is the distance between the spectrum and the centroid of each class. As an additional transformation, specifically used in recalculating presented SIMCA discriminating powers, feature scaling (unity-based normalization) was applied, a technique that brings all values within the range from 0 to 1, where the smallest value becomes 0, the biggest becomes 1, and all other values are spread in between, calculated by the following formula:

$$X' = \frac{X - X_{min}}{X_{max} - X_{min}} \tag{2}$$

where X is the selected value, X' is the resulting normalized value, X_{min} is the smallest (minimum) and X_{max} is the biggest (maximum) values within each discriminating power table. All MVA analyses were performed using commercially available multivariate analysis software, Pirouette (version 4.5, Infometrix, Bothell, WA, USA).

After conducting the listed MVA above, prominent WABs were chosen for distinguishing the effects from sound and aquagrams were generated for illustrating the spectral patterns of the averaged datasets in a simple manner:

$$A'_{\lambda} = \frac{A_{\lambda} - \mu_{\lambda}}{\sigma_{\lambda}} \tag{3}$$

where λ is the selected wavelength, A'_{λ} is the resulting wavelength value in the aquagram, A_{λ} is the absorbance after applying SNV preprocessing, μ_{λ} is the mean for all values at the specific wavelength and σ_{λ} is the standard deviation of the same wavelength.

Assignments for the main WAMACS of the 1st water overtone are provided in Table 5 and used for characterization and interpretation of the changes in water molecular structure of the tested samples.

Table 5. Water matrix coordinates (WAMACS) in the 1st water overtone and their assignments. All assignments are based on Tsenkova 2009 [15], unless otherwise indicated.

WAMACS	Assignment	Significance/Phenomena in Biological and Aqueous Systems for Which the WAMACS Was Found Important
C1: 1336–1348 nm	ν3, H_2O asymmetric stretching vibration, proton hydration [28]	Self-organization [29], water activity [46], germination [47].
C2: 1360–1366 nm	Water solvation shell, OH-$(H_2O)_{1,2,4}$, Ion hydration, proton hydration [46]	Water vapor/moisture absorbance bands [41,46], self-organization [29], water activity [46], viability [48], germination [47], firmness [49], hardness [50], solubility [29]
C3: 1370–1376 nm	ν1 + ν3, symmetric and asymmetric stretching vibration Ion hydration, proton hydration [46]	
C4: 1380–1388 nm	Water solvation shell, OH-$(H_2O)_{1,4}$ and/or superoxide- tetrahydrate, O_2-$(H_2O)_4$ Ion hydration, proton hydration [46]	

Table 5. *Cont.*

WAMACS	Assignment	Significance/Phenomena in Biological and Aqueous Systems for Which the WAMACS Was Found Important
C5: 1398–1418 nm	Water confined in the local field of ions (1396–1403 nm) [32] 1st overtone of the free OH group trapped in the hydrophobic interior [51]	Water activity [46], drying and dehydration [52], expulsion of cellular water, damage [53,54]
	Free water molecules and free OH-(S0)	Moisture content [55,56], water activity [46], seed vitality [57]
C6: 1421–1430 nm	Water hydration, H-OH bend and O . . . O	Protein hydration, protein fibrillation [58,59], water activity [46,60], damage and defects [61–63], amorphous phase [64–69], density [65]
C7: 1432–1444 nm	Water molecules with 1 hydrogen bond (S1)	Phase transition, sugar-water interaction [70,71], hardness [50], seed vitality [55], protection against dehydration [72]
C8: 1448–1454 nm	$\nu 2 + \nu 3$, Water solvation shell, OH-$(H_2O)_{4,5}$ Bulk water [46]	Water activity [46,60], viral infection in plants [73], damage [53]
C9: 1458–1468 nm	Water molecules with 2 hydrogen bonds (S2)	Water-protein interaction [58,74,75], firmness [49],
C10: 1472–1482 nm	Water molecules with 3 hydrogen bonds (S3)	Semi-crystalline phase [64–69], firmness [49]
C11: 1482–1495 nm	Water molecules with 4 hydrogen bonds (S4)	Damage/preservation (1496 nm) [53,72], firmness [49]
C12: 1506–1516 nm	$\nu 1$, $\nu 2$, symmetrical stretching, strongly bound water	Structural water, preservation/damage [53,61,76,77], seed viability [48,78]

Author Contributions: Conceptualization, A.S., S.S. and R.T.; methodology, A.S., J.M. and R.T.; software, A.S.; validation, A.S., K.T. and N.T.; formal analysis, A.S.; investigation, A.S., K.T., N.T. and J.M.; resources, S.S. and R.T.; data curation, A.S., S.S. and R.T.; writing—original draft preparation, A.S. and J.M.; writing—review and editing, A.S., J.M. and R.T.; visualization, A.S.; supervision, J.M., S.S. and R.T.; project administration, S.S. and R.T.; funding acquisition, S.S. and R.T. All authors have read and agreed to the published version of the manuscript.

Funding: This research received no external funding.

Institutional Review Board Statement: Not applicable.

Informed Consent Statement: Not applicable.

Data Availability Statement: The data presented in this study are available on request from the corresponding author. The data are currently not publicly available due to the organization of the local repository that will be open to public in future.

Conflicts of Interest: The authors declare no conflict of interest.

Sample Availability: Samples of the waters are available from the corresponding authors on reasonable request.

References

1. Acuña-González, E.; Ibarra, D.; Benavides, J. Effects of sound elements on growth, viability and protein production yield in *Escherichia coli*. *J. Chem. Technol. Biotechnol.* **2019**, *94*, 1100–1113. [CrossRef]
2. López-Ribera, I.; Vicient, C.M. Drought tolerance induced by sound in Arabidopsis plants. *Plant Signal. Behav.* **2017**, *12*, e1368938. [CrossRef] [PubMed]
3. Khait, I.; Obolski, U.; Yovel, Y.; Hadany, L. Sound perception in plants. *Semin. Cell Dev. Biol.* **2019**, *92*, 134–138. [CrossRef] [PubMed]

4. Fernandez-Jaramillo, A.A.; Duarte-Galvan, C.; Garcia-Mier, L.; Jimenez-Garcia, S.N.; Contreras-Medina, L.M. Effects of acoustic waves on plants: An agricultural, ecological, molecular and biochemical perspective. *Sci. Hortic.* **2018**, *235*, 340–348. [CrossRef]
5. Xiujuan, W.; Bochu, W.; Yi, J.; Chuanren, D.; Sakanishi, A. Effect of sound wave on the synthesis of nucleic acid and protein in chrysanthemum. *Colloids Surf. B Biointerfaces* **2003**, *29*, 99–102. [CrossRef]
6. Zhang, C.-Y.; Liu, J.; Wang, M.-Y.; Liu, W.-J.; Jia, N.; Yang, C.-Q.; Hu, M.-L.; Liu, Y.; Ye, X.-Y.; Zhou, R.-B.; et al. Protein Crystallization Irradiated by Audible Sound: The Effect of Varying Sound Frequency. *Cryst. Growth Des.* **2019**, *19*, 258–267. [CrossRef]
7. Yi, J.; Bochu, W.; Xiujuan, W.; Chuanren, D.; Toyama, Y.; Sakanishi, A. Influence of sound wave on the microstructure of plasmalemma of chrysanthemum roots. *Colloids Surf. B Biointerfaces* **2003**, *29*, 109–113. [CrossRef]
8. Sarvaiya, N.; Kothari, V. Effect of audible sound in form of music on microbial growth and production of certain important metabolites. *Microbiology* **2015**, *84*, 227–235. [CrossRef]
9. Kothari, V.; Sarvaiya, N. Audible Sound in Form of Music Can Influence Microbial Growth, Metabolism and Antibiotic Susceptibility. *J. Appl. Biotechnol. Bioeng.* **2017**, *2*, 227–235. [CrossRef]
10. Zhang, C.-Y.; Wang, Y.; Schubert, R.; Liu, Y.; Wang, M.-Y.; Chen, D.; Guo, Y.-Z.; Dong, C.; Lu, H.-M.; Liu, Y.-M.; et al. Effect of Audible Sound on Protein Crystallization. *Cryst. Growth Des.* **2016**, *16*, 705–713. [CrossRef]
11. Russo, C.; Russo, A.; Gulino, R.; Pellitteri, R.; Stanzani, S. Effects of different musical frequencies on NPY and Ghrelin secretion in the rat hypothalamus. *Brain Res. Bull.* **2017**, *132*, 204–212. [CrossRef]
12. Halbert, J.D.; van Tuyll, D.R.; Purdy, C.; Hao, G.; Cauthron, S.; Crookall, C.; Babak, B.; Topolski, R.; Al-Hendy, A.; Kapuku, G.K. Low Frequency Music Slows Heart Rate and Decreases Sympathetic Activity. *Music Med.* **2018**, *10*, 180–185. [CrossRef]
13. Tsuda, A.; Nagamine, Y.; Watanabe, R.; Nagatani, Y.; Ishii, N.; Aida, T. Spectroscopic visualization of sound-induced liquid vibrations using a supramolecular nanofibre. *Nat. Chem.* **2010**, *2*, 977–983. [CrossRef]
14. Hotta, Y.; Fukushima, S.; Motoyanagi, J.; Tsuda, A. Photochromism in sound-induced alignment of a diarylethene supramolecular nanofibre. *Chem. Commun.* **2015**, *51*, 2790–2793. [CrossRef]
15. Tsenkova, R. Aquaphotomics: Dynamic spectroscopy of aqueous and biological systems describes peculiarities of water. *J. Near Infrared Spectrosc.* **2009**, *17*, 303–313. [CrossRef]
16. Muncan, J.; Tsenkova, R. Aquaphotomics—From Innovative Knowledge to Integrative Platform in Science and Technology. *Molecules* **2019**, *24*, 2742. [CrossRef]
17. *ISO 16:1975*; Acoustics—Standard Tuning Frequency (Standard Musical Pitch). International Organization for Standardization ISO: Geneva, Switzerland, 1975. Available online: https://www.iso.org/standard/3601.html (accessed on 7 September 2022).
18. Palmblad, S. *A = 432: A Superior Tuning or Just a Different Intonation? How Tuning Standards Affects Emotional Response, Timbre and Sound Quality in Music*; Högskolan I Skövde: Skövde, Sweden, 2018.
19. Calamassi, D.; Pomponi, G.P. Music Tuned to 440 Hz Versus 432 Hz and the Health Effects: A Double-blind Cross-over Pilot Study. *Explore* **2019**, *15*, 283–290. [CrossRef]
20. Aravena, P.C.; Almonacid, C.; Mancilla, M.I. Effect of music at 432 Hz and 440 Hz on dental anxiety and salivary cortisol levels in patients undergoing tooth extraction: A randomized clinical trial. *J. Appl. Oral Sci.* **2020**, *28*, e20190601. [CrossRef]
21. Di Nasso, L.; Nizzardo, A.; Pace, R.; Pierleoni, F.; Pagavino, G.; Giuliani, V. Influences of 432 Hz Music on the Perception of Anxiety during Endodontic Treatment: A Randomized Controlled Clinical Trial. *J. Endod.* **2016**, *42*, 1338–1343. [CrossRef]
22. Calamassi, D.; Lucicesare, A.; Pomponi, G.P.; Bambi, S. Music tuned to 432 Hz versus music tuned to 440 Hz for improving sleep in patients with spinal cord injuries: A double-blind cross-over pilot study. *Acta Bio Medica Atenei Parm.* **2020**, *91*, e2020008.
23. Kopka, M. The influence of music tuned to 440 Hz & 432 Hz on the perceived arousal. In *Musik & Marken*; Springer: Berlin, Germany, 2022; pp. 227–245.
24. Muehsam, D.; Ventura, C. Life rhythm as a symphony of oscillatory patterns: Electromagnetic energy and sound vibration modulates gene expression for biological signaling and healing. *Glob. Adv. Health Med.* **2014**, *3*, 40–55. [CrossRef] [PubMed]
25. Gelman, A.; Stern, H. The Difference Between "Significant" and "Not Significant" is not Itself Statistically Significant. *Am. Stat.* **2012**, *60*, 328–331. [CrossRef]
26. Jamasb, S.; Collins, S.D.; Smith, R.L. Correction of instability in ion-selective field effect transistors (ISFET's) for accurate continuous monitoring of pH. In Proceedings of the 19th Annual International Conference of the IEEE Engineering in Medicine and Biology Society. 'Magnificent Milestones and Emerging Opportunities in Medical Engineering' (Cat. No. 97CH36136), Chicago, IL, USA, 30 October–2 November 1997; Volume 5, pp. 2337–2340.
27. Kato, Y.; Munćan, J.; Tsenkova, R.; Kojić, D.; Yasui, M.; Fan, J.-Y.; Han, J.-Y. Aquaphotomics reveals subtle differences between natural mineral, processed and aged water using temperature perturbation near-infrared spectroscopy. *Appl. Sci.* **2021**, *11*, 9337. [CrossRef]
28. Kojić, D.; Tsenkova, R.; Tomobe, K.; Yasuoka, K.; Yasui, M. Water confined in the local field of ions. *ChemPhysChem* **2014**, *15*, 4077–4086. [CrossRef]
29. Muncan, J.; Kovacs, Z.; Pollner, B.; Ikuta, K.; Ohtani, Y.; Terada, F.; Tsenkova, R. Near infrared aquaphotomics study on common dietary fatty acids in cow's liquid, thawed milk. *Food Control* **2020**, *122*, 107805. [CrossRef]
30. Headrick, J.M.; Diken, E.G.; Walters, R.S.; Hammer, N.I.; Christie, R.A.; Cui, J.; Myshakin, E.M.; Duncan, M.A.; Johnson, M.A.; Jordan, K.D. Spectral signatures of hydrated proton vibrations in water clusters. *Science* **2005**, *308*, 1765–1769. [CrossRef]

31. Weber, J.W.; Kelley, J.A.; Nielsen, S.B.; Ayotte, P.; Johnson, M.A. Isolating the spectroscopic signature of a hydration shell with the use of clusters: Superoxide tetrahydrate. *Science* **2000**, *287*, 2461–2463. [CrossRef]
32. Bázár, G.; Kovacs, Z.; Tanaka, M.; Furukawa, A.; Nagai, A.; Osawa, M.; Itakura, Y.; Sugiyama, H.; Tsenkova, R. Water revealed as molecular mirror when measuring low concentrations of sugar with near infrared light. *Anal. Chim. Acta* **2015**, *896*, 52–62. [CrossRef]
33. van de Kraats, E.B.; Munćan, J.; Tsenkova, R.N. Aquaphotomics—Origin, concept, applications and future perspectives. *Substantia* **2019**, *3*, 13–28.
34. Tsenkova, R. Aquaphotomics: Water in the biological and aqueous world scrutinised with invisible light. *Spectrosc. Eur.* **2010**, *22*, 6–10.
35. Mizuse, K.; Fujii, A. Tuning of the Internal Energy and Isomer Distribution in Small Protonated Water Clusters $H^+(H_2O)_{4-8}$: An Application of the Inert Gas Messenger Technique. *J. Phys. Chem. A* **2012**, *116*, 4868–4877. [CrossRef]
36. Xantheas, S.S. Ab initio studies of cyclic water clusters $(H_2O)n$, n = 1–6. III. Comparison of density functional with MP2 results. *J. Chem. Phys.* **1995**, *102*, 4505. [CrossRef]
37. Robertson, W.H.; Diken, E.G.; Price, E.A.; Shin, J.-W.; Johnson, M.A. Spectroscopic determination of the OH^- solvation shell in the $OH^- \cdot (H_2O)n$ clusters. *Science* **2003**, *299*, 1367–1372. [CrossRef]
38. Tsenkova, R.; Munćan, J.; Pollner, B.; Kovacs, Z. Essentials of Aquaphotomics and Its Chemometrics Approaches. *Front. Chem.* **2018**, *6*, 363. [CrossRef]
39. Segtnan, V.H.; Šašić, Š.; Isaksson, T.; Ozaki, Y. Studies on the structure of water using two-dimensional near-infrared correlation spectroscopy and principal component analysis. *Anal. Chem.* **2001**, *73*, 3153–3161. [CrossRef]
40. Büning-Pfaue, H. Analysis of water in food by near infrared spectroscopy. *Food Chem.* **2003**, *82*, 107–115. [CrossRef]
41. Tsenkova, R.; Kovacs, Z.; Kubota, Y. Aquaphotomics: Near infrared spectroscopy and water states in biological systems. In *Membrane Hydration*; DiSalvo, E.A., Ed.; Springer: Cham, Switzerland, 2015; pp. 189–211.
42. Wold, S.; Esbensen, K.; Geladi, P. Principal component analysis. *Chemom. Intell. Lab. Syst.* **1987**, *2*, 37–52. [CrossRef]
43. Wold, S.; Sjostrom, M. SIMCA: A Method for Analyzing Chemical Data in Terms of Similarity and Analogy. In *Chemometrics: Theory and Application*; American Chemical Society: Washington, DC, USA, 1977; pp. 243–282.
44. Barnes, R.J.; Dhanoa, M.S.; Lister, S.J. Standard Normal Variate Transformation and De-trending of Near-Infrared Diffuse Reflectance Spectra. *Appl. Spectrosc.* **1989**, *43*, 772–777. [CrossRef]
45. Savitzky, A.; Golay, M.J.E. Smoothing and Differentiation of Data by Simplified Least Squares Procedures. *Anal. Chem.* **1964**, *36*, 1627–1639. [CrossRef]
46. Malegori, C.; Muncan, J.; Mustorgi, E.; Tsenkova, R.; Oliveri, P. Analysing the water spectral pattern by near-infrared spectroscopy and chemometrics as a dynamic multidimensional biomarker in preservation: Rice germ storage monitoring. *Spectrochim. Acta Part A Mol. Biomol. Spectrosc.* **2022**, *265*, 120396. [CrossRef]
47. Nugraha, D.T.; Zaukuu, J.-L.Z.; Bósquez, J.P.A.; Bodor, Z.; Vitalis, F.; Kovacs, Z. Near-Infrared Spectroscopy and Aquaphotomics for Monitoring Mung Bean (*Vigna radiata*) Sprout Growth and Validation of Ascorbic Acid Content. *Sensors* **2021**, *21*, 611. [CrossRef]
48. Kandpal, L.M.; Lohumi, S.; Kim, M.S.; Kang, J.-S.; Cho, B.-K. Near-infrared hyperspectral imaging system coupled with multivariate methods to predict viability and vigor in muskmelon seeds. *Sens. Actuators B Chem.* **2016**, *229*, 534–544. [CrossRef]
49. Vanoli, M.; Lovati, F.; Grassi, M.; Buccheri, M.; Zanella, A.; Cattaneo, T.M.P.; Rizzolo, A. Water spectral pattern as a marker for studying apple sensory texture. *Adv. Hortic. Sci.* **2018**, *32*, 343–352.
50. Hong, B.H.; Rubenthaler, G.L.; Allan, R.E. Wheat pentosans. II. Estimating kernel hardness and pentosans in water extracts by near-infrared reflectance. *Cereal Chem.* **1989**, *66*, 374–377.
51. Zhang, L.; Noda, I.; Czarnik-Matusewicz, B.; Wu, Y. Multivariate estimation between mid and near-infrared spectra of hexafluoroisopropanol-water mixtures. *Anal. Sci.* **2007**, *23*, 901–905. [CrossRef] [PubMed]
52. Gowen, A.A. Water and Food Quality. *Contemp. Mater.* **2012**, *1*, 31–37. [CrossRef]
53. Gowen, A.A.; Tsenkova, R.; Esquerre, C.; Downey, G.; O'Donnell, C.P. Use of near infrared hyperspectral imaging to identify water matrix co-ordinates in mushrooms (*Agaricus bisporus*) subjected to mechanical vibration. *J. Near Infrared Spectrosc.* **2009**, *17*, 363–371. [CrossRef]
54. Esquerre, C.; Gowen, A.A.; O'Donnell, C.P.; Downey, G. Water absorbance pattern of physically-damaged mushrooms stored at ambient conditions. *J. Near Infrared Spectrosc.* **2009**, *17*, 353–361. [CrossRef]
55. Phetpan, K.; Udompetaikul, V.; Sirisomboon, P. In-line near infrared spectroscopy for the prediction of moisture content in the tapioca starch drying process. *Powder Technol.* **2019**, *345*, 608–615. [CrossRef]
56. Achata, E.; Esquerre, C.; O'Donnell, C.; Gowen, A. A study on the application of near infrared hyperspectral chemical imaging for monitoring moisture content and water activity in low moisture systems. *Molecules* **2015**, *20*, 2611–2621. [CrossRef]
57. He, X.; Feng, X.; Sun, D.; Liu, F.; Bao, Y.; He, Y. Rapid and nondestructive measurement of rice seed vitality of different years using near-infrared hyperspectral imaging. *Molecules* **2019**, *24*, 2227. [CrossRef]
58. Tsenkova, R.N.; Iordanova, I.K.; Toyoda, K.; Brown, D.R. Prion protein fate governed by metal binding. *Biochem. Biophys. Res. Commun.* **2004**, *325*, 1005–1012. [CrossRef]
59. Chatani, E.; Tsuchisaka, Y.; Masuda, Y.; Tsenkova, R. Water molecular system dynamics associated with amyloidogenic nucleation as revealed by real time near infrared spectroscopy and aquaphotomics. *PLoS ONE* **2014**, *9*, e101997. [CrossRef]

60. Heiman, A.; Licht, S. Fundamental baseline variations in aqueous near-infrared analysis. *Anal. Chim. Acta* **1999**, *394*, 135–147. [CrossRef]
61. Šakota Rosić, J.; Munćan, J.; Mileusnić, I.; Kosić, B.; Matija, L. Detection of protein deposits using NIR spectroscopy. *Soft Mater.* **2016**, *14*, 264–271. [CrossRef]
62. Cheng, J.; Guo, W.; Du, R.; Zhou, Y. Optical properties of different kiwifruit cultivars (*Actinidia deliciosa* and *Actinidia chinensis*) and their correlation with internal quality. *Infrared Phys. Technol.* **2022**, *123*, 104113. [CrossRef]
63. Cho, J.-S.; Bae, H.-J.; Cho, B.-K.; Moon, K.-D. Qualitative properties of roasting defect beans and development of its classification methods by hyperspectral imaging technology. *Food Chem.* **2017**, *220*, 505–509. [CrossRef]
64. Fujimoto, T.; Kobori, H.; Tsuchikawa, S. Prediction of wood density independently of moisture conditions using near infrared spectroscopy. *J. Near Infrared Spectrosc.* **2012**, *20*, 353–359. [CrossRef]
65. Tsuchikawa, S.; Hirashima, Y.; Sasaki, Y.; Ando, K. Near-infrared spectroscopic study of the physical and mechanical properties of wood with meso- and micro-scale anatomical observation. *Appl. Spectrosc.* **2005**, *59*, 86–93. [CrossRef]
66. Fujimoto, T.; Yamamoto, H.; Tsuchikawa, S. Estimation of wood stiffness and strength properties of hybrid larch by near-infrared spectroscopy. *Appl. Spectrosc.* **2007**, *61*, 882–888. [CrossRef]
67. Rambo, M.K.D.; Ferreira, M.M.C. Determination of cellulose crystallinity of banana residues using near infrared spectroscopy and multivariate analysis. *J. Braz. Chem. Soc.* **2015**, *26*, 1491–1499. [CrossRef]
68. Tsuchikawa, S.; Murata, A.; Kohara, M.; Mitsui, K. Spectroscopic monitoring of biomass modification by light-irradiation and heat treatment. *J. Near Infrared Spectrosc.* **2003**, *11*, 401–405. [CrossRef]
69. Wu, Y.-Q.; Tsuchikawa, S.; Hayashi, K. Application of near infrared spectroscopy to assessments of colour change in plantation-grown Eucalyptus grandis wood subjected to heat and steaming treatments. *J. Near Infrared Spectrosc.* **2005**, *13*, 371–376. [CrossRef]
70. Lane, R.A.; Buckton, G. The novel combination of dynamic vapour sorption gravimetric analysis and near infra-red spectroscopy as a hyphenated technique. *Int. J. Pharm.* **2000**, *207*, 49–56. [CrossRef]
71. Luner, P.E.; Seyer, J.J. Assessment of crystallinity in processed sucrose by near-infrared spectroscopy and application to lyophiles. *J. Pharm. Sci.* **2014**, *103*, 2884–2895. [CrossRef] [PubMed]
72. Kuroki, S.; Tsenkova, R.; Moyankova, D.; Muncan, J.; Morita, H.; Atanassova, S.; Djilianov, D. Water molecular structure underpins extreme desiccation tolerance of the resurrection plant Haberlea rhodopensis. *Sci. Rep.* **2019**, *9*, 3049. [CrossRef] [PubMed]
73. Naidu, R.A.; Perry, E.M.; Pierce, F.J.; Mekuria, T. The potential of spectral reflectance technique for the detection of Grapevine leafroll-associated virus-3 in two red-berried wine grape cultivars. *Comput. Electron. Agric.* **2009**, *66*, 38–45. [CrossRef]
74. Hayati, R.; Munawar, A.A.; Marliah, A. Rapid quantification of rice (*Oryza sativa*) qualities based on adaptive near infrared spectroscopy. *IOP Conf. Ser. Earth Environ. Sci.* **2021**, *922*, 012020. [CrossRef]
75. Ma, L.; Cui, X.; Cai, W.; Shao, X. Understanding the function of water during the gelation of globular proteins by temperature-dependent near infrared spectroscopy. *Phys. Chem. Chem. Phys.* **2018**, *20*, 20132–20140. [CrossRef]
76. Munćan, J.; Mileusnić, I.; Šakota Rosić, J.; Vasić-Milovanović, A.; Matija, L. Water Properties of Soft Contact Lenses: A Comparative Near-Infrared Study of Two Hydrogel Materials. *Int. J. Polym. Sci.* **2016**, *2016*, 1–8. [CrossRef]
77. Esquerre, C.; Gowen, A.A.; O'Donnell, C.P.; Downey, G. Initial Studies on the Quantitation of Bruise Damage and Freshness in Mushrooms Using Visible-Near-Infrared Spectroscopy. *J. Agric. Food Chem.* **2009**, *57*, 1903–1907. [CrossRef]
78. Tigabu, M.; Odén, P.C. Discrimination of viable and empty seeds of Pinus patula Schiede & Deppe with near-infrared spectroscopy. *New For.* **2003**, *25*, 163–176.

molecules

MDPI

Article

Investigation of Water Interaction with Polymer Matrices by Near-Infrared (NIR) Spectroscopy

Vanessa Moll, Krzysztof B. Beć, Justyna Grabska and Christian W. Huck *

Institute of Analytical Chemistry and Radiochemistry, University of Innsbruck, 6020 Innsbruck, Austria
* Correspondence: christian.w.huck@uibk.ac.at

Abstract: The interaction of water with polymers is an intensively studied topic. Vibrational spectroscopy techniques, mid-infrared (MIR) and Raman, were often used to investigate the properties of water–polymer systems. On the other hand, relatively little attention has been given to the potential of using near-infrared (NIR) spectroscopy (12,500–4000 cm^{-1}; 800–2500 nm) for exploring this problem. NIR spectroscopy delivers exclusive opportunities for the investigation of molecular structure and interactions. This technique derives information from overtones and combination bands, which provide unique insights into molecular interactions. It is also very well suited for the investigation of aqueous systems, as both the bands of water and the polymer can be reliably acquired in a range of concentrations in a more straightforward manner than it is possible with MIR spectroscopy. In this study, we applied NIR spectroscopy to investigate interactions of water with polymers of varying hydrophobicity: polytetrafluoroethylene (PTFE), polypropylene (PP), polystyrene (PS), polyvinylchloride (PVC), polyoxymethylene (POM), polyamide 6 (PA), lignin (Lig), chitin (Chi) and cellulose (Cell). Polymer–water mixtures in the concentration range of water between 1–10%(w/w) were investigated. Spectra analysis and interpretation were performed with the use of difference spectroscopy, Principal Component Analysis (PCA), Median Linkage Clustering (MLC), Partial Least Squares Regression (PLSR), Multivariate Curve Resolution Alternating Least Squares (MCR-ALS) and Two-Dimensional Correlation Spectroscopy (2D-COS). Additionally, from the obtained data, aquagrams were constructed and interpreted with aid of the conclusions drawn from the conventional approaches. We deepened insights into the problem of water bands obscuring compound-specific signals in the NIR spectrum, which is often a limiting factor in analytical applications. The study unveiled clearly visible trends in NIR spectra associated with the chemical nature of the polymer and its increasing hydrophilicity. We demonstrated that changes in the NIR spectrum of water are manifested even in the case of interaction with highly hydrophobic polymers (e.g., PTFE). Furthermore, the unveiled spectral patterns of water in the presence of different polymers were found to be dissimilar between the two major water bands in NIR spectrum ($\nu_s + \nu_{as}$ and $\nu_{as} + \delta$).

Keywords: near-infrared spectroscopy; NIR; polymer; water; polymer-water interaction; hydrophilic; hydrophobic; chemometrics; data analysis

Citation: Moll, V.; Beć, K.B.; Grabska, J.; Huck, C.W. Investigation of Water Interaction with Polymer Matrices by Near-Infrared (NIR) Spectroscopy. *Molecules* **2022**, *27*, 5882. https://doi.org/10.3390/molecules27185882

Academic Editors: Roumiana Tsenkova and Jelena Muncan

Received: 11 August 2022
Accepted: 7 September 2022
Published: 10 September 2022

1. Introduction

The interaction of water with different polymers has been an intensively studied research field [1–3], especially in recent years, with biocompatible polymers being one of the main focuses [4,5]. It has been demonstrated that the biocompatibility of a polymer is affected by its interaction with water [4]; furthermore, water–polymer interactions play a key role in biological processes [1,6]. The effect of moisture on commercially used polymers is also of high interest in material science and industrial applications. For example, an excess of water may cause swelling and, subsequently, changes of mechanical and chemical properties of polymers [1]. For these reasons, considerable attention has been diverted into investigations of the interaction of polymers with water, with a focus both on its phenomenological manifestations in various conditions as well as on its physicochemical background. With respect to the former, one of the promising concepts proposes to distinguish different species of water molecules in terms of their interaction strength with a polymer into strongly-bound, loosely-bound and free water species [1,4,6,7]. On the other hand, the so called "hydrophobic interactions" are often considered to be an important property of a material, appearing due to the interactions between water molecules being stronger than between water and the molecules of the hydrophobic material [8]. Hydrophobic interactions are highly dependent on various factors, e.g., temperature, size and shape of the interacting particles [8,9], among others. Insights into the underlying physicochemical properties of the interactions occurring between a polymer and water, including molecular structure effects, have been examined using various approaches. In these studies, diverse spectroscopic (e.g., vibrational, dielectric, nuclear magnetic resonance, etc. [7,10–14]) techniques, mass spectrometry [1], X-ray diffraction [15], differential scanning calorimetry [1,6,12] or gel-permeation chromatography [10] have been found to be helpful. Often, the experimental studies were combined with methods of computational chemistry to provide deepened physical insights [16,17].

Vibrational spectroscopic techniques, MIR and Raman, were often used to derive both phenomenological and molecular insights into the effects of the interactions between water and polymers [12,14,18–20]. In contrast, NIR spectroscopy has not yet attracted similar attention in the studies of this problem. This spectroscopic technique offers unique suitability for this purpose [21,22], as the intensity change in water absorption is known to mirror the change in the chemical environment of water molecules [11,23]. Spectral bands in NIR spectroscopy manifest unique sensitivity towards the chemical environment and hydrogen bonding [21,24,25]. The positions and intensities of NIR bands, primarily arising from combinations and overtones of C-H, O-H and N-H stretching vibrations, are intrinsically related to the properties of hydrogen bonding existing in the investigated system [12,13]. Because of the profound influence of specific interactions on mechanical and electrical anharmonicity of the partner molecules [26], NIR spectra provide information on the properties of hydrogen-bonded complexes that is unavailable in MIR or Raman spectra [27]. Consequently, NIR spectroscopy provides exclusive opportunities for the investigation of molecular structure and interactions [21,25]. These effects manifested in NIR spectra can be utilized to investigate the interaction of the hydrogen-bonding centers, present in the polymer, with water and provide insight into the interaction behavior of these species [11,21,25]. Therefore, NIR spectroscopy has been demonstrated to provide valuable information for the characterization of polymers and their composites [22,28].

Physical principles underlying NIR spectroscopy make it also very well suited for the analysis of aqueous systems in a practical sense. NIR bands of water feature relatively weaker intensities, in contrast to very strong bands of water in the MIR region [21,29]. This makes it much easier to examine both the bands of water and the polymer in the NIR spectra, particularly over a wider range of water concentrations in the sample [21]. Although less of a critical hindrance than it appears in MIR spectroscopy, the water bands in NIR spectra can still obscure (i.e., mask) the signal of other constituents present in the sample [21,23]. In certain applications this remains to be an unwanted effect, for which developing effective mitigation methods would be helpful. Even though the removal of water bands from vibrational spectra has been studied for years, there is still very little knowledge of universal reach gathered in this area. This specific problem was almost exclusively investigated using the MIR technique [29,30]. A considerable focus has been directed at the suppression of the ro-vibrational structure of water vapor, as atmospheric water is the source of a common interference in MIR spectroscopy. The need for effective removal of water bands was identified relatively early in the field of the applications of NIR spectroscopy, with most of the proposed approaches to alleviate this problem being chemometric methods [23,31,32] and wavenumber selection methods [33]. Some attempts were made by using the refinement [23,31] of the Orthogonal Signal Correction method [34]. For example, the Regional Orthogonal Signal Correction was one of the approaches proposed, in combination with Moving Window Partial Least Squares Regression, to remove interfering water signals from NIR spectra [23]. Other well-known spectral transformation techniques were also evaluated for this purpose. For the investigation of the phosphorus and nitrogen concentration in fresh leaves [32], a non-linear Least Squares Spectral Matching technique was introduced [35], where the spectrum of a fresh leave was approximated by a nonlinear combination of the leaf-water spectrum and a dry sample spectrum. Nevertheless, no practically applicable method of universal reach could be established, due to major limitations in the transferability to other data sets, accuracy, overfitting [32] and noteworthy complexity for the user, because individual calculations and sample-tailored solutions were necessary for each specific case. Owing to single, purpose-driven NIR spectroscopic studies of these effects, the knowledge gathered so far remains fragmentary; little attention has been given to systematic studies of series of compounds of relatively similar character but with gradually varying key properties affecting their interaction with water.

In this study, we investigated polymer–water interactions and the manifestation of this phenomenon in NIR spectra by applying a systematic approach and employing a synergistic set of methods and techniques. We attempted to provide a more universal reach and deeper insights into the problem of water bands obscuring the signal of the analyzed compound in NIR spectra. For this purpose, polymers of varying hydrophilicity were investigated by diffuse reflectance NIR measurements: polytetrafluoroethylene (PTFE), polypropylene (PP), polystyrene (PS), polyvinylchloride (PVC), polyoxymethylene (POM), polyamide 6 (PA), lignin (Lig), chitin (Chi) and cellulose (Cell). Pure polymers as well as polymer–water mixtures in the concentration range of 1–10% (w/w) of water were analyzed. Spectra analysis and interpretation were performed with the use of difference spectroscopy, Principal Component Analysis (PCA), Median Linkage Clustering (MLC), Partial Least Squares Regression (PLSR), Multivariate Curve Resolution Alternating Least Squares (MCR-ALS) and Two-Dimensional Correlation Spectroscopy (2D-COS). Additionally, from the obtained data, aquagrams were constructed and interpreted with aid of the conclusions drawn from the conventional approaches. By simultaneous use of synergistic tools, generalized trends in the spectral manifestation of the interaction of water with polymers, including the dependencies on chemical nature and hydrophobicity, were obtained. In addition to physicochemical insights, these conclusions provide better understanding of the effects of water–solid matrix interactions, which often play a meaningful role in various applications of NIR spectroscopy.

2. Materials and Methods

2.1. Samples and Data Aquisition

2.1.1. Polymer Samples

The polymer samples were acquired as standards for synthetic, non-water-soluble, polymers from the suppliers present at the commercial market (Saudi Basic Industries Corporation SABIC, INOVYN, INEOS Styrolution, Euro OTC Pharmas GmbH, Sigma Aldrich). Cellulose (synthetic), lignin (kraft), chitin (from shrimp shells), PTFE and PVC were derived as practical grade powder, with an approximate particle size of 100 µm. PP, PS, PA and POM samples were acquired as pellets from different manufacturers. The polymer pellets were separately milled with the centrifugal mill ZM 200 (Retsch, Verder Scientific, Haan, Germany) while being cooled with liquid nitrogen to prevent temperature-induced changes. The centrifugal mill was equipped with a sieve with the pore size selected to obtain the particle diameter of approximately 250 µm. Deionized water was prepared by a Milli-Q® Reference (Merck KGaA, Darmstadt, Germany), with a conductance of 18.2 MΩcm. To ensure reproducibility, the polymer powders were completely dried in the drying chamber, at 50 °C and with a pressure of 200 mbar. An hour before measuring, the polymers were equilibrated to room temperature and stored in a desiccator until measurement.

2.1.2. NIRFlex N-500 FT-NIR Spectrometer

Measurements were performed with the NIRFlex N-500 FT-NIR spectrometer (BÜCHI Labortechnik AG, Flawil, Switzerland) with the attachment for solid sample measurements and a spinner add-on, which enables spatial averaging of the sample spot during the spectra measurement. The NIRFlex N-500 is equipped with a HeNe laser as a high-precision wavelength reference, a polarization interferometer with TeO_2 wedges and a tungsten halogen lamp for sample irradiation. Measurements were performed in diffuse reflection mode; 64 scans were accumulated per single spectrum, with an optical resolution of 8 cm^{-1}, in the wavenumber region of 10,000–4000 cm^{-1}. Cylindrical cuvettes for reflection measurements of solid samples, made of optical glass, with a volume of approximately 12 mL, were purchased from Hellma (Müllheim, Germany).

2.1.3. Data Acquisition

All polymers were directly weighted and prepared in the measuring cells. The amount of each individual polymer was constant throughout all measurements. Respectively, 1%, 3%, 5%, 7% or 10% deionized water (*w*/*w*) was added. Afterwards, the polymer–water mixtures were stirred for approximately 165 s with disposal spatulas, to ensure homogenous distribution of water in the polymer matrices. A metal stamp with a Teflon-foil ring was used to seal the measuring cells, to prevent water evaporation and ensure constant measurement conditions, by pressing the polymer–water mixtures to the ground of the cuvettes. The preparation of the samples and their placement in the measurement cell was repeated six times for each polymer–water mixture and each concentration level, in order to monitor the reproducibility of the procedure; the spectra measurements were done in triplicate. This procedure was performed for all polymers, with the exception of PTFE. Since PTFE is highly hydrophobic, it repels water completely and is not mixable with water at all. Therefore, we measured nine spectra of PTFE, with approximately 10% of water (water was the bottom layer). These spectra were then averaged, in order to overcome the variances in spectral intensity due to variation of the thickness of the water layer. At this stage, PLSR analysis was used to identify outliers in the measured spectral dataset; for the identified sample outliers, the measurements were repeated.

2.2. Chemometric Methods–Spectra Processing and Analysis

The collected raw spectra were transferred into the Unscrambler® X Version 10.5 (CAMO Software, Oslo, Norway). Before spectral analysis, firstly the spectra were recalculated from reflectance R into absorbance A, by applying a negative common logarithm (log 1/R). A linear offset correction was then used as a pretreatment method; it enables direct comparison of all measurements and polymers. For most of the analysis methods, the spectral dataset was averaged to one spectrum per concentration, except for PCA and PLSR analysis, where no sample averaging was used. All plots were generated with OriginPro® 2020. Noteworthily, the spectra below 4500 cm^{-1} should be considered less reliable, as the complete absorption phenomenon occurred for several samples. However, this region was not used for the purpose of this study, nor are any discussions in this work based on this fragment of spectra. Nonetheless, throughout this manuscript, full spectral data are presented (i.e., in the region of 10,000–4000 cm^{-1}), as they may be found useful by the readers for qualitative (i.e., rough) assessment.

2.2.1. Principal Component Analysis (PCA) and Median Linkage Clustering (MLC)

PCA and MLC were performed with the Unscrambler® X Version 10.5. The polymer–water mixture spectra, pretreated by linear offset correction, were used for this purpose. Full-cross-validation by means of the leave-one-out (LOO) approach was performed, and for determining the latent variables in the PCA approach, a nonlinear iterative partial least squares algorithm (NIPALS) was utilized. As the MLC method, a hierarchical clustering with a squared Euclidean distance measurement and the number of eight clusters (corresponding to the eight polymers used in this study), was used.

2.2.2. Partial Least Squares Regression (PLSR)

PLSR was carried out with the Unscrambler® X Version 10.5. The linear offset was applied to correct and normalize the spectra prior the generation of the PLSR models. A full-cross-validation by means of the LOO approach was conducted, and an NIPALS algorithm was used for determining the latent variables in the PLSR procedure.

2.2.3. Difference Spectroscopy

Difference spectroscopy was conducted manually; all calculations were carried out with Microsoft® 365 Excel®. For this purpose, the averaged, linear offset corrected spectra were used. The polymer difference spectra were generated by firstly scaling the water spectrum individually for each polymer–water mixture spectrum. The peak maximum of the combination water band, located at 5180 cm^{-1}, was utilized as the scaling reference point. At 5180 cm^{-1}, the intensity of the water band was scaled to the intensity of the water peak in each polymer–water mixture spectra, by dividing the intensity of the sample spectra by the intensity of the pure water spectrum. The scaling factor generated this way was used to multiply the water spectrum at each wavelength, which subsequently was subtracted from the respective polymer–water mixture spectrum. The water difference spectra were generated in an analogous procedure, by subtraction of the pure polymer spectrum from the mixture spectra, with individual scaling wavelengths for each polymer. The following reference points in the spectra of polymers were selected for this purpose: PTFE at 5944 cm^{-1} PP at 5796 cm^{-1}, PS at 5952 cm^{-1}, PVC at 5828 cm^{-1}, POM at 5968 cm^{-1}, PA at 5828 cm^{-1}, lignin at 5964 cm^{-1}, chitin at 5800 cm^{-1} and cellulose at 5604 cm^{-1}.

2.2.4. Multivariate Curve Resolution Alternating Least Squares (MCR-ALS)

A multivariate curve resolution (MCR) analysis was performed with the Unscrambler® X Version 10.5. The polymer–water spectra pretreated by linear offset correction were used, and the averaged pure water and polymer spectra were provided as a Y-reference. Two components were selected in this procedure to match the chemical rank of binary mixtures. Constraints were set to non-negativity for concentrations and spectra. The MCR procedure was performed using an alternating least squares algorithm (i.e., MCR-ALS). In order to compare the resulting spectra with the experimental gathered spectra, a SNV transformation had to be performed on both spectra sets.

2.2.5. Two-Dimensional Correlation Spectroscopy (2D-COS)

A 2D-COS analysis was accomplished using the extension 2D Correlation Spectroscopy Analysis, available in OriginPro® 2020. This software enables calculation of synchronous and asynchronous 2D-COS spectra. The averaged spectra of the pure polymer and the polymer–water mixture spectra were selected as dynamic spectra, with the concentrations as perturbations. The average dynamic spectrum was used as the reference. Subsequently, the synchronous and asynchronous 2D-COS plots were calculated for all polymers. Note, for better comparison, in this work, the synchronous plots are presented in an identical scale of intensity (z-axis) for all polymers. The intensity axis was chosen in a way so that all relevant information is easily accessible and the correlation strength is directly comparable. The intensities of the asynchronous plots on the other hand are scaled individually, because the intensity ranges are much less comparable between different systems, and uniform scaling would compromise the accessibility to the individual information on each sample.

2.2.6. Aquagrams

Aquagrams generally display water patterns exclusively for the overtone water band, which is not comprehensive enough to describe the dissimilarities of the investigated polymer–water systems. Therefore, aquagrams in this study were expanded to include also the second major water band, the combination band. Wavelengths of interest were selected by a comparison of all normalized polymer spectra. For the normalization, the averaged polymer–water mixture spectra were used. Firstly, an SNV transformation was performed in the Unscrambler® X Version 10.5 as pretreatment, and afterwards, the normalized absorbance $A^{n}_{\smile}$ for each spectrum and, respectively, each polymer was calculated regarding Equation (1) in Microsoft® 365 Excel®. Where $A_{\smile}$ is the SNV transformed absorption spectrum, $\mu_{\smile}$ is the mean spectrum of the regarding polymer and $\sigma_{\smile}$ is the standard deviation for the regarding polymer spectra after SNV transformation [36]. The selected wavenumbers were consequently plotted in an extended aquagram, representing both water bands.

$$A^{n}_{\smile} = \frac{A_{\smile} - \mu_{\smile}}{\sigma_{\smile}} \quad (1)$$

3. Results

3.1. General Features of the NIR Spectra of Polymer–Water Systems

The averaged NIR spectra of the polymer–water mixtures, additionally corrected by applying a linear offset of the baseline, are displayed in Figure 1. Note, the two major NIR bands of water have a complex internal structure, resulting from overlapping contributions from different species, and their exact nature is a matter of intensive and long-lasting discussions [37,38]. These bands originate primarily from combination vibrations, respectively, $\nu_s + \nu_{as}$ in the case of the peak observed at ca. 6900 cm^{-1} and $\nu_{as} + \delta$ for the band at ca. 5200 cm^{-1}. However, in the case of the former one, a meaningful component of the OH stretching overtone ($2\nu_{OH}$) is present as well. Despite that contribution to the intensity being lesser, it is commonly accepted in literature to refer to the ca. 6900 cm^{-1} band of water as the "overtone band". The band observed at ca. 5200 cm^{-1} is described as the "combination band", which precisely reflects its nature. For clarity, that commonly accepted, albeit not entirely precise, naming convention for those spectral features will be adopted in this work.

In Figure 1, spectra of the samples containing a varying water content are clearly differentiable for all polymers, with some variances manifested in the spectra of dissimilar polymers, which can be easily noticed. Interestingly, it can be noted that the variation in water content also influences the intensity of the polymer bands. This effect tends to grow with rising hydrophilicity for all investigated materials. Furthermore, it is not suppressed upon performing a linear offset correction or Standard Normal Variate (SNV) treatments, indicating that polymer–water interactions may be responsible for these intensity variations. In general, the biopolymers notably differ from the synthetic polymers, as they show more constant changes in the NIR spectra of the samples with varying water content. Moreover, clear red- and blueshifts of the water bands for different polymers and water concentrations are observed. In the case of hydrophobic polymers, the appearance of the spectra is distinctly influenced by the amount of added water. One the one hand, a low water content in the polymer matrix leads to strongly shifted and deformed water bands. On the other hand, when more water is added to the sample, the appearance of the water bands gets less deviated from that of bulk water. For example, PP shows a pronounced shift of the combination band of water for the sample spectrum containing 1% of water. On the contrary, the spectrum of the sample containing 10% water reveals a water band at the position very similar to that of bulk water.

However, hydrophobic polymers are anticipated to only weakly interact with water. Indicating, that only a small amount of water interacts with the polymer, and the addition of more water results in the presence of free bulk water. This is also supported by the finding that water band shifts get more uniform with increasing hydrophilicity of the samples. The water bands in the presence of biopolymers show almost completely constant shifts through all concentration levels. Interestingly, both major water bands show a dissimilar behavior in the presence of different polymers. For instance, blue- and redshifts for the same sample are manifested in the NIR spectra, e.g., for PA, a blueshift is observable for the overtone band of water, whereas a slight redshift is present for the combination band. Moreover, wavenumber shifts are much more pronounced for the combination band than for the overtone water band.

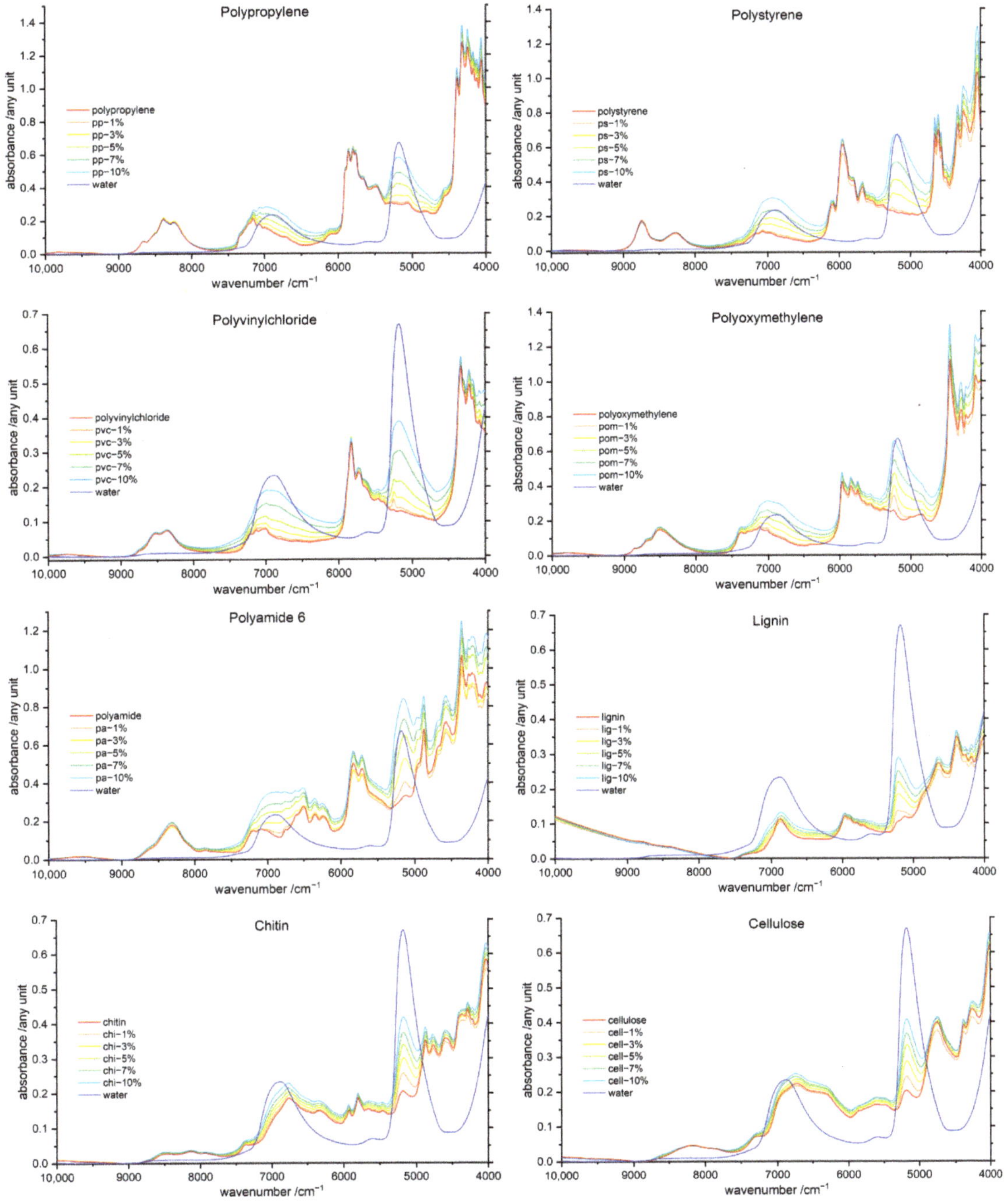

Figure 1. Averaged NIR absorbance spectra of the polymer–water mixtures after linear offset correction, in the range of 1–10% (*w*/*w*) water and the pure water spectra (dark blue) for comparison. The polymers are ordered according to increasing hydrophilicity, with the least hydrophilic polymer, polypropylene (**upper left** corner), to the most hydrophilic polymer, cellulose (**lower right** corner).

3.2. Band Assignment

As presented in Figure 1, most of the polymers show strong and specific polymer bands in the wavenumber region of 9000–8000 cm^{-1}, between 7500–7000 cm^{-1}, in the region of 6500–5500 cm^{-1} and near 4500 cm^{-1}. Additionally, more hydrophilic polymers show peaks in the vicinity of both major water bands. Especially for the combination band of water, the polymer spectra reveal a signal growing in intensity with rising hydrophilicity, which most likely indicates the presence of trace water bound to hydrophilic polymers, even for dried samples. Biopolymers are highly hydrophilic and therefore always contain bound water [11]. The overtone band of water displays a peak maximum at approximately 6900 cm^{-1} in this case, even though both water bands arise due to combinations of vibrational modes. In Table 1, we provided the assignments for the major polymer and water vibrations.

Table 1. Wavenumber assignments of relevant polymer and water groups [39].

Wavenumber/cm^{-1}	Assignment	Polymer/Water
10,000–9000	3 ν (OH); hydrogen-bonded	
8600–8200 [21,39] 8250 [21]	3 ν (CH_3 [21,39], CH_2 [39]) 2 ν + 2 δ (CH_3, CH_2)	all
7200–7000	2 ν (free OH) 2 ν + δ (CH_3, CH_2)	Lig, Chi, Cell all
7200–6800 [25]	$ν_s$ + $ν_{as}$ (OH)	water
7000–6200	2 ν (OH); hydrogen-bonded ν (OH) + ν (CH)	all
6900 [40]	2 ν CH + δ CH	all
6700–6500	2 ν (NH); free	PA, Chi
6600–6300	2 ν (NH); hydrogen-bonded	
6500	2 ν (OH); carbohydrates, polyphenols, . . . ; hydrogen-bonded	Lig, Chi, Cell
6200	ν (CH_3, CH_2)	all
6000–5600	2 ν (CH_3, CH_2) $ν_s$ + 2 δ (CH_3, CH_2)	
5300–5000 [25] 5200 [11,39,40]	$ν_{as}$ + δ (OH)	water
5280 [11]	Hydrogen-bonded water	water
5190 [11,39]	$ν_{as}$ + δ (OH) water molecule trapped in Polymer	Cell + water
5150 [28]	$ν_{as}$ + δ (OH); water molecule trapped in Polymer	PA + water
4900–4600	ν + δ (NH)	PA, Chi
4500	ν (CH_3, CH_2)	all
4400–4200	ν + δ (CH_3, CH_2)	all

ν—stretching; δ—bending vibration; $ν_{s/as}$—symmetric/asymmetric; 2—first overtone; 3—second overtone.

3.3. Principal Component Analysis (PCA) and Median Linkage Clustering (MLC)

A PCA and a hierarchical MLC method were utilized for a general inspection of the spectral set and analysis of the distribution of the samples to verify the consistency of the experimental conditions. Furthermore, these methods also enabled us to gain an overview of the trend related to the polymer hydrophilicity in the samples containing different concentrations of water. For this purpose, a PCA and a hierarchical MLC were respectively performed for the pure polymers, as well as for each individual concentration level of water in polymer –water samples. Exemplary PCA scores and an MLC dendrogram for the pure polymers are illustrated in Figure 2. The figures presenting the PCA score plots and MLC dendrograms for the entire concentration range of water (1–10%) added to the polymer (w/w) are displayed in the Supplementary Material (Figures S1 and S2, respectively).

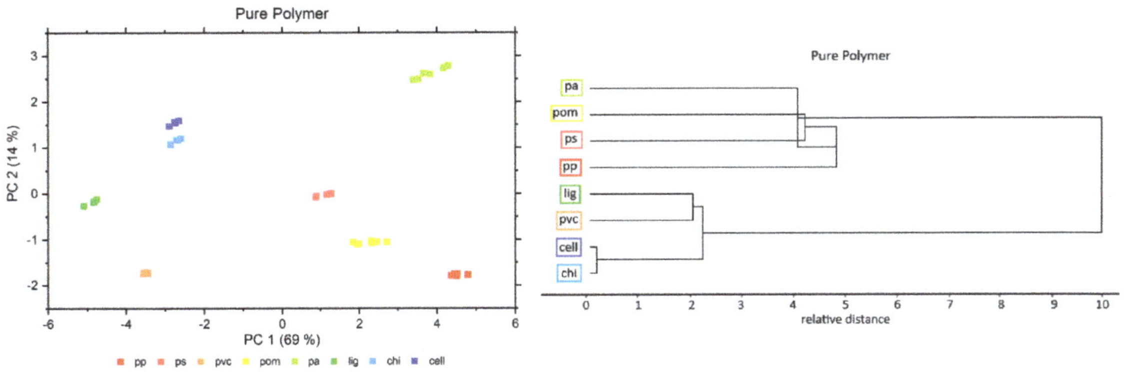

Figure 2. PCA scores (**left**) and MLC dendrogram (**right**) for the pure polymers after linear offset correction. The PCA scores and MLC dendrograms for the entire concentration range of water (1–10%) added to the polymer (w/w) are displayed in the Supplementary Materials (Figures S1 and S2, respectively).

The PCA scores in Figure 2 reveal perfectly separated groups for each individual polymer, without greater variance in between the repetition measurements of a single polymer. Cellulose and chitin are aligned relatively close to each other, but still, both polymers are easily differentiable. This reflects the high similarity of cellulose and chitin, which only differ in one functional group. Additionally, lignin is located near to chitin and cellulose, which may be interpreted as the relatively greater similarity of the biopolymers in comparison to all other polymers. The comparison of the PCA scores for the pure polymers and the water–polymer systems with 1–10% water (w/w) revealed no significant changes in the distribution of the samples, as presented in Figure S1.

The MLC analysis revealed the presence of two major groups in between the investigated polymers (Figures 2 and S2). Interestingly, the first major cluster consisted of three biopolymers and PVC, with chitin and cellulose forming a subcluster and lignin and PVC another subcluster. The second major cluster includes the remaining synthetic polymers. This grouping corresponds well to the PCA scores plotted in Figure 2.

3.4. Partial Least Squares Regression (PLSR)

A PLSR was performed for all samples in order to validate that the observed spectral variations were indeed well-correlated with the concentration of water in the sample. On the example of PP and cellulose, the resulting scores, regression coefficients for factor 1 and prediction performances of the cross-validation are displayed in Figure 3. The PLSR metrics obtained for all polymers investigated in this study and the regression coefficients for factor 1–3 are provided in the Supplementary Material (Figures S3–S5).

A clear separation of the different water contents and the pure polymers can be observed in the scores plots in Figure 3. Minor tendencies for sample clustering are apparent and should be accounted to the variations in the sample preparation process or unavoidable external conditions, e.g., the temperature and humidity. However, these effects are nearly negligible and not expected to interfere with the main investigation of this study. For all polymers, a high quality of the model fit was obtained in the PLSR procedure; an R^2 of at least 0.93 or higher was obtained in each case. This clearly indicates that the water concentration levels manifested in the NIR spectra were indeed near the nominal values intended for the prepared sample. No other effects of random or polymer-specific character, resulting, for example, from a potential vaporization or different distribution of liquid water in granulated polymer matrix, occurred in the sample set that could introduce spectral changes other than those directly correlated with water concentration. For all polymers within the first two factors, at least 98% of the variation in the NIR spectra was explained by 98% of the variation in the water concentration. Interestingly, the regression coefficients also showed resemblance to the water spectrum itself, conforming that water is the main inductor for changes in the spectra and for grouping of the samples in the scores plot (Figure 3).

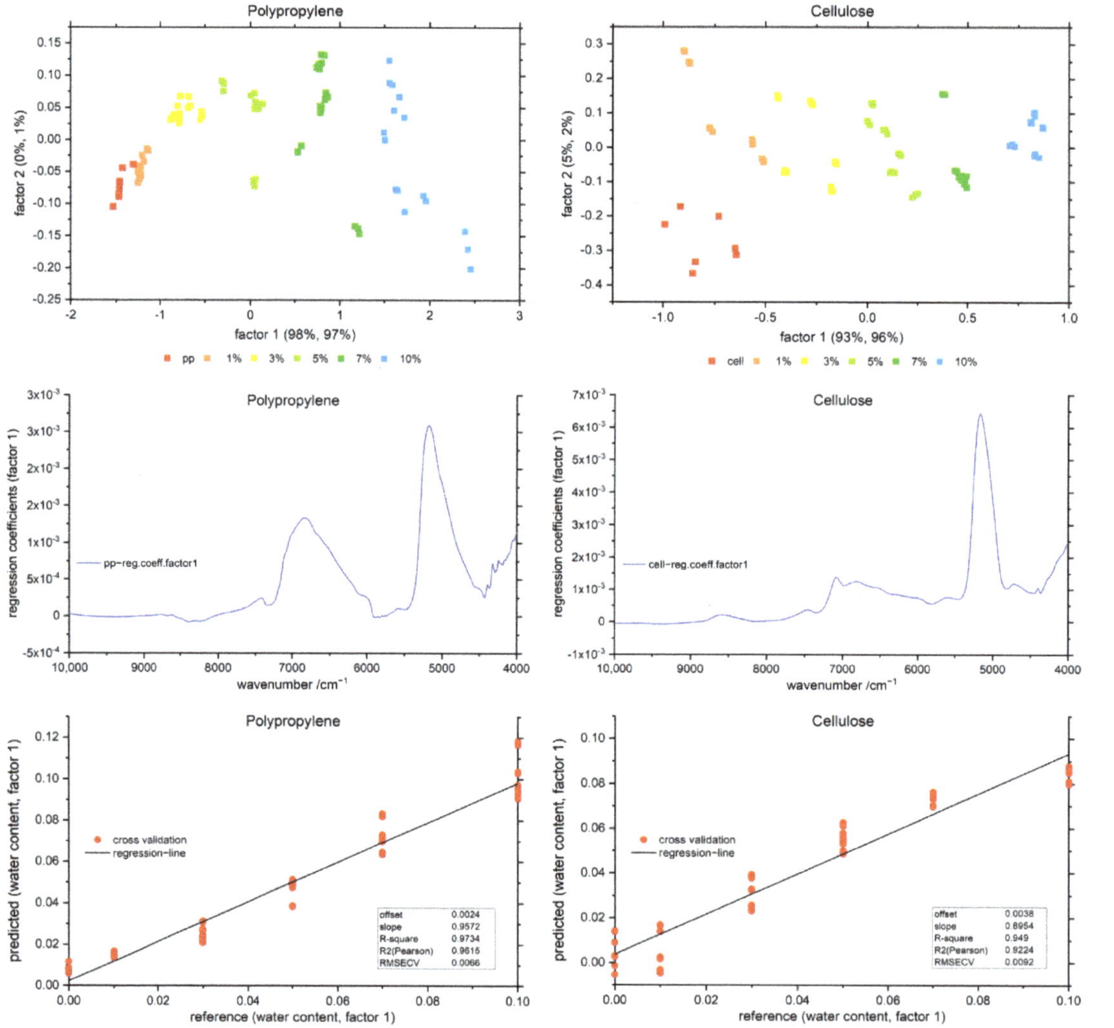

Figure 3. PLSR scores (**top**), regression coefficients (**middle**) and predicted vs. reference (**bottom**) for polypropylene (**left**) and cellulose (**right**) polymer–water mixtures, after linear offset correction. The scores, regression coefficients and predicted vs. reference of all polymers in comparison are displayed in the Supplementary Materials (Figures S3–S5).

3.5. *Difference Spectroscopy*

3.5.1. Water difference Spectra

A difference spectroscopy approach was applied to elucidate the NIR line shape of the water component present in the samples. In the procedure, the spectra of the pure polymers were subtracted from the spectra of polymer–water mixtures after the treatments to normalize spectral sets were applied as described in Section 2.2.3. In Figure 4, the line shapes resolved for the water component in the presence of PP and cellulose are displayed, while the results of this procedure for the remaining six polymer–water systems are provided in the Supplementary Materials (Figure S6).

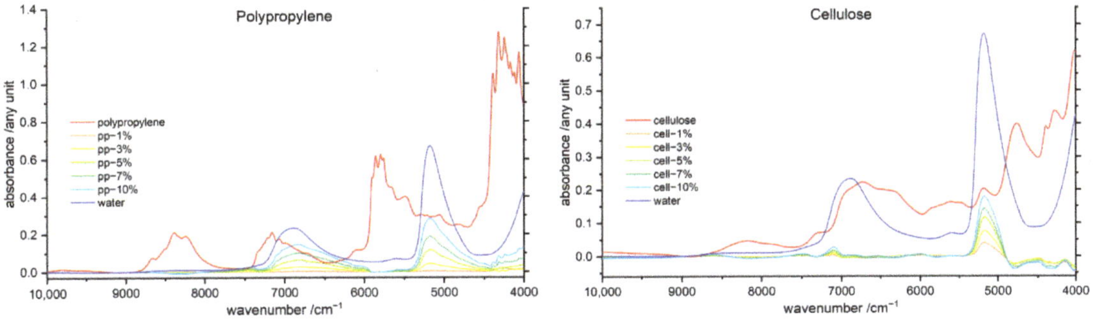

Figure 4. Water difference spectra of the polymer–water mixtures after linear offset correction and subtraction of the polymer spectra, in the range of 1–10% (*w*/*w*), with, respectively, the pure water (dark blue) and polymer (red) spectra for comparison, of PP (**left**) and cellulose (**right**). The water difference spectra of all investigated polymers are displayed in the Supplementary Materials (Figure S6).

The water difference spectra revealed significantly different shapes of the water bands for each individual polymer. However, the extent of band change neither followed hydrophilicity, nor was it related to the chemical nature of the polymer, indicating that another effect was in play causing the observed specificity. Interestingly, the water spectrum of the 1% PP–water mixture in Figure 4 is nearly featureless, with only a very shallow and broad peak at the combination water band; this is also noticeable in the raw spectrum in Figure 1. Furthermore, Figure S6 reveals that the water bands arose only with rising hydrophilicity of the polymer matrix. This effect was clearly present in the spectra and related to the polymer hydrophilicity. Interestingly, these spectra evidence the presence of strongly bonded water molecules observed in hydrophobic matrices such as PP (specifically, steadily increasing intensity and broadened shape of both water bands). However, the spectra of the systems involving hydrophilic polymers such as cellulose reveal that, rather, weakly interacting water species are present in such matrices at low concentrations (specifically, narrow, blue-shifted overtone band of water at ca. 7100 cm^{-1}). This observation suggests that the formation of strongly-interacting bulk-like water domains is promoted in hydrophobic matrices such as PP. At the same time, in the cellulose matrix, apparently the formation of bulk-like water is not promoted at low concentrations. This might occur because the hydrophilic matrix attracts more water molecules than hydrophobic surfaces of polymers such as PP. Consequently, a hydrophilic matrix creates a more competitive environment for binding water molecules, and bulk-like water domains are less easily formed at very low concentration of water in the matrix.

A separate note should be made about the inconsistency of the intensity change observed between the water overtone and combination band in the cellulose matrix being not uniform. The intensity of the overtone band with water concentration increases less rapidly than it is observed for the combination band. This seems to be plausible, as the electrical anharmonicity of hydrogen-bonded species has a profound effect in the intensities of overtone bands [26,27].

Moreover, PP, PS, PVC and POM reveal a highly specific behavior, with the water bands being profoundly asymmetric. For these systems, the presence of differently interacting water species is manifested in the NIR spectra. On the one hand, the water molecules weakly interacting with moderately hydrophilic polymer can be identified by the appearance of a water band for the combination band and overtone band. Furthermore, the existence of a broadened absorption feature extending towards lower wavenumbers (i.e., a broad band shoulder) reveals the presence of self-interacting water, i.e., bulk-like water domains. In the case of PP and PS, the revealed water bands are significantly widened, together with the additional extension towards lower wavenumbers; this indicates the presence of two different bulk-like water domains. This suggests that these polymer matrices effectively create two different chemical environments for water molecules. It is also possible that physical properties and morphology of the particles of these polymers are in play here; for instance, the less-developed areas of the hydrophobic surface of these polymers might lead to a faster evaporation of water from the polymer surface. Surprisingly, the lignin–water system also reveals a pronounced water band component observed at the low wavenumber shoulder of the combination water band. This suggests that lignin only weakly interacts with water, which promotes the organization of self-associated domains of water resembling bulk water. Noteworthily, the PA–water system interrupts this trend, which might be stemming from the chemical nature of this polymer. On the other hand, the water spectra for chitin and cellulose are relatively uniform. These effects can be observed for both water bands, and therefore, polymer–water interactions are strongly manifested in the NIR spectra. Note, in the case of the lignin–water system, the overtone water band is distorted by the subtraction procedure, and therefore, the water component of this sample should be considered less reliable.

Furthermore, distinct wavenumber shifts of both water bands occur in the presence of different polymers. The shift is especially noticeable for the overtone water band; the respective band shifts for each polymer are listed in Table 2. The biopolymers show, in this wavenumber region, profoundly broadened and strongly shifted water bands.

Table 2. By difference spectroscopy, we revealed wavenumber shifts of the overtone and combination water band in the concentration range of 1–10% of water (*w*/*w*) for the investigated polymers. Note, wavenumber shifts for lignin are given in brackets, because the experimental data may be considered less reliable.

Polymer	Shifts for Overtone Water Band/cm^{-1}	Shifts for Combination Water Band/cm^{-1}
Polypropylene	6796–6836	5180/not shifted
Polystyrene	6812–6852	5248–5176
Polyvinylchloride	6808–6842	5256–5180
Polyoxymethylene	6822–6826	5228–5204
Polyamide 6	6828–6840	5140–5164
(Lignin)	(7084–7064)	(5224–5208)
Chitin	7048–7024	5176–5164
Cellulose	7100–7120	5180–5172

3.5.2. Polymer Difference Spectra

With the aim to elucidate the variations in NIR spectra of the polymers, which can potentially occur as the effect of the interaction with water, the difference spectroscopy approach was applied as well to resolve the line shape associated with the polymer component. In this case, the spectrum of pure water was subtracted from the spectra of the water–polymer samples in the subtraction procedure. PTFE was the most hydrophobic polymer included in our study; the interaction between water and PTFE should be distinctively low. Furthermore, it has no meaningful absorption in the NIR region. Therefore, PTFE offers favorable properties for the validation of the use of difference spectroscopy in this study (Figure 5). The figure additionally displays the difference spectra of the cellulose–

water system, as it constitutes the most hydrophilic polymer examined in this study.

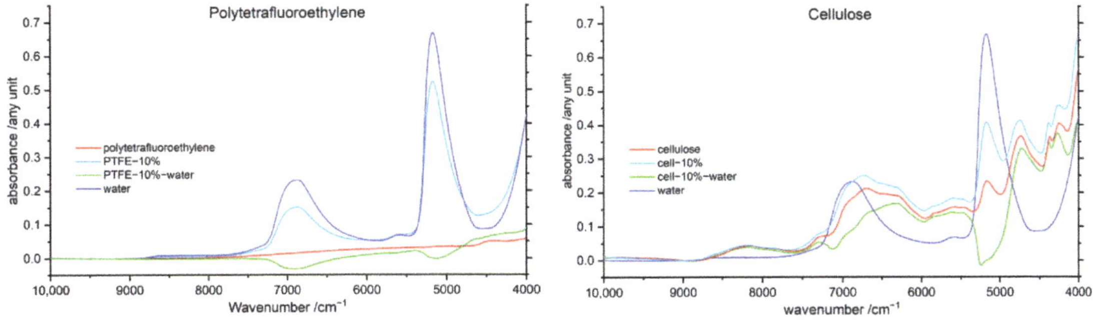

Figure 5. Polymer difference spectra of the 10% polymer–water mixtures after linear offset correction and subtraction of the water spectrum, with, respectively, the pure water (dark blue) and polymer (red) spectra for comparison of PTFE (**left**) and cellulose (**right**).

The resolved polymer component spectrum of the averaged 10% PTFE–water system in Figure 5 shows two broad negative features in the wavelength region of both water bands. A similar result was obtained for cellulose but with even more pronounced adverse features. The most probable reason of this is the presence of several OH groups in cellulose and likely also the relatively higher content of strongly bound inherent water molecules persisting in dried cellulose. Therefore, cellulose is highly interacting with water molecules. In NIR spectra, hydrogen-bonded species feature lower band intensities [26,27]; consequently, the spectrum of water bound strongly to cellulose differs from that of bulk water. This effect in combination with the dissimilar behavior of both major water bands, described in Section 3.1, confines the applicability of the polymer difference spectroscopy notably. Because of these limitations, the MCR-ALS study (Section 3.6) was conducted to provide independent, and potentially less affected by imperfections of the method itself, insights into the components of the NIR spectra associated with each of the interacting species. On the other hand, the results of difference spectroscopy clearly evidence the manifestation of polymer–water interactions in the spectra, even for highly hydrophobic polymers, i.e., PTFE. Therefore, for effectively revealing NIR peaks of the polymer masked by water bands, the polymer–water interactions should be considered. Especially biopolymers or other plant materials strongly interact with water. These highly hydrophilic and potentially hygroscopic materials always contain water by nature.

3.6. Multivariate Curve Resolution Alternating Least Squares (MCR-ALS)

An MCR-ALS analysis provides decomposition of the polymer–water mixture spectra into the resolved spectral curves associated with each of the components, i.e., in this case, water and the polymer spectra. The resolved curves are presented in Figure 6 for PP and cellulose, while the results for all eight investigated polymers are provided in the Supplementary Materials (Figure S7).

In general, the MCR-ALS polymer spectra are very similar to the experimental spectra measured for the pure polymers, indicating physical representativeness of the resolved curves. Consequently, the resolved spectral curve of the water component accurately reflects the true absorption profile of water existing in polymer matrix. In the case of PP, the resolved polymer component is almost undistinguishable from the spectrum measured for the pure polymer. In the case of the remaining polymers, the MCR-ALS curves show some minor deviations, almost exclusively located in the wavenumber regions of both water bands. However, these deviations form a trend. Especially in the vicinity of the combination water band, the resolved curves reveal a water band growing in intensity with rising hydrophilicity of the polymer. Noteworthy, for highly hydrophilic chitin and cellulose, the MCR-ALS spectra are surprisingly similar to the experimental spectra of pure polymers. The highest changes are obtainable for the hydrophilic polymers POM, PA and lignin. In contrast, the resolved water component curves for both water bands highly diverge from the experimental NIR spectrum of bulk water. Moreover, significant changes in band-shape and additionally band shifts are observed. While the absolute band intensities of the resolved MCR-ALS line shapes are not representative because of SNV treatment, the analysis of the intensities of the two major water bands remains legitimate in relative sense. Interestingly, the resolved water bands indicate diminished intensity of the combination band and enhanced intensity of the overtone band of water in comparison with those of bulk water for synthetic polymers. However, for the biopolymer matrices, an opposite trend in relative intensities of water bands can be noticed.

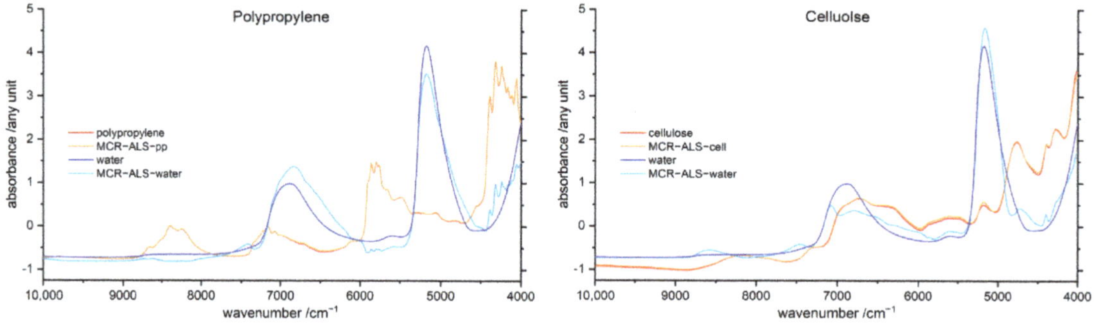

Figure 6. MCR-ALS polymer (orange) and water spectra (light blue) of polypropylene (**left**) and cellulose (**right**), additionally the NIR absorbance spectra of the pure polymer (red) and pure water (dark blue) are shown. The reference spectra as well as the resolved curves were normalized using an SNV transformation. The MCR-ALS polymer and water spectra of the remaining six polymers are displayed in the Supplementary Materials (Figure S7).

Furthermore, in the resolved water curves, the overtone band diverges (in shape and position of peak maximum) more substantially from the experimental water spectrum than it occurs for the combination band of water. In the case of lignin and cellulose, the resolved component spectra may be considered less reliable, because a splitting of the overtone MCR-ALS water band into two peaks was observed. Analogous to the water difference spectra discussed in Section 3.5.1, for PP, PS, PVC and POM, a low wavenumber shoulder of the water band component was revealed for the water overtone and combination band, indicating strong interactions between the water and polymer matrix. Therefore, the presence of both strongly and weakly interacting water can be evidenced from the MCR-ALS water curves.

3.7. Two-Dimensional Correlation Spectroscopy (2D-COS)

The NIR spectra of polymer–water systems were also analyzed with help of the 2D-COS approach, as it is known to be superior in the deconvolution ability of spectra [41], as well as in elucidating the effects of intermolecular interactions. The exemplary 2D-COS spectra of PP and cellulose are displayed in Figure 7, while the synchronous and asynchronous 2D-COS spectra of all investigated polymers are provided in the Supplementary Materials (Figure S8).

It is immediately noticeable that both systems show a distinctly different correlation pattern. The synchronous 2D-COS plots reveal the presence of only positive cross peaks, which is expected, considering that the investigated sample set features increasing water concentration. In the synchronous 2D-COS of PP in Figure 7 intense diagonal peaks for both water bands are observed, indicating a high magnitude of spectral changes associated with water addition at these wavelengths. Moreover, peak shapes also reflect the broadening of the water bands with increasing water content. The observed cross-peaks on the other hand show the high extent of correlation between both water bands, as a similar increase of intensities of both bands occurs with the addition of water.

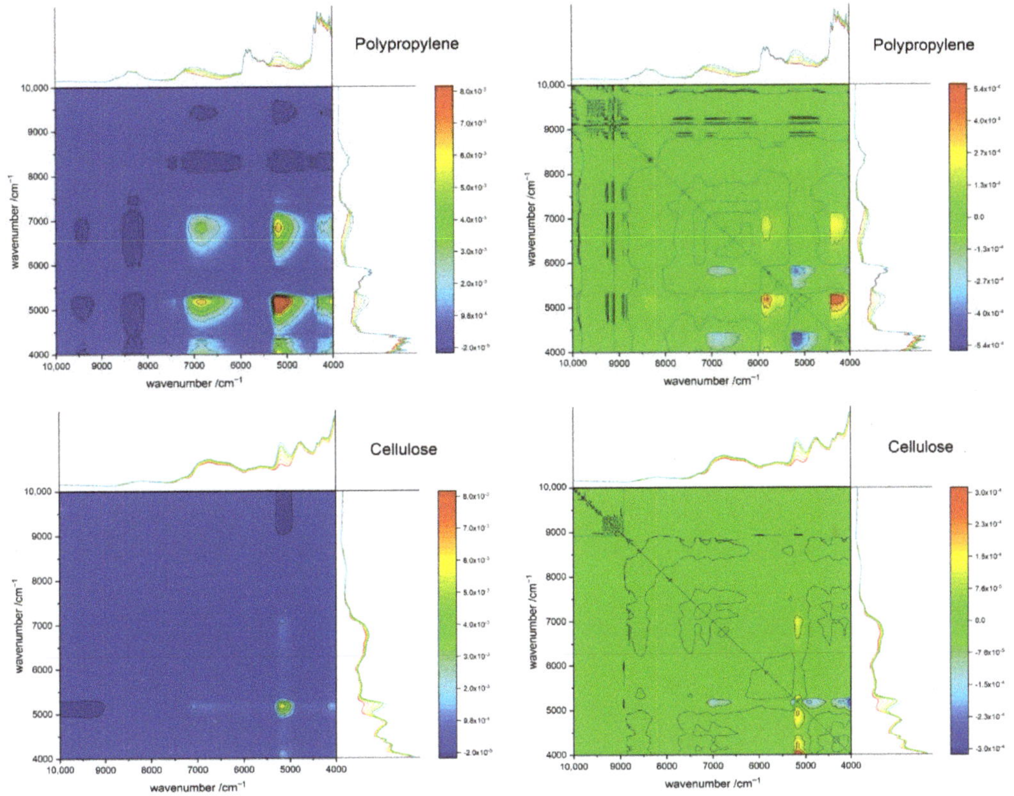

Figure 7. Synchronous (**left**) and asynchronous (**right**) 2D-COS spectra of the polymer–water mixtures after linear offset correction, in the ranges from 0–10% water (w/w), of PP (**left**) and cellulose (**right**). Note, the intensity scale of the synchronous 2D-COS spectra is the same for all polymers. The remaining 2D-COS spectra are displayed in the Supplementary Materials (Figure S8).

Figure S8 reveals visible interactions of the synthetic polymers with water below 4500 cm^{-1}. Furthermore, in the case of the hydrophilic polymers POM and PA, additional interactions of polymer with water are visible in the wavenumber region of 6500–5500 cm^{-1}. Interestingly, the biopolymers reveal a completely dissimilar correlation pattern, in contrast to the other investigated polymers. Much less profound correlations are observed for these systems, despite their high hydrophilicity. This might result from a relatively higher content of strongly bound water present in the biopolymer matrix even in nominally similar state of dryness as the other examined polymers. As already mentioned in Section 3.5.2, hydrogen-bonded species lead to lower band intensities in the NIR spectra [26,27]. Therefore, the spectral pattern of the water component changes less radically with increasing water content than it appears for less hydrophilic polymers. In other words, the interaction opportunities that the hydrophilic biopolymer matrix creates for water molecules seemingly shows similarities with the one that molecules of water find in a bulk state. All remaining polymers used in this study, on the other hand, show strong interactions of the polymer vibrations with the water bands. The asynchronous spectra in Figure S8 reveal that the sequence of intensity changes between both water bands is dissimilar for polymers of diverging hydrophilicity. In the case of the non-hydrophilic PP, both water bands show the same behavior. Conversely, for polymers of low hydrophilicity, PS and PVC, the overtone water band reacts more rapidly to the increase in water content. In contrast, for hydrophilic polymers, the overtone band of water reacts less rapidly than the combination water band. The latter effect appears to be less profound for POM and is more decisive for the biopolymers.

3.8. Aquagrams

An aquagram is a unique way for rescaling the spectral intensity at selected key wavenumbers and presenting the data with magnified differences that are less perceptible in absolute scale. For better representation of the polymers, we displayed the normalized spectra of each polymer in both water regions. Wavenumbers of interest were selected by comparison of the transformed polymer spectra; the detailed information about this procedure is given in Methods Section 2.2.6. In Figure 8, the aquagrams obtained for PP and cellulose are displayed as the examples, and the remaining aquagrams of all investigated polymers are provided in the Supplementary Materials (Figure S9).

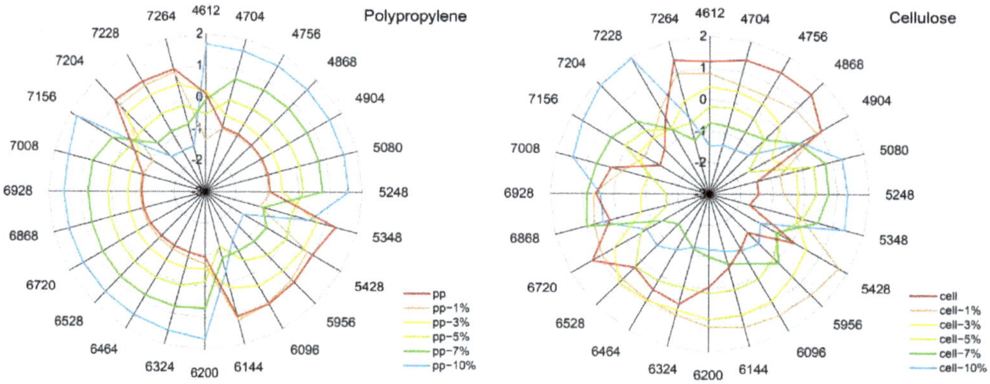

Figure 8. Aquagrams of both water regions for the polymer-water mixtures after SNV and standardization, in the ranges from 0–10% water (w/w), of PP (**left**) and cellulose (**right**). Aquagrams of all investigated polymers are displayed in the Supplementary Materials (Figure S9).

While useful for assessing intensity trends of large sets of data at glance, aquagrams are less suited to present an exhaustive cross-section of complex spectral variations. However, when analyzed together with the results provided by the methods discussed in previous sections, a deeper interpretation of the information encoded in aquagrams becomes possible. In general, aquagrams remain in agreement with the information derived from the other methods used in this study, while also revealing unique insights. In the case of hydrophobic to slightly hydrophilic polymers, the water component is highly dominant in the aquagrams, as it can be observed in Figure 8 for PP. At most of the meaningful wavenumbers selected for the aquagrams, a profound increase of the intensity of water bands with rising water content is reflected. Whereas there appear to be spectral regions where the polymer itself has higher contributions to the aquagram than water. Moreover, shifts of the water-dominated areas, i.e., water band shifts, can be easily monitored in the aquagrams. Interestingly, in the case of hydrophilic polymers, the aquagrams become highly complex, reflecting a convoluted spectral pattern associated with the changing water concentration in these systems. The characteristic water bands are not as similar to bulk water in the aquagrams, as they are manifested in the systems constituting more hydrophobic polymers. Hence, aquagrams can immediately identify the systems where a high degree of interaction with water occurs.

4. Discussion

4.1. Polymer Hydrophilicity as the Background for the NIR Spectral Trend in Polymer–Water Systems

The concept of hydrophilicity and hydrophobicity is very useful for the comparison of functional groups [42], as well as for capturing the relationship between polymer structure, properties or polymer solubility [9]. It is also frequently used as a physical property for block copolymers [43] and other nanostructures. However, this concept shows its limits when too dissimilar polymers are compared [42]. Despite the concept of hydrophobicity frequently being mentioned in literature, it is still challenging to quantify hydrophobicity in a definitive manner. Polymers are large macromolecules, while the concept of hydrophobicity applies best for single functional groups or small, rigid molecules [9,42].

The hydrophobicity of a polymer directly influences the interaction with solvents and, thus, the solubility or self-assembly behavior in the solution phase [9,43]. Natural and synthetic polymers feature various hydrophilicity levels and therefore interact differently with water. These interactions distinctly influence the physical properties of water and the polymers [1]. Nonetheless, the polymers used in this study may be approximately ordered with respect to their hydrophilicity as shown in Figure 9 [9,44,45]. This opens the question of whether NIR spectra that are sensitive to intermolecular interactions in a specific way (as discussed in Section 1) can bring new insights into the state of water in a well-defined chemical environment that features a gradually changing hydrophobicity.

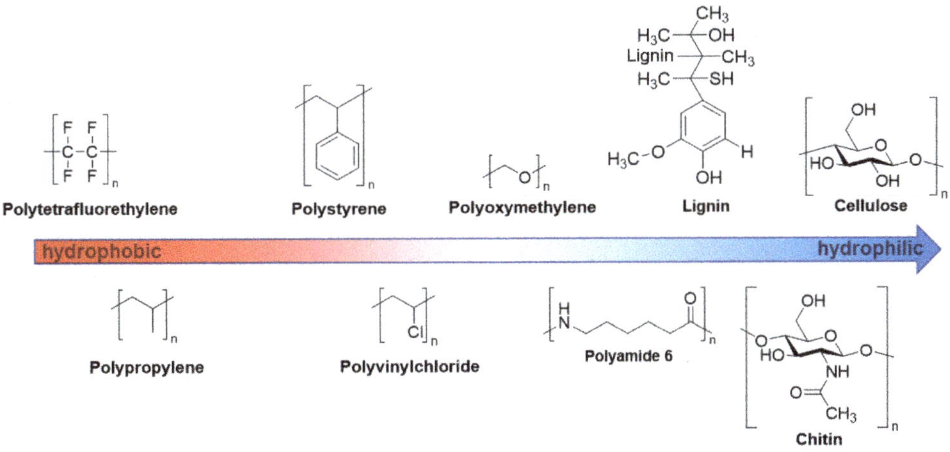

Figure 9. Approximate order of hydrophilicity of the polymers used in this study. From the most hydrophobic (**left**) to the most hydrophilic (**right**) polymers: Polytetrafluoroethylene, polypropylene, polystyrene, polyvinylchloride, polyoxymethylene, polyamide 6, lignin, chitin and cellulose.

4.2. General Discussion and Comparison of the Information Derived from Synergistic Methods

Each method used in this study contributes to clarifying the interaction of water with polymers of varying hydrophilicity. The MCR-ALS analysis separates (i.e., deconvolutes) the investigated NIR spectra of polymer–water systems into the spectral components, i.e., water and polymer spectra. The application of this method unveils resolved water curves clearly affected by the interactions of water and polymers. Furthermore, the resolved spectra of water in Figure 6 are surprisingly similar to the regression coefficients in Figure 3. Moreover, distinct band shifts and a dissimilar behavior of both water bands was revealed. The MCR-ALS analysis provides the averaged resolved component spectra of water and polymer from the investigated water–polymer mixtures in the concentration range of 1–10% water in the sample (w/w). Therefore, this method delivers a centralization of induced changes by the interaction of varying water contents with polymer samples, manifesting in the water bands in the presence of different polymers.

On the other hand, the water difference spectra show more detailed changes correlated to varying water content and dissimilarities among different polymers. Interestingly, this method evidenced the presence of strongly bonded water molecules observed in hydrophobic matrices. Contrarily, the spectra of hydrophilic polymers revealed that rather weakly interacting water species are present in such matrices at low concentrations. Therefore, water difference spectra suggest that the formation of strongly-interacting bulk-like water domains is promoted in hydrophobic matrices. A hydrophilic matrix attracts more water molecules than hydrophobic surfaces. Consequently, hydrophilic polymers create a more competitive environment for binding water molecules, and bulk-like water domains are less easily formed at very low concentration of water in the matrix.

Both methods revealed polymers of low to moderate hydrophilicity, i.e., PP, PS, PVC and POM, to create a special chemical environment for water molecules in NIR. The resolved water spectra reveal trends of spectral changes of the combination and overtone band of water roughly corresponding to the hydrophilicity of the polymer matrix, albeit with specific features associated with the chemical nature of the polymer. Furthermore, a broadened absorption feature towards lower wavenumbers for both water bands appear in hydrophobic polymer matrices. The former effect identifies a weak interaction of water and the polymer, while the latter reveals the presence of strongly interacting water, i.e., self-interacting water.

Comparing the resolved water difference spectra (Figure S6) with MCR-ALS, deconvolution (Figure S7) reveals that there are three diverse behaviors present among polymers of varying hydrophobicity with water. Firstly, in polymer matrices of very weak hydrophilicity, i.e., PP and PS, water molecules tend to form bulk-like water domains rather than being attracted to the polymer surface. Therefore, in this case, water bands resemble those of pure liquid water. However, for PS, probably additional sterically driven captivation of water molecules is present. The second case is formed for polymers of low or medium hydrophilicity, i.e., PVC and POM, which weakly interact with water. Therefore, also for these samples, additional bulk-like water domains are formed. Thirdly, for hydrophilic polymers which strongly interact with water, i.e., PA, chitin and cellulose, no clear manifestation of bulk water domains can be seen in the spectra. Interestingly, lignin forms an exception in this trend. It should be noted that the actual hydrophilicity of lignin is difficult to estimate owing to its complex structure (Figure 9). Therefore, the molecular environment created for water molecules by lignin may promote a relatively stronger formation of bulk-water domains at low water concentration levels, effectively resembling the features of nominally more hydrophobic polymers. Further investigations are needed to provide insights into this phenomenon; however, these findings reveal a high sensitivity of water towards its chemical environment and attribute it to the interaction of water with the polymer matrices.

Furthermore, the application of the 2D-COS approach revealed that the sequence of intensity changes between both major water bands is dissimilar for polymers of diverging hydrophilicity. In the presence of very weak hydrophilic polymers, i.e., PP, both water bands manifest the same behavior. For polymer matrices of weak hydrophilicity, PS and PVC, the intensity of the overtone water band reacts more rapidly to the increase in water content than it occurs for the combination water band. Contrarily, for hydrophilic polymers, the overtone band of water reacts less rapidly. Moreover, this behavior is less profound for POM and PA, but it is more decisive for highly hydrophilic polymers, i.e., lignin, chitin and cellulose. This effect is also noticeable for biopolymer matrices in water difference spectra. The intensity of the overtone band increases less rapidly with an increasing water concentration in the matrix than is observed for the intensity of the combination band.

By rescaling the intensities of the NIR spectra, aquagrams provide the ability to highlight spectral changes of largely different magnitude, which would be difficult to trace in absolute scale of spectral intensity. Therefore, not only intensity variations of great magnitudes are displayed, but also, small changes in the NIR spectra can be easily monitored, by using aquagrams. While aquagrams are very useful to extract intensity trends occurring in large datasets while displaying those at glance, they are less suited for the comprehensive presentation of spectral variations and their interpretation, e.g., band shifts and changes in band shape cannot be easily followed in this form of presentation. However, when used in combination with other methods of spectral analysis, aquagrams can help in identifying the spectral regions of interest for elucidating the spectral pattern associated with the change in water concentration in the matrix. In this study, the application of aquagrams jointly with the other approaches to analyze the behavior of water in polymer matrices of varying hydrophobicity and chemical nature showed the usefulness of aquagrams for rapid qualitative assessment of the matrix property. Polymer–water systems of weak interaction strength therefore show the profound increase of the intensity of water bands and rather smooth patterns displayed in aquagrams. Contrarily, for hydrophilic polymers, aquagrams become highly convoluted and reflect the complex interaction of the polymer–water systems. Furthermore, water band shifts are immediately noticeable in the aquagrams. Therefore, the aquagrams can, at a glance, reveal the varying complexity of the matrix as it creates different environments for water molecules. This information seems helpful for screening large spectral sets with the purpose of identifying the systems of particular interest for molecular studies of the interactions of water with various chemical environments.

5. Conclusions

In this study, we unveiled trends associated with the chemical nature of the polymer and its increasing hydrophilicity, which are specifically manifested in NIR spectra. The results obtained with several independent methods provide confirmatory conclusions, with each method also providing unique findings. The MCR-ALS method and water difference spectroscopy revealed that polymers of varying hydrophilicity manifest three major dissimilar behaviors. Firstly, polymers of very low hydrophilicity feature non-attracting behavior towards water, and therefore, bulk-like water domains are formed more easily in the sample. Secondly, the polymers of low or medium hydrophilicity weakly interact with water, and additionally, bulk-like water domains are formed. Thirdly, hydrophilic polymers strongly interact with water; therefore, no clear evidence of bulk water domains is present in the NIR spectra of polymer–water systems. Of particular interest is the dissimilar spectral manifestation of both major water bands, located at ca. 6900 cm^{-1} and 5200 cm^{-1} ($\nu_s + \nu_{as}$ and $\nu_{as} + \delta$) in the presence of diverse polymers. Some polymers show simultaneous blue- and redshifts for both major water bands. Furthermore, wavenumber shifts are much more pronounced for the overtone water band (6900 cm^{-1}) than they are for the combination band (5200 cm^{-1}).

The 2D-COS analysis revealed that the sequence of intensity changes of the water bands is dissimilar for polymers of varying hydrophilicity. While for polymers of weak hydrophilicity, the overtone water band reacts more rapidly to the increase in water content than the combination band; this trend is opposite for hydrophilic polymers. The experimental findings by difference spectroscopy proved that even highly hydrophobic polymers (e.g., PTFE) interact with water, and these interactions manifest themselves in the water component of the NIR spectra. Hydrophilicity, therefore, is not exhaustive enough to describe the interaction of a polymer with water. Taking into account the chemical specificity of the matrix in describing spectral effects of the water–substance interactions is necessary for successful removing of the water contributions in NIR spectra. The analysis of the polymer–water mixtures also confirmed that the sensitivity of water towards its chemical environment is a major factor clearly manifested in NIR spectra. Moreover, with increasing hydrophilicity of the matrix, in NIR spectra the amplitude and complexity of spectral variations resulting from water–matrix interactions are enhanced. The 2D-COS investigations confirmed that strong hydrogen-bonding leads to a diminished band intensity of the interacting species in NIR spectra [26,27].

Finally, aquagrams are a unique way for rescaling the data and showing wavelength-specific phenomena. Water band shifts are immediately noticeable in the aquagrams. When compared with the other methods used in this study, the usefulness of aquagrams for rapid assessment of the interaction strength of water with the sample matrix was shown.

Furthermore, when compared with the outcomes of the MCR-ALS procedure, aquagrams seem capable of highlighting effects, which could not be easily derived in difference spectra.

Supplementary Materials: The following supporting information can be downloaded at: https://www.mdpi.com/article/10.3390/molecules27185882/s1. Figure S1: PCA Scores; Figure S2: MLC Dendrograms; Figure S3: PLSR Scores; Figure S4: PLSR Regression Coefficients; Figure S5: PLSR Predicted vs. Reference; Figure S6: Water Difference Spectra; Figure S7: MCR-ALS; Figure S8: 2D-COS; Figure S9: Aquagrams.

Author Contributions: Conceptualization, V.M., K.B.B. and C.W.H.; methodology, K.B.B.; software, V.M.; validation, V.M. and K.B.B.; formal analysis, V.M.; investigation, V.M.; resources, C.W.H.; data curation, V.M. and J.G.; writing—original draft preparation, V.M.; writing—review and editing, K.B.B., J.G. and C.W.H.; visualization, V.M.; supervision, K.B.B. and C.W.H.; project administration, C.W.H.; funding acquisition, J.G. and C.W.H. All authors have read and agreed to the published version of the manuscript.

Funding: The authors cordially acknowledge the support from the Tsuki no Shizuku Foundation, Japan. The Foundation covered the article processing charges for this publication.

Institutional Review Board Statement: Not applicable.

Informed Consent Statement: Not applicable.

Data Availability Statement: Not applicable.

Conflicts of Interest: The authors declare no conflict of interest.

Sample Availability: Samples are not available.

References

1. Hatakeyama, H.; Hatakeyama, T. Interaction between water and hydrophilic polymers. *Thermochim. Acta* **1998**, *308*, 3–22. [CrossRef]
2. Hsu, S.L.; Patel, J.; Zhao, W. Vibrational spectroscopy of polymers. In *Molecular Characterization of Polymers*; Elsevier: Amsterdam, The Netherlands, 2021; pp. 369–407. ISBN 9780128197684.
3. Jellinek, H.H.G. (Ed.) *Water Structure at the Water-Polymer Interface: Proceedings of a Symposium held on March 30 and April 1, 1971, at the 161st National Meeting of the American Chemical Society*; Springer US: Boston, MA, USA, 1972; ISBN 978-1-4615-8683-8.
4. Yasoshima, N.; Ishiyama, T.; Gemmei-Ide, M.; Matubayasi, N. Molecular Structure and Vibrational Spectra of Water Molecules Sorbed in Poly(2-methoxyethylacrylate) Revealed by Molecular Dynamics Simulation. *J. Phys. Chem. B* **2021**, *125*, 12095–12103. [CrossRef] [PubMed]
5. Arif, U.; Haider, S.; Haider, A.; Khan, N.; Alghyamah, A.A.; Jamila, N.; Khan, M.I.; Almasry, W.A.; Kang, I.-K. Biocompatible Polymers and their Potential Biomedical Applications: A Review. *Curr. Pharm. Des.* **2019**, *25*, 3608–3619. [CrossRef] [PubMed]
6. Tanaka, M.; Motomura, T.; Ishii, N.; Shimura, K.; Onishi, M.; Mochizuki, A.; Hatakeyama, T. Cold crystallization of water in hydrated poly(2-methoxyethyl acrylate) (PMEA). *Polym. Int.* **2000**, *49*, 1709–1713. [CrossRef]
7. Koguchi, R.; Jankova, K.; Hayasaka, Y.; Kobayashi, D.; Amino, Y.; Miyajima, T.; Kobayashi, S.; Murakami, D.; Yamamoto, K.; Tanaka, M. Understanding the Effect of Hydration on the Bio-inert Properties of 2-Hydroxyethyl Methacrylate Copolymers with Small Amounts of Amino- or/and Fluorine-Containing Monomers. *ACS Biomater. Sci. Eng.* **2020**, *6*, 2855–2866. [CrossRef]
8. Southall, N.T.; Dill, K.A.; Haymet, A.D.J. A View of the Hydrophobic Effect. *J. Phys. Chem. B* **2002**, *106*, 521–533. [CrossRef]
9. Foster, J.C.; Akar, I.; Grocott, M.C.; Pearce, A.K.; Mathers, R.T.; O'Reilly, R.K. 100th Anniversary of Macromolecular Science Viewpoint: The Role of Hydrophobicity in Polymer Phenomena. *ACS Macro Lett.* **2020**, *9*, 1700–1707. [CrossRef]
10. Sato, K.; Kobayashi, S.; Kusakari, M.; Watahiki, S.; Oikawa, M.; Hoshiba, T.; Tanaka, M. The Relationship Between Water Structure and Blood Compatibility in Poly(2-methoxyethyl Acrylate) (PMEA) Analogues. *Macromol. Biosci.* **2015**, *15*, 1296–1303. [CrossRef]
11. Christy, A.A. Chemistry of Desiccant Properties of Carbohydrate Polymers as Studied by Near-Infrared Spectroscopy. *Ind. Eng. Chem. Res.* **2013**, *52*, 4510–4516. [CrossRef]
12. Tanaka, M.; Hayashi, T.; Morita, S. The roles of water molecules at the biointerface of medical polymers. *Polym. J.* **2013**, *45*, 701–710. [CrossRef]
13. Ryabov, Y.E.; Feldman, Y.; Shinyashiki, N.; Yagihara, S. The symmetric broadening of the water relaxation peak in polymer–water mixtures and its relationship to the hydrophilic and hydrophobic properties of polymers. *J. Chem. Phys.* **2002**, *116*, 8610. [CrossRef]
14. Malik, M.I.; Mays, J.; Shah, M.R. (Eds.) *Molecular Characterization of Polymers*; Elsevier: Amsterdam, The Netherlands, 2021; ISBN 9780128197684.
15. Mastai, Y.; Rudloff, J.; Cölfen, H.; Antoniette, M. Control over the structure of ice and water by block copolymer additives. *ChemPhysChem* **2002**, *3*, 119–123. [CrossRef]

16. Liu, Y.; Liu, X.; Duan, B.; Yu, Z.; Cheng, T.; Yu, L.; Liu, L.; Liu, K. Polymer-Water Interaction Enabled Intelligent Moisture Regulation in Hydrogels. *J. Phys. Chem. Lett.* **2021**, *12*, 2587–2592. [CrossRef]
17. Dong, W.; Yan, M.; Zhang, M.; Liu, Z.; Li, Y. A computational and experimental investigation of the interaction between the template molecule and the functional monomer used in the molecularly imprinted polymer. *Anal. Chim. Acta* **2005**, *542*, 186–192. [CrossRef]
18. Taylor, L.S.; Langkilde, F.W.; Zografi, G. Fourier transform Raman spectroscopic study of the interaction of water vapor with amorphous polymers. *J. Pharm. Sci.* **2001**, *90*, 888–901. [CrossRef]
19. Schmidt, P.; Dybal, J.; Trchová, M. Investigations of the hydrophobic and hydrophilic interactions in polymer–water systems by ATR FTIR and Raman spectroscopy. *Vib. Spectrosc.* **2006**, *42*, 278–283. [CrossRef]
20. Maeda, Y.; Kitano, H. The structure of water in polymer systems as revealed by Raman spectroscopy. *Spectrochim. Acta Part A Mol. Biomol. Spectrosc.* **1995**, *51*, 2433–2446. [CrossRef]
21. Beć, K.B.; Grabska, J.; Huck, C.W. Near-Infrared Spectroscopy in Bio-Applications. *Molecules* **2020**, *25*, 2948. [CrossRef]
22. Bokobza, L. Some Applications of Vibrational Spectroscopy for the Analysis of Polymers and Polymer Composites. *Polymers* **2019**, *11*, 1159. [CrossRef]
23. Du Yi, P.; Liang, Y.Z.; Kasemsumran, S.; Maruo, K.; Ozaki, Y. Removal of interference signals due to water from in vivo near-infrared (NIR) spectra of blood glucose by region orthogonal signal correction (ROSC). *Anal. Sci.* **2004**, *20*, 1339–1345. [CrossRef]
24. Schwanninger, M.; Rodrigues, J.C.; Fackler, K. A Review of Band Assignments in near Infrared Spectra of Wood and Wood Components. *J. Near Infrared Spectrosc.* **2011**, *19*, 287–308. [CrossRef]
25. Czarnecki, M.A.; Beć, K.B.; Grabska, J.; Hofer, T.S.; Ozaki, Y. Overview of Application of NIR Spectroscopy to Physical Chemistry. In *Near-Infrared Spectroscopy*; Ozaki, Y., Huck, C., Tsuchikawa, S., Engelsen, S.B., Eds.; Springer: Singapore, 2021; pp. 297–330. ISBN 978-981-15-8647-7.
26. Schuler, M.J.; Hofer, T.S.; Morisawa, Y.; Futami, Y.; Huck, C.W.; Ozaki, Y. Solvation effects on wavenumbers and absorption intensities of the OH-stretch vibration in phenolic compounds—Electrical- and mechanical anharmonicity via a combined DFT/Numerov approach. *Phys. Chem. Chem. Phys.* **2020**, *22*, 13017–13029. [CrossRef] [PubMed]
27. Futami, Y.; Ozaki, Y.; Hamada, Y.; Wojcik, M.J.; Ozaki, Y. Frequencies and absorption intensities of fundamentals and overtones of NH stretching vibrations of pyrrole and pyrrole–pyridine complex studied by near-infrared/infrared spectroscopy and density-functional-theory calculations. *Chem. Phys. Lett.* **2009**, *482*, 320–324. [CrossRef]
28. Lachenal, G.; Ozaki, Y. Advantages of near infrared spectroscopy for the analysis of polymers and composites. *Macromol. Symp.* **1999**, *141*, 283–292. [CrossRef]
29. Zhang, X.; He, A.; Guo, R.; Zhao, Y.; Yang, L.; Morita, S.; Xu, Y.; Noda, I.; Ozaki, Y. A new approach to removing interference of moisture from FTIR spectrum. *Spectrochim. Acta Part A Mol. Biomol. Spectrosc.* **2022**, *265*, 120373. [CrossRef]
30. Margenot, A.J.; Calderón, F.J.; Parikh, S.J. Limitations and Potential of Spectral Subtractions in Fourier-Transform Infrared Spectroscopy of Soil Samples. *Soil Sci. Soc. Am. J.* **2016**, *80*, 10–26. [CrossRef]
31. Chen, D.; Hu, B.; Shao, X.; Su, Q. Removal of major interference sources in aqueous near-infrared spectroscopy techniques. *Anal. Bioanal. Chem.* **2004**, *379*, 143–148. [CrossRef]
32. Ramoelo, A.; Skidmore, A.K.; Schlerf, M.; Mathieu, R.; Heitkönig, I.M. Water-removed spectra increase the retrieval accuracy when estimating savanna grass nitrogen and phosphorus concentrations. *ISPRS J. Photogramm. Remote Sens.* **2011**, *66*, 408–417. [CrossRef]
33. Yoon, G.; Amerov, A.K.; Jeon, K.J.; Kim, Y.-J. Determination of glucose concentration in a scattering medium based on selected wavelengths by use of an overtone absorption band. *Appl. Opt.* **2002**, *41*, 1469–1475. [CrossRef]
34. Wold, S.; Antti, H.; Lindgren, F.; Öhman, J. Orthogonal signal correction of near-infrared spectra. *Chemom. Intell. Lab. Syst.* **1998**, *44*, 175–185. [CrossRef]
35. Gao, B.-C.; Goetzt, A.F. Retrieval of equivalent water thickness and information related to biochemical components of vegetation canopies from AVIRIS data. *Remote Sens. Environ.* **1995**, *52*, 155–162. [CrossRef]
36. Tsenkova, R.; Munćan, J.; Pollner, B.; Kovacs, Z. Essentials of Aquaphotomics and Its Chemometrics Approaches. *Front. Chem.* **2018**, *6*, 363. [CrossRef]
37. Tan, J.; Sun, Y.; Ma, L.; Feng, H.; Guo, Y.; Cai, W.; Shao, X. Knowledge-based genetic algorithm for resolving the near-infrared spectrum and understanding the water structures in aqueous solution. *Chemom. Intell. Lab. Syst.* **2020**, *206*, 104150. [CrossRef]
38. Czarnik-Matusewicz, B.; Pilorz, S. Study of the temperature-dependent near-infrared spectra of water by two-dimensional correlation spectroscopy and principal components analysis. *Vib. Spectrosc.* **2006**, *40*, 235–245. [CrossRef]
39. Sandorfy, C.; Buchet, R.; Lachenal, G. Principles of Molecular Vibrations for Near-Infrared Spectroscopy. In *Near-Infrared Spectroscopy in Food Science and Technology*; Ozaki, Y., McClure, W.F., Christy, A.A., Eds.; John Wiley & Sons, Inc.: Hoboken, NJ, USA, 2006; pp. 11–46, ISBN 9780470047705.
40. Beganović, A.; Moll, V.; Huck, C.W. Comparison of Multivariate Regression Models Based on Water- and Carbohydrate-Related Spectral Regions in the Near-Infrared for Aqueous Solutions of Glucose. *Molecules* **2019**, *24*, 2696. [CrossRef]
41. Pazderka, T.; Kopecky, V., Jr. 2D Correlation Spectroscopy and Its Application in Vibrational Spectroscopy Using Matlab. Institute of Physics, Faculty of Mathematics and Physics, Charles University: Prague, Czech Republic, 2008; pp. 978–998.

42. Dharmaratne, N.U.; Jouaneh, T.M.M.; Kiesewetter, M.K.; Mathers, R.T. Quantitative Measurements of Polymer Hydrophobicity Based on Functional Group Identity and Oligomer Length. *Macromolecules* **2018**, *51*, 8461–8468. [CrossRef]
43. Figg, C.A.; Carmean, R.N.; Bentz, K.C.; Mukherjee, S.; Savin, D.A.; Sumerlin, B.S. Tuning Hydrophobicity To Program Block Copolymer Assemblies from the Inside Out. *Macromolecules* **2017**, *50*, 935–943. [CrossRef]
44. Piao, C.; Winandy, J.E.; Shupe, T.F. From Hydrophilicity to Hydrophobicity: A Critical Review: Part I. Wettability and Surface Behavior. *Wood Fiber Sci.* **2010**, *42*, 490–510.
45. Hou, X.; Deem, P.T.; Choy, K.-L. Hydrophobicity study of polytetrafluoroethylene nanocomposite films. *Thin Solid Films* **2012**, *520*, 4916–4920. [CrossRef]

molecules

Article

Analysis of Vicinal Water in Soft Contact Lenses Using a Combination of Infrared Absorption Spectroscopy and Multivariate Curve Resolution

Shoichi Maeda [1], Shunta Chikami [1], Glenn Villena Latag [1], Subin Song [1], Norio Iwakiri [2] and Tomohiro Hayashi [1,3,*]

1 Department of Material Science and Engineering, School of Materials and Chemical Technology, Tokyo Institute of Technology, 4259 Nagatsuta-Cho Midori-Ku, Yokohama 226-8502, Japan; maeda.s.am@m.titech.ac.jp (S.M.); chikami.s.aa@m.titech.ac.jp (S.C.); latag.g.aa@m.titech.ac.jp (G.V.L.); song.s.ad@m.titech.ac.jp (S.S.)
2 Life Science Products Division, NOF Corporation, Yebisu Garden Place Tower, 20-3 Ebisu 4-Chome, Shibuya-Ku, Tokyo 150-6019, Japan; norio_iwakiri@nof.co.jp
3 The Institute for Solid State Physics, The University of Tokyo, 5-1-5, Kashiwanoha, Kashiwa 277-0882, Japan
* Correspondence: tomo@mac.titech.ac.jp; Tel.: +81-45-924-5400

Abstract: In this paper, we propose a new spectroscopic method to explore the behavior of molecules near polymeric molecular networks of water-containing soft materials such as hydrogels. We demonstrate the analysis of hydrogen bonding states of water in the vicinity of hydrogels (soft contact lenses). In this method, we apply force to hydrated contact lenses to deform them and to modulate the ratio between the signals from bulk and vicinal regions. We then collect spectra at different forces. Finally, we extracted the spectra of the vicinal region using the multivariate curve resolution-alternating least square (MCR-ALS) method. We report the hydration states depending on the chemical structures of hydrogels constituting the contact lenses.

Keywords: infrared absorption spectroscopy; molecular vibration; soft contact lenses; water; multivariate curve resolution; hydrogel; soft material

Citation: Maeda, S.; Chikami, S.; Latag, G.V.; Song, S.; Iwakiri, N.; Hayashi, T. Analysis of Vicinal Water in Soft Contact Lenses Using a Combination of Infrared Absorption Spectroscopy and Multivariate Curve Resolution. *Molecules* **2022**, *27*, 2130. https://doi.org/10.3390/molecules27072130

Academic Editors: Roumiana Tsenkova and Jelena Muncan

Received: 17 February 2022
Accepted: 23 March 2022
Published: 25 March 2022

1. Introduction

Water in the vicinity of material surfaces has been studied in many systems since it has significant impacts on various interfacial phenomena such as chemical reaction, adsorption, friction, and adhesion [1,2]. In the field of biomaterials, water at biomaterial surfaces plays a critical role in determining the response to protein molecules, cells, and tissues [3–5]. Soft contact lenses are biodevices consisting of polymer hydrogels that contain water molecules inside and also on their surfaces [6–8]. Thus, the structure of water in the vicinities of soft contact lenses (SCLs) has been widely studied by a lot of methods, such as sum-frequency generation spectroscopy (SFG) and infrared spectroscopy (IR) [9,10]. However, the OH stretching signal of the vicinal water, which is present at the interface between materials and water, is not accurately and selectively analyzed by conventional methods. For example, sum-frequency generation (SFG) spectroscopy enables us to measure the molecules only in the region where the inversion symmetry is broken. However, it cannot measure the whole interfacial region with several layers of interfacial molecules. As for attenuated total reflection (ATR) infrared (IR) absorption spectroscopy, it measures both interface and bulk regions due to the long evanescent field's decay length (several hundred nm) [11,12]. Therefore, a method is required to analyze structures of vicinal water, whose property is different from bulk [13,14].

Here, we apply the algorithm of multivariate curve resolution-alternating least squares (MCR-ALS) to resolve overlapping OH stretching signals of water molecules into two components, namely bulk and vicinal water. MCR-ALS is a model-free or soft-modeling method that extracts pure component contributions from multicomponent components [15]. All that is needed to perform an analysis with MCR-ALS is matrix data of raw measurement results that contain a mixture of the components. MCR-ALS can provide information on the concentration and spectral profile of each component. Thus far, MCR-ALS has been successfully used to analyze data obtained from a variety of analytical techniques, including mass spectrometry [16–18], spectroscopic techniques [10,19,20], and cyclic voltammetry [21–23].

In this study, a straightforward method for measuring the vibrational spectra of the vicinal water of water-containing soft materials, such as SCLs, has been developed by combining attenuated total reflection-infrared spectroscopy (ATR-IR) with controlled pressure and the MCR-ALS method. Multiple ATR-IR spectra with varying signal ratios of bulk and vicinal water were obtained through dehydrating the SCLs by changing the pressure applied to the SCLs. Using the MCR-ALS method to the ATR-IR spectra of water in the vicinity of SCLs, the OH stretching signals were resolved into two components (i.e., bulk and vicinal water). We attempted the comparison of the spectra of the vicinal water of four different SCLs. This comparison shows that the difference in spectra depends on the composition of the materials that compose the SCLs. Moreover, it was found that there is a material dependence of the spectra of vicinal water. In this paper, we also discussed the relationship between the degree of fouling and the spectral shapes of the vicinal water in poly(hydroxyethyl methacrylate) (PHEMA)-based SCLs and silicone-based SCLs.

2. Materials and Methods

2.1. *Soft Contact Lenses (SCLs)*

The SCLs analyzed in this work are summarized in Table 1. The SCLs (PHEMA-based) of nonionic and anionic hydrogel used for were omafilcon A (Group II) and ocufilcon D (Group IV), commercially available as Proclear® 1 day (CooperVision Inc., San Ramon, CA, USA) and Menicon® 1 DAY (Menicon Co., Ltd., Nagoya, Japan), respectively. In addition, the SCLs (silicone-based) of nonionic hydrogel (Group V) used were delefilcon A and somofilcon A, commercially available as DAILIES TOTAL 1® (Alcon Inc., Geneva, Switzerland) and clariti® 1 day (CooperVision Inc., San Ramon, CA, USA), respectively.

Table 1. SCLs used in the experiments.

Trade Name	USAN Name	FDA Category (Group)	Constituent Monomers
Proclear® 1 day	omafilcon A	II	HEMA, MPC
Menicon® 1 DAY	ocufilcon D	IV	HEMA, MAA
DAILIES TOTAL 1®	delefilcon A	V	silane, NNDMAA
clariti® 1 day	somofilcon A	V	silane, NVP

USAN = U.S. Adopted Names; FDA = Food and Drug Administration; Group II = high water (≥50%), nonionic; Group IV = high water (≥50%), ionic; Group V = silicone-based; HEMA = hydroxyethyl methacrylate, MPC = 2-Methacryloyloxyethyl phosphorylcholine, MAA = methacrylic acid, NNDMAA = N,N-dimethylacrylamide; NVP = N-vinylpyrrolidone.

2.2. *Attenuated Total Reflection—Infrared Spectroscopy (ATR-IR)*

The IR absorption spectra of hydrated SCLs were measured by Fourier-transform infrared (FTIR) absorption spectrometer (FT/IR-4600, JASCO Inc., Tokyo, Japan) equipped with a diamond prism for an ATR configuration. The measurements were performed at room temperature, and the measurement chamber was constantly purged by pure nitrogen gas. The intensity of the evanescent field generated in the vicinity of the prism surface decreases exponentially away from the surface. The decay length of the evanescent wave, d is expressed as Equation (1):

$$d = \frac{\lambda}{2\pi n_1 \sqrt{\sin^2\theta - \left(\frac{n_2}{n_1}\right)^2}} \quad (1)$$

where n_1, n_2, λ, and θ are the refractive indices of the diamond prism and sample, the wavelength of the infrared light, and the incident angle, respectively. All spectra were collected in the regions from 4000 to 500 cm^{-1} with a resolution of 4 cm^{-1}, and 300 spectra were averaged to acquire a final spectrum. In this work, we focus on the region between 3800 and 2800 cm^{-1} (region of OH stretching mode), where the theoretical penetration depth ranges between 416.3 and 570.0 nm.

The background spectrum on the prism without the solution was taken first, and then 10 µL of the filling solution was put onto the prism to obtain the spectrum of the bulk water. After that, a piece of the SCLs cut into 5 × 5 mm^2 surrounded by a plastic wall was placed in the solution on the prism, then the pressure-controlled ATR-IR measurements were performed by pressing down the SCLs with a plate from the top, shown in Figure 1. In this configuration (Figure 1), we can minimize the drying of the SCLs during the measurements. In that case, the ATR-IR spectra include three different signal components, i.e., (i) bulk, (ii) water near the polymer networks of the SCLs (vicinal water), and (iii) interfacial water between the prism and SCLs. The contribution of (i) decreases, whereas the contribution of (ii) increases when the pressure to hold down the SCLs is increased due to dehydration of SCLs (Figure 2). The ATR-IR spectra, which consist of bulk and the vicinal water between the SCLs and the prism, were collected t at different pressures [Pressure 1 to Pressure 4 (ranging between 26 and 157 kPa), with the latter having the highest pressure exerted]. We optimized the applying pressure to avoid irreversible damage to the SCLs through this process. We checked that there is no damage to the SCLs from the recovery of the shape of the SCLs by optical microscopy and the reproducibility of the ATR-IR spectra.

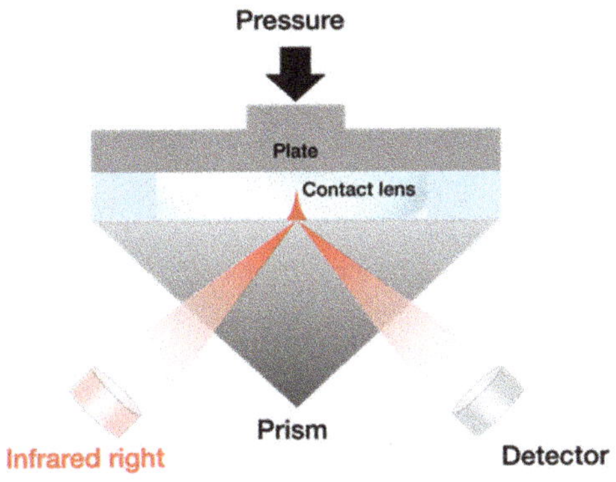

Figure 1. Schematic illustration of the pressure-controlled ATR-IR method.

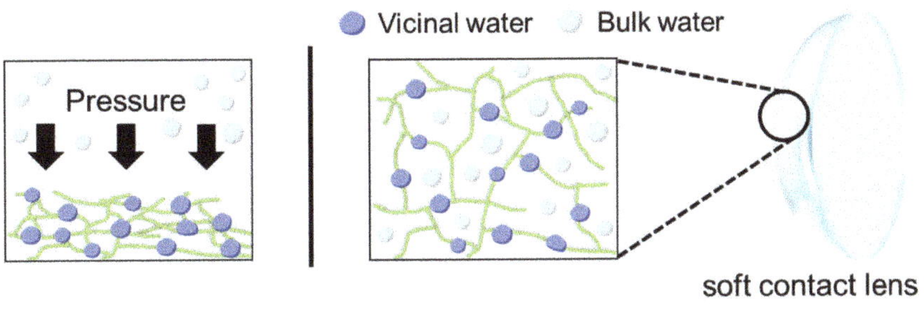

Figure 2. The dehydration process of SCLs by applying pressure.

2.3. Multivariate Curve Resolution—Alternating Least Squares (MCR-ALS)

The MCR-ALS process was performed in two steps with MATLAB 2021b using the MCR-ALS package developed by Jaumot et al. [24,25]. The data of all ATR-IR spectra in the region between 3800 and 2800 cm^{-1} (OH stretching band) were imported into MATLAB. The initial estimation was calculated by a principal component analysis to separate the spectrum into two pure components at the first step of the MCR-ALS method with the non-negativity restrictions. At the second step of the MCR-ALS process, the difference spectra were calculated to remove the components of (iii). The data from the calculation of the difference spectra can be arranged in a data matrix **D** ($r \times c$), the r rows of which are the number of the difference spectra and the c columns of which are the number of absorbance wavelengths. The MCR-ALS decomposition of matrix **D** is carried out according to Equation (2):

$$\mathbf{D} = \mathbf{C}\mathbf{S}^T + \mathbf{E} \tag{2}$$

where **C** ($r \times n$), $\mathbf{S^T}$ ($n \times r$), and **E** ($r \times c$) are the matrix that describes how the n chemical species' contribution in the spectroscopically active process varies in the different r rows of the data matrix, the matrix that describes how the spectra of n species changes in the c columns of the data matrix (pure spectra profiles) estimated by the initial estimation in the first step of the MCR-ALS method, and the residuals matrix with the data variance that cannot be explained by the product $\mathbf{CS^T}$, respectively. This relationship is shown in Figure 3. The bulk and vicinal water spectra were estimated from the initial estimation analysis in this study. Then, we apply the MCR-ALS method to extract spectra of two components from the difference spectra of mixtures of bulk water and vicinal water.

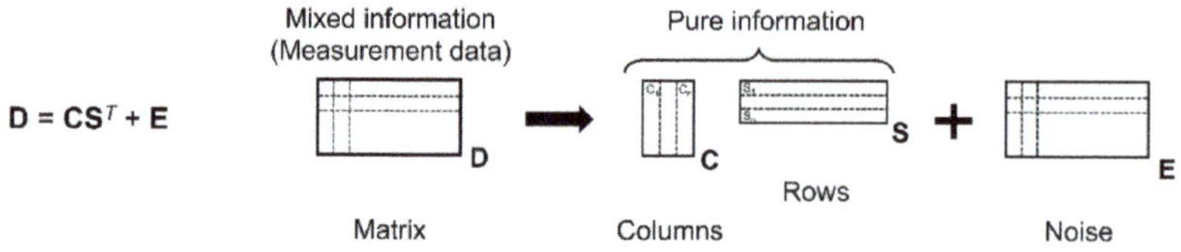

Figure 3. A principle of multivariate curve resolution (MCR).

3. Results and Discussion

Figure 4a displays typical ATR-IR spectra of contact lenses in the whole measurement range with applying pressure 4 (157 kPa). Depending on the monomers constituting the SCLs, the spectral shapes in the fingerprint region (1500–500 cm^{-1}) are different. Figure 4b shows the spectra measured under different pressure (clariti® 1 day). With increasing the pressure (Pressure 1 to Pressure 4), the signal in the fingerprint region increases, whereas the intensity in the O-H stretching region decreases. This indicates that the application of pressure induces the dehydration of SCLs in the measuring region. Figure 4c shows the spectra in the OH stretching region under different pressure (clariti® 1 day). Together with the decrease in the intensity, the spectral shape also changed, indicating that the ratio between the vicinal and bulk water changes depending on the applying pressure. As the applied pressure increased, the dehydration of SCLs progressed.

We applied the MCR-ALS method to the spectra in the OH stretching region to separate the spectral components of bulk and vicinal water. Figure 5a displays the results of ATR-IR spectra, and Figure 5b displays the concentration of bulk and vicinal water obtained by the MCR-ALS method. We successfully resolved the overlapping ATR-IR spectra of bulk and vicinal water. The peaks in the region between 2900 and 3000 cm^{-1} are assigned to CH stretching modes. Since these modes are not included in the spectrum of bulk water, these modes are extracted together with the components of the vicinal water in the MCR-ALS process.

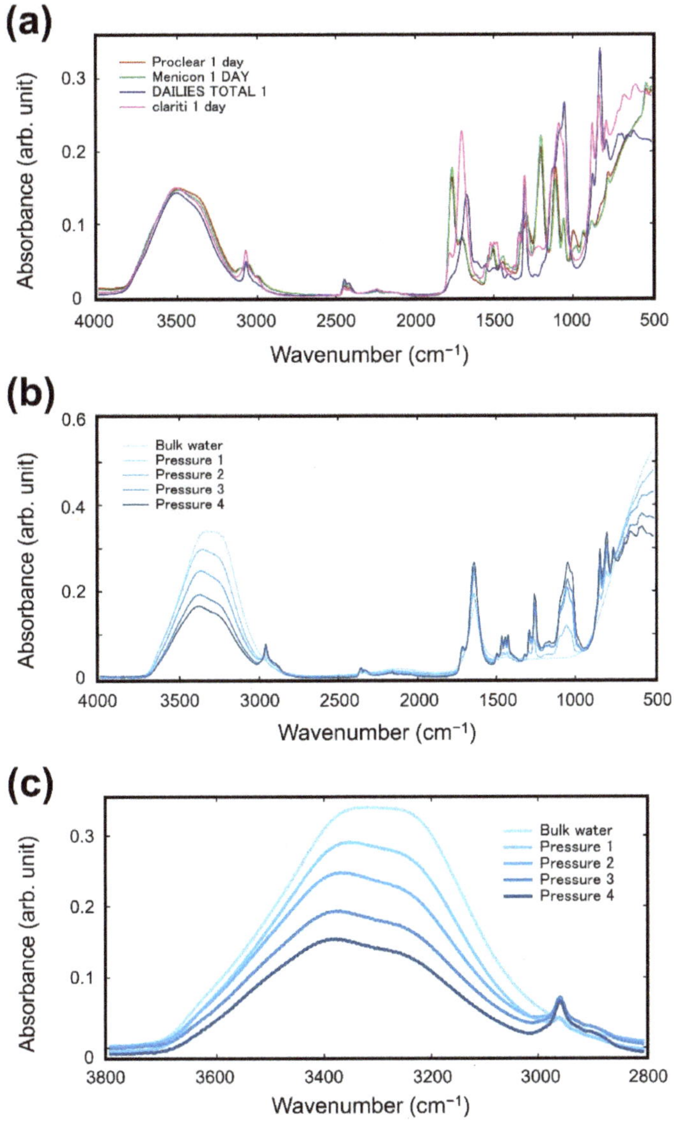

Figure 4. (**a**) ATR-IR spectra of the SCLs in the whole measuring range with applying pressure 4; (**b**) ATR-IR spectra in the whole measurement region under different pressures. (clariti® 1 day) (**c**) ATR-IR spectra in the region of the OH stretching band under different pressures (clariti® 1 day).

The MCR-ALS process also provides the ratio of the components (in this case bulk and vicinal water). Figure 5b showed that the ratio of the vicinal water increases, whereas that of bulk water decreased with the increase of the pressure, which is reasonable considering the process of dehydration under the application of pressure.

Figure 6 shows the spectra of bulk water and vicinal water of each sample in the OH stretching region. The spectra in the OH stretching region reflect the state of hydrogen bonding states of the vicinal water determined by water–water and water–SCLs interactions. The spectra of the vicinal water of PHEMA- and silicone-based SCLs were different from that of bulk water. This indicates that the hydrogen bonding state of the vicinal water is different from that of bulk water due to the water-SCLs interaction.

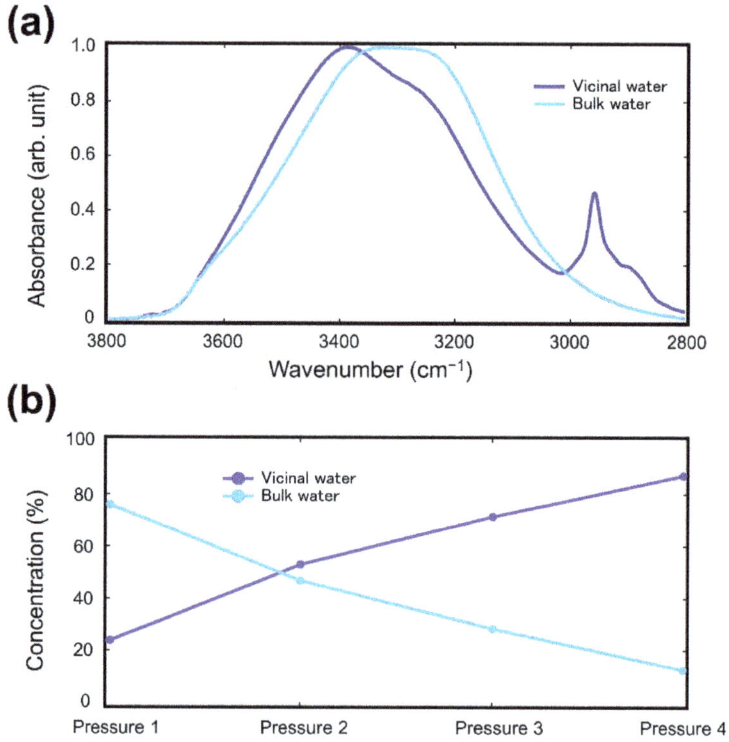

Figure 5. The results of (**a**) ATR-IR spectra and (**b**) concentration ratio by MCR-ALS analysis (clariti® 1 day).

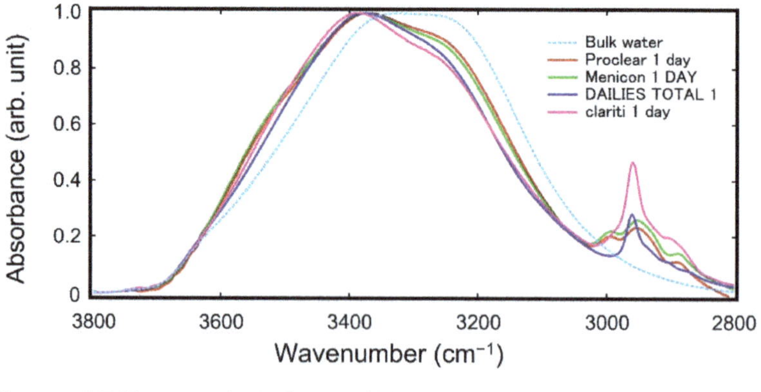

Figure 6. ATR-IR spectra of vicinal water of SCLs in the OH stretching region obtained by the MCR-ALS method. Proclear 1 day and Menicon 1 DAY are PHEMA-based SCLs, and DAILIES TOTAL 1 and clariti 1 day are silicone-based SCLs.

We performed the peak fitting to deconvolute the spectra into pure components to extract more information from these spectra. Figure 7 shows the results of the peak fitting of the spectra of the vicinal water for PHEMA and silicone-based SCLs. For the fitting, we checked the second derivative of each spectrum to find the position of the peaks in the O-H stretching region. For all spectra, we found four major components at around 3200, 3400, 3500, and 3600 cm^{-1}, and we performed the fitting of the spectra with the four peaks by optimizing the positions of the peaks.

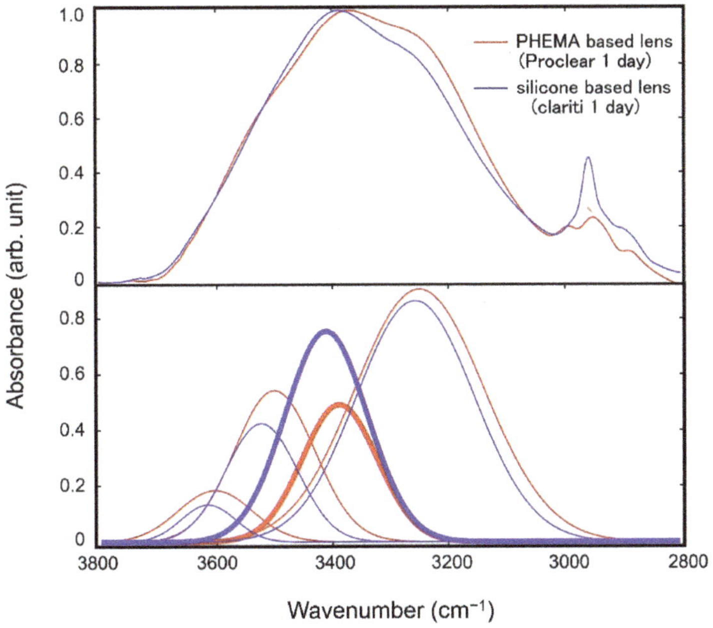

Figure 7. The results of the peak fitting of the spectra of the vicinal water for PHEMA (Proclear 1 day) and silicone-based (clarity® 1 day) SCLs. The peaks for the CH stretching modes in the region between 3000 and 2900 cm^{-1} were removed by assuming peaks for the modes in the fittings.

According to the previous works on the analyses of water in the vicinity of polymeric materials by IR absorption spectroscopy [12], water can be classified into three categories: water that is tightly hydrogen-bonded to polymers, water which is weakly bound to polymers, and water which has no hydrogen bond with polymers and has a bulk water-like structure. These three types in the classification are often denoted as non-freezing (strongly bound) (peak at around 3600 cm^{-1}), freezing bound (weakly bound) (3400 cm^{-1}), and freezing (free) (3200 cm^{-1}) water, respectively.

The most prominent difference is found for the intensity of freezing bound water at around 3400 cm^{-1}. Freezing bound water has flexible mobility and fewer water clusters than bulk water, playing an essential role in anti-fouling properties by acting as a water barrier when proteins and cells adsorb onto polymers [26–28]. Freezing bound water has been observed in blood compatible polymers such as poly(2-methoxyethyl acrylate) (PMEA), poly(ethyleneeglycol) (PEG), and poly(2-methacryloyloxyethyl phosphorylcholine) (PMPC) [12]. In general, it is well-known that the amounts of protein adsorbed on SCLs are less for silicon-based SCLs than PHEMA-based ones [8]. Our results show that the peak tops of the vicinal water spectra of silicone-based SCLs with higher protein resistance are at around 3400 cm^{-1}, indicating agreement with the above-mentioned previous findings on blood-compatible polymeric materials.

We are currently measuring the amount of protein adsorption on SCLs quantitatively and correlating the spectra of the vicinal water with the degree of the SCLs' protein resistance. Furthermore, we will also attempt to connect the water structure with the degree of amenity during the usage of SCLs since the vicinal water contributes to friction between an eye surface and SCLs.

4. Conclusions

In this work, we proposed a method to analyze the behavior of water in the vicinity of water-absorbing soft materials such as hydrogels by using conventional ATR-IR absorption spectroscopy by applying various pressures to modulate the ratio between interface and bulk components. Then, we extract these spectral components using the MCR-ALS method from the set of measured spectra. Our results showed that the spectral shapes of the OH-stretching band, which reflects the hydrogen bonding state of the vicinal water, are different depending on the chemical structure of polymers constituting contact lenses. We found that our method can effectively explore the hydration states of materials functioning in water, such as porous materials, hollow fibers, and other soft materials.

The modulation to the ratio of vicinal and bulk components is not limited to the pressure used in this work. When we employ the ATR-IR configuration, the concentration of samples or the surface-prism distance can be possible modulation to change the ratio between bulk and interface components. We are currently evaluating various interfaces using these modulations, which will be published elsewhere.

Author Contributions: Conceptualization, T.H. and N.I.; methodology, S.M., S.S. and T.H.; software, S.M., S.C., S.S, G.V.L. and T.H.; writing—original draft preparation, S.M., G.V.L. and T.H.; writing—review and editing, N.I. and T.H.; project administration, T.H. All authors have read and agreed to the published version of the manuscript.

Funding: This work was supported by the JSPS KAKENHI grant (Grant Number JP21H05511, JP20H05210, and JP19H02565). This work was performed under the "Five-star Alliance" Research Program in "NJRC Mater. & Dev.".

Institutional Review Board Statement: Not applicable.

Informed Consent Statement: Not applicable.

Data Availability Statement: Our research activities are summarized in http://lab.spm.jp/.

Acknowledgments: We thank Kazue Taki for the administration of this project.

Conflicts of Interest: The authors declare no conflict of interest.

References

1. Björneholm, O.; Hansen, M.H.; Hodgson, A.; Liu, L.M.; Limmer, D.T.; Michaelides, A.; Pedevilla, P.; Rossmeisl, J.; Shen, H.; Tocci, G.; et al. Water at interfaces. *Chem. Rev.* **2016**, *116*, 7698–7726. [CrossRef] [PubMed]
2. Hayashi, T. Water at interfaces: Its Behavior and Roles in Interfacial Phenomena. *Chem. Lett.* **2021**, *50*, 1173–1180. [CrossRef]
3. Vogler, E.A. Structure and reactivity of water at biomaterial surfaces. *Adv. Colloid Interface Sci.* **1998**, *74*, 69–117. [CrossRef]
4. Patel, A.; Mequanint, K. Hydrogel biomaterials. In *Biomedical Engineering—Frontiers and Challenges*; Reza, F.R., Ed.; In Tech: London, UK, 2011; pp. 275–296.
5. Ratner, B.D.; Latour, R.A. Role of water in biomaterials. In *Biomaterials Science*; Academic Press: Cambridge, MA, USA, 2020; pp. 77–82.
6. Garrett, Q.; Laycock, B.; Garrett, R.W. Hydrogel lens monomer constituents modulate protein sorption. *Investig. Ophthalmol. Vis. Sci.* **2000**, *41*, 1687–1695.
7. Garrett, Q.; Garrett, R.W.; Milthorpe, B.K. Lysozyme sorption in hydrogel contact lenses. *Investig. Ophthalmol. Vis. Sci.* **1999**, *40*, 897–903.
8. Luensmann, D.; Jones, L. Protein deposition on contact lenses: The past, the present, and the future. *Contact Lens Anterior Eye* **2012**, *35*, 53–64. [CrossRef]
9. Kim, S.H.; Opdahl, A.; Marmo, C.; Somorjai, G.A. AFM and SFG studies of pHEMA-based hydrogel contact lens surfaces in saline solution: Adhesion, Friction, and the Presence of Non-Crosslinked Polymer Chains at the Surface. *Biomaterials* **2002**, *23*, 1657–1666. [CrossRef]
10. Ahmed, M.; Singh, A.K.; Mondal, J.A. Hydrogen-bonding and vibrational coupling of water in a hydrophobic hydration shell as observed by Raman-MCR and isotopic dilution spectroscopy. *Phys. Chem. Chem. Phys.* **2016**, *18*, 2767–2775. [CrossRef]
11. Nagasawa, D.; Azuma, T.; Noguchi, H.; Uosaki, K.; Takai, M. Role of interfacial water in protein adsorption onto polymer brushes as studied by sfg spectroscopy and QCM. *J. Phys. Chem. C* **2015**, *119*, 17193–17201. [CrossRef]

12. Morita, S.; Tanaka, M.; Ozaki, Y. Time-resolved in situ ATR-IR observations of the process of sorption of water into a poly (2-methoxyethyl acrylate) film. *Langmuir* **2007**, *23*, 3750–3761. [CrossRef]
13. Bai, M.Y.; Ku, F.Y.; Shyu, J.F.; Hayashi, T.; Wu, C.C. Evaluation of polyacrylonitrile nonwoven mats and silver-gold bimetallic nanoparticle-decorated nonwoven mats for potential promotion of wound healing In Vitro and In Vivo and bone growth In Vitro. *Polymers* **2021**, *13*, 516. [CrossRef] [PubMed]
14. Leng, C.; Sun, S.; Zhang, K.; Jiang, S.; Chen, Z. Molecular level studies on interfacial hydration of zwitterionic and other antifouling polymers in situ. *Acta Biomater.* **2016**, *40*, 6–15. [CrossRef] [PubMed]
15. Ardila, J.A.; Funari, C.S.; Andrade, A.M.; Cavalheiro, A.J.; Carneiro, R.L. Cluster analysis of commercial samples of Bauhinia spp. using HPLC-UV/PDA and MCR-ALS/PCA without peak alignment procedure. *Phytochem. Anal.* **2015**, *26*, 367–373. [CrossRef] [PubMed]
16. Pere-Trepat, E.; Lacorte, S.; Tauler, R. Solving liquid chromatography mass spectrometry coelution problems in the analysis of environmental samples by multivariate curve resolution. *J. Chromatogr. A* **2005**, *1096*, 111–122. [CrossRef]
17. Dantas, C.; Tauler, R.; Miguel, M.; Ferreira, C. Exploring In Vivo violacein biosynthesis by application of multivariate curve resolution on fused UV-VIS absorption, fluorescence, and liquid chromatography-mass spectrometry data. *Anal. Bioanal. Chem.* **2013**, *405*, 1293–1302. [CrossRef]
18. Sinanian, M.M.; Cook, D.W.; Rutan, S.C.; Wijesinghe, D.S. Multivariate curve resolution-alternating least squares analysis of high-resolution liquid chromatography-mass spectrometry data. *Anal. Chem.* **2016**, *88*, 11092–11099. [CrossRef]
19. Spegazzini, N.; Ruisanchez, I.; Larrechi, M.S. MCR-ALS for sequential estimation of FTIR-ATR spectra to resolve a curing process using global phase angle convergence criterion. *Anal. Chim. Acta* **2009**, *642*, 155–162. [CrossRef]
20. Bortolato, S.A.; Olivieri, A.C. Chemometric processing of second-order liquid chromatographic data with UV-Vis and fluorescence detection. A comparison of multivariate curve resolution and parallel factor analysis 2. *Anal. Chim. Acta* **2014**, *842*, 11–19. [CrossRef]
21. Johnson, J.A.; Gray, J.H.; Rodeberg, N.T.; Wightman, R.M. Multivariate curve resolution for signal isolation from fast-scan cyclic voltammetric data. *Anal. Chem.* **2017**, *89*, 10547–10555. [CrossRef]
22. Diaz-Cruz, M.S.; Mendieta, J.; Tauler, R.; Esteban, M. Multivariate curve resolution of cyclic voltammetric data: Application to the Study of the Cadmium-Binding Properties of Glutathione. *Anal. Chem.* **1999**, *71*, 4629–4636. [CrossRef]
23. Torres, M.; Diaz-Cruz, J.M.; Arino, C.; Grabaric, B.S.; Tauler, R.; Esteban, M. Multivariate curve resolution analysis of voltammetric data obtained at different time windows: Study of the System Cd^{2+}–Nitrilotriacetic Acid. *Anal. Chim. Acta* **1998**, *371*, 23–37. [CrossRef]
24. Tauler, R. Multivariate curve resolution applied to second order data. *Chemom. Intell. Lab. Syst.* **1995**, *30*, 133–146. [CrossRef]
25. Jaumot, J.; Gargallo, R.; de Juan, A.; Tauler, R. A graphical user-friendly interface for MCR-ALS: A New Tool for Multivariate Curve Resolution in MATLAB. *Chemom. Intell. Lab. Syst.* **2005**, *76*, 101–110. [CrossRef]
26. Tanaka, M.; Hayashi, T.; Morita, S. The roles of water molecules at the biointerface of medical polymers. *Polym. J.* **2013**, *45*, 701–710. [CrossRef]
27. Tanaka, M.; Morita, S.; Hayashi, T. Role of interfacial water in determining the interactions of proteins and cells with hydrated materials. *Colloids Surf. B Biointerfaces* **2021**, *198*, 111449. [CrossRef]
28. Hayashi, T.; Tanaka, M.; Yamamoto, S.; Shimomura, M.; Hara, M. Direct observation of interaction between proteins and blood-compatible polymer surfaces. *Biointerphases* **2007**, *2*, 119–125. [CrossRef] [PubMed]

molecules

MDPI

Article

Intermolecular Interaction of Tetrabutylammonium and Tetrabutylphosphonium Salt Hydrates by Low-Frequency Raman Observation

Yasuhiro Miwa [1], Tomoki Nagahama [1], Harumi Sato [1], Atsushi Tani [1,*] and Kei Takeya [2]

[1] Graduate School of Human Development and Environment, Kobe University, 3-11 Tsurukabuto, Nada, Kobe 657-8501, Japan; 186d415d@stu.kobe-u.ac.jp (Y.M.); tomo.n.0820.shu@gmail.com (T.N.); hsato@tiger.kobe-u.ac.jp (H.S.)

[2] Institute for Molecular Science (IMS), 38 Nishigonaka, Myodaiji, Okazaki 444-8585, Japan; takeya@ims.ac.jp

* Correspondence: tani@carp.kobe-u.ac.jp

Abstract: Semi-clathrate hydrates are attractive heat storage materials because the equilibrium temperatures, located above 0 °C in most cases, can be changed by selecting guest cations and anions. The equilibrium temperatures are influenced by the size and hydrophilicity of guest ions, hydration number, crystal structure, and so on. This indicates that intermolecular and/or interionic interaction in the semi-clathrate hydrates may be related to the variation of the equilibrium temperatures. Therefore, intermolecular and/or interionic interaction in semi-clathrate hydrates with quaternary onium salts was directly observed using low-frequency Raman spectroscopy, a type of terahertz spectroscopy. The results show that Raman peak positions were mostly correlated with the equilibrium temperatures: in the semi-clathrate hydrates with higher equilibrium temperatures, Raman peaks around 65 cm^{-1} appeared at a higher wavenumber and the other Raman peaks at around 200 cm^{-1} appeared at a lower wavenumber. Low-frequency Raman observation is a valuable tool with which to study the equilibrium temperatures in semi-clathrate hydrates.

Keywords: semi-clathrate hydrate; intermolecular interaction; interionic interaction; low-frequency Raman; equilibrium temperature

Citation: Miwa, Y.; Nagahama, T.; Sato, H.; Tani, A.; Takeya, K. Intermolecular Interaction of Tetrabutylammonium and Tetrabutylphosphonium Salt Hydrates by Low-Frequency Raman Observation. *Molecules* **2022**, *27*, 4743. https://doi.org/10.3390/molecules27154743

Academic Editor: Stefano Materazzi

Received: 5 July 2022
Accepted: 20 July 2022
Published: 25 July 2022

1. Introduction

Semi-clathrate hydrate compounds formed from host water molecules and guest molecules have a similar structure to clathrate hydrate typified by methane hydrate. They have a hydrogen-bonded cage structure that surrounds a guest cation, and one of the water molecules is replaced with a guest anion. Due to having empty cages and mild formation conditions under atmospheric pressure (the equilibrium temperature is above 0 °C), semi-clathrate hydrates have potential for use in gas separation and storage as well as for latent heat storage materials [1–3]. In terms of practical use, semi-clathrate hydrates with greater gas storage capacity and phase change at an adaptive temperature are required [4,5], and it is desired to freely select the combination of ions as guest substances [6].

A large number of the guest substances, i.e., combinations of various cations and anions, have been reported [7–11]. Among them, tetrabutylammonium (TBA) salts and tetrabutylphosphonium (TBP) salts, which are quaternary onium salts, are well known as ionic guest substances. In tetrabutylammonium bromide (TBAB) semi-clathrate hydrate, bromide anions displace part of the host water molecules and form cage structures with them. Meanwhile, the butyl groups of TBA cations occupy four partially broken cages. A cage is composed of water molecules in several different patterns, and the total cage structure is defined by the combination of these cages. For this reason, even for the same guest substance, the crystal structure of semi-clathrate hydrate may differ depending on the cage structure of the surrounding water molecules. For example, TBAB hydrates have two main crystal structures depending on hydration number (TBAB·26H_2O and TBAB·38H_2O) with different equilibrium temperatures (12.0 and 9.5 °C) and dissociation enthalpies (150.7 and 219.4 kJ/mol), respectively [12,13]. In addition, the hydrates encapsulating guest substances with different combinations of TBA/TBP cations and halide anions (bromide/chloride) have inherent enthalpies and equilibrium temperatures; tetrabutylammonium chloride (TBAC) hydrate has a dissociation enthalpy of 156 kJ/mol and an equilibrium temperature of 15.1 °C [14], and tetrabutylphosphonium chloride (TBPC) hydrate has a dissociation enthalpy of 164.7 kJ/mol and an equilibrium temperature of 10.3 °C [15]. Tetrabutylphosphonium bromide (TBPB) hydrates also have two crystal structures depending on the hydration number (TBPB·32H_2O and TBPB·38H_2O) [16,17]. Their dissociation enthalpies are 184.0 kJ/mol for TBPB·32H_2O and 211.8 kJ/mol for TBPB·38H_2O, and their equilibrium temperatures are 9.1 and 9.2 °C, respectively [18].

Thus, the equilibrium temperature and the dissociation enthalpy are greatly different in each guest substance. The cause of the difference in the equilibrium temperature between anion species such as bromide and chloride ions is currently estimated to be the size of the ionic radius of the anion [19], that is, the size of the partial molar volume of the anion [20]. Though other inferences about the shape of the anion, the fit of the cation into the cage, and the hydrophilicity have also been considered as reasons for the differences in the equilibrium temperatures [6,8,10,21], no view to understand the difference in equilibrium temperatures from the intermolecular interactions between ions or between guest and host molecules has yet been formulated.

Intermolecular interactions are strongly associated with phase change materials because the change in the binding force directly affects the equilibrium temperatures of materials. The energy of this intermolecular interaction corresponds to the terahertz region (THz) between infrared waves and microwaves. In other words, spectroscopy in the THz region can reveal intermolecular interactions such as lateral and translational vibration binding energies instead of intramolecular bending and stretching vibrations which reflect the conformation of guest molecules. For example, several studies were conducted on the higher order structure of proteins, hydration of polymers, and discrimination of crystal polymorph of pharmaceutical products [22–24]. In general, the terahertz region often refers to the 0.1–10 THz range. Low-frequency Raman spectroscopy, known as a type of terahertz spectroscopy, used in this study, covered the region of 3.3–330 cm^{-1} (corresponding to 0.1–10 THz) below the fingerprint region. Practically, intermolecular interactions during phase change were investigated. For example, terahertz spectroscopic observation of carbamazepine revealed that intermolecular interaction changed during solid and glass transitions [25]. In the observation of the change in the low-frequency Raman spectra upon the melting of ion liquids, the structural change of the substances was discussed in terms of intermolecular binding strength [26]. These studies suggest that the direct observation of intermolecular binding forces in semi-clathrate hydrates could provide a correlation with equilibrium temperatures.

The simple structure of clathrate hydrates of Xe hydrate and tetrahydrofuran (THF) hydrate was investigated using low-frequency Raman spectroscopy [27–29]. They showed two Raman peaks at around 210 cm^{-1} and below 100 cm^{-1}. The peak around 210 cm^{-1} was attributed to the host water framework. The other peak below 100 cm^{-1} was related to the localized anharmonic motions of guest atoms and host lattice phonons, which was discussed in Xe hydrate. In addition, molecular dynamics simulation for methane hydrate estimated the degree of rotation and vibration as translational rattling motions of molecules in the low-frequency region [30]. According to these studies, intermolecular interactions, especially between guest/guest or guest/host molecules in semi-clathrate hydrates, mainly appeared near or below 100 cm^{-1}. Nevertheless, semi-clathrate hydrates below 100 cm^{-1} were not investigated, although the Raman spectra of genuine clathrate hydrates were observed below 100 cm^{-1} as described above. In addition, Raman measurements of semi-clathrate hydrates in the THz region of 100–300 cm^{-1} were performed only for TBAB hydrate [31]. Therefore, we investigated the low-frequency Raman spectra, particularly of less than 300 cm^{-1} with several quaternary onium salts and their semi-clathrate hydrates to reveal the intermolecular interaction between guest/guest and guest/host molecules that may have a considerable influence on the equilibrium temperatures.

2. Results and Discussion

2.1. Semi-Clathrate Hydrates, Clathrate Hydrates, and Ice

Figure 1 shows the Raman spectra at 263 K in the 15–300 cm^{-1} region of TBAB hydrate (hydration number was 26), THF hydrate and ice with H_2O or D_2O. This spectral region contains common or unique features among semi-clathrate hydrate, clathrate hydrate, and ice, all of which are composed of water molecule networks. In the region from 100–300 cm^{-1}, the TBAB hydrate (H_2O) had an apparent peak at 261 cm^{-1} and a broad one around 191 cm^{-1}. The peak at 261 cm^{-1} is related to TBA cations and the peak around 191 cm^{-1} is attributed to the intermolecular hydrogen stretching O-O vibration mode, which is in good agreement with the previous Raman investigations [31,32]. TBAB hydrate (D_2O) revealed a peak at 261 cm^{-1} which was the same position of the TBAB hydrate (H_2O) and a peak around 189 cm^{-1} which was slightly shifted to a lower wavenumber from 191 cm^{-1} in TBAB hydrate (H_2O). On the other hand, THF hydrate and ice showed a peak around 200 cm^{-1}, reflecting the O-O vibration mode [28]. The peaks in THF hydrate were observed at 208 cm^{-1} for the H_2O hydrate and 203 cm^{-1} for the D_2O hydrate and the peaks in ice were observed at 214 cm^{-1} for H_2O ice and 208 cm^{-1} for D_2O ice. The peaks in all the deuterated samples around 200 cm^{-1} shifted to a lower wavenumber. The peak around 191 cm^{-1} in TBAB hydrate was much broader than that in THF hydrate and ice. These results indicate that the peak position and broadness of O-O vibration modes apparently depend on the materials with hydrogen-bonded networks and their hydrogen isotope in water molecules.

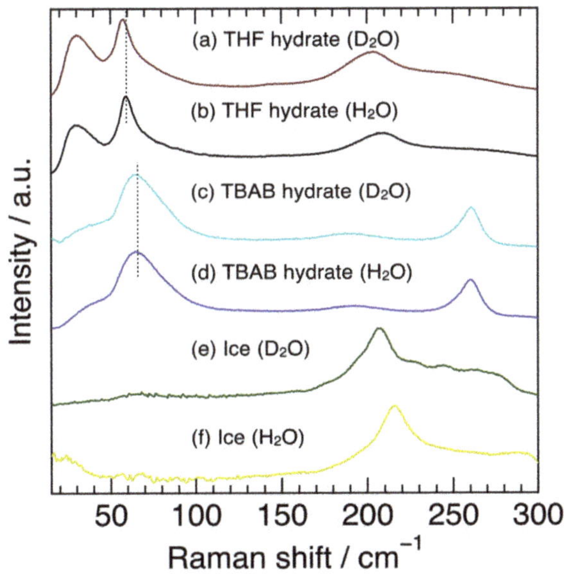

Figure 1. Raman spectra for THF hydrate, TBAB hydrate, and ice with H_2O or D_2O. The dotted vertical lines around 65 cm^{-1} from (a–d) were used to make it easier to see a peak shift.

In the region below 100 cm^{-1}, TBAB hydrate (H_2O) had a broad peak around 67 cm^{-1} and THF hydrate (H_2O) had a sharp peak at 59 cm^{-1}, although no clear peak was observed in ice. The sharp peak of THF hydrate was attributed to the host water framework in structure-II clathrate hydrate [28]. The Raman and inelastic neutron scattering (INS) spectra of Xe hydrate (Structure-I) also have a similar peak at 60 cm^{-1}, which is considered to be based on the water framework [27]. Furthermore, the Raman spectrum of liquid water shows weak peaks at 53 and 73 cm^{-1} [33]. Isotope effects on the peak position were also observed in THF hydrate (59.0 cm^{-1} for the H_2O hydrate and 57.4 cm^{-1} for the D_2O hydrate), while they were not clearly observed in TBAB hydrate. Though the broader peak in TBAB hydrate might mask the isotope effect, the peak in TBAB hydrate may be attributed to not only the water framework but also to other factors. Subbotin et al. reported that the phonon density of states in this region was different between semi-clathrate hydrate and genuine clathrate hydrate [34]. Furthermore, the shift of the peak position around 67 cm^{-1} was not observed between 173 K and 273 K, although the peak near 191 cm^{-1}, intermolecular hydrogen stretching O-O vibration mode, shifted to a higher wavenumber with decreasing temperature. These results reinforce that factors other than the water molecule framework itself affected the characteristics of the peak around 67 cm^{-1} in TBAB hydrate.

The Raman spectra of tetrabutylammonium and tetrabutylphosphonium salts and their hydrates (H_2O) are summarized in Figure 2. For the spectra of the hydrates, single peak spectra around 65 cm^{-1} were simulated by fitting and are indicated in Figure 2.

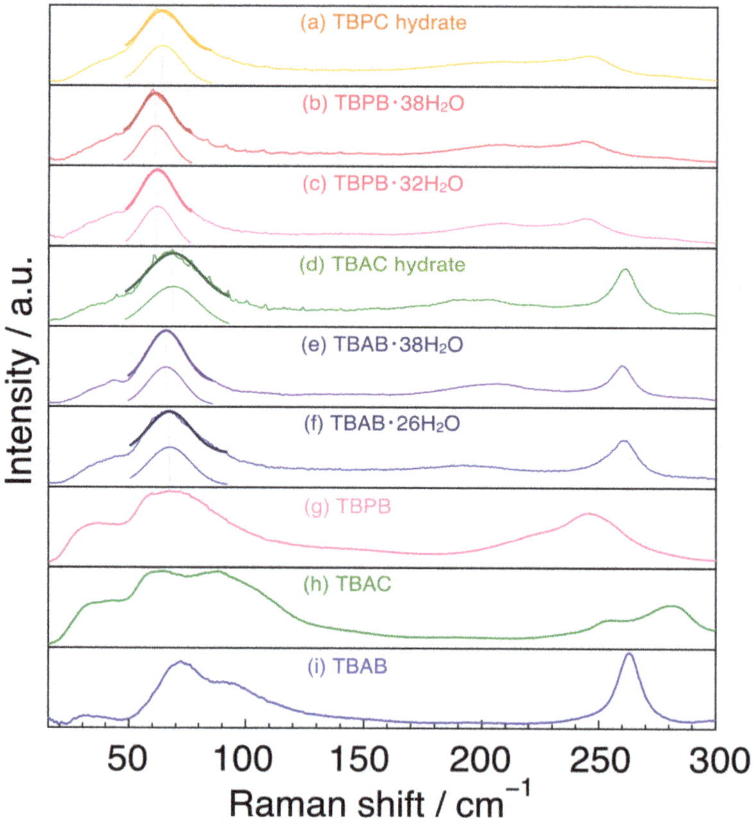

Figure 2. Raman spectra for tetrabutylammonium and tetrabutylphosphonium salts and their hydrates. (a) TBPC hydrate; (b) TBPB·38H_2O; (c) TBPB·32H_2O; (d) TBAC hydrate; (e) TBAB·38H_2O; (f) TBAB·26H_2O; (g) TBPB; (h) TBAC and (i) TBAB. The solid thick lines around 65 cm^{-1} are single peak spectra simulated by fitting.

2.2. Tetrabutylammonium and Tetrabutylphosphonium Salts

First, we focused on the spectra of the three salts. In the region of 150–300 cm^{-1}, TBAB had only one peak at 263 cm^{-1}, whereas TBPB and TBAC had two peaks at around 220 cm^{-1} and at 247 cm^{-1} in TBPB and at 255 and 280 cm^{-1} in TBAC. In the 50–150 cm^{-1} region, undistinguished peaks were observed in all the salt samples. TBAB had a main peak at 71 cm^{-1} and another peak around 92 cm^{-1} with about half of the intensity of the main peak. These two peaks had a similar line width. TBAC had broad peaks around 59 and 83 cm^{-1} together with a smaller peak at around 110 cm^{-1}, and TBPB had broad peak(s) around 68 cm^{-1}.

The two main peaks in TBAC were a little far apart from each other in comparison with those in TBAB and TBPB, which was possibly caused by the mobility of anion [35]. Besides, the peak intensity around 83 cm^{-1} in TBAC was comparatively large rather than that around 92 cm^{-1} in TBAB, which was also considered to be due to the difference of anions. Similar trends were also observed in the THz infrared absorption spectra in the liquid state of TBAB and TBAC [36]. Quantum calculations for TBAB in this wavenumber region revealed four main infrared active peaks at 46, 57, 80, and 93 cm^{-1} and corresponding Raman active peaks at similar positions [37]. In comparison with the simulated Raman peaks, the peak positions observed in this study were slightly shifted to lower wavenumber in all cases. It is noteworthy that the clearly visible peak around 70 cm^{-1} was attributed to the translation of the anion along with a degree of flexing and rotation of the alkyl chains, related to the cation–anion interaction [37].

2.3. Tetrabutylammonium and Tetrabutylphosphonium Salt Hydrates: Around 240–265 cm^{-1}

In the range of 240–265 cm^{-1}, TBAB and TBAC hydrates had a sharp peak at 261 cm^{-1}, whereas TBPB and TBPC hydrates had a broad peak around 245 cm^{-1}. The peak in TBA hydrates was attributed to a stretching lattice vibration mode in the cation [38], indicating that the peak in TBP hydrates is caused by the same motion. The sharp peak of the TBA ion may be due to the fact that the TBA ion has only a trans conformation, while the TBP ion has both trans and gauche conformations, as reported by Kobori et al. who investigated the conformations in the comparison of tetrabutylphosphonium hydroxide (TBPOH) hydrate and tetrabutylammonium fluoride (TBAF) hydrate [20]. In addition, Muromachi et al. [17] reported that TBP ions distorted the cage structure by pushing the cage more strongly than TBA ions because of the larger bond length between carbon and phosphonium than that between carbon and nitrogen. This is another reason for the broader peak observed in TBP hydrate.

2.4. Tetrabutylammonium and Tetrabutylphosphonium Salt Hydrates: Around 200 cm^{-1}

All peaks were weak and broad in comparison with those in the THF hydrate and ice as shown in Figure 1. Peak tops appeared at 193 cm^{-1} for TBAB·26H_2O, 195 cm^{-1} for TBAC hydrate, 203 cm^{-1} for TBAB·38H_2O, 205 cm^{-1} for TBPC hydrate, 208 cm^{-1} for both TBPB·32H_2O and TBPB·38H_2O. The peak positions of the TBA salt hydrates were at a lower wavenumber than those of the TBP ones. Besides, the TBAB hydrate with higher hydration number (TBAB·38H_2O) had a peak at a higher wavenumber than TBAB·26H_2O, although TBPB hydrates with different hydration numbers had peaks at the same position. As described before, these peaks around 200 cm^{-1} were attributed to intermolecular hydrogen stretching O-O vibration mode. In comparison with the peaks in liquid water and solid ice, all peaks in the semi-clathrate hydrates were observed between the peaks of liquid water (175 cm^{-1}) and solid ice (213 cm^{-1}) [33,39].

The differences in the peak positions were first considered in terms of the bonding distance of the water framework. The neighbor distance between oxygen atoms in water molecules was obtained for the three following hydrates using the reported crystal structures [14,17,40]. The average O-O length is 2.76 Å for TBAB·38H_2O and TBPB·38H_2O, whereas it is 2.80 Å for TBAC·30H_2O, which is slightly longer than that in the bromide hydrates. The variation of the neighbor O-O length in TBAC hydrate was also larger than that in the two bromide hydrates. According to reference [41], the distribution of the O-O length in solid ice is concentrated between 2.7 and 2.8 Å with a maximum at 2.76 Å, whereas the distribution in liquid water is much broader (2.5–3.2 Å) with a longer average distance (2.81 Å). Though the average O-O lengths in these bromide hydrates were closer to that in the solid ice, the observed peaks in the hydrates appeared around 200 cm^{-1}, which is a lower wavenumber than for ice. Similarly, though the average O-O length in TBAC·30H_2O was closer to that in the liquid water, the observed peak was around 195 cm^{-1}, with a higher wavenumber than the liquid water peak. These results mean that this perspective is insufficient to explain the differences of the peak position around 200 cm^{-1} among the hydrates.

Then, we focused on the tetrahedrality of water molecules in the hydrates. The peak position in this region was reflected by the degree of deformation of the tetrahedral unit and the shift to a lower wavenumber indicated a deformation of the tetrahedral unit [42]. All the peaks in the hydrates were located at a lower wavenumber than that in solid ice, indicating that the tetrahedrality of water molecules deformed in the hydrates rather than in ice. In comparison with the TBA and TBP salt hydrates, peaks at lower wavenumbers in the TBA hydrates than in the TBP hydrates suggested that tetrahedrality was more deformed in the TBA hydrates. In particular, TBAB·26H_2O and TBAC hydrates, whose peaks were located below 200 cm^{-1}, could be highly deformed. The deformation of the tetrahedral units is considered to be related to the presence of soft hydrogen bonds, i.e., water-like hydrogen bonds [31]. This could be the reason why TBAB·26H_2O and TBAC hydrates had relatively higher equilibrium temperature.

The small difference in the peak positions near 200 cm^{-1} in the hydrates could be also affected by the charge distribution of onium ions because the motion of water molecules in the hydrates was influenced by the charge distribution. Based on molecular orbital simulation [21], the charge density on phosphonium was concentrated in the TBP ion rather than that of nitrogen in the TBA ion. In other words, the positive charge in the TBA ion was distributed compared to the TBP ion. This implies that the water molecules surrounding the center cation interact with phosphonium and move less easily in TBP hydrates. This may also cause the peaks near 200 cm^{-1}, at a relatively high wavenumber in the TBP hydrates.

All these results indicate that the vibrational peaks between water molecules in the hydrates could be used to discuss the water molecule network including influences by guest cations, although the intensity of the peaks themselves was smaller than that of ice or clathrate hydrate. In contrast, the effect of guest anions was less pronounced.

2.5. *Tetrabutylammonium and Tetrabutylphosphonium Salt Hydrates: Below 100 cm^{-1}*

The fitting results of the peak position around 65 cm^{-1} and their full width at half maximum (FWHM) in six semi-clathrate hydrates are summed up in Figure 3. The peaks of the TBA series are located at about 65–69 cm^{-1} and those of the TBP series at 61–64 cm^{-1}. The FWHM of the TBP series was relatively narrower than that of the TBA series. TBAC and TBPC hydrates had a wider FWHM than TBAB and TBPB hydrates, respectively. TBAB·26H_2O had a wider FWHM than TBAB·38H_2O, which is related to the lower hydration number. Similar results were observed in TBPB·32H_2O and TBPB·38H_2O. As discussed in Section 2.1, the peak around 65 cm^{-1} in TBAB·26H_2O was attributed to not only the water molecule framework but also other factors such as guest anions and cations. This is supported by the variation of the peak position and FWHM in six semi-clathrate hydrates as shown in Figure 3.

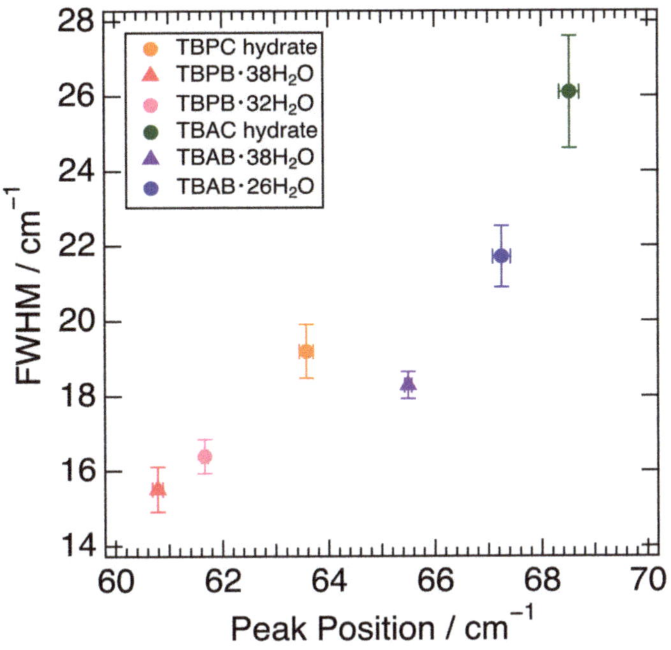

Figure 3. Relationship between peak position and FWHM in six semi-clathrate hydrates. Markers are explained in the legend.

Figure 3 shows that the differences in the peak positions largely depend on the cations. In the comparison of TBAB·38H_2O and TBPB·38H_2O, which have the same crystal structure and hydration number, the interionic distance of TBAB was 5.703 Å [40] and closer than that of TBPB, 5.837 Å [17]. This is one of the reasons why TBA salt hydrates have peaks at relatively higher wavenumbers. Although another reason may be a lower mass in the ammonium ion than in the phosphonium one, the difference is small and would not affect the peak position effectively. In addition, one of the more intriguing factors is the charge dispersion of the onium ions. As mentioned above, the charge distribution of TBA ions was relatively delocalized compared to that of TBP ions. This indicates that the cation–anion interaction was expected to be stronger in the TBA salt hydrates because a study on quaternary phosphonium/ammonium ionic liquids (ILs) showed that the cation–anion interaction was stronger in the dispersive ammonium ILs than in the phosphonium ILs [43]. This also causes the peaks in TBA salt hydrates at a comparatively higher wavenumber.

The influence of the anions may also have been observed in this region due to the mass of the anions; among the same cations, the hydrates with Cl ions showed peaks at a higher wavenumber than those with Br ions. The smaller ionic radius of the Cl ion is also responsible for the shorter interionic distance, which may affect the peak position at a higher wavenumber. Since the anions were incorporated into the water molecule network, the interionic interaction affected the stability of the cages. This implies that the peaks related to interionic interaction at a higher wavenumber are related to a higher equilibrium temperature. It is consistent with the fact that the hydrates with Cl ions have relatively high equilibrium temperatures among the same cations as shown in Section 1.

A peak shift to a low wavenumber was observed around 65 cm^{-1} in the hydrates in comparison with the salt samples. This peak shift was due to hydration, which is in agreement with several studies using the terahertz region [44,45]. The cations were isolated by the hydrogen bonding of water molecules, which increased the interionic distance and lowered the binding energy. In the case of TBAB, the interionic distance actually increased from 4.905 Å [46] for TBAB to 5.703 Å [40] for TBAB $38H_2O$. Another reason may be that hydration restricts the motion of the ions. Therefore, the spectra observed in the hydrates were generally similar without the significant differences observed between the ILs of TBAB and TBAC. The ratio of the average frequency of the peak positions in TBAB and TBAC ILs is 0.70 [36].

As for the differences in FWHM, crystal structures and hydration numbers affect the FWHM; tetragonal bromide hydrate, TBAB·$26H_2O$, expressed a wider peak than the orthorhombic hydrate, TBAB·$38H_2O$, and the hydrate with a lower hydration number, TBPB·$32H_2O$, had a wider peak than that with a higher hydration number, TBPB·$38H_2O$. This is probably due to the fact that the higher hydration number in the orthorhombic hydrates reduced the number of ionic guests per unit cell [8], i.e., the influence of cation–anion interactions. It was noted that the FWHM was even smaller for THF hydrate (clathrate hydrate), which had no ionic interaction as shown in Figure 1. For further investigation, a simulation study was necessary to clarify the main causes behind the differences in FWHM.

2.6. Raman Peaks and Equilibrium Temperatures in Semi-Clathrate Hydrates

Low-frequency Raman observation of the six semi-clathrate hydrates revealed the peak shift was related with interionic distance, hydration number, and guest ion species. We found the trend that for a higher hydration number, with bromide ion as an anion, and/or TBP ion as a cation, (a) Raman peaks of around 65 cm^{-1} shifted to a lower wavenumber, (b) Raman peaks around 200 cm^{-1} shifted to a higher wavenumber, and (c) Raman peaks around 65 cm^{-1} became narrower. The positions of these peaks were generally inversely correlated. This may be because the peak around 200 cm^{-1} mainly reflected the interaction between water molecules and the peak around 65 cm^{-1} mainly reflected the interaction between the ions.

Interestingly, in most cases of the semi-clathrate hydrates with a higher equilibrium temperature among all the samples, (a) Raman peaks of around 65 cm^{-1} appeared at a higher wavenumber and a (b) Raman peak around 200 cm^{-1} appeared at a lower wavenumber. This means that low-frequency Raman observations are valuable as a tool to study the equilibrium temperature in semi-clathrate hydrates. For further investigation from the physicochemical aspect, molecular simulation should be performed to understand the attribution of the peaks at the low-frequency region.

3. Materials and Methods

3.1. Preparation of Semi-Clathrate Hydrates

The chemicals used in this study are listed in Table 1. According to the previous reports, the aqueous solutions were prepared with a composition in the range of mass percent concentration w = 0.32–0.40 (w = 0.40 for TBAB·$26H_2O$ [12], w = 0.32 for TBAB·$38H_2O$ [13], w = 0.34 for TBAC hydrate [14], w = 0.37 for TBPB·$32H_2O$ [47], w = 0.30 for TBPB·$38H_2O$ [17], w = 0.36 for TBPC hydrate [15]) using ultrapure water. Once the initial crystal nuclei were formed by cooling the aqueous solutions at −20 °C, semi-clathrate hydrates were formed by maintaining the samples at 3 °C for at least 3 days. THF hydrate was also prepared as a reference of a genuine clathrate hydrate by the same procedure using an THF aqueous solution adjusted to w = 0.19. In addition, to observe the isotope effect, TBAB hydrate (hydration number was 26) and THF hydrates with D_2O were prepared according to the same procedure using the aqueous solutions with the same molar ratio as those of H_2O. The salt samples shown in Table 1 were also prepared by keeping them dry with nitrogen gas to avoid further hydration just before Raman measurements.

Table 1. Information on chemical compound.

Chemical Name	Source	Mass Fraction Purity
Tetrabutylammonium Bromide	Wako Pure Chemical Industries Ltd.	98+%
Tetrabutylammonium Chloride	Tokyo Chemical Industry Co., Ltd.	98%
Tetrabutylphosphonium Bromide	Wako Pure Chemical Industries Ltd.	95+%
Tetrabutylphosphonium Chloride	Iolitec Ionic Liquids Technologies GmbH	95+%
Ultrapure water	homemade by ADVANTEC RFU464TA	resistivity is 18.2 MΩ cm
Deuterium oxide	Cambridge Isotope Laboratories, Inc.	D, 99.9%

Two observation methods of Raman and equilibrium temperature were used to confirm the hydrate samples had the desired hydration number, especially for the different hydration numbers of TBAB hydrates ($26H_2O$ and $38H_2O$) and TBPB ones ($32H_2O$ and $38H_2O$). For TBAB hydrates, based on the previous studies on the ordinary Raman spectra of the hydrates [31], we confirmed the hydration number of 26 or 38. We observed slightly different spectra both in the C-H stretching modes of the butyl groups (2700–3050 cm^{-1}) and in CH_2 bending modes of the alkyl groups (around 1320 and 1455 cm^{-1}), which were comparable to those in the previous study [31]. For TBPB hydrates, we confirmed the hydration numbers using the equilibrium temperature observed by increasing the temperature of the thermostatic bath carefully, because no clear differences in the Raman spectra emerged. The other hydrates were also recognized as the desired semi-clathrate hydrates by the same method.

3.2. Low-Frequency Raman Measurements

For the Raman scattering study, the particle samples were placed into aluminum pans on the temperature control stage (THMS600, Linkam, Salfords, UK) with liquid nitrogen. The semi-clathrate hydrates were measured at a temperature in the range of 173–273 K. The THF hydrates and water ices were measured only at 263 K. The salt samples were measured at room temperature.

Low-frequency Raman measurements were performed using LabRAM HR Evolution (HORIBA, Kyoto, Japan). The wavenumber calibration was performed on a Si plate with a Raman line at 520.7 cm^{-1}. The spectral resolution was 0.5 cm^{-1} and wavelength of the laser was 532 nm. The laser beam had a power of about 100 mW. Scans were performed 10 times and the exposure time was 15 s. The background noise was separately acquired and subtracted from the original spectrum to obtain the Raman spectrum from the samples.

3.3. Spectrum Processing

For discussion, the observed spectrum was divided into two wavenumber ranges of below 100 cm^{-1} and 100–300 cm^{-1}. The common features of the peaks below 100 cm^{-1} in the semi-clathrate hydrates were a large broad peak at around 65 cm^{-1} and a tiny broad one below 50 cm^{-1}. The weak peak below 50 cm^{-1} appeared on the tilt background and showed no apparent peak top, meaning that it was difficult to identify the peak accurately. Therefore, we focused on the peak around 65 cm^{-1} in further discussions. To evaluate the peak position and FWHM, we assumed the constant base line from 47–50 cm^{-1} to 80–90 cm^{-1} to decrease the influence from the broad peak below 50 cm^{-1} and performed fitting with a single gaussian peak after subtraction with the base line. We attempted to evaluate peak position and FWHM with several different base lines, indicating that the peak position was the same whereas the FWHM was slightly changed. In all cases, we confirmed that the correlation of the FWHM with the samples did not change. Since these parameters depend on the fitting model, we considered the relative differences of the peak position and FWHM in the discussion. We postulated a gaussian peak for the peak around 65 cm^{-1} because a gaussian function was used for fitting the main peak in the spectral analysis of the low-wavenumber region in the case of alkylimidazolium-based ILs and alkylammonium-based ILs [36,48].

4. Conclusions

Low-frequency Raman observation was performed with tetrabutylammonium and tetrabutylphosphonium salt hydrates as well as tetrabutylammonium and tetrabutylphosphonium salts. The spectra revealed that Raman peaks appeared in three wavenumber regions. In the range of 240–265 cm^{-1}, Raman peaks due to a stretching lattice vibration mode in the cation were narrow and apparent in TBA salt hydrates and broad in TBP salt hydrates. In the range around 200 cm^{-1}, Raman peaks, attributed to the O-O stretching vibration between water molecules, appeared below 200 cm^{-1}, i.e., at a lower wavenumber in the TBAB·26H_2O and TBAC hydrate. In the range around 65 cm^{-1}, Raman peaks, affected by not only the water framework but the contribution of guest substances as well, were observed at a higher wavenumber in the TBAB·26H_2O and TBAC hydrate. The trends in the peak shift were opposite in these two peaks. Furthermore, these two hydrates with higher equilibrium temperatures suggested that the equilibrium temperature in the semi-clathrate hydrates was related with the peak positions of the peak around 65 cm^{-1} and 200 cm^{-1}. In designing a semi-clathrate hydrate, the direct observation of low-frequency Raman peaks could be used as an indicator of the equilibrium temperature of the hydrate.

Author Contributions: Conceptualization, Y.M. and A.T.; methodology, Y.M. and T.N.; formal analysis, Y.M.; investigation, Y.M.; resources, H.S.; writing—original draft preparation, Y.M.; writing—review and editing, A.T., H.S. and K.T.; visualization, Y.M.; supervision, A.T. and H.S.; project administration, A.T. and K.T.; funding acquisition, A.T. and K.T. All authors have read and agreed to the published version of the manuscript.

Funding: This research was funded by JSPS KAKENHI (JP17H06456 and JP17H03535) and by JST SPRING (JPMJFS2126).

Institutional Review Board Statement: Not applicable.

Informed Consent Statement: Not applicable.

Data Availability Statement: The data presented in this study are openly available in figshare at 10.6084/m9.figshare.20364387.v1.

Acknowledgments: This work was carried out by the joint research program of Molecular Photoscience Research Center, Kobe University (R03023; R04034).

Conflicts of Interest: The authors declare no conflict of interest.

References

1. Shimada, W.; Ebinuma, T.; Oyama, H.; Kamata, Y.; Takeya, S.; Uchida, T.; Nagao, J.; Narita, H. Separation of Gas Molecule Using Tetra-*n*-butyl Ammonium Bromide Semi-Clathrate Hydrate Crystals. *Jpn. J. Appl. Physics* **2003**, *42*, L129. [CrossRef]
2. Veluswamy, H.P.; Kumar, R.; Linga, P. Hydrogen storage in clathrate hydrates: Current state of the art and future directions. *Appl. Energy* **2014**, *122*, 112–132. [CrossRef]
3. Wang, X.; Dennis, M. Characterisation of thermal properties and charging performance of semi-clathrate hydrates for cold storage applications. *Appl. Energy* **2016**, *167*, 59–69. [CrossRef]
4. Schüth, F. Technology: Hydrogen and Hydrates. *Nature* **2005**, *434*, 712–713. [CrossRef] [PubMed]
5. Hashimoto, H.; Yamaguchi, T.; Ozeki, H.; Muromachi, S. Structure-driven CO_2 selectivity and gas capacity of ionic clathrate hydrates. *Sci. Rep.* **2017**, *7*, 17216. [CrossRef]
6. Muromachi, S.; Takeya, S. Design of Thermophysical Properties of Semiclathrate Hydrates Formed by Tetra-*n*-butylammonium Hydroxybutyrate. *Ind. Eng. Chem. Res.* **2018**, *57*, 3059–3064. [CrossRef]
7. Mcmullan, R.; Jeffrey, G.A. Hydrates of the Tetra *n*-butyl and Tetra *i*-amyl Quaternary Ammonium Salts. *J. Chem. Phys.* **1959**, *31*, 1231–1234. [CrossRef]
8. Dyadin, Y.A.; Udachin, K.A. Clathrate polyhydrates of peralkylonium salts and their analogs. *J. Struct. Chem.* **1987**, *28*, 394–432. [CrossRef]
9. Rodionova, T.V.; Terekhova, I.S.; Villevald, G.V.; Karpova, T.D.; Manakov, A.Y. Calorimetric and PXRD studies of ionic clathrate hydrates of tetrabutylammonium carboxylates in binary $(C_4H_9)_4NC_nH2_{n+1}CO_2–H_2O$ (n = 0–3) systems. *J. Therm. Anal. Calorim.* **2017**, *128*, 1165–1174. [CrossRef]
10. Muromachi, S.; Kamo, R.; Abe, T.; Hiaki, T.; Takeya, S. Thermodynamic stabilization of semiclathrate hydrates by hydrophilic group. *RSC Adv.* **2017**, *7*, 13590–13594. [CrossRef]

11. Muromachi, S.; Takeya, S. Thermodynamic Properties and Crystallographic Characterization of Semiclathrate Hydrates Formed with Tetra-*n*-butylammonium Glycolate. *ACS Omega* **2019**, *4*, 7317–7322. [CrossRef] [PubMed]
12. Rodionova, T.V.; Komarov, V.Y.; Villevald, G.V.; Karpova, T.D.; Kuratieva, N.V.; Manakov, A.Y. Calorimetric and Structural Studies of Tetrabutylammonium Bromide Ionic Clathrate Hydrates. *J. Phys. Chem. B* **2013**, *117*, 10677–10685. [CrossRef] [PubMed]
13. Oyama, H.; Shimada, W.; Ebinuma, T.; Kamata, Y.; Takeya, S.; Uchida, T.; Nagao, J.; Narita, H. Phase diagram, latent heat, and specific heat of TBAB semiclathrate hydrate crystals. *Fluid Phase Equilibria* **2005**, *234*, 131–135. [CrossRef]
14. Rodionova, T.V.; Komarov, V.Y.; Villevald, G.; Aladko, L.S.; Karpova, T.; Manakov, A.Y. Calorimetric and Structural Studies of Tetrabutylammonium Chloride Ionic Clathrate Hydrates. *J. Phys. Chem. B* **2010**, *114*, 11838–11846. [CrossRef]
15. Sakamoto, H.; Sato, K.; Shiraiwa, K.; Takeya, S.; Nakajima, M.; Ohmura, R. Synthesis, characterization and thermal-property measurements of ionic semi-clathrate hydrates formed with tetrabutylphosphonium chloride and tetrabutylammonium acrylate. *RSC Adv.* **2011**, *1*, 315–322. [CrossRef]
16. Dyadin, Y.A.; Udachin, K.A. Clathrate formation in water-peralkylonium salts systems. *J. Incl. Phenomema* **1984**, *2*, 61–72. [CrossRef]
17. Muromachi, S.; Takeya, S.; Yamamoto, Y.; Ohmura, R. Characterization of tetra-*n*-butylphosphonium bromide semiclathrate hydrate by crystal structure analysis. *CrystEngComm* **2014**, *16*, 2056–2060. [CrossRef]
18. Suginaka, T.; Sakamoto, H.; Iino, K.; Takeya, S.; Nakajima, M.; Ohmura, R. Thermodynamic properties of ionic semiclathrate hydrate formed with tetrabutylphosphonium bromide. *Fluid Phase Equilibria* **2012**, *317*, 25–28. [CrossRef]
19. Aladko, L.S.; Dyadin, Y.A.; Rodionova, T.V.; Terekhova, I.S. Clathrate Hydrates of Tetrabutylammonium and Tetraisoamylammonium Halides. *J. Struct. Chem.* **2002**, *43*, 990–994. [CrossRef]
20. Kobori, T.; Muromachi, S.; Yamasaki, T.; Takeya, S.; Yamamoto, Y.; Alavi, S.; Ohmura, R. Phase Behavior and Structural Characterization of Ionic Clathrate Hydrate Formed with Tetra-*n*-butylphosphonium Hydroxide: Discovery of Primitive Crystal Structure. *Cryst. Growth Des.* **2015**, *15*, 3862–3867. [CrossRef]
21. Shimada, J.; Shimada, M.; Sugahara, T.; Tsunashima, K.; Tani, A.; Tsuchida, Y.; Matsumiya, M. Phase Equilibrium Relations of Semiclathrate Hydrates Based on Tetra-*n*-butylphosphonium Formate, Acetate, and Lactate. *J. Chem. Eng. Data* **2018**, *63*, 3615–3620. [CrossRef]
22. Falconer, R.J.; Markelz, A.G. Terahertz Spectroscopic Analysis of Peptides and Proteins. *J. Infrared Millim. Terahertz Waves* **2012**, *33*, 973–988. [CrossRef]
23. Lipiäinen, T.; Fraser-Miller, S.J.; Gordon, K.C.; Strachan, C.J. Direct comparison of low- and mid-frequency Raman spectroscopy for quantitative solid-state pharmaceutical analysis. *J. Pharm. Biomed. Anal.* **2018**, *149*, 343–350. [CrossRef] [PubMed]
24. Kojima, S.; Mori, T.; Shibata, T.; Kobayashi, Y. Broadband Terahertz Time-Domain and Low-Frequency Raman Spectroscopy of Crystalline and Glassy Pharmaceuticals. *Pharm. Anal. Acta* **2015**, *6*, 1000401. [CrossRef]
25. Zeitler, J.A.; Taday, P.F.; Pepper, M.; Rades, T. Relaxation and crystallization of amorphous carbamazepine studied by terahertz pulsed spectroscopy. *J. Pharm. Sci.* **2007**, *96*, 2703–2709. [CrossRef]
26. Chen, H.K.; Srivastava, N.; Saha, S.; Shigeto, S. Complementing Crystallography with Ultralow-Frequency Raman Spectroscopy: Structural Insights into Nitrile-Functionalized Ionic Liquids. *ChemPhysChem* **2016**, *17*, 93–97. [CrossRef]
27. Adichtchev, S.V.; Belosludov, V.R.; Ildyakov, A.V.; Malinovsky, V.K.; Manakov, A.Y.; Subbotin, O.S.; Surovtsev, N.V. Low-Frequency Raman Scattering in a Xe Hydrate. *J. Phys. Chem. B* **2013**, *117*, 10686–10690. [CrossRef]
28. Takasu, Y.; Iwai, K.; Nishio, I. Low Frequency Raman Profile of Type II Clathrate Hydrate of THF and Its Application for Phase Identification. *J. Phys. Soc. Jpn.* **2003**, *72*, 1287–1291. [CrossRef]
29. Prasad, P.S.R.; Prasad, K.S.; Thakur, N.K. Laser Raman spectroscopy of THF clathrate hydrate in the temperature range 90–300 K. *Spectrochim. Acta Part A Mol. Biomol. Spectrosc.* **2007**, *68*, 1096–1100. [CrossRef]
30. Hiratsuka, M.; Ohmura, R.; Sum, A.K.; Yasuoka, K. Molecular vibrations of methane molecules in the structure I clathrate hydrate from *ab initio* molecular dynamics simulation. *J. Chem. Phys.* **2012**, *136*, 044508. [CrossRef]
31. Chazallon, B.; Ziskind, M.; Carpentier, Y.; Focsa, C. CO_2 Capture Using Semi-Clathrates of Quaternary Ammonium Salt: Structure Change Induced by CO_2 and N_2 Enclathration. *J. Phys. Chem. B* **2014**, *118*, 13440–13452. [CrossRef] [PubMed]
32. Jin, Y.; Nagao, J. Change in the Stable Crystal Phase of Tetra-*n*-butylammonium Bromide (TBAB) Hydrates Enclosing Xenon. *J. Phys. Chem. C* **2013**, *117*, 6924–6928. [CrossRef]
33. Okajima, H.; Ando, M.; Hamaguchi, H. Formation of "Nano-Ice" and Density Maximum Anomaly of Water. *Bull. Chem. Soc. Jpn.* **2018**, *91*, 991–997. [CrossRef]
34. Subbotin, O.S.; Gets, K.V.; Bozhko, Y.Y.; Belosludov, V.R.; Zhdanov, R.K. Theoretical investigation of thermodynamic properties of tetrabutylammonium bromide ionic clathrate hydrate. *J. Phys. Conf. Ser.* **2019**, *1359*, 012053. [CrossRef]
35. Funkner, S.; Niehues, G.; Schmidt, D.A.; Heyden, M.; Schwaab, G.; Callahan, K.M.; Tobias, D.J.; Havenith, M. Watching the Low-Frequency Motions in Aqueous Salt Solutions: The Terahertz Vibrational Signatures of Hydrated Ions. *J. Am. Chem. Soc.* **2012**, *134*, 1030–1035. [CrossRef]
36. Reichenbach, J.; Ruddell, S.A.; González-Jiménez, M.; Lemes, J.; Turton, D.A.; France, D.J.; Wynne, K. Phonon-like Hydrogen-Bond Modes in Protic Ionic Liquids. *J. Am. Chem. Soc.* **2017**, *139*, 7160–7163. [CrossRef]
37. Burnett, A.D.; Kendrick, J.; Russell, C.; Christensen, J.; Cunningham, J.E.; Pearson, A.R.; Linfield, E.H.; Davies, A.G. Effect of Molecular Size and Particle Shape on the Terahertz Absorption of a Homologous Series of Tetraalkylammonium Salts. *Anal. Chem.* **2013**, *85*, 7926–7934. [CrossRef]

38. Jin, Y.; Kida, M.; Nagao, J. Phase Transition of Tetra-*n*-butylammonium Bromide Hydrates Enclosing Krypton. *J. Chem. Eng. Data* **2016**, *61*, 679–685. [CrossRef]
39. Walrafen, G.E.; Chu, Y.C.; Piermarini, G.J. Low-Frequency Raman Scattering from Water at High Pressures and High Temperatures. *J. Phys. Chem.* **1996**, *100*, 10363–10372. [CrossRef]
40. Shimada, W.; Shiro, M.; Kondo, H.; Takeya, S.; Oyama, H.; Ebinuma, T.; Narita, H. Tetra-*n*-butylammonium bromide-water (1/38). *Acta Crystallogr. Sect. C Cryst. Struct. Commun.* **2005**, *61*, o65–o66. [CrossRef]
41. Belosludov, V.R.; Gets, K.V.; Zhdanov, R.K.; Malinovsky, Y.V.; Bozhko, Y.Y.; Belosludov, R.V.; Surovtsev, N.V.; Subbotin, O.S.; Kawazoe, Y. The Nano-Structural Inhomogeneity of Dynamic Hydrogen Bond Network of TIP4P/2005 Water. *Sci. Rep.* **2020**, *10*, 7323. [CrossRef] [PubMed]
42. Funke, S.; Sebastiani, F.; Schwaab, G.; Havenith, M. Spectroscopic fingerprints in the low frequency spectrum of ice (Ih), clathrate hydrates, supercooled water, and hydrophobic hydration reveal similarities in the hydrogen bond network motifs. *J. Chem. Phys.* **2019**, *150*, 224505. [CrossRef] [PubMed]
43. Carvalho, P.J.; Ventura, S.P.M.; Batista, M.L.S.; Schröder, B.; Gonçalves, F.; Esperança, J.; Mutelet, F.; Coutinho, J.A.P. Understanding the impact of the central atom on the ionic liquid behavior: Phosphonium vs ammonium cations. *J. Chem. Phys.* **2014**, *140*, 064505. [CrossRef]
44. Pan, T.; Li, S.; Zou, T.; Yu, Z.; Zhang, B.; Wang, C.; Zhang, J.; He, M.; Zhao, H. Terahertz spectra of L-phenylalanine and its monohydrate. *Spectrochim. Acta—Part A Mol. Biomol. Spectrosc.* **2017**, *178*, 19–23. [CrossRef]
45. Otaki, T.; Tanabe, Y.; Kojima, T.; Miura, M.; Ikeda, Y.; Koide, T.; Fukami, T. In situ monitoring of cocrystals in formulation development using low-frequency Raman spectroscopy. *Int. J. Pharm.* **2018**, *542*, 56–65. [CrossRef] [PubMed]
46. Wang, Q.; Habenschuss, A.; Xenopoulos, A.; Wunderlich, B. Mesophases of Alkylammonium Salts. VI. The Crystal Structures of Tetra-*n*-butylammonium Bromide and Iodide. *Mol. Cryst. Liq. Cryst. Sci. Technol. Sect. A Mol. Cryst. Liq. Cryst.* **1995**, *264*, 115–129. [CrossRef]
47. Mayoufi, N.; Dalmazzone, D.; Delahaye, A.; Clain, P.; Fournaison, L.; Fürst, W. Experimental Data on Phase Behavior of Simple Tetrabutylphosphonium Bromide (TBPB) and Mixed CO_2 + TBPB Semiclathrate Hydrates. *J. Chem. Eng. Data* **2011**, *56*, 2987–2993. [CrossRef]
48. Iwata, K.; Okajima, H.; Saha, S.; Hamaguchi, H. Local Structure Formation in Alkyl-imidazolium-Based Ionic Liquids as Revealed by Linear and Nonlinear Raman Spectroscopy. *Acc. Chem. Res.* **2007**, *40*, 1174–1181. [CrossRef]

molecules

MDPI

Article

Aquaphotomic Study of Effects of Different Mixing Waters on the Properties of Cement Mortar

Jelena Muncan [1,†], Satoshi Tamura [2,*,†], Yuri Nakamura [2], Mizuki Takigawa [3], Hisao Tsunokake [3] and Roumiana Tsenkova [1,*]

1 Aquaphotomics Research Department, Graduate School of Agricultural Science, Kobe University, Kobe 657-8501, Japan
2 Technical Department, ISOL Technica Corporation, Kyoto 606-0022, Japan
3 Institute of Engineering, Graduate School of Engineering, Division of Urban Engineering, Osaka Metropolitan University, Osaka 599-8531, Japan
* Correspondence: s-tamura@isol-technica.co.jp (S.T.); rtsen@kobe-u.ac.jp (R.T.)
† These authors contributed equally to this work.

Abstract: The mixing water used for cement concrete has a significant effect on the physical properties of the material after hardening; however, other than the upper limit for the mixed impurities, not enough consideration has been given to the functions and characteristics of water at the molecular level. In this study, we investigated the effect of four different types of water (two spring-, mineral waters, tap water and distilled water) on the drying shrinkage of the hardened cement by comparing the material properties of the concrete specimens and analyzing the molecular structure of the water and cement mortar using aquaphotomics. The near infrared (NIR) spectra of waters used for mixing were acquired in the transmittance mode using a high-precision, high-accuracy benchtop spectrometer in the range of 400–2500 nm, with the 0.5 nm step. The NIR spectra of cement paste and mortar were measured in 6.2 nm increments in the wavelength range of 950 nm to 1650 nm using a portable spectrometer. The measurements of cement paste and mortar were performed on Day 0 (immediately after mixing, cement paste), 1 day, 3 days, 7 days, and 28 days after mixing (cement mortar). The spectral data were analyzed according to the aquaphotomics' multivariate analysis protocol, which involved exploration of raw and preprocessed spectra, exploratory analysis, discriminating analysis and aquagrams. The results of the aquaphotomics' analysis were interpreted together with the results of thermal and drying shrinkage measurements. Together, the findings clearly demonstrated that the thermal and drying shrinkage properties of the hardened cement material differed depending on the water used. Better mechanical properties were found to be a result of using mineral waters for cement mixing despite minute differences in the chemical content. In addition, the aquaphotomic characterization of the molecular structure of waters and cement mortar during the initial hydration reaction demonstrated the possibility to predict the characteristics of hardened cement at a very early stage. This provided the rationale to propose a novel evaluation method based on aquaphotomics for non-invasive evaluation and monitoring of cement mortar.

Keywords: cement concrete; mortar; water; water molecular structure; drying shrinkage; aquaphotomics; near infrared spectroscopy

Citation: Muncan, J.; Tamura, S.; Nakamura, Y.; Takigawa, M.; Tsunokake, H.; Tsenkova, R. Aquaphotomic Study of Effects of Different Mixing Waters on the Properties of Cement Mortar. *Molecules* **2022**, *27*, 7885. https://doi.org/10.3390/molecules27227885

Academic Editor: Stefano Materazzi

Received: 9 August 2022
Accepted: 6 November 2022
Published: 15 November 2022

1. Introduction

Cement concrete is composed of cement, water, fine aggregate (sand), coarse aggregate (gravel), and admixture. The hydration reaction of cement starts immediately when it comes into the contact with water, and cement hydrates are formed as the cement gradually hardens. Generally, the material properties of cement concrete and the quality of cement depend on the weight ratio of water to cement (water–cement ratio, *w/c* ratio) [1–5]. This number *w/c* is in inverse correlation with the concrete strength: the smaller the *w/c* ratio, the greater the strength, durability and watertightness [3]. The *w/c* ratio is linked to the spacing between the cement particles in the cement paste—if the spacing is smaller, the process of filling in the gaps between cement particles by cement hydrates is faster and the links created by the hydrates are stronger, hence the stronger the concrete [3]. Another important aspect related to the water-to-binder (or water-to-cement) ratio is the microstructure, and especially the nanoscale characteristics [6]. For example, the dense microstructure provides the excellent mechanical properties and long-term service performance to ultra-high performance concrete (UHPC), an advanced cement-based [7,8]. The UHPC mixtures usually have a low water-to-binder ratio, and a higher content of cement and silica fume particles [8], which, as research studies showed, mainly play the filling role, and the hydration degree of cement is only around 30–35% [9]. On the other hand, a high water-to-binder ration leads to high risks for cracking due to autogenous shrinkage, which is closely related to mechanical properties and durability [6]. The incorporation of various organic or inorganic modifiers in cement is another method of effectively influencing the water-to-binder ratio due to the modified binder properties, which can lead to improved volume stability and water resistance [10]. Therefore, it is important to control the water–cement ratio in order to provide resistance to neutralization (carbonation-reaction with the carbon dioxide from the atmosphere) and infiltration of salt (chloride damage) into cement concrete—the two main causes of chemo-mechanical changes and deterioration of the durability of the concrete structure [5].

The shrinkage of cement concrete is a phenomenon that can occur in any concrete structure, and cracks and dimensional changes due to shrinkage can greatly affect the state of stress in the structure and various performance parameters, including durability. The cement shrinkage is one of the classical research subjects in concrete engineering; the elucidation of the mechanism of shrinkage, theoretical and various other models and prediction methods have been proposed [11–20]. The shrinkage behavior is associated rather with the microscale thermodynamic properties such as hydration, pore-structure formation, and the water status in micropores [20], than with the macroscale properties such as the *w/c* ratio [21]. This is because the shrinkage behavior cannot always be evaluated only by the *w/c* ratio. In order to explain the microscale aspects of the drying shrinkage principle, several theories concerning the water status in micropores have been proposed to explain the mechanism that causes drying shrinkage: capillary tension theory (caused by the water meniscus), disjoining pressure theory (caused by water films in narrow pores), surface tension theory (surface energy change caused by water desorption), and interlayer water transfer theory [20–28].

Since the size of the micropores in cement matrix varies greatly, the water status can be quite different, and the theories explaining the shrinkage behavior are usually combined to provide an explanation for the behavior at various levels of relative humidity (RH) [20]. Capillary tension and disjoining pressure are considered to be the predominant mechanisms in the mid to high humidity range, and surface tension and interlayer water transfer in the low humidity range [20]. However, there is currently no unified theory that can explain the shrinkage behavior of hardened cement over the entire humidity range. Since water, fine aggregate, and coarse aggregate in cement concrete are generally collected and procured locally at the place where cement concrete is manufactured, the physical properties of the materials, composition, and curing conditions (environmental conditions) can vary greatly. This makes it additionally difficult, considering the great many number of variables, to efficiently investigate the microscopic mechanisms causing the shrinkage, and to understand the shrinkage behavior of hardened cement. Therefore, there is a great need for the establishment of a universal and comprehensive analysis method that can take into consideration all these aspects.

Given the background explained above, and especially the role of water in the shrinkage process, it is evidently necessary to examine various chemical and physical properties of water because they will directly influence the physical properties of cement concrete after hardening. In regards to the conditions that water should satisfy in order to be used for the production of cement concrete, the standards such as JIS A 5308—Ready-Mixed

Concrete Appendix C [29] and ASTM Designation C94-96—Standard Specification for Ready-Mixed Concrete [30], only specify that the water used should be clean potable water. However, even the sludge and well water are sometimes used, and there are no specific requirements other than the upper limit of harmful substances such as impurities and chloride ions [30,31].

In recent years, various types of "functional water" have been developed, that is, waters whose functionality is supposedly enhanced to serve a specific purpose for health and well-being [32,33], or other purposes in medicine and agriculture [34–39]. In the science of cement materials, studies have demonstrated that the use of "functional water", for example magnetically treated water or hydrogen nano-bubble water, can effectively improve the compressive strength, workability, and watertightness of cement concrete, even reducing the needed amount of cement in the mix [40–48]. However, since the mechanism of action of "functional water" on the physical properties of the hardened cement has not been investigated at the molecular level, the effectiveness of "functional water" cannot be quantitatively evaluated for full-scale practical use and warrants further investigations [48,49].

The methods used to date to investigate the cement hydration include isothermal calorimetry, thermal analyses, monitoring of chemical shrinkage, in situ quantitative X-ray diffraction, nuclear magnetic resonance spectroscopy (NMR), quasi-elastic neutron scattering (QENS), and small angle neutron scattering (SANS). They have proven useful for comparing the hydration of different cements, and especially in combination, they can provide insights into the hydration process that cannot be obtained by any one method alone. However, all of them monitor the overall progress of hydration, without providing more insight into the nature of the occurring chemical reactions or resolving the details of particular underlaying mechanisms [50]. In particular, they cannot be exploited on a massive scale in practical applications.

In this study, aquaphotomic near infrared (NIR) spectroscopy [51] is proposed as a suitable method for the characterization of both mixing water and cement mortar. This method is based on the utilization of the light–water interaction, which provides the information about the state of the water molecular network within the material, and indirectly about the material itself by analysis of the NIR spectra [52]. The aquaphotomics' science and technology have been gaining worldwide attention in recent years due to the noninvasiveness, ease of use, wide field of applications, and novel discoveries [52–54]. Further, considerable efforts have been invested in the developments of spectral preprocessing [55] and chemometrics techniques [56–61] for analysis of NIR spectra that contributed to the better understanding of the water molecular structure. Aquaphotomics has been providing a basic understanding of the water molecular network-related functionalities and new technical solutions for water and food quality monitoring, biometrics, biological diagnosis, biological monitoring, and water quality monitoring in waterworks facilities, but construction materials such as hardened cement have not been explored enough [52].

Therefore, in this study, the effects of four different types of water on the physical properties of the hardened cement were investigated. For the purpose of this work, the focus will be placed only on the drying shrinkage characteristics of the hardened cement, while other properties such as the compressive and bending strength, elastic modulus and others will be the object of further investigations. The results of this research will demonstrate that using the same cement components, but different waters for mixing, despite their negligible differences in mineral components, leads to different drying shrinkage properties of the produced cement. Further, using aquaphotomics for the characterization of waters, it will be demonstrated that the different water molecular structure is the reason for this because it dictates the different formation of cement matrix in the paste and mortar. The entire process can be monitored immediately upon the mixing of cement, which is used to predict the cement hardness at a very early stage and also monitored throughout the course of the cement hardening.

2. Results and Discussion

2.1. Mineral Content of Waters Used for Preparation of Cement

The results of the Inductively Coupled Plasma Mass Spectrometry (ICP-MS) analysis are presented in Table 1 for all the water samples used as mixing waters in preparation of the cement. Distilled water (W_{dist}) was water from which minerals were removed, although trace amounts of Ca and Mg were still detected. The other three types of water had a higher mineral content compared to W_{dist}. Mineral waters from the shallow source ($W_{shallow}$) and mineral water obtained by mixing two mineral waters from shallow and deep source (W_{mix}) had higher contents of Na, Si, and Ca compared to the Osaka city tap (W_{tap}) water.

Table 1. Mineral content of the waters used for preparation of cement mortar. W_{mix} water has the highest mineral content, followed by $W_{shallow}$ and W_{tap}.

Contained Elements (ppm)	W_{dist}	W_{tap}	$W_{shallow}$	W_{mix}
Li	0.000	0.000	0.000	0.000
B	0.000	0.014	0.057	0.540
Na	0.000	13.220	17.340	39.300
Mg	0.002	2.074	4.364	12.105
Al	0.000	0.014	0.000	0.006
Si	0.000	2.870	24.400	20.570
K	0.000	2.234	1.679	3.094
Ca	0.107	11.315	11.555	28.750
Ti	0.000	0.000	0.000	0.000
Mn	0.000	0.000	0.001	0.108
Fe	0.000	0.013	0.001	0.006
Cu	0.000	0.000	0.006	0.000
Zn	0.000	0.003	0.012	0.002
Sr	0.000	0.526	0.133	0.273
Ag	0.000	0.000	0.000	0.000
Ba	0.000	0.012	0.019	0.046

Minerals that have a relatively high content are highlighted in the Table 1 and the comparison of their amount in waters used for cement preparation is shown in Figure 1. The Si content is particularly high in mineral waters compared to W_{tap} and W_{dist}. In addition, the content of Na, Mg, and Ca in W_{mix} is more than twice the amount in W_{tap} and $W_{shallow}$. Even though there are large differences in the content of the five minerals (Na, Mg, Si, K, and Ca) (Figure 1), this is not considered relevant in the usual practice, and all four waters satisfy the tolerable limits of constituents according to the standards for most countries [62].

To conclude, according to the contemporary standards for mixing water, each of the four waters can readily be used for preparation of cement concrete. The existence of differences in constituents would not be considered relevant or of any consequence for the properties of concrete.

2.2. Aquaphotomic Characterization of Mixing Water

The characterization of mixing waters was performed using aquaphotomics' NIR spectroscopy. The NIR spectra of mixing waters, acquired in the range 400–2500 nm, at a controlled temperature of 25 °C were trimmed to a region of 1300–1600 nm that corresponds to the first overtone of water stretching vibrations, which typically has a maximum around 1450 nm (Figure 2). The NIR spectra of waters are broad and the differences between the individual spectra are very small. In order to extract and emphasize the differences between the mixing waters' spectra, the use of multivariate data analysis is required.

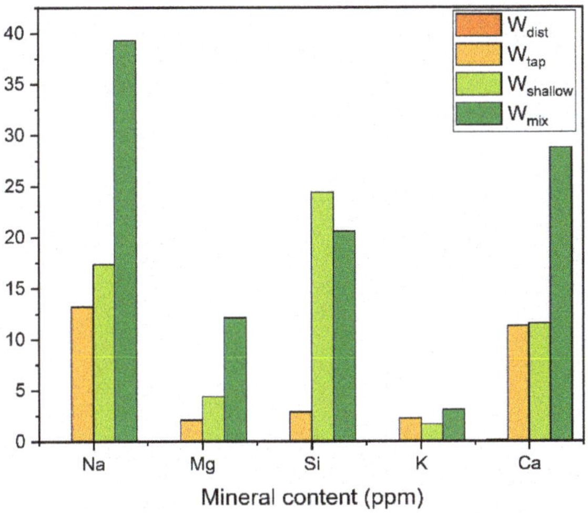

Figure 1. Major differences in mineral content of waters used for cement preparation.

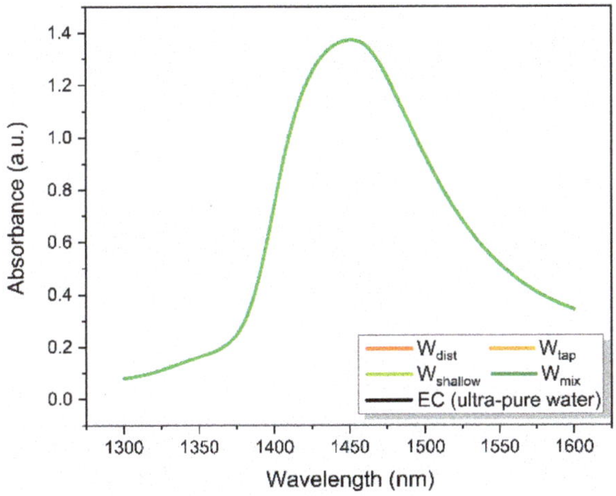

Figure 2. Raw absorbance spectra of mixing waters used for preparation of cement.

Therefore, the spectra were analyzed according to the protocol of the aquaphotomic spectral analysis [63]. Difference spectra, Principal Component Analysis (PCA) [64], Soft Modeling of Class Analogies (SIMCA) [65], and Partial Least Squares Regression (PLSR) Analysis (using temperature and consecutive irradiation as dependent variables) were performed (results not presented) in order to find the representative water absorbance bands—water matrix coordinates (WAMACS) [51]. The WAMACS are then used to depict the characteristic water spectral patterns (WASPs) of mixing waters on aquagrams [63,66] related to the respective functionalities. The selection of WAMACS was performed as described in the recent literature [63,67], by choosing the most consistently repeating and most influential absorbance bands in the entire performed analysis.

The calculated aquagrams of four mixing waters are presented in Figure 3, with 15 radial axes defined by the chosen WAMACS, displaying normalized absorbance values after the correction of spectra by standard normal variate (SNV) transformation [68] to cancel the potential baseline effects. The aquagrams of mixing waters demonstrate succinctly their water spectral patterns, compared to the ultra-pure water (labeled as EC, zero line on the graph, Figure 3).

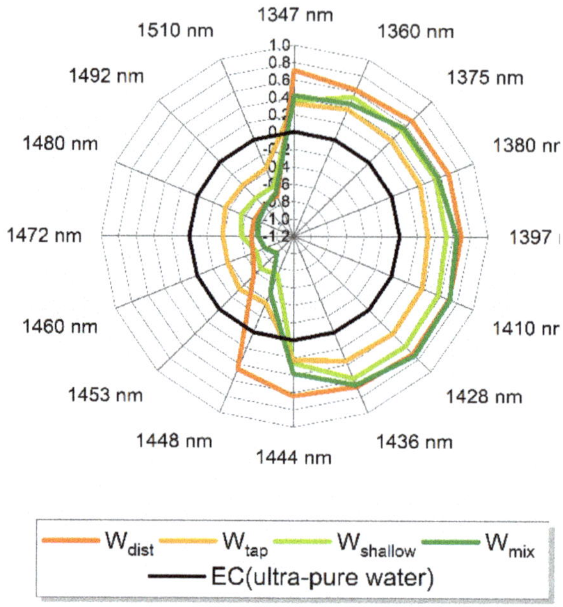

Figure 3. Aquagrams of various mixing waters used for preparation of cement.

Each radial axis on the aquagram, i.e., wavelength corresponds to the absorption of particular water molecular species. The resulting aquagrams present the water absorbance spectral patterns of each examined water and effectively convey the differences in their molecular structure. The wavelengths presented can be attributed to the absorbance bands of the following water species: 1347 nm represents OH group asymmetric stretching vibration ν_3 and is the common band for all proton hydrates, 1360 nm is water solvation shell OH-$(H_2O)_n$ where n = 1, 2, or 4; 1375 nm is attributed to combination of symmetric and asymmetric stretching vibration $\nu_1 + \nu_3$; 1380 nm is water solvation shell OH-$(H_2O)_n$ where n = 1, 4 or superoxide tetrahydrate O_2-$(H_2O)_4$; 1397 nm is water confined in the local field of ions; 1410 nm corresponds to free water molecules (S_0); 1428 nm is hydration water–hydroxide and OH-$(H_2O)_4$ water shell; 1436 nm and 1444 nm are absorbance bands of protonated water dimer (Zundel Cation) and water dimers (S_1); bands 1448 nm and 1453 nm can be assigned to solvation shells OH-$(H_2O)_n$, where n = 4, 5; 1460 nm to water molecules with two hydrogen bonds (S_2), 1472 and 1480 nm to water molecules with three hydrogen bonds (S_3), 1492 nm to water molecules with all four hydrogen bonds (S_4); 1510 nm to the combination of symmetric stretching and bending vibrations $\nu_1 + \nu_2$; and strongly bound water [51,69–73].

In simple words, the bands located at the right side of the aquagram (1347–1444 nm) can be said to encompass the absorbance bands of free water, quasi-free water, weakly hydrogen-bonded water, and water involved in the hydration of solutes (solvation shells), while the left side of the aquagram (1444 nm to 1510 nm) represents absorbance bands of hydrogen-bonded water. Compared to the pure water, the spectral patterns of all mixing waters demonstrate higher absorbance at the right side of the aquagram, showing much higher ability for solvation. The water molecular structure of these waters resembles the ones that could be observed at increased temperatures. The largest differences in spectral patterns between the four types of waters can be found in the region of 1428 to 1460 nm, in particular at 1448 nm—bands that can be attributed to the absorption of water molecules in solvation shells, which feature four or five water molecules.

These results demonstrate that, regarding the composition, despite what seems to be negligible amounts of ions, the mixing waters do not have the same molecular structure, and they are quite different compared to the ultra-pure water, and furthermore, even the W_{dist} shows a distinctive spectral pattern. It could be said that, compared to the spectral pattern of pure water at 25 °C, all the examined waters demonstrate the molecular structure that would correspond to the molecular structure of pure water at higher temperatures [74]. This especially can be of significance with respect to the solvation ability.

2.3. *Aquaphotomic Characterization of Cement Mortar*

2.3.1. Raw and Transformed near Infrared Spectra of Cement Mortar

Raw NIR spectra acquired for the mortar on the day it is prepared (cement paste, Day 0) and during the process of setting and hardening (cement mortar, after 1, 3, and 7 days) are presented in Figure 4a.

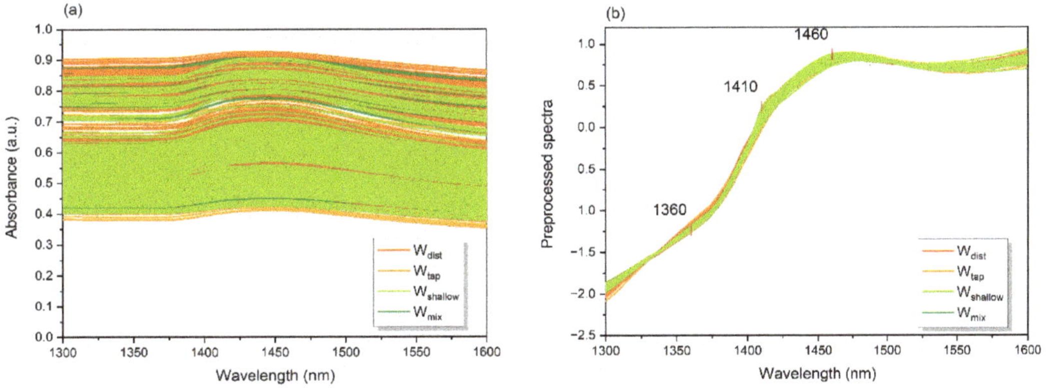

Figure 4. Near infrared spectra of cement paste and mortar samples created using different waters: (**a**) Raw absorbance spectra; (**b**) Preprocessed spectra using linear detrend correction and standard normal variate transformation.

The absorbance spectra demonstrate large baseline effects due to the influence of scatter and are mainly overlapped, making it difficult to observe differences depending on the water used in the mixing of the concrete. However, the broad band centered around 1450 nm, corresponding to the first overtone of water stretching vibrations, can still be observed.

To emphasize the chemical information in the spectra, the transformation using the linear detrend correction and SNV transformation [68] was performed and the spectra after correction are presented in Figure 4b. The pre-processing eliminated the baseline differences efficiently and at three places in the spectra interesting features appeared—at 1360 nm, 1410 nm, and 1460 nm. At these specific places, some differences in the spectra of mortar could be observed even with the naked eye. All three bands are, as mentioned before, well-known water absorbance bands that can be attributed to solvation shells, free water molecules, and water molecules with two hydrogen bonds.

This suggests the importance of these water molecular structures for the description of the process of change in cement mortar over time, and as a function of the molecular structure of water used for mixing. To explore these differences further, the multivariate analysis tools were employed.

2.3.2. Principal Component Analysis (PCA) of Cement Mortar

The exploratory analysis in the form of PCA [75] was applied on the spectral data separated in four datasets according to the type of water used for mixing. The separation was performed with the aim to take the full advantage of pre-processing using detrend and SNV and correct the baseline effects appropriately, since the origin of scatter is physical in nature, and therefore may vary between the different mortars. The smoothing using Savitzky-Golay 2nd order polynomial filter [76] and 21-point window size was also performed to eliminate the noise from the spectra.

The majority of variance (more than 95%) in each dataset was captured by the first two principle components PC1 and PC2. The PC1-PC2 scores plots of PCA analyses are presented in Figure 5, for mortar created using W_{dist} (Figure 5a), W_{tap} (Figure 5b), $W_{shallow}$ (Figure 5c) and W_{mix} (Figure 5d), where the scores are colored depending on the day of the spectral acquisition. In all four cases, the first two principal components explained more than 95% of variations in the datasets (Table 2) and the patterns of scores corresponding to the different days (the day of cement paste preparation—Day 0 and cement mortar after 1, 3, and 7 days) could be well-distinguished in the PC1-PC2 spaces.

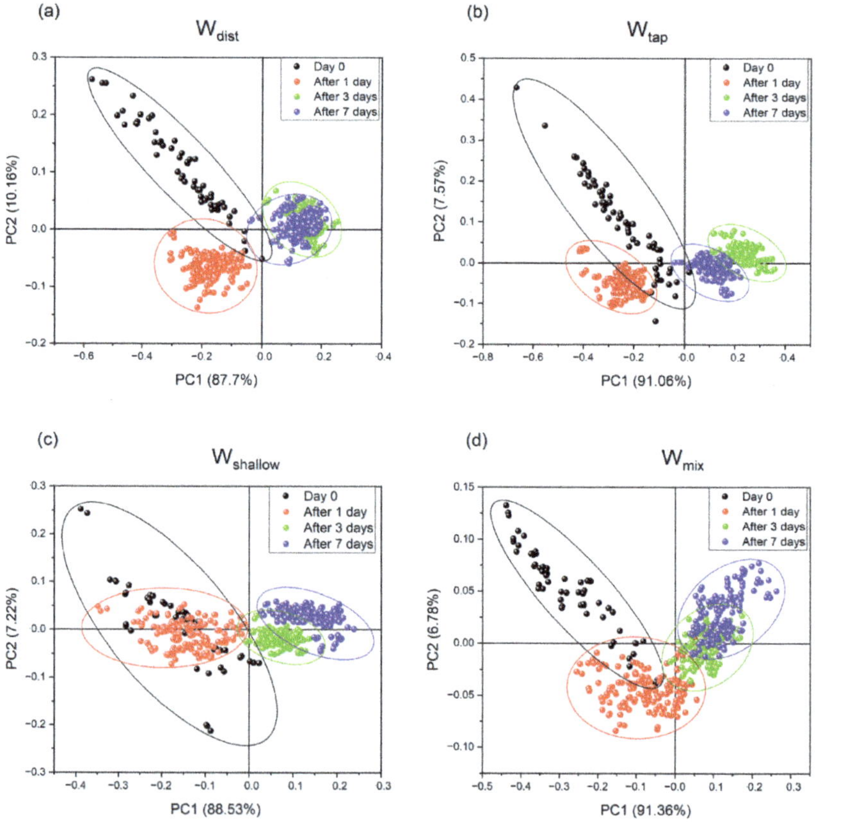

Figure 5. Transformation and the projection of the original spectral data into the space defined by two orthogonal principal components (PC1 and PC2) that retained more than 95% of original variance. PC1-PC2 scores plots of PCA analysis show changes in cement mortar prepared with different mixing water: (**a**) W_{dist}, (**b**) W_{tap}, (**c**) $W_{shallow}$, and (**d**) W_{mix}. According to the results of the analysis, the PC1 axis can be related to the changes in water of cement as the time progresses from Day 0 to 7, while the PC2 axis describes changes in water during first 24 h.

Table 2. The percentage of explained variance by two first principal components from the results of PCA analyses performed on four separate datasets of cement mortar depending on the mixing water.

Mixing Water	PC1 (%)	PC2 (%)	PC1 and PC2 (%)
W_{dist}	87.7	10.16	97.86
W_{tap}	91.06	7.57	98.63
$W_{shallow}$	88.53	7.22	95.75
W_{mix}	91.36	6.78	98.14

While so far in the analysis the minute quantities in ions and their differences between mixing waters might have seem negligible, and even the water spectral patterns similar, from the PC1-PC2 score plots it now becomes evident that the use of different waters for the mixing of cement results in quite different characteristics during the cement setting. First, it can be noticed that the spreading of the scores differs, and it is largest on Day 0 in cement paste, immediately after the mixing, suggesting large differences across the cement paste. However, after the mortar is set and left to harden, the differences diminish over time, suggesting that the water in cement paste is still in a variety of states, compared to the subsequent days. The scores corresponding to the Day 0 are for all water types located in the negative part of PC1 and mostly positive part of PC2, with the exception of $W_{shallow}$, whose scores are located neutrally along the zero line of PC2. This clearly indicates that cement paste created with $W_{shallow}$ is very different compared to others, while the smaller spreading of the scores may indicate more uniform characteristics of cement paste.

The pattern of changes along time, as the cement is aging, can be observed mostly along the PC1. This means that the PC1 describes the transformation of water in the cement during this process. Especially in regards to the time trend, the differences increase. The scores corresponding to the spectra acquired after 1 day are, in the case of all waters, located in the negative parts of both PC1 and PC2, except again in the case of $W_{shallow}$. It seems that in the case of $W_{shallow}$, the cement mortar is not changed much during first 24 h, as can be observed from Figure 5c—the scores of Day 0 almost coincide with the scores after 1 day.

The scores corresponding to the age of 3 and 7 days in all four cases are located in the positive part of PC1, but there are particular differences among the waters. The most well-defined groups of scores for 3- and 7-days age can be observed for W_{tap} (Figure 5b), suggesting that changes still take place in this cement. On the contrary, in the scores of W_{dist} (Figure 5a), the groups of scores corresponding to the 3rd and 7th day coincide, indicating very small changes after 3 days. The scores corresponding to these days of cement age in the cases of $W_{shallow}$ and W_{mix} water partially overlap; however, the time trend is the opposite compared to the W_{tap}, where the scores corresponding to the 7 days are located more closely to the Day 0 scores. From these observations, it can be concluded that the waters used for mixing cement mortar influence the uniformity of the mixture (cement paste, Day 0) and the behavior during the aging of the cement mortar during the first 7 days. The time trend of the changes is mostly described by first two principal components, but the changes during the first 24 h are mainly described by the PC2. The loadings of PC1 and PC2 are presented in Figure 6 for all four datasets.

From the loadings' plots, the first thing to observe is the very similar shape of PC1 loadings for all four examined cases, and the occurrence of almost the same bands: the negative peaks at 1391 nm and 1397 nm, and positive peaks at 1472 and 1478 nm. The first two may be attributed to the, so-called, trapped water while the latter ones to the water molecules with three hydrogen bonds. Looking at the position of scores at the scores' plots (Figure 5) and relating it to the sign of the observed peaks, it can be concluded that from the Day 0 during the first 24 h there is an increase in trapped water, but from that day onwards, the water in cement after 3 and 7 days is characterized by increased amount of water that is hydrogen–bonded. This may also account for the loss in the spreading of the scores on the 3rd and the 7th day, because the hydrogen bonded water is not easily changed.

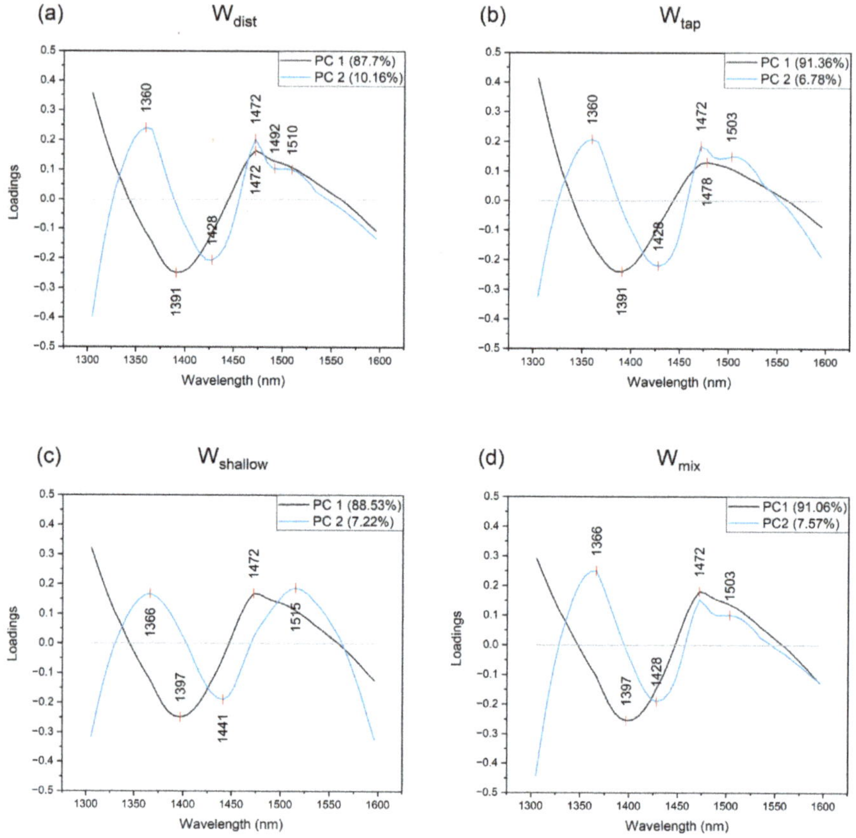

Figure 6. PC1 and PC2 loadings plots of PCA analysis describe changes in the water molecular structure during hardening of cement mortar prepared with different mixing water: (**a**) W_{tap}, (**b**) W_{mix}, (**c**) W_{dist}, and (**d**) $W_{shallow}$.

The differences in bands 1391 nm and 1397 nm may be in the nature of ions or the confinement which entrap single water molecules, while the differences in 1472 and 1478 nm may be due to the isomerism of water molecular species with three hydrogen bonds. In the study of wood stiffness and strength properties, by Fujimoto, Yamamoto and Tsuchikawa 2007, the band located at 1476 nm was related to the semi-crystalline regions in cellulose [77]. The bands in our work (1472 nm, 1478 nm) may also indicate that the state of water in the cement matrix is semi-crystalline as the cement ages to the 3rd and 7th day. The confined water observed at 1391 nm or 1397 nm can also be understood as an interlayer between the sheets of calcium hydroxide $Ca(OH)_2$, similar to the findings of Kondo et al. 2021 for the hydration and dehydration of $Mg(OH)_2$ [78]. In any case, this entire process can be described as a transformation of weakly hydrogen bonded water to hydrogen bonded water, and as such, to use analogy with temperature it could be compared to the cooling of water within the cement matrix, which is consistent with the release of heat during the reaction of cement hydration [50].

On the other hand, the loadings of PC2, which is more related to the changes during the first 24 h, and therefore to the initial reaction of cement hydration, demonstrate somewhat different shapes depending on the water used in mixing. The common features are positive peaks at 1360 and 1366 nm, both of which correspond to water solvation shells, and a positive peak at 1472 nm, and again the water molecules bonded with three hydrogen bonds. Here, similarly, the difference in the position of the bands of solvation shells might be due to the differences in ions present in the waters, and their solvation. Or more likely, it is due to the different coordination number; Kondo et al. 2021 have reported band 1362 nm to correspond to OH-coordinated with 1 or 2 Mg^{2+} on the corner and edge of the $Mg(OH)_2$ surface, while 1368 to OH-coordinated with 3 Mg^{2+}. Having this in mind, the bands observed in PC2 loadings could be related to the Ca^{2+} ions. It is interesting to notice that there is a report of the absorbance band at 1366 nm, as related to the absorbance of a compound highly correlated with hardness [79]. This report was about the hardness of wheat, modeled based on the water extracts of whole wheat flours. Using selected treatments, it was established that the active compound was not a protein, lipid, hemicellulose, nor sugar. Based on the findings of this report, it may be concluded the band 1366 nm is very likely a water absorbance band related in general to hardness. Since the entire process of cement curing is about the loss of moisture and consequent hardening of cement, the observed absorbance band can be related to the hardness of cement mortar.

The negative peak common for loadings of PC2 for W_{dist}, W_{tap} and W_{mix} appears at 1428 nm, while in the case of $W_{shallow}$ at 1441 nm. The first one is assigned to hydroxide and hydration water, while the second one to the water dimer [51]. The importance of band 1428 nm, found to be related to amorphous regions in cellulose matrix of the wood and its stiffness and strength [77], may indicate not only the different state of water, but also the macro-scale properties of cement mortars made using W_{tap}, W_{mix} and W_{dist}. Particular differences occur at the region of hydrogen bonded water, where positive peaks and/or shoulders could be observed at 1503 nm in the case of W_{tap} and W_{mix}, at 1492 and 1510 nm for W_{dist} and 1515 nm for $W_{shallow}$. Looking again, together at the position of scores and sign of the peaks on loading plots, the process of cement hydration during the first 24 h can be described as a transformation of hydrogen-bonded water (>1492 nm) and water participating in ion solvation (1360 nm) to, in most cases, hydration water (1428 nm). The $W_{shallow}$ should be excluded from this explanation, as the PC2 in this case is not related to the changes in the aging of cement; it only describes some variations within the groups of scores for each of the days. It is interesting to note, however, that water dimers were the water species connected to preservation of biological structures during the complete desiccation of resurrection plants, and were related to the glassy state of water due to the sugar–water interaction [80]. This finding may indicate the existence of that type of glassy structure of water in the mortar made by $W_{shallow}$.

2.3.3. Soft Modeling of Class Analogies (SIMCA) of Cement Mortar

SIMCA analysis was performed on datasets of cement paste and mortar spectral data and separated according to the type of water used. Each dataset, after separation, was first smoothed using the Savitzky–Golay 2nd order polynomial filter (21 points) and baseline corrected using linear fit and SNV transformation, considering that each spectral dataset can have specific baseline variations. Following the pre-processing, each dataset was subjected to SIMCA analysis in order to discriminate between different days when the spectra were acquired, specifically on the day when the cement paste was first prepared (Day 0), and after leaving the mortar to cure (After 1 day, 3 days, and 7 days).

The results of the analysis, first presented in Table 3, demonstrate that irrespectively of the water used for cement preparation, the discrimination accuracy between the spectra of cement mortar acquired on different days was higher than 90%, and the interclass distances were larger than three, demonstrating very good, reliable separation [81,82] and indicating large changes in cement over time. However, the trends in the values of interclass distances were quite different depending on the water used in mixing, especially for the 3rd and 7th day, which implies differences in the hardening of mortar over time.

To investigate which variables, i.e., wavelengths in the spectra carried most information with regards to their discrimination with respect to different days, the discriminating powers of SIMCA analysis were plotted in Figure 7 and compared.

Table 3. SIMCA analysis results: discrimination accuracy and values of interclass distance compared to Day 0.

Water	Interclass Distance Compared to the Day 0			Discrimination Accuracy (%)
	After 1 Day	After 3 Days	After 7 Days	
W_{tap}	10.392	6.342	5.191	91.03
W_{dist}	9.511	4.977	6.312	93.53
$W_{shallow}$	9.807	4.539	4.030	94.12
W_{mix}	8.945	6.471	7.204	98.18

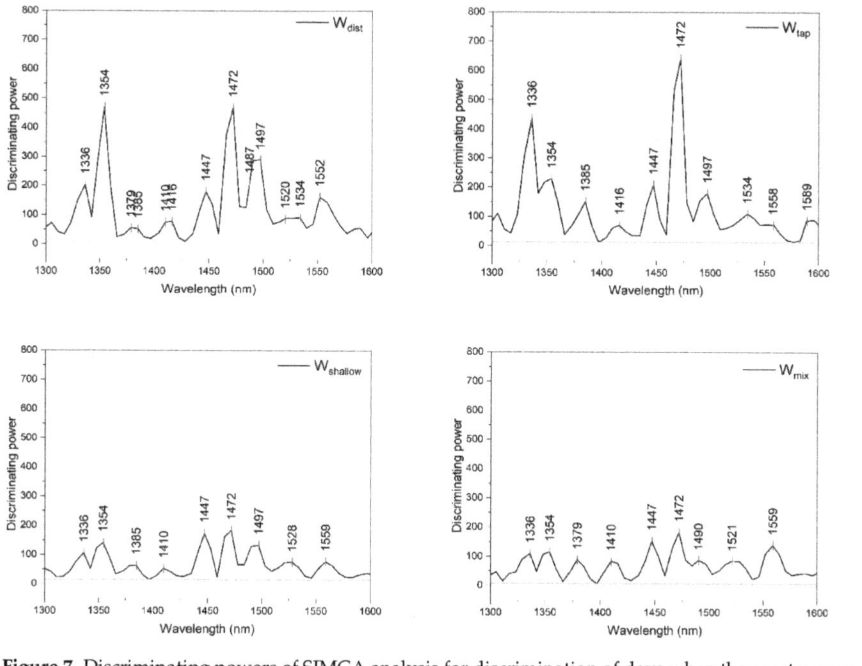

Figure 7. Discriminating powers of SIMCA analysis for discrimination of days when the spectra were acquired from paste and mortar prepared using 4 different waters.

The discriminating powers of SIMCA demonstrated one particular band with the highest discriminating power in all four cases of analyses, located at 1472 nm, corresponding to water molecules with three hydrogen bonds. The influential bands from all four models are similar, especially in the area of weakly hydrogen bonded water, however, with a different degree of influence in different models. The differences in discriminating powers are mostly in the area of hydrogen-bonded water and strongly bound water, which indicates differences in the water bound to cement components, i.e., the cement matrix differences as well.

It is also interesting to mention the difference in the magnitude of discriminating powers—in the case of $W_{shallow}$ and W_{mix}, the magnitude of discriminating powers does not cross 200, while in comparison, discriminating power values for W_{dist} and W_{tap} are about 500 and higher. The influence of the bands is rather uniform for all indicated bands in the case of $W_{shallow}$ and W_{mix}, which indicates balanced changes over time in mortar created using these waters.

Next, SIMCA analysis was performed with another objective. The dataset was split according to the day of acquisition of the spectra to Day0, and after 1, 3, and 7 days and data were analyzed by SIMCA to discriminate between mortars prepared using different mixing waters. Despite rather small values of interclass distances between the classes, the discrimination of different mortars according to the age was successful, with a discrimination accuracy higher than 82.64% (Table 4).

Table 4. SIMCA analysis results: discrimination accuracy and values of interclass distance between mortars prepared by different waters on the day of preparation and after 1, 3, and 7 days.

Day	Interclass Distance Range Min to Max	Discrimination Accuracy (%)
Day 0	0.319–0.606	82.64
After 1 day	0.244–2.056	88.33
After 3 days	0.256–1.589	94.36
After 7 days	0.244–1.013	91.68

In this case also, the discriminating powers of SIMCA analyses (Figure 8) were inspected for the most influential variables. The inspection of discriminating powers demonstrated which absorbance bands were most important for the discrimination between mortars on each of the examined days.

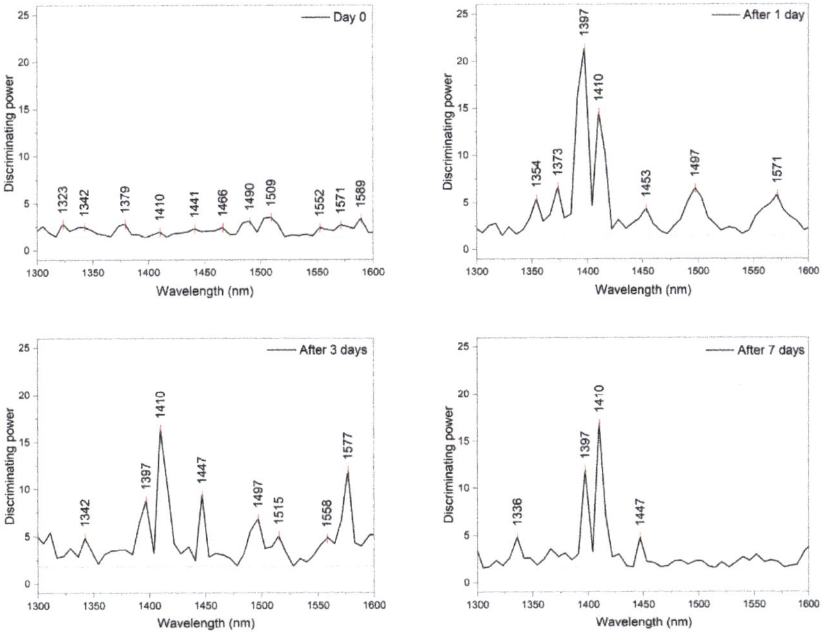

Figure 8. Discriminating powers of SIMCA analysis for discrimination of different mortars, on separate days during the process of setting cement concrete.

On the Day 0, there are many influential bands, demonstrating lots of differences in the water structure immediately upon mixing: particularly important are the bands at 1490 nm and 1509 nm, which can be attributed to water molecules with four hydrogen bonds and strongly bound water. Moreover, three important bands appear in the area of strongly bound water at 1552, 1571, and 1589 nm. In general, bands above 1500 nm can be assigned to the 1st overtone of the ice-like clusters of water, highly organized molecular structures expected around hydrated macromolecules [83–85]. Fujimoto et al. 2007 reported the similar, very closely located bands, 1548 nm and 1592 nm, to be related to crystalline regions in the cellulose matrix of the wood [77]. In the area of weakly hydrogen-bonded water, bands 1323 nm, which can be assigned to water monomers or bulk water [86,87], and band 1379 nm, which corresponds to solvation shells of water, appear significant. On subsequent days, the most differences between the mortars prepared with different water types could be explained by the differences at 1397 nm—trapped water depending on the ion concentration and 1410 nm—free water species that increase in water with the increase in temperature. These two bands become dominant for discrimination, especially after 7 days.

2.3.4. Aquagrams of Cement Mortar

Based on the entirety of the previous analysis, the absorbance bands that appeared consistently and had importance in the interpretation of results were summarized and 18 of them had been selected for representation on aquagram, to describe succinctly the water spectral patterns of cement paste and mortar over the time of investigation and depending on the water used for mixing. These absorbance bands and their tentative assignments with some remarks are provided in Table 5.

Table 5. Tentative assignments of the absorbance bands found to be important during analysis of cement spectral data. The wavelengths given in the parentheses in the assignments' column are the band positions from the cited literature and recalculated from wavenumbers or calculated overtones from fundamental frequencies reported in the original source.

Absorbance Band [nm]	Assignment/Remark
1342	(1342.6 nm, 1st overt. of 3724 cm^{-1}) proton hydrates [$H+\cdot(H_2O)_3$]—H_2O asymmetric stretch, 1st overt. [83] WAMACS C1: 1336–1348 nm: 1st overtone ν_3 asymmetric stretch [51]
1354	(1353.18 nm, 1st over. of 3695 cm^{-1}) two to four nonbonded OH stretches in 2 to 11 member cluster of hydrated proton [83] (1353.55 nm, 1st overt. of 3694 cm^{-1}) free OH stretch ($OH-\cdot(H_2O)_2$) [88]
1366	(1366.12 nm, 1st overt. of 3660 cm^{-1})—proton hydrates [$H+\cdot(H_2O)_2$]—H_2O asymmetric stretch [83] (1366.12 nm 1st overt. of 3660 cm^{-1}) OH-stretch in ($OH-\cdot(H_2O)_2$) [88] (1366.1 nm) Dangling -OH (non-hydrogen-bonded), 1st overt. [89] (1362 nm (7339 cm^{-1})) OH-coordinated with 1 or 2 Mg^{2+} on the corner and edge of the $Mg(OH)_2$ surface [78] (1368 nm (7306 cm^{-1})) OH-coordinated with 3 Mg^{2+} [78] (1366 nm)—absorbance band of a compound highly correlated with hardness [79] WAMACS C2: 1360–1366 nm—water solvation shell $OH-(H_2O)_{1,2,4}$ [51]
1379	WAMACS C3: 1370–1376 nm—combination symmetric asymmetric stretch $\nu_1+\nu_3$ [51]or WAMACS C4: 1380–1388 nm—water solvation shell $OH-(H_2O)_{1,4}$ [51] (1374 nm)—-OH group of $Ca(OH)_2$ [90] (1373–1375 nm)—-OH of portlandite phase; this band is useful for diagnosis of the initiation of hydration process [90] (1379.31 nm, 1st overt. of 3625 cm^{-1})—proton oscillation, H_2O symmetric stretch in $H+\cdot(H_2O)_6$ [83]
1385	(1383.13 nm 1st overt. of 3615 cm^{-1})—H_2O symmetric stretch in $H+\cdot(H_2O)_5$ [83] (1383.13 nm, 1st overt. of 3615 cm^{-1}) Interwater/Double donor stretch ($OH-$ $(H_2O)_4$) [88] (1385.12 nm, 1st overt. of 3609.8 cm^{-1}) H_2O symmetric stretch in proton hydrate $H+(H_2O)_4$ [91] (1385.50 nm, 1st over. of 3608.8 cm^{-1}) H_2O symmetric stretch in proton hydrate $H+(H_2O)_4$ [92] WAMACS C4: 1380–1388 nm—water solvation shell $OH-(H_2O)_{1,4}$ [51]
1391	(1391.21 nm 1st overt. of 3594 cm^{-1}) H_2O symmetric stretch in proton hydrate $H+(H_2O)_4$ [91,92] or trapped water 1396–1403 nm [69]
1397	(1396.6 nm, 1st overt. of 3580 cm^{-1}) proton hydrates [$H+\cdot(H_2O)_3$]—H_3O+ free-OH stretch, 1st overt. [83] (1397 nm (7158 cm^{-1}))—1st overtone of the free OH group trapped in the hydrophobic interior [93] WAMACS C5: water confined in the local field of ions 1396–1403 nm [52,69] (1397.23 nm (7157 cm^{-1}))—interlayer $OH-$ (stacked between sheets of $Mg(OH)_2$) [78]

Table 5. *Cont.*

Absorbance Band [nm]	Assignment/Remark
1410	1st overt. band of the OH stretching mode of free OH monomer [94] (1410.6 nm)—water species with no hydrogen bonds S_0 [95] WAMACS C5: 1398–1418 nm—free water molecules S_0
1428	(1428.6 nm) isolated H_3O+ -OH stretch vibration, 1st overt. [96] 1st overtone of the fundamental OH stretching vibration in water; the water molecules are condensed in one or more layers on sorption sites in the amorphous region; related to stiffness and strength [77]
1441	WAMACS C7: 1432–1444 nm—water molecules with 1 hydrogen bond S_1
1447	(1447 nm (6910 cm^{-1}))—1st overt. of O−H stretching of the water OH hydrated to other water molecules (bulk state) [97] (1447.18 nm (6910 cm^{-1}))—OH group involved in the OH· · · OH hydrogen bonding [98] (1447.18 nm, 1st overt. of 3445 cm^{-1})—stretching modes of surface H_2O molecules or to an envelope of hydrogen-bonded surface OH groups [99] (1450.11 nm, 1st overt. of 3448 cm^{-1})—OH stretching vibrations of the water lattice in the hydrated calcium silicates and aluminosilicates (C-S-H and C-A-S-H) [90] WAMACS C8: 1448–1454 nm—solvation shell OH-$(H_2O)_{4,5}$
1460	WAMACS C9: 1458–1468 nm—water molecules with 2 hydrogen bonds S_2
1472	(1470 nm)—chemically bound water in the hydrated calcium silicate phases [90] WAMACS C10: 1472–1482 nm—water molecules with 3 hydrogen bonds S_3
1490	WAMACS C11: 1482–1495 nm—water molecules with 4 hydrogen bonds S_4
1503	(1503.3 nm 1st overt. of 3326 cm^{-1})—OH stretching vibrations of hydrogen bonded water molecules participating in the crystal structure [100] (1503.3 nm 1st overt. of 3326 cm^{-1})—OH stretching vibration in Ice III [101] (1503.3 nm 1st overt. of 3326 cm^{-1})—strong intermolecular hydrogen bond [102] (1503.3 nm 1st overt. of 3326 cm^{-1})—water stretching vibrations in minerals, in connection with hydrogen defects (incorporation of hydrogen (protonation)) [103–108]
1515	WAMACS C12: 1506–1516 nm—combination of symmetric stretching and bending vibration $\nu1 + \nu2$, strongly bound water [51]
1534	(1534.21 nm, 1st overt. of 3259 cm^{-1})—hydrogen bonded hydroxyl groups (-O-$H^{\delta+}$· · · $O^{\delta-}$-) [109] (1534.21 nm, 1st overt. of 3259 cm^{-1})—the H-O stretching vibrations of the absorbent water [110] (1534.21 nm (6518 cm^{-1}))—1st over. of hydrogen bonded O-H stretching [111] (1534.21 nm, 1st overt. of 3259 cm^{-1})—one of the 3 water stretching bands observed in carbonate mineral huanghoite by Raman spectroscopy (the other two being 1435 nm (3484 cm^{-1}) and 1393 nm (3589 cm^{-1})) [103] (1534.21 nm, 1st overt. of 3259 cm^{-1})—sesquihydrate crystallite [112] (hydrate whose solid contains 3 molecules of water of crystallization per two molecules) (1534 nm)—one of 3 wavelengths used in multiple linear regression for predicting bread loaf volume (1506, 1534 and 1618 nm); measurement of some parameter related to volume independent of protein [113]
1559	(1557 nm) ionic bound water molecules 1st overt. [114] (1560 nm (3205 cm^{-1}))—strongly hydrogen bonded water, water coordinated to cations [115] (1560 nm)—hydrogen bonded water [116] (1560 nm (6410 cm^{-1})) crystalline water ice feature [117]

The calculated aquagrams presented in Figures 9 and 10, using these 18 bands as radial axes, give a comparative overview of water spectral patterns (WASPs) of cement paste and mortar. First, aquagrams shown in Figure 9 present how WASPs for each cement mortar evolves over time for each mixing water separately, while aquagrams in Figure 10 show how WASPs of mortars created using different waters compare at a particular cement age (days).

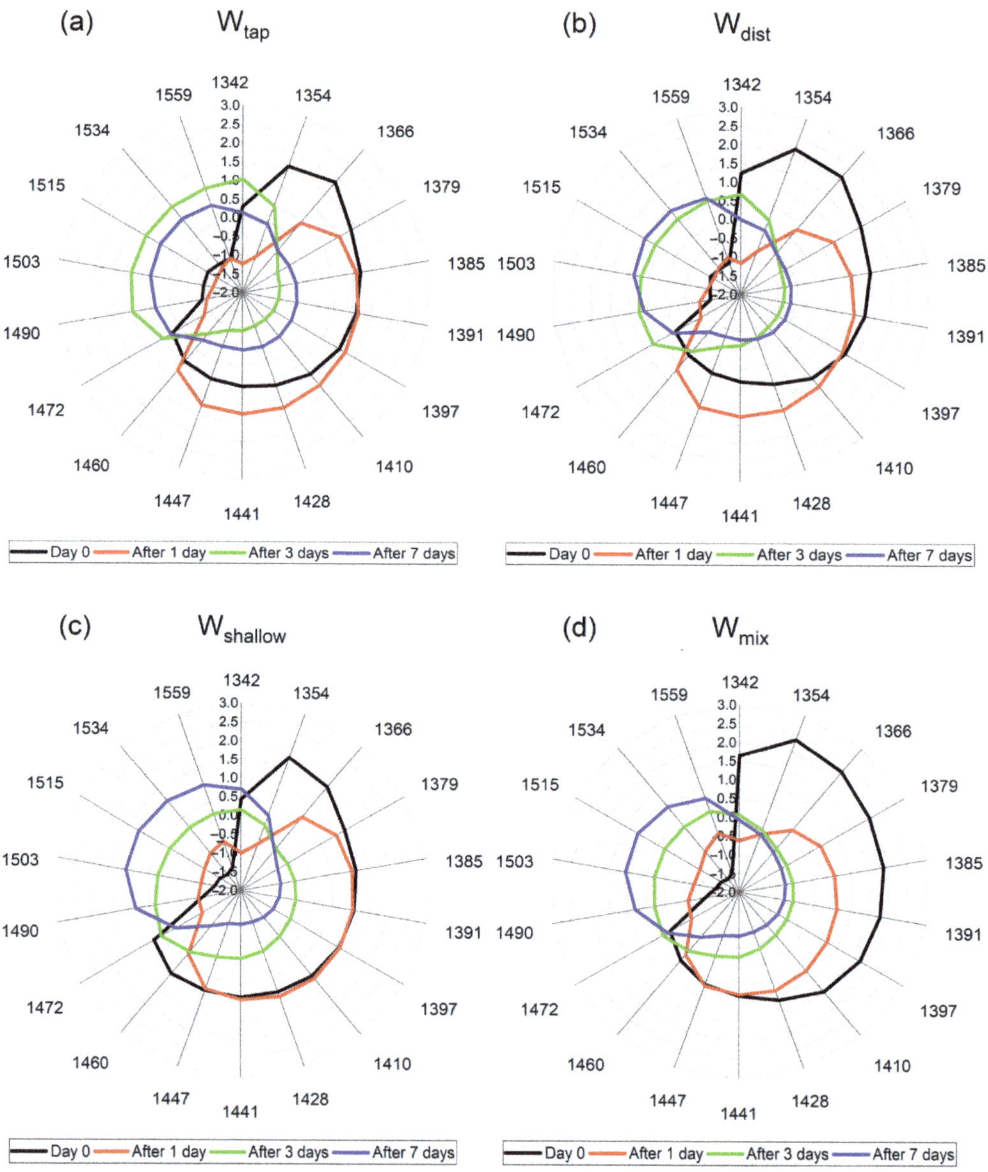

Figure 9. Aquagrams of cement paste and mortar according to the water used for cement mixing: (**a**) W_{tap}, (**b**) W_{dist}, (**c**) $W_{shallow}$, and (**d**) W_{mix} water. The aquagrams demonstrate the differences in water spectral patterns (WASPs) of cement mortar at different points in time: at Day 0—immediately after mixing of cement paste, and when the mortar was removed from the frame and aged 1 day, 3 days, and 7 days. The aquagrams are colored according to the corresponding measurement day.

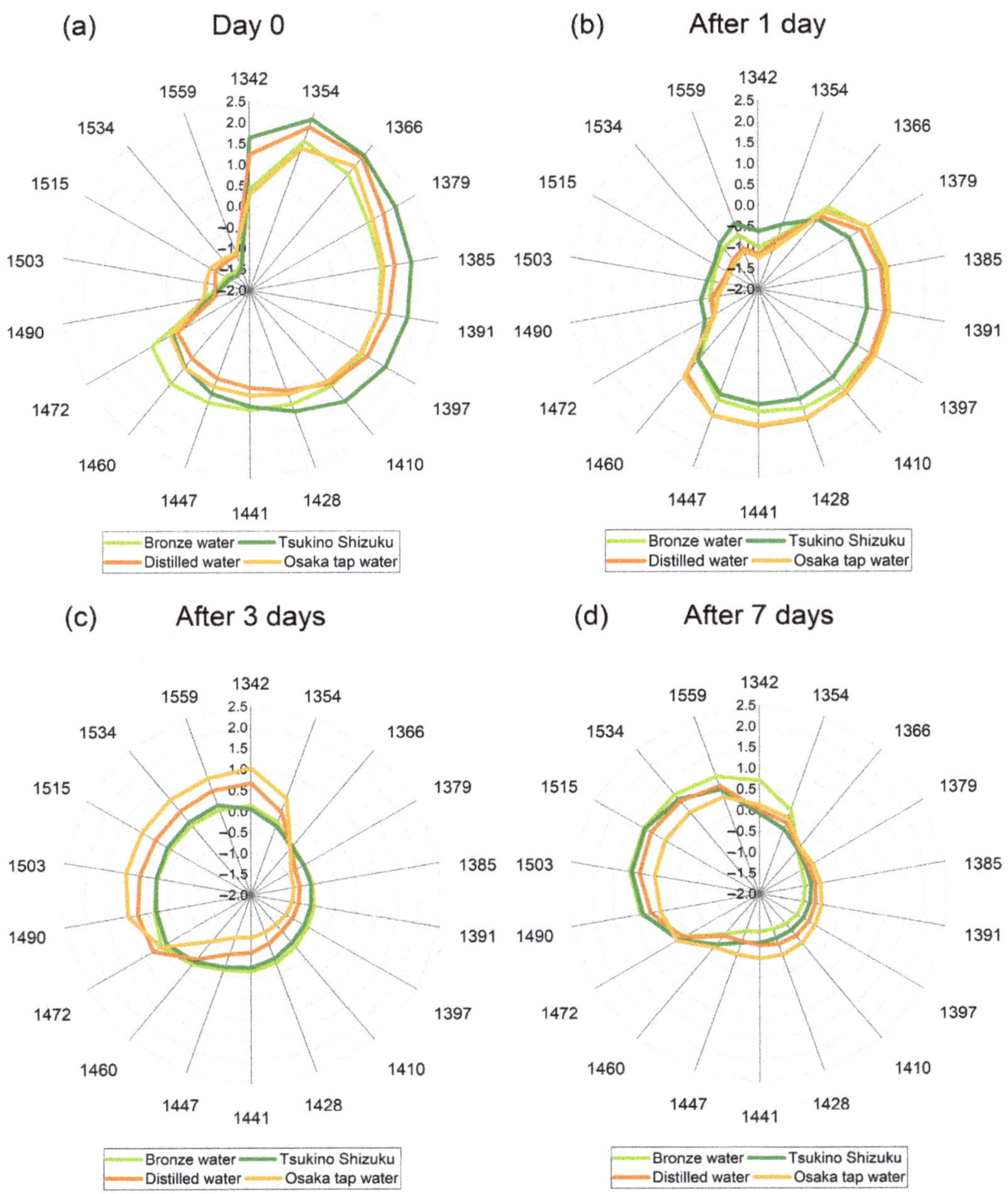

Figure 10. Aquagrams of cement paste and mortar grouped according to the time points when the measurements were performed: (**a**) Day 0—immediately after mixing of cement paste, (**b**) one day after the mortar was removed from the frame and left to cure, (**c**) three days after the mortar was removed from the frame and left to cure, and (**d**) seven days after the mortar was removed from the frame and left to age. The aquagrams demonstrate the differences in water spectral patterns (WASPs) of cement mortar depending on the water used for mixing, and the aquagram profiles are colored accordingly.

From the aquagrams presented in Figure 9, the common trend can be observed for changes from cement paste and mortar with time regardless of water used for mixing. In general, the spectral pattern of water in cement paste is located in the right part of aquagrams, ending at 1472 nm, and with time it moves to the left part, demonstrating that the process of change in the cement during curing is characterized by the transformation of proton hydrates, solvation shells, free and quasi-free water, hydration water, and some small water clusters bonded with 1 to 3 hydrogen bonds. The differences in the cement paste can be better observed from Figure 10a, where it can be observed that W_{mix} water and W_{dist} provide more proton hydrates in cement paste (1342–1354 nm); W_{mix} water seems to provide more free and weakly bound water species (1379–1428 nm), while $W_{shallow}$, in particular, results in more hydrogen-bonded water clusters.

The change in WASPs from cement paste (Day 0) and cement mortar aged 1 day, seem to be particularly different between the waters. During this 24 h, the transformation of the water molecular network is radical, where the major water species reduced during this process are proton hydrates and solvation shells (1342–1379 nm). However, in the case of $W_{shallow}$ and W_{mix} water (Figure 9c,d), these species are lost at the expense of the increased amount of water bonded to the elements of cement matrix (1503–1559 nm), while in the case of W_{tap} and W_{dist}, there is a increase in free water, hydration water, solvation shells/surface water, and small water clusters (1410–1460 nm).

The aquagrams comparing the state of mortar after 1 day given at Figure 10b especially demonstrate this difference in the area of strongly bound water. The water species that are initially lost (1342–1379 nm) are the species with the highest energy and highest mobility, such as water vapor, or the so-called moisture [72].

On the other hand, among the bands of strongly bound water, a 1534 nm absorbance band of water was demonstrated to carry the information about the specific volume [113]. The drying shrinkage as a phenomenon is closely related to the moisture loss and to the changes in volume; thus, our findings may indicate the possibility to directly measure those properties and at the same time relate them to the specific water spectral patterns.

Another interesting feature that can be observed from Figure 9, is that the spectral pattern of mortar in the case of $W_{shallow}$ does not change at all in the region of 1385–1447 nm. This lack of change in the cement during first 24 h agrees with what was earlier observed during the PCA analysis. Since the bands 1391 nm, 1397 nm, 1428 nm, and 1447 nm are all related to water species that are in some kind of interaction with the material—either confined, or participating in hydration, solvation, or adsorption, this may indicate that mortar made with $W_{shallow}$ does not really change some elements of the created cement matrix during this time. W_{tap} and W_{dist} mortars, particularly, demonstrate higher absorbance after 1 day at these absorbance bands, corresponding to the absorbance of water species that have less mobility and energy compared to the moisture, but still with lots of ability to participate in chemical reactions.

The WASPs at later days (after 3 and 7) demonstrate quite similar profiles for all mortars, with increasing absorbance at the bands of hydrogen-bonded water and water bonded to elements of cement (1470–1559 nm). This type of water can be considered to be an integral part of the cement and cannot be changed or lost to drying, unless the cement matrix itself is damaged. This agrees with the observations about the non-evaporable water content differences—it was reported that they become less pronounced in three types of Portland cement (different chemical composition of cement) at later ages, and further that the relationship between the non-evaporable water and degree of hydration appears to be dependent upon the chemical composition [118]. Therefore, even though the cement components did not change at all, it may be that the chemical content and hence water molecular structure of the mixing waters contributed to this.

When it comes to the loss of this strongly bound water, as already said, it might happen only due to the damage of the matrix that is binding it, and this may be the case with the mortar made with W_{tap}, where, in contrast to all other mortars, the WASPs for the 3rd and 7th day are reversed, with lower absorbance corresponding to the 7th day. This may be the case of cracks in the cement internal structure, where the elements of cement matrix are being broken and the water which was bound, is being released. This can explain the increase in free water that can be observed in Figure 10d, where the highest absorbance in the region 1397–1460 nm can be observed for exactly W_{tap} mortar.

In summary, from the aquagrams, it was observed that WASPs in the first 24 h could be divided in two groups, where $W_{shallow}$ and W_{mix} water mortars were similar, and W_{tap} and W_{dist} mortars were similar. This may result in similar properties of the mortars on the macroscale. $W_{shallow}$ mortar was particularly specific in the terms that it demonstrates stability during first 24 h, while W_{tap} mortar was specific in the terms that it demonstrated opposite change between the 3rd and 7th day of curing. These results, which demonstrate differences at such a detailed scale in the water molecular matrix of the paste and mortar, practically from the very start when paste is mixed, with further research may result in the prediction of mortar properties at the earliest possible stage.

2.4. Characterization of the Internal Temperature Change and Thermal Strain in Cement Paste

In ordinary Portland-hydrated cement paste there are four major compounds: tricalcium silicate (C_3S), dicalcium silicate (C_2S), tricalcium aluminate (C_3A) and tetracalcium aluminoferrite (C_4AF); both C_3S and C_2S react with water (H) to form calcium silicate hydrate (C-S-H) and the portlandite, also called calcium hydroxyde (CH) [119,120].

The process of cement hydration is an exothermic reaction and the temperature rise in mass concrete pours [121]. The measured values of internal temperature in cement pastes made by W_{tap}, W_{dist}, $W_{shallow}$, and W_{mix} water are presented in Figure 11a and demonstrated that this temperature increase is similar for all pastes up to 24 h after casting. The well-known stages of hydration in Portland cement can be observed: (I) initial reaction, (II) period of slow reaction, (III) acceleration period, and (IV) deceleration period. Generally, the hydration reaction starts when cement comes into the contact with water, and the internal temperature of the cement paste rises for a certain period as the cement hardens. However, for the first few hours immediately after casting, the cement paste goes through the setting process where the fluidity is gradually lost, which is different from the above-mentioned hardening process. As shown in Figure 11a, the internal temperature of the cement paste rises and then drops immediately after casting, and then after about 2 h it starts rising again.

There are distinctive differences in the values of internal temperature of paste in the phases I and II, depending on the water used for preparation. In phase I, the paste made with W_{dist} shows the fastest increase and the highest temperature during the initial reaction of cement with water. In phase II, the temperature values are quite different between all the pastes, but in particular between the cement made with W_{dist} and W_{mix} water, demonstrating differences in this stage of cement hydration with respect to the water used. Important point to take into consideration is that the internal temperature at the start of measurement is already different for each cement paste. Therefore, to be able to grasp real change in the internal temperature compared to the initial temperature of the paste, the temperature difference during phases III and IV is plotted in Figure 11b.

The results shown in Figure 11b indicate that the amount of released heat is at its maximum 12.25 h after casting for W_{mix} water, 12.8 h for W_{dist} and $W_{shallow}$, and 13.25 h for W_{tap}. This suggests that the progression of hydration reaction happens at a different speed depending on the water used, and it is especially different in the case of W_{tap}. The maximum heat generation was the largest for the W_{dist}, followed by $W_{shallow}$, W_{tap}, and W_{mix}.

The hardened cement paste has different thermal expansion properties, which leads to different volumetric changes that generate internal stress causing the cracking of concrete at the micro- or macro-scale [90,122,123]. The thermal expansion coefficients (TEC) are affected by the water contents in a hardened cement paste, especially the free water content, which is why TEC have large values in the early hydration ages [124]. The TEC of a compacted material is smaller than that of a porous material [125].

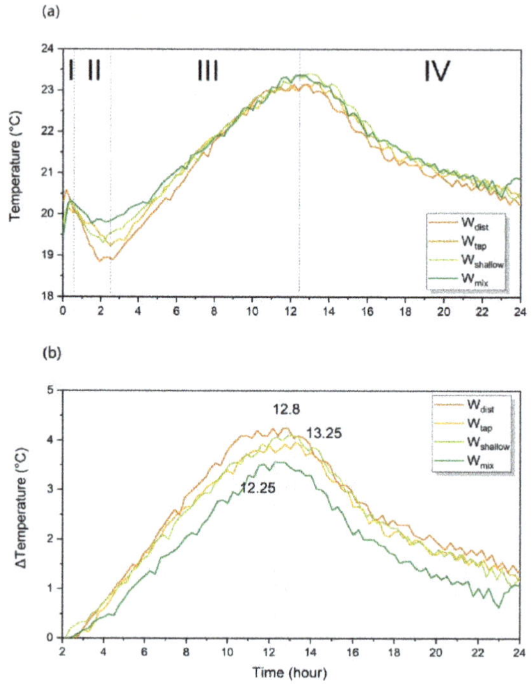

Figure 11. (**a**) Internal temperature of the cement paste specimens during first 24 h; (**b**) the trend of the change in the internal temperature of cement paste during phases III and IV.

The measured values of thermal expansion during 24 h after casting are plotted in Figure 12. The thermal strain was larger in the cases of W_{dist} and W_{tap}, which were quite similar, but different compared to the thermal strain recorded in mortar made by $W_{shallow}$ and W_{mix} water (Figure 12). The grouping strongly resembles grouping two-by-two that can be observed in the WASPs of mortars after 1 day (Figure 10b). Given the above background, it can be expected that hardened paste created by $W_{shallow}$ and W_{mix} water have a less porous, more compact structure.

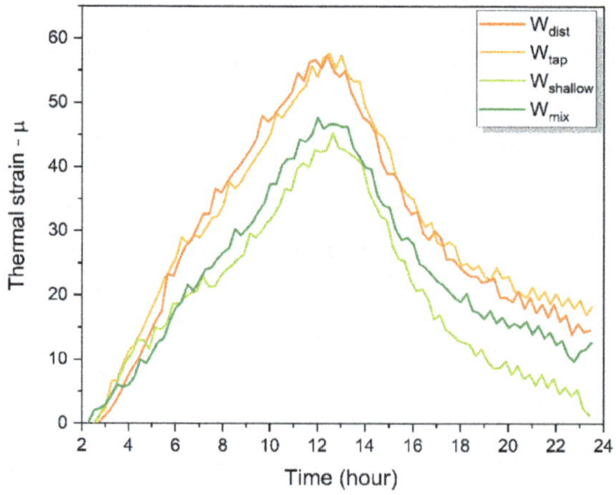

Figure 12. The time trend of thermal strain of cement paste.

2.5. Characteristics of Drying Shrinkage Strain

Drying shrinkage is defined as the volumetric change of concrete induced by the loss and redistribution of moisture, which can lead to the formation of cracks within the concrete and influence important properties such as durability, deformation, and stress distribution [126–128]. It is therefore desirable to reduce drying shrinkage; the techniques proposed so far are to apply low shrinkage cement or cement with low hydration heat [129]. It is also reported that drying shrinkage is more pronounced in specimens with rapid moisture loss [130]; therefore, slowing down this process could help in the reduction of drying shrinkage. As this study already pointed out, this may be achieved by the adequate choice of water for the preparation of cement.

The results of the drying shrinkage strain measurements performed over the period of 91 days after casting demonstrate considerably reduced drying shrinkage strain in specimens prepared with $W_{shallow}$ and W_{mix} water (Figure 13a). The worst performance can be observed in cement prepared with the W_{tap}, followed by W_{dist}. The drying shrinkage strain properties already demonstrated the same result even only 7 days after casting (Figure 13b). The drying shrinkage strain was about the same for $W_{shallow}$ and W_{mix} water, and W_{dist} and W_{tap} followed in increasing order. Similar to the results of thermal stress, grouping two-by-two can also be observed here in Figure 13, which closely matches the pattern observed in WASPs of cement paste given in Figure 10b.

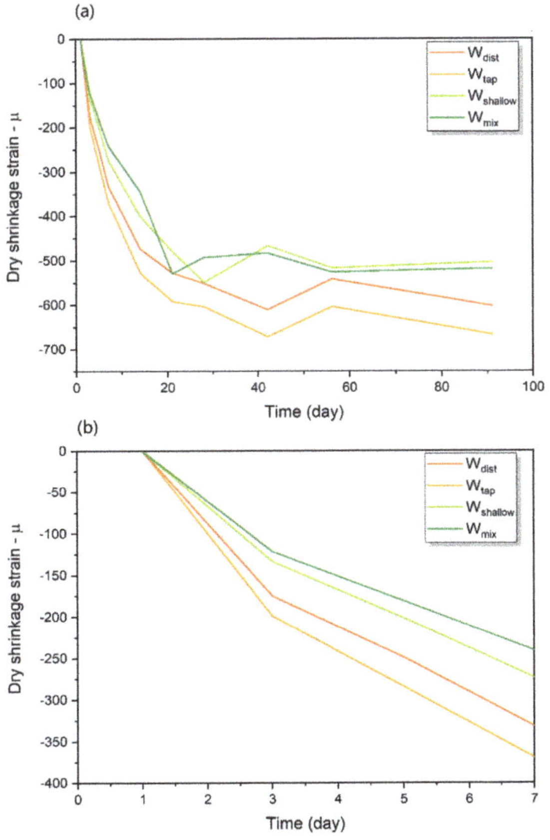

Figure 13. Drying shrinkage strain: (**a**) in time period up to Day 91; (**b**) in time period up to Day 7.

To understand the reason why the drying shrinkage strains of $W_{shallow}$ and W_{mix} water were smaller, the results of the water component analysis and spectral patterns of cement paste and mortar were taken into consideration.

First, the water composition analysis demonstrated that the Si content was considerably higher in $W_{shallow}$ and W_{mix}, compared to the W_{dist} and W_{tap}, as shown in Table 1 and Figure 1. $W_{shallow}$ and W_{mix} water also contained a large amount of sodium. Generally, when $Ca(OH)_2$ produced by the hydration reaction of cement comes into contact with silicate compounds such as $Na_2O{\cdot}SiO_2$ at the initial stage, $CaO{\cdot}SiO_2$ crystals are formed. This is understood to improve the watertightness of the hardened cement, and the application of silicate compounds is used for improving the properties of cement concrete [131–133]. In this study, it can be concluded that Si and Na in the $W_{shallow}$ and W_{mix} water affected the crystal structure of cement mortar, and the suppression performance against drying shrinkage might have improved as a result. The water spectral patterns of cement paste 24 h after setting, indeed demonstrate an increase in strongly bound, crystalline water (Figure 10b, region 1490–1559 nm). The spectral patterns of mortar 7 days after casting also demonstrate the same for $W_{shallow}$ and W_{mix} mortars compared to the W_{dist} and W_{tap} mortar (Figure 10d).

Further, since $W_{shallow}$ demonstrated the best drying shrinkage characteristics, it is of interest to notice that the spectral pattern of cement paste after 24 h (Figure 10b) was particularly different, demonstrating no changes in absorbance in the region of 1385–1447 nm, while the W_{mix} paste demonstrated no changes in absorbance in the narrower region of 1441–1447 nm. In contrast, the cement paste created with W_{tap} and W_{dist} demonstrated an increased amount of water species absorbing in these regions. The water species that are initially lost (1342–1379 nm), the so-called moisture [72], in the case of $W_{shallow}$ and W_{mix} water (Figure 9c,d), led to the increased amount of water bonded to the elements of cement matrix (1503–1559 nm), while in the case of W_{tap} and W_{dist}, to increase in free water, hydration water, solvation shells/surface water, and small water clusters (1410–1460 nm). Considering the resulting drying shrinkage properties, this indicates that this particular water molecular structure might be especially important to monitor during the early age of cement. In this respect, this study has made considerable progress in pinpointing the exact absorbance bands corresponding to specific water structures within cement paste and mortar that can serve as WAMACs, i.e., the coordinates at which the absorbance of water in concrete can be measured and provide the information about the state of water within cement matrix and how it is related to the current state and future properties of produced concrete.

To conclude, it is clear that even a small difference in the water composition used for the cement mortar affects the molecular structures of the water inside the cement mortar and lead to different mechanical properties. The difficulties of relating single components to a specific function were overcome by using water spectral pattern as an integrative multidimensional marker, displayed on aquagram and mirroring even a small perturbation to the water molecular matrix in each mixture. These research findings may be interpreted within the existing framework of current understanding, but for the first time the state of the water in cement was described using a water spectral pattern, where numbers were used instead of the vague and broad terms such as capillary water, adsorbed water, interlayer water, and others. This provides a strong basis for the development of a universal method for the characterization of cement paste, mortar, and concrete from an aspect of hydration and allows quantitative comparisons and the optimal choice of cement materials and water for mixing with possibilities for early prediction of cement quality by using non-invasive monitoring.

3. Materials and Methods

3.1. Water Samples

Four types of water were used for the preparation of the cement: tap water from the Osaka city municipal supply, distilled water, and two spring mineral waters (Table 6).

Mineral spring waters were first filtered using activated charcoal to remove the impurities, and then using an antibacterial filter.

Table 6. Summary of the water samples used in this study.

Water	Collection Site	Characteristics
W_{dist}	—	High purity Wdist purified by ion exchange method and followed by distillation
W_{tap}	Osaka City, Osaka Prefecture, Japan	Tap water collected mainly from the surface water of Lake Biwa and purified at a water treatment facility
$W_{shallow}$	Water from the shallow underground source located at the dept of 40 m	Natural hot spring Yunosato, Hashimoto City, Wakayama Prefecture, Japan (https://www.spa-yunosato.com/yunosato_eng/ accessed on 1 November 2022)
W_{mix}	Water that is a blend of two types of spring waters (90% water from the shallow source located at 50 m depth and 10% water from the deep source at 1187 m depth)	Natural hot spring Yunosato, Hashimoto City, Wakayama Prefecture, Japan (https://www.spa-yunosato.com/yunosato_eng/ accessed on 1 November 2022);

The mineral content of all four water types was determined by inductively coupled plasma mass spectroscopy (ICP-MS). The component analysis was conducted by the Metal team at Kyoto Municipal Institute of Industrial Technology and Culture (http://tc-kyoto.or.jp/about/organization/kinzoku/detail.html accessed on 14 November 2020).

3.2. Cement and Fine Aggregate (Sand)

For the preparation of cement, Ordinary Portland cement (OPR) was used. The main components are CaO, SiO_2, Al_2O_3, and Fe_2O_3, but since the content ratio differs depending on the manufacturing plant, the quality of Portland cement is standardized by JIS (Japanese Industrial Standards) R5210 "Portland cement". As an example, Table 7 shows the standard for the chemical composition contained in cement. The density of the cement used was 3.15 g/cm^3. Australian standard sand conforming to ISO 679 was used as the fine aggregate. Table 8 shows the chemical composition of standard sand, and Table 9 shows an example of its physical properties, respectively.

Table 7. An example of the quality of Portland cement (chemical composition).

Chemical Name	Maximum Content Allowed (%)
MgO	5.0
SO_3	3.5
Ignition Loss	5.0
Total alkali content	0.75

Table 8. An example of the chemical composition of standard sand.

Chemical Name	Content (%)
SiO_2	98.4
Al_2O_3	0.4
Fe_2O_3	0.4
CaO	0.2
MgO	0.00
Na_2O	0.01
K_2O	0.01

Table 9. An example of the physical properties of standard sand.

Property	Value
Specific gravity in oven-dried condition	2.64
Sater absorption rate	0.42%
Unit volume mass	1.76 kg/L
Solid content	66.7%

3.3. *Preparation of Hardened Cement Specimens*

The specimens were prepared at the Osaka Metropolitan University (formerly Osaka City University) Graduate School of Engineering, Department of Urban Design and Engineering. The specimens produced were cement paste and cement mortar. The mixing ratio of cement paste and cement mortar was determined according to JIS R 5201, the "Physical testing methods for cement" [134].

Cement paste is a mixture composed of water and cement with a mass ratio of water to cement of 1:2. Cement mortar is a mixture composed of water, cement, and fine aggregate, and the mass ratio of water, cement, and sand is 1:2:6. In order to minimize the influence of temperature when mixing the materials, water, cement, and fine aggregate were left in a curing room at the constant temperature one day before the mixing of materials. The mixing of cement paste and cement mortar was carried out in accordance with JIS R 5201, the "Physical testing methods for cement" [134], as follows:

1. Add water and cement to the container for mixing.
2. Mix at a low speed for 30 s.
3. Add fine aggregate.
4. Mix at a high speed for 30 s.
5. Scrape the mortar adhering to the walls and bottom of the mixing container (Stop for 90 s).
6. Mix at high speed for 60 s and then take out.

For cement paste, the procedure ends with step 2. The cement paste was left in a plastic beaker for subsequent measurements (Figure 14). After casting in steel formwork, the surface of the cement mortar specimens was covered with a wrap, and the specimens were left in a curing room at a constant temperature of 20 °C ± 2 °C and humidity of 60 ± 5%. The formwork was removed the next day, and the specimens were placed in the curing room at the constant temperature and in the air atmosphere.

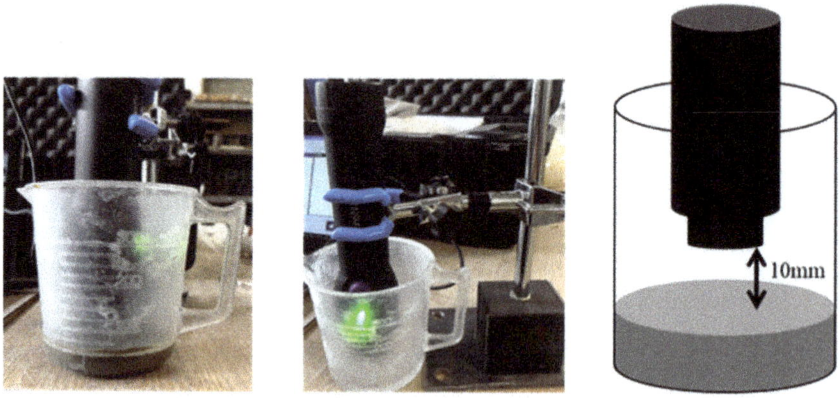

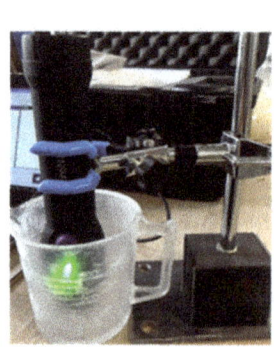

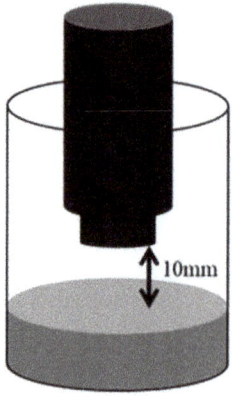

Figure 14. Spectral measurement immediately after mixing (cement paste).

3.4. NIR Spectroscopy

3.4.1. NIR Spectroscopy Measurement of Water Samples

The water used in this study was analyzed at the Aquaphotomics Research Department, Graduate School of Agricultural Science, Kobe University. The NIR spectra of the water samples were measured with the FOSS XDS spectrometer equipped with a Rapid Liquid Analyzed (RLA) module (FOSS NIRSystems, Inc., Höganäs, Sweden) using a quartz cuvette (optical path length 1 mm). The spectra were acquired in the transmittance mode, with the resolution of 0.5 nm in the spectral range 400–2500 nm. Each recorded spectrum was an average of 32 co-added spectra. The water samples were prepared in triplicates, and each sample was measured with 5 consecutive scans. The experiment was performed at 25 °C, keeping the temperature of the sample holder at this temperature throughout the measurements using circulating water bath. The order of measurements was randomized, but after every 5 samples, the sample of ultra-pure water (MilliQ, Millipore, Molsheim, France) was scanned. The temperature of the samples was monitored and logged during the experiment.

3.4.2. NIR Spectroscopy Measurement of Cement Paste and Mortar

Measurement of cement specimens was carried out at the Graduate School of Engineering, Department of Urban Design and Engineering, Osaka Metropolitan University. Using a portable, handheld NIR spectrometer (MicroNIR OnSite-W, VIAVI Solutions Inc. Milpitas, CA, USA), the spectrum was measured in 6.2 nm increments in the wavelength range of 950 nm to 1650 nm. The measurement was taken on Day 0 (immediately after mixing, cement paste), 1 day, 3 days, 7 days, and 28 days after mixing (cement mortar).

The NIR spectrometer was fixed as shown in Figure 14 to measure the specimen immediately after mixing. The measurements were performed with a gap of approximately 10 mm between the cement paste surface and the NIR spectrometer. The mortar specimens were measured as presented schematically in Figure 15 at particularly chosen measurement points. The spectral measurements were acquired at 5 points on the right and left surface of the specimen, with 3 consecutive measurements each. These measurements were performed 1 day, 3 days, 7 days, and 28 days after mixing.

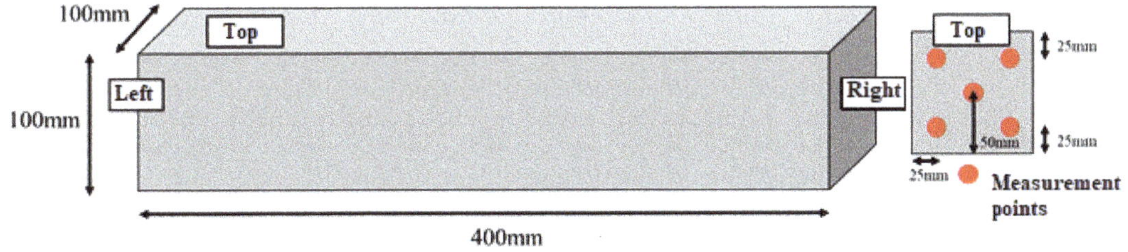

Figure 15. Measurements of cement mortar specimens.

3.5. Aquaphotomic Spectral Data Analysis

3.5.1. Water Characterization

The characterization of mixing waters was performed using aquaphotomics NIR spectroscopy. The NIR spectra of mixing waters, acquired in the range 400–2500 nm, at controlled temperature of 25 °C were trimmed to region of 1300–1600 nm that corresponds to first overtone of water stretching vibrations which typically has a maximum around 1450 nm.

The spectra were analyzed according to the protocol of aquaphotomic spectral analysis [63]. Difference spectra, Principal Component Analysis (PCA) [64], Soft Modeling of Class Analogies (SIMCA) [65] and Partial Least Squares Regression (PLSR) Analysis (using temperature and consecutive irradiation as dependent variables) were performed (results not presented) in order to find the representative water absorbance bands—water matrix coordinates (WAMACS) [51] that can be used to depict the characteristic water spectral patterns (WASPs) of mixing waters on aquagrams [63,66]. The selection of WAMACS was performed as described in the recent literature [63,67], by choosing the consistently repeating and most influential absorbance bands in the entire performed analysis. This resulted in selection of 15 wavelengths to serve as WAMACS and create aquagrams.

The aquagram shows the average normalized absorbance of the spectra of various samples at selected 15 wavelengths associated with the various molecular structures of water which define radial axes of the graph. Microsoft Office Excel 2013 (Microsoft Co., Redmond, WA, USA) was used for aquagram calculations.

3.5.2. Cement Paste and Mortar Characterization

The spectral data were converted to pseudo-absorbance (logT^{-1} where T is the transmittance). In order to investigate the first overtone of the OH stretching vibration, the wavelength range of the measured spectrum was limited to 1300 to 1600 nm.

The exploratory analysis in the form of Principal Component Analysis (PCA) [75] was applied on the spectral data separated in four datasets according to the type of water used for mixing, and corrected for baseline effects using detrend and standard normal variate transformation [135] after the smoothing to eliminate the noise from the spectra (Savitzky-Golay 2nd order polynomial filter [76] and 21-point window size).

Soft Modeling of Class Analogies (SIMCA) [65] is a supervised pattern recognition technique, used in the study to discriminate between the mortars created by different mixing waters and the age of the mortars.

Aquagrams of the cement paste and mortar were prepared following the same procedure as described in the Section 3.5.1, with the difference that spectral data were preprocessed using smoothing, linear detrend and standard normal variate transformation, and 18 wavelengths were selected to be presented on aquagrams.

3.6. *Physical Test Method for Cement Mortar*

All the tests were conducted at the Graduate School of Engineering, Department of Urban Design and Engineering, Osaka Metropolitan University.

3.6.1. Temperature Change and Thermal Strain

The specimens were prepared using cement paste for this test. A strain gauge with a temperature measurement function was used to reduce the influence of surrounding environmental conditions such as temperature. In order to place the strain gauge near the center of the specimen, a jig with the strain gauge attached was installed in the formwork in advance, and then cement paste was placed in the formwork. A schematic representation of the jig with the attached strain gauge is presented in Figure 16a. This jig was fixed to the bottom of a cylindrical formwork with a diameter of 50 mm and a height of 100 mm using an adhesive (Figure 16b). The final formwork for experimental measurements before the cement paste was poured in is shown in photographs in Figure 16c.

The cement paste was then placed in formwork and left in the air in a constant temperature curing room with a temperature of 20 $\pm$ 2 °C and a humidity of 60 $\pm$ 5%.

The measurement of the thermal change of the cement paste was started immediately using the digital micron strain gauge, contact type (Mitutoyo ABSOLUTE, Mitutoyo Corporation, Kawasaki, Japan). The measurements were performed every 15 min until approximately 24 h after the cement paste was placed.

3.6.2. Dry Shrinkage Test

The drying shrinkage strain test was performed in accordance with JIS A 1129-2 "Methods of measurement for length change of mortar and concrete—Part 2: Method with contact-type strain gauge." The measuring instrument used was the digital micron strain gauge (contact-type gauge), shown in Figure 17.

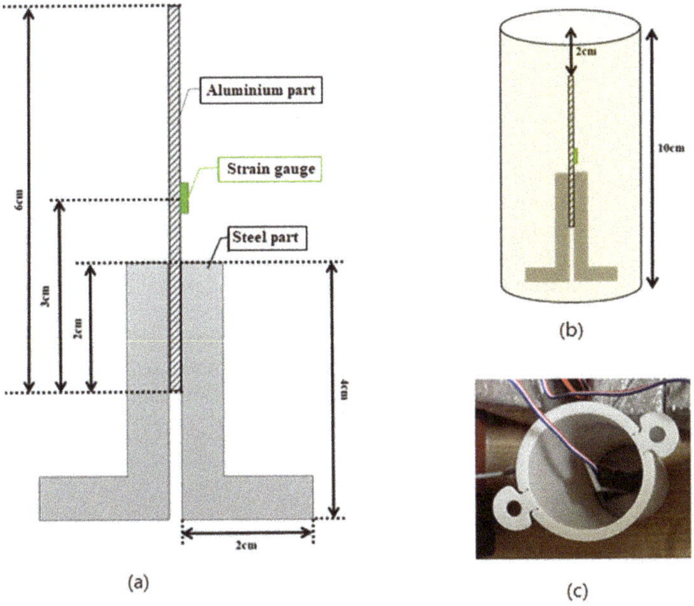

Figure 16. Measurements of the thermal changes of the cement paste; the method of fixing the strain gauge: (**a**) schematic representation of attached strain gauge, (**b**) arrangement of the jig in the formwork, and (**c**) experimental setup.

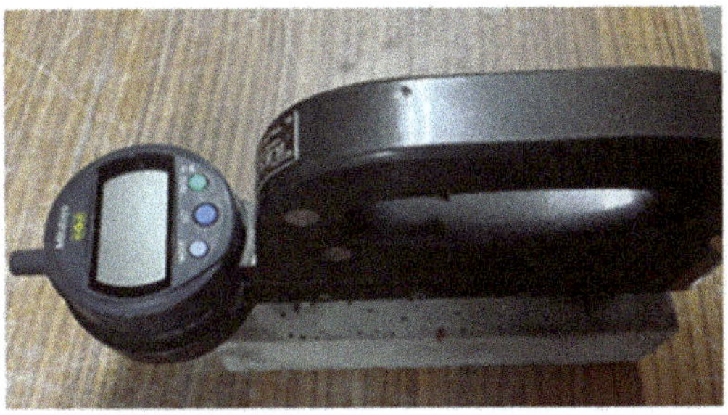

Figure 17. Measurement of length change of mortar using digital micron strain gauge (contact-type gauge).

The specimens were produced using a regular right prism formwork with dimensions of 40 mm × 40 mm × 160 mm. After taking them out of the formwork, a gauge plug was attached to the side of each specimen. Figure 17 shows the position of the gauge plug attachment. The specimens were then left to stand in the air in a constant temperature curing room with a temperature of 20 ± 2 °C and a humidity of 60 ± 5%.

This test was performed with the aim to calculate the rate of the shrinkage of the specimen using the measured length between the gauge plugs. The measurements of the length between the gauge plugs were performed on the day 1 (when taking the specimens out of the formwork) and 3 days, 5 days, 7 days, 14 days, 21 days, 28 days, 42 days, 56 days, and 91 days after casting. The rate of the length change was calculated using the following equation:

$$\varepsilon = \frac{X_i - X_0}{L_0} \times 10^6 \quad (1)$$

where ε is the drying shrinkage strain or change in length ($\times 10^{-6}$), L_0 is the base length (length between gauge plugs), X_i is the measured value of the specimen i day(s) after casting, and X_0 is the measured value of the specimen immediately after casting.

4. Conclusions

This research study conducted an aquaphotomic near infrared spectral analysis to investigate the effects of the different types of water on the shrinkage characteristics of the hardened cement. The aquaphotomic characterization of mixing waters and monitoring of cement mortar was performed immediately after mixing, and after 1, 3 and 7 days of curing in air. The change in internal temperature and thermal strain in cement paste were measured during first 24 h after mixing, and the dry shrinkage strain was measured up to the period of 91 days.

The research results demonstrated that the measured mechanical properties of the hardened cement material differed depending on the water used. Specifically, based on the results of the analyses, the following conclusions were drawn:

1. The results of the standard analysis of mineral constituents in four mixing waters demonstrated small differences considered negligible and irrelevant for the cement production according to the standards for the most countries. However, aquaphotomics' characterization demonstrated that mixing waters have a higher solvation ability compared to the pure water and the largest differences between the four types of waters were found at the 1448 nm water absorbance band, assigned to the absorption of water molecules in solvation shells with four or five water molecules.
2. The PCA analysis of cement paste and mortar created by different mixing waters demonstrated that the major variation in the spectra can be described by only two principal components, related to the changes of cement mortar during curing (in terms of days) and to the changes during early hydration reaction in the first 24 h. The most important water absorbance bands for the description of changes during curing were identified at 1391, 1397, 1472, and 1478 nm. The first two can be attributed to the absorbance of the confined water molecules in the interlayer between the crystal lattice, while the latter two to water molecular species with three hydrogen bonds indicated the semi-crystalline state of cement. For the description of the initial hydration reaction, the most important absorbance bands were found at 1360 and 1366 nm assigned to water solvation shells around ions, located at the edge and the corners of crystal lattices, and at 1472 nm, the water molecules bonded with three hydrogen bonds. There are indications that first two bands could be related to the hardness, which agrees well with the understanding of cement curing as the process of hardening of cement. The process of cement curing was described as a transformation of weakly hydrogen-bonded water to hydrogen-bonded water, which agrees with the release of heat during the reaction of cement hydration. Despite the common absorbance bands present in developed PCA models, each cement mortar demonstrated a specific time evolution depending on the water used for its preparation.
3. The results of the SIMCA discriminating analysis confirmed that it is possible to discriminate the age of cement mortar with an accuracy higher than 90%, and to discriminate between mortars made with different mixing waters with accuracy higher than 82%. The discriminating powers of SIMCA demonstrated the importance of the absorbance band of 1472 nm (water molecules with three hydrogen bonds) for discrimination. The differences were found mostly in the area of hydrogen-bonded water and strongly bound water, which indicates differences in the water bound to cement components, i.e., the cement matrix differences as well.
4. The entirety of aquaphotomics analysis discovered 18 water absorbance bands: 1342, 1354, 1366, 1379, 1385, 1391, 1397, 1410, 1428, 1441, 1447, 1460, 1472, 1490, 1503, 1515, 1534, and 1559 nm as absorbance bands that could be used to measure the state of water directly and the state of cement mortar during curing indirectly, over time. These

absorbance bands can be considered as WAMACS, i.e., Water Matrix Coordinates and their combination was used to depict Water Spectral Patterns—WASPs of cement mortar in aquagrams. The aquagrams revealed that $W_{shallow}$ and W_{mix} water mortars were similar, and W_{tap} and W_{dist} mortars were similar, indicating similar properties of the mortars on the macroscale. The aquagrams demonstrated differences at such a detailed scale in the water molecular matrix of the paste and mortar, practically from the very start when paste is mixed, providing a possibility for the prediction of mortar properties at the earliest possible stage.

5. The measured values of thermal strain revealed that $W_{shallow}$ and W_{mix} water mortars were similar, and W_{tap} and W_{dist} mortars were similar, strongly resembling grouping two-by-two, which is observed in the WASPs of mortars. Judging by the WASPs, it was concluded that hardened paste created by $W_{shallow}$ and W_{mix} water has a less porous and more compact structure. The results of the drying shrinkage strain measurements performed over the period of 91 days after casting demonstrate considerably reduced drying shrinkage strain in specimens prepared with $W_{shallow}$ and W_{mix} water. The drying shrinkage strain was about the same for the $W_{shallow}$ and W_{mix} cement mortar, and W_{dist} and W_{tap} followed in increasing order. Similar to the results of thermal stress, grouping two-by-two was also observed in drying shrinkage properties closely matching the pattern observed in WASPs of cement paste.

In summary, using aquaphotomics, it was demonstrated that four waters used for cement mixing had significantly different molecular structure, which influenced the cement hydration and curing, causing differences in water molecular dynamics after casting that resulted in different mechanical properties, specifically, in thermal and drying shrinkage of produced cement mortar. The mineral waters could be considered as a better choice to be used in the mixing of cement because they provide better shrinkage behavior.

Understanding the mechanisms of cement hydration intersects both scientific and practical interests. This study is, in this sense, a pioneering one, since for the first time, a novel, completely non-invasive, non-destructive, and rapid method based on aquaphotomics is presented and evaluated for this purpose. From scientific aspects, this research presented a novel way to describe the chemical and microstructural phenomena that characterize cement hydration by directly following the changes in the molecular structure of water within the cement, in a very detailed manner, with defined water molecular species and their functionality explained. From practical aspects, this study demonstrated the need to update the current standards regarding the water that can be used for mixing concrete, by demonstrating the impact the molecular structure of water has on shrinkage behavior. Further, this also provides a basis for development of a precise quantitative method that allows for rapid assessment and comparisons of the cement concrete at the very place where the production is performed.

Finally, this study is not without limitations: the focus was only on investigating four types of water and how they are related to shrinkage properties. The shrinkage is not the only concerned property to evaluate the overall performance of cement concrete, and further aquaphotomics studies will be directed at also evaluating strength and permeability. Another limitation is that the link between the water spectral patterns and the resulting mechanical properties was made primarily qualitatively, by comparison. This can be overcome by better experimental design, with spectral acquisition and reference measurements performed simultaneously, which will allow the development of quantitative prediction models and discovery of direct correlation patterns between particular water species and the measured mechanical properties.

Author Contributions: Conceptualization, S.T., Y.N., J.M. and R.T.; methodology, S.T., J.M., R.T., M.T. and H.T.; software, M.T., S.T. and J.M.; validation, M.T., H.T. and J.M.; formal analysis, M.T., S.T., H.T. and J.M.; investigation, M.T., S.T. and J.M.; resources, S.T., Y.N., H.T. and R.T.; data curation, S.T., J.M. and R.T.; writing—original draft preparation, S.T.; writing—review and editing, S.T., Y.N., J.M. and R.T.; visualization, M.T., S.T. and J.M.; supervision, H.T. and R.T.; project administration, S.T., Y.N. and R.T.; funding acquisition, S.T., Y.N. and R.T. All authors have read and agreed to the published version of the manuscript.

Funding: This research received no external funding.

Institutional Review Board Statement: Not applicable.

Informed Consent Statement: Not applicable.

Data Availability Statement: All data used in this study are available from the corresponding author on reasonable request.

Acknowledgments: The authors gratefully acknowledge Naomi Shima for her valuable support with language editing.

Conflicts of Interest: The authors declare no conflict of interest.

Sample Availability: Samples of all materials and water used in the study are available from the corresponding authors on reasonable request.

References

1. Popovics, S.; Ujhelyi, J. Contribution to the Concrete Strength versus Water-Cement Ratio Relationship. *J. Mater. Civ. Eng.* **2008**, *20*, 459–463. [CrossRef]
2. Popovic, S. Analysis of the concrete strength versus water cement ratio relationship. *ACI Mater. J.* **1990**, *87*, 517–529.
3. Bentz, D.P.; Aïtcin, P.-C. The Hidden Meaning of Water- Cement Ratio. *Concr. Int.* **2008**, *30*, 51–54.
4. Kohno, K.; Tazava, E.; Monji, T. *Atarashii Konkurîto Kougaku*, 1st ed.; Asakura Shoten: Tokyo, Japan, 1987.
5. Lee, H.J.; Kim, D.G.; Lee, J.H.; Cho, M.S. A Study for Carbonation Degree on Concrete using a Phenolphthalein Indicator and Fourier-Transform Infrared Spectroscopy. *Int. J. Civ. Environ. Eng.* **2012**, *6*, 95–101.
6. He, Z.; Han, X.; Zhang, M.; Yuan, Q.; Shi, J.; Zhan, P. A novel development of green UHPC containing waste concrete powder derived from construction and demolition waste. *Powder Technol.* **2022**, *398*, 117075. [CrossRef]
7. Ting, L.; Qiang, W.; Shiyu, Z. Effects of ultra-fine ground granulated blast-furnace slag on initial setting time, fluidity and rheological properties of cement pastes. *Powder Technol.* **2019**, *345*, 54–63. [CrossRef]
8. Li, J.; Wu, Z.; Shi, C.; Yuan, Q.; Zhang, Z. Durability of ultra-high performance concrete—A review. *Constr. Build. Mater.* **2020**, *255*, 119296. [CrossRef]
9. Mo, Z.; Wang, R.; Gao, X. Hydration and mechanical properties of UHPC matrix containing limestone and different levels of metakaolin. *Constr. Build. Mater.* **2020**, *256*, 119454. [CrossRef]
10. Ma, C.; Chen, G.; Shi, J.; Zhou, H.; Ren, W.; Du, Y. Improvement mechanism of water resistance and volume stability of magnesium oxychloride cement: A comparison study on the influences of various gypsum. *Sci. Total Environ.* **2022**, *829*, 154546. [CrossRef]
11. Rougelot, T.; Skoczylas, F.; Burlion, N. Water desorption and shrinkage in mortars and cement pastes: Experimental study and poromechanical model. *Cem. Concr. Res.* **2009**, *39*, 36–44. [CrossRef]
12. Pichler, C.; Lackner, R.; Mang, H.A. A multiscale micromechanics model for the autogenous-shrinkage deformation of early-age cement-based materials. *Eng. Fract. Mech.* **2007**, *74*, 34–58. [CrossRef]
13. Hua, C.; Acker, P.; Ehrlacher, A. Analyses and models of the autogenous shrinkage of hardening cement paste: I. Modelling at macroscopic scale. *Cem. Concr. Res.* **1995**, *25*, 1457–1468. [CrossRef]
14. Xi, Y.; Jennings, H.M. Shrinkage of cement paste and concrete modelled by a multiscale effective homogeneous theory. *Mater. Struct.* **1997**, *30*, 329–339. [CrossRef]
15. Liu, J.; Shi, C.; Ma, X.; Khayat, K.H.; Zhang, J.; Wang, D. An overview on the effect of internal curing on shrinkage of high performance cement-based materials. *Constr. Build. Mater.* **2017**, *146*, 702–712. [CrossRef]
16. Comité Euro-International du Béton. *Model Code 1990*; Comité Euro-International du Béton: Paris, France, 1991; pp. 87–109.
17. Bazant, Z.P.; Baweja, S. Creep and shrinkage prediction model for analysis and design of concrete structures—Model B3—Northwestern Scholars. *Mater. Constr.* **1995**, *28*, 357–365.
18. Shimomura, T.; Maekawa, K. Drying shrinkage model or concrete based on micromechanism in concrete. *Doboku Gakkai Ronbunshu* **1995**, *1995*, 35–45. [CrossRef]
19. Zhu, Y.; Ishida, T.; Maekawa, K. Multi-scale constitutive model or concrete based on thermodynamic states of moisture in micro-pores. *Doboku Gakkai Ronbunshu* **2004**, *2004*, 241–260. [CrossRef]

20. Ishida, T.; Luan, Y. An Enhanced model for shrinkage behavior based on early age hydration and moisture state in pore structure. *J. Jpn. Soc. Civ. Eng. Ser. E2* **2012**, *68*, 422–436. [CrossRef]
21. Montanari, L.; Amirkhanian, A.N.; Suraneni, P.; Weiss, J. Design Methodology for Partial Volumes of Internal Curing Water Based on the Reduction of Autogenous Shrinkage. *J. Mater. Civ. Eng.* **2018**, *30*, 04018137. [CrossRef]
22. Lura, P.; Jensen, O.M.; Van Breugel, K. Autogenous shrinkage in high-performance cement paste: An evaluation of basic mechanisms. *Cem. Concr. Res.* **2003**, *33*, 223–232. [CrossRef]
23. Tang, S.; Huang, D.; He, Z. A review of autogenous shrinkage models of concrete. *J. Build. Eng.* **2021**, *44*, 103412. [CrossRef]
24. Powers, T.C. The thermodynamics of volume change and creep. *Matér. Constr.* **1968**, *1*, 487–507. [CrossRef]
25. Shimomurat, T.; Maekawa, K. Analysis of the drying shrinkage behaviour of concrete using a micromechanical model based on the micropore structure of concrete. *Mag. Concr. Res.* **2015**, *49*, 303–322. [CrossRef]
26. Beltzung, F.; Wittmann, F.H. Role of disjoining pressure in cement based materials. *Cem. Concr. Res.* **2005**, *35*, 2364–2370. [CrossRef]
27. Maruyama, I. Origin of Drying Shrinkage of Hardened Cement Paste: Hydration Pressure. *J. Adv. Concr. Technol.* **2010**, *8*, 187–200. [CrossRef]
28. Feldman, R.H. Sorption and Length-Change Scanning Isotherms of Methanol and Water on Hydrated Portland Cement. In Proceedings of the Fifth International Symposium on the Chemistry of Cement, National Research Council Canada, Tokyo, Japan, 7–11 October 1968; Volume 3, pp. 53–66.
29. Japanese Standards Association (JSA). *Japanese Industrial Standards (JIS) A 5308, Ready-Mixed Concrete*; Japanese Standards Association: Tokyo, Japan, 2019; p. 7.
30. ASTM C94. Standard Specification for Ready-Mixed Concrete; ASTM International: West Conshohocken, PA, USA, 1996.
31. Japanese Standards Association (JSA). *Japanese Industrial Standard (JIS) R 5210 Portland Cement*; Japanese Standards Association: Tokyo, Japan, 2019; Volume 1607, p. 5.
32. Maheshwari, R.K.; Rani, B.; Rani, B.; Maheshwari, R.; Garg, A.; Prasad, M. Bottled Water—A Global Market Overview Bottled Water—A Global Market Overview. *Bull. Environ. Pharmacol. Life Sci.* **2012**, *1*, 1–4.
33. Brei, V.A. How is a bottled water market created? *Wiley Interdiscip. Rev. Water* **2018**, *5*, e1220. [CrossRef]
34. Kubota, M.; Nishimoto, Y. *Koredewakaru Mizu no Kisotishiki*; Maruzen Corp.: Tokyo, Japan, 2003.
35. Toda, M. *Shohokaramanabu Kinousui*; Nihon Sangyo Senjou Kyougikai, Kougyo Chousakai Corp.: Tokyo, Japan, 2002.
36. Al-Haq, M.I.; Sugiyama, J.; Isobe, S. Applications of Electrolyzed Water in Agriculture & Food Industries. *Food Sci. Technol. Res.* **2005**, *11*, 135–150. [CrossRef]
37. Teixeira da Silva, J.A.; Dobránszki, J. Impact of magnetic water on plant growth. *Environ. Exp. Biol.* **2014**, *12*, 137–142.
38. Johnson, K.E.; Sanders, J.J.; Gellin, R.G.; Palesch, Y.Y. The effectiveness of a magnetized water oral irrigator (Hydro Fioss®) on plaque, calculus and gingival health. *J. Clin. Periodontol.* **1998**, *25*, 316–321. [CrossRef]
39. Hafizi, L.; Gholizadeh, M.; Karimi, M.; Hosseini, G.; Mostafavi-Toroghi, H.; Haddadi, M.; Rezaiean, A.; Ebrahimi, M.; Meibodi, N.E. Effects of magnetized water on ovary, pre-implantation stage endometrial and fallopian tube epithelial cells in mice. *Iran. J. Reprod. Med.* **2014**, *12*, 243. [PubMed]
40. Kim, Y.-H.; Park, Y.; Bae, S.; Kim, S.Y.; Han, J.-G. Compressive Strength Evaluation of Ordinary Portland Cement Mortar Blended with Hydrogen Nano-Bubble Water and Graphene. *J. Nanosci. Nanotechnol.* **2019**, *20*, 647–652. [CrossRef] [PubMed]
41. Grzegorczyk-Frańczak, M.; Barnat-Hunek, D.; Andrzejuk, W.; Zaburko, J.; Zalewska, M.; Łagód, G. Physical Properties and Durability of Lime-Cement Mortars Prepared with Water Containing Micro-Nano Bubbles of Various Gases. *Materials* **2021**, *14*, 1902. [CrossRef] [PubMed]
42. Kim, W.K.; Hong, G.; Kim, Y.H.; Kim, J.M.; Kim, J.; Han, J.G.; Lee, J.Y. Mechanical Strength and Hydration Characteristics of Cement Mixture with Highly Concentrated Hydrogen Nanobubble Water. *Materials* **2021**, *14*, 2735. [CrossRef]
43. Kim, W.K.; Kim, Y.H.; Hong, G.; Kim, J.M.; Han, J.G.; Lee, J.Y. Effect of Hydrogen Nanobubbles on the Mechanical Strength and Watertightness of Cement Mixtures. *Materials* **2021**, *14*, 1823. [CrossRef]
44. Abdel-Magid, T.I.M.; Hamdan, R.M.; Abdelgader, A.A.B.; Omer, M.E.A.; Ahmed, N.M.R.A. Effect of Magnetized Water on Workability and Compressive Strength of Concrete. *Procedia Eng.* **2017**, *193*, 494–500. [CrossRef]
45. Prabakaran, E.; Vijayakumar, A.; Rooby, J.; Nithya, M. A comparative study of polypropylene fiber reinforced concrete for various mix grades with magnetized water. *Mater. Today Proc.* **2021**, *45*, 123–127. [CrossRef]
46. Zhang, Z.; Li, B.; Song, N.; Venkatesh, S.; Jagannathan, P.; Prasath Kumar, V.R. An Experimental Study on the Effect of Magnetized Water on Mechanical Properties of Concrete. *IOP Conf. Ser. Mater. Sci. Eng.* **2020**, *912*, 032081. [CrossRef]
47. Lal, P.; Kavitha, P.E. Modified Magnetized Water Concrete Using Nanosilica. *Lect. Notes Civ. Eng.* **2021**, *97*, 421–431. [CrossRef]
48. Mohammadnezhad, A.; Azizi, S.; Sousanabadi Farahani, H.; Tashan, J.; Habibnejad Korayem, A. Understanding of the Magnetizing Process of Water and its Effects on Properties of Cementitious Composites—A Critical Review. *SSRN Electron. J.* **2022**, 47. [CrossRef]
49. Takigawa, M.; Konaka, T.; Tsunokake, H.; Tamura, S. Basic research on the effects of various mixed water on the physical characteristics or mortar. In Proceedings of the Reiwa 3th annual Meeting of the Japan Society of Civil Engineers, Tokyo, Japan, 6–10 September 2021.
50. Bullard, J.W.; Jennings, H.M.; Livingston, R.A.; Nonat, A.; Scherer, G.W.; Schweitzer, J.S.; Scrivener, K.L.; Thomas, J.J. Mechanisms of cement hydration. *Cem. Concr. Res.* **2011**, *41*, 1208–1223. [CrossRef]

51. Tsenkova, R. Aquaphotomics: Dynamic spectroscopy of aqueous and biological systems describes peculiarities of water. *J. Near Infrared Spectrosc.* **2009**, *17*, 303–313. [CrossRef]
52. Muncan, J.; Tsenkova, R. Aquaphotomics-From Innovative Knowledge to Integrative Platform in Science and Technology. *Molecules* **2019**, *24*, 2742. [CrossRef] [PubMed]
53. Tsenkova, R.; Muncan, J.; Kovacs, Z. Aquaphotomics. In *Handbook of Near-Infrared Analysis*; Ciurczak, E.W., Igne, B., Workman, J., Jr., Burns, D.A., Eds.; CRC Press: Boca Raton, Florida, USA, 2022; p. 917. ISBN 9781138576483.
54. van de Kraats, E.B.; Munćan, J.; Tsenkova, R.N. Aquaphotomics—Origin, concept, applications and future perspectives. *Substantia* **2019**, *3*, 13–28. [CrossRef]
55. Roger, J.; Mallet, A.; Marini, F. Preprocessing NIR Spectra for Aquaphotomics. *Molecules* **2022**, *27*, 6795. [CrossRef]
56. Tan, J.; Sun, Y.; Ma, L.; Feng, H.; Guo, Y.; Cai, W.; Shao, X. Knowledge-based genetic algorithm for resolving the near-infrared spectrum and understanding the water structures in aqueous solution. *Chemom. Intell. Lab. Syst.* **2020**, *206*, 104150. [CrossRef]
57. Cui, X.; Sun, Y.; Cai, W.; Shao, X. Chemometric methods for extracting information from temperature-dependent near-infrared spectra. *Sci. China Chem.* **2019**, *62*, 583–591. [CrossRef]
58. Shao, X.; Cui, X.; Liu, Y.; Xia, Z.; Cai, W. Understanding the molecular interaction in solutions by chemometric resolution of near−infrared spectra. *ChemistrySelect* **2017**, *2*, 10027–10032. [CrossRef]
59. Cui, X.; Zhang, J.; Cai, W.; Shao, X. Chemometric algorithms for analyzing high dimensional temperature dependent near infrared spectra. *Chemom. Intell. Lab. Syst.* **2017**, *170*, 109–117. [CrossRef]
60. Shao, X.; Cui, X.; Wang, M.; Cai, W. High order derivative to investigate the complexity of the near infrared spectra of aqueous solutions. *Spectrochim. Acta Part A Mol. Biomol. Spectrosc.* **2019**, *213*, 83–89. [CrossRef]
61. Su, T.; Sun, Y.; Han, L.; Cai, W.; Shao, X. Revealing the interactions of water with cryoprotectant and protein by near–infrared spectroscopy. *Spectrochim. Acta Part A Mol. Biomol. Spectrosc.* **2022**, *266*, 120417. [CrossRef] [PubMed]
62. Babu, G.R.; Reddy, B.M.; Ramana, N.V. Quality of mixing water in cement concrete. A review. *Mater. Today Proc.* **2018**, *5*, 1313–1320. [CrossRef]
63. Tsenkova, R.; Munćan, J.; Pollner, B.; Kovacs, Z. Essentials of Aquaphotomics and Its Chemometrics Approaches. *Front. Chem.* **2018**, *6*, 363. [CrossRef]
64. Martens, H.; Martens, M. *Multivariate Analysis of Quality: An Introduction*; Wiley: Chichester, UK, 2001; ISBN 9780471974284.
65. Wold, S.; Sjostrom, M. SIMCA: A Method for Analyzing Chemical Data in Terms of Similarity and Analogy. In *Chemometrics: Theory and Application*; Kowalski, B.R., Ed.; American Chemical Society at New York University: New York, NY, USA, 1977; pp. 243–282.
66. Tsenkova, R. Aquaphotomics: Water in the biological and aqueous world scrutinised with invisible light. *Spectrosc. Eur.* **2010**, *22*, 6–10.
67. Kovacs, Z.; Muncan, J.; Veleva, P.; Oshima, M.; Shigeoka, S.; Tsenkova, R. Aquaphotomics for monitoring of groundwater using short-wavelength near-infrared spectroscopy. *Spectrochim. Acta Part A Mol. Biomol. Spectrosc.* **2022**, *279*, 121378. [CrossRef] [PubMed]
68. Rinnan, Å.; Nørgaard, L.; van den Berg, F.; Thygesen, J.; Bro, R.; Engelsen, S.B. Data Pre-Processing. In *Infrared Spectroscopy for Food Quality Analysis and Control*; Sun, D.-W., Ed.; Academic Press: Cambridge, MA, USA, 2009; ISBN 9780123741363.
69. Kojić, D.; Tsenkova, R.; Tomobe, K.; Yasuoka, K.; Yasui, M. Water confined in the local field of ions. *ChemPhysChem* **2014**, *15*, 4077–4086. [CrossRef] [PubMed]
70. Muncan, J.; Kovacs, Z.; Pollner, B.; Ikuta, K.; Ohtani, Y.; Terada, F.; Tsenkova, R. Near infrared aquaphotomics study on common dietary fatty acids in cow's liquid, thawed milk. *Food Control* **2020**, *122*, 107805. [CrossRef]
71. Gowen, A.A.; Tsenkova, R.; Esquerre, C.; Downey, G.; O'Donnell, C.P. Use of near infrared hyperspectral imaging to identify water matrix co-ordinates in mushrooms (*Agaricus bisporus*) subjected to mechanical vibration. *J. Near Infrared Spectrosc.* **2009**, *17*, 363–371. [CrossRef]
72. Malegori, C.; Muncan, J.; Mustorgi, E.; Tsenkova, R.; Oliveri, P. Analysing the water spectral pattern by near-infrared spectroscopy and chemometrics as a dynamic multidimensional biomarker in preservation: Rice germ storage monitoring. *Spectrochim. Acta Part A Mol. Biomol. Spectrosc.* **2022**, *265*, 120396. [CrossRef]
73. Tsenkova, R.N.; Iordanova, I.K.; Toyoda, K.; Brown, D.R. Prion protein fate governed by metal binding. *Biochem. Biophys. Res. Commun.* **2004**, *325*, 1005–1012. [CrossRef]
74. Kovacs, Z.; Pollner, B.; Bazar, G.; Muncan, J.; Tsenkova, R. A Novel Tool for Visualization of Water Molecular Structure and Its Changes, Expressed on the Scale of Temperature Influence. *Molecules* **2020**, *25*, 2234. [CrossRef] [PubMed]
75. Geladi, P.; Dåbakk, E. Computational Methods and Chemometrics in Near Infrared Spectroscopy. In *Encyclopedia of Spectroscopy and Spectrometry*, 2nd ed.; Lindon, J.C., Ed.; Academic Press: Cambridge, MA, USA, 1999; pp. 386–391. [CrossRef]
76. Savitzky, A.; Golay, M.J.E. Smoothing and Differentiation of Data by Simplified Least Squares Procedures. *Anal. Chem.* **1951**, *36*, 1627–1639. [CrossRef]
77. Fujimoto, T.; Yamamoto, H.; Tsuchikawa, S. Estimation of wood stiffness and strength properties of hybrid larch by near-infrared spectroscopy. *Appl. Spectrosc.* **2007**, *61*, 882–888. [CrossRef] [PubMed]
78. Kondo, A.; Kurosawa, R.; Ryu, J.; Matsuoka, M.; Takeuchi, M. Investigation on the Mechanisms of Mg(OH)2Dehydration and MgO Hydration by Near-Infrared Spectroscopy. *J. Phys. Chem. C* **2021**, *125*, 10937–10947. [CrossRef]

79. Hong, B.H.; Rubenthaler, G.L.; Allan, R.E. Wheat pentosans. II. Estimating kernel hardness and pentosans in water extracts by near-infrared reflectance. *Cereal Chem.* **1989**, *66*, 374–377.
80. Kuroki, S.; Tsenkova, R.; Moyankova, D.P.; Muncan, J.; Morita, H.; Atanassova, S.; Djilianov, D. Water molecular structure underpins extreme desiccation tolerance of the resurrection plant Haberlea rhodopensis. *Sci. Rep.* **2019**, *9*, 3049. [CrossRef]
81. Blomquist, G.; Johansson, E.; Söderström, B.; Wold, S. Data analysis of pyrolysis—Chromatograms by means of simca pattern recognition. *J. Anal. Appl. Pyrolysis* **1979**, *1*, 53–65. [CrossRef]
82. Kvalheim, O.M.; Karstang, T.V. SIMCA—Classification by means of disjoint cross validated principal components models. In *Multivariate Pattern Recognition in Chemometrics: Illustrated by Case Studies*; Brereton, R.G., Ed.; Elsevier: Amsterdam, The Netherlands, 1992; Volume 9, pp. 209–248.
83. Headrick, J.M.; Diken, E.G.; Walters, R.S.; Hammer, N.I.; Christie, R.A.; Cui, J.; Myshakin, E.M.; Duncan, M.A.; Johnson, M.A.; Jordan, K.D. Spectral signatures of hydrated proton vibrations in water clusters. *Science* **2005**, *308*, 1765–1769. [CrossRef]
84. Mizuse, K.; Fujii, A. Tuning of the Internal Energy and Isomer Distribution in Small Protonated Water Clusters H + (H_2O) 4–8: An Application of the Inert Gas Messenger Technique. *J. Phys. Chem. A* **2012**, *116*, 4868–4877. [CrossRef]
85. Bázár, G.; Romvári, R.; Szabó, A.; Somogyi, T.; Éles, V.; Tsenkova, R. NIR detection of honey adulteration reveals differences in water spectral pattern. *Food Chem.* **2016**, *194*, 873–880. [CrossRef]
86. Kurashige, J.; Takaoka, K.; Takasago, M. State of Dissolved Water in Triglycerides as Determined by Fourier Transform Infrared and Near Infrared Spectroscopy. *J. Jpn. Oil Chem. Soc.* **1991**, *40*, 549–553. [CrossRef]
87. Hofmann, D.W.M.; Kuleshova, L.; D'Aguanno, B.; Di Noto, V.; Negro, E.; Conti, F.; Vittadello, M. Investigation of water structure in Nafion membranes by infrared spectroscopy and molecular dynamics simulation. *J. Phys. Chem. B* **2009**, *113*, 632–639. [CrossRef] [PubMed]
88. Robertson, W.H.; Diken, E.G.; Price, E.A.; Shin, J.-W.; Johnson, M.A. Spectroscopic determination of the OH- solvation shell in the OH-.(H2O)n clusters. *Science* **2003**, *299*, 1367–1372. [CrossRef] [PubMed]
89. Davis, J.G.; Gierszal, K.P.; Wang, P.; Ben-Amotz, D. Water structural transformation at molecular hydrophobic interfaces. *Nature* **2012**, *491*, 582–585. [CrossRef] [PubMed]
90. Abd. el.aleem, S.; Heikal, M.; Morsi, W.M. Hydration characteristic, thermal expansion and microstructure of cement containing nano-silica. *Constr. Build. Mater.* **2014**, *59*, 151–160. [CrossRef]
91. Okumura, M.; Yeh, L.I.; Myers, J.D.; Lee, Y.T. Infrared spectra of the solvated hydronium ion: Vibrational predissociation spectroscopy of mass-selected $H_3O+\cdot(H_2O)n\cdot(H_2)m$. *J. Phys. Chem.* **1990**, *94*, 3416–3427. [CrossRef]
92. Yeh, L.I.; Okumura, M.; Myers, J.D.; Price, J.M.; Lee, Y.T. Vibrational spectroscopy of the hydrated hydronium cluster ions $H_3O+\cdot(H_2O)n$ (n = 1, 2, 3). *J. Chem. Phys.* **1989**, *91*, 7319–7330. [CrossRef]
93. Zhang, L.; Noda, I.; Czarnik-Matusewicz, B.; Wu, Y. Multivariate estimation between mid and near-infrared spectra of hexafluoroisopropanol-water mixtures. *Anal. Sci.* **2007**, *23*, 901–905. [CrossRef]
94. Iwahashi, M.; Suzuki, M.; Katayama, N.; Matsuzawa, H.; Czarnecki, M.A.; Ozaki, Y.; Wakisaka, A. Molecular self-assembling of butan-1-ol, butan-2-ol, and 2-methylpropan-2-ol in carbon tetrachloride solutions as observed by near-infrared spectroscopic measurements. *Appl. Spectrosc.* **2000**, *54*, 268–276. [CrossRef]
95. Maeda, H.; Ozaki, Y.; Tanaka, M.; Hayashi, N.; Kojima, T. Near Infrared Spectroscopy and Chemometrics Studies of Temperature-Dependent Spectral Variations of Water: Relationship between Spectral Changes and Hydrogen Bonds. *J. Near Infrared Spectrosc.* **1995**, *3*, 191–201. [CrossRef]
96. Shin, J.-W.; Hammer, N.I.; Diken, E.G.; Johnson, M.A.; Walters, R.S.; Jaeger, T.D.; Duncan, M.A.; Christie, R.A.; Jordan, K.D. Infrared Signature of Structures Associated with the $H+(H_2O)n$ (n = 6 to 27) Clusters. *Science* **2004**, *304*, 1137–1140. [CrossRef] [PubMed]
97. Sagawa, N.; Shikata, T. Hydration Behavior of Poly(ethylene oxide)s in Aqueous Solution As Studied by Near-Infrared Spectroscopic Techniques. *J. Phys. Chem. B* **2013**, *117*, 10883–10888. [CrossRef] [PubMed]
98. Czarnecki, M.A.; Morisawa, Y.; Katsumoto, Y.; Takaya, T.; Singh, S.; Sato, H.; Ozaki, Y. Solvent effect on the competition between weak and strong interactions in phenol solutions studied by near-infrared spectroscopy and DFT calculations. *Phys. Chem. Chem. Phys.* **2021**, *23*, 19188–19194. [CrossRef] [PubMed]
99. Gotić, M.; Musić, S. Mössbauer, FT-IR and FE SEM investigation of iron oxides precipitated from $FeSO_4$ solutions. *J. Mol. Struct.* **2007**, *834–836*, 445–453. [CrossRef]
100. Frost, R.L.; Dickfos, M.J.; Čejka, J. Raman spectroscopic study of the uranyl carbonate mineral zellerite. *J. Raman Spectrosc.* **2008**, *39*, 582–586. [CrossRef]
101. Bertie, J.E.; Whalley, E. Infrared spectra of ices II, III, and V in the range 4000 to 350 cm^{-1}. *J. Chem. Phys.* **1964**, *40*, 1646–1659. [CrossRef]
102. Solcaniova, E.; Kovac, S. Hydrogen Bonding in Phenols. IV. Intramolecular OH... n Hydrogen Bonds of Some Alkyl Derivatives. *Chem. Zvesti* **1969**, *691*, 687–691.
103. Frost, R.L.; Scholz, R.; Lõpez, A. Raman and infrared spectroscopic characterization of the arsenate-bearing mineral tangdanite–and in comparison with the discredited mineral clinotyrolite. *J. Raman Spectrosc.* **2015**, *46*, 920–926. [CrossRef]
104. Rémazeilles, C.; Refait, P. Fe(II) hydroxycarbonate $Fe_2(OH)_2CO_3$ (chukanovite) as iron corrosion product: Synthesis and study by Fourier Transform Infrared Spectroscopy. *Polyhedron* **2009**, *28*, 749–756. [CrossRef]

105. Litasov, K.; Ohtani, E. Systematic Study Of Hydrogen Incorporation Into Fe-bearing Wadsleyite and Water Storage Capacity Of The Transition Zone. *AIP Conf. Proc.* **2008**, *987*, 113. [CrossRef]
106. Walker, A.M.; Demouchy, S.; Wright, K. Computer modelling of the energies and vibrational properties of hydroxyl groups in α- and β-Mg_2SiO_4. *Eur. J. Mineral.* **2006**, *18*, 529–543. [CrossRef]
107. Shi, G.A.; Saboktakin, M.; Stavola, M.; Pearton, S.J. "Hidden hydrogen" in as-grown ZnO. *Appl. Phys. Lett.* **2004**, *85*, 5601. [CrossRef]
108. Herklotz, F.; Chaplygin, I.; Lavrov, E.V.; Neiman, A.; Reeves, R.J.; Allen, M.W. Bistability of a hydrogen defect with a vibrational mode at 3326 cm^{-1} in ZnO. *Phys. Rev. B* **2019**, *99*, 115203. [CrossRef]
109. Som, T.; Karmakar, B. Structure and properties of low-phonon antimony glasses and nano glass-ceramics in K_2O–B_2O_3–Sb_2O_3 system. *J. Non. Cryst. Solids* **2010**, *356*, 987–999. [CrossRef]
110. Wei, J.; Zhao, L.; Peng, S.; Shi, J.; Liu, Z.; Wen, W. Wettability of urea-doped TiO_2 nanoparticles and their high electrorheological effects. *J. Sol-Gel Sci. Technol.* **2008**, *47*, 311–315. [CrossRef]
111. Cai, C.B.; Tao, Y.Y.; Wang, B.; Wen, M.Q.; Yang, H.W.; Cheng, Y.J. Investigating the adsorption process of isoamyl alcohol vapor onto silica gel with near-infrared process analytical technology. *Spectrosc. Lett.* **2014**, *48*, 190–197. [CrossRef]
112. Kakuda, H.; Okada, T.; Hasegawa, T. Temperature-Induced Molecular Structural Changes of Linear Poly(ethylene imine) in Water Studied by Mid-Infrared and Near-Infrared Spectroscopies. *J. Phys. Chem. B* **2009**, *113*, 13910–13916. [CrossRef]
113. Rubenthaler, G.L.; Pomeranz, Y. Near-Infrared reflectance spectra of hard red winter wheats varying widely in protein content and breadmaking potential. *Cereal Chem.* **1987**, *64*, 407–411.
114. Awatani, T.; Midorikawa, H.; Kojima, N.; Ye, J.; Marcott, C. Morphology of water transport channels and hydrophobic clusters in Nafion from high spatial resolution AFM-IR spectroscopy and imaging. *Electrochem. Commun.* **2013**, *30*, 5–8. [CrossRef]
115. Frost, R.L.; Erickson, K.L.; Čejka, J.; Reddy, B.J. A Raman spectroscopic study of the uranyl sulphate mineral johannite. *Spectrochim. Acta Part A Mol. Biomol. Spectrosc.* **2005**, *61*, 2702–2707. [CrossRef]
116. Wenz, J.J. Influence of steroids on hydrogen bonds in membranes assessed by near infrared spectroscopy. *Biochim. Biophys. Acta—Biomembr.* **2021**, *1863*, 183553. [CrossRef] [PubMed]
117. Mastrapa, R.M.E.; Moore, M.H.; Hudson, R.L.; Ferrante, R.L.; Brown, R.H.; Mastrapa, R.M.E.; Moore, M.H.; Hudson, R.L.; Ferrante, R.L.; Brown, R.H. Proton Irradiation of Crystalline Water Ice: Timescales for Amorphization in the Kuiper Belt. *DPS* **2005**, *37*, 745.
118. Parrott, L.J.; Geiker, M.; Gutteridge, W.A.; Killoh, D. Monitoring Portland cement hydration: Comparison of methods. *Cem. Concr. Res.* **1990**, *20*, 919–926. [CrossRef]
119. Sha, W.; O'Neill, E.A.; Guo, Z. Differential scanning calorimetry study of ordinary Portland cement. *Cem. Concr. Res.* **1999**, *29*, 1487–1489. [CrossRef]
120. Alarcon-Ruiz, L.; Platret, G.; Massieu, E.; Ehrlacher, A. The use of thermal analysis in assessing the effect of temperature on a cement paste. *Cem. Concr. Res.* **2005**, *35*, 609–613. [CrossRef]
121. Swaddiwudhipong, S.; Chen, D.; Zhang, M.H. Simulation of the exothermic hydration process of Portland cement. *Adv. Cem. Res.* **2015**, *14*, 61–69. [CrossRef]
122. Fu, Y.F.; Wong, Y.L.; Tang, C.A.; Poon, C.S. Thermal induced stress and associated cracking in cement-based composite at elevated temperatures—Part I: Thermal cracking around single inclusion. *Cem. Concr. Compos.* **2004**, *26*, 113–126. [CrossRef]
123. Shui, Z.H.; Zhang, R.; Chen, W.; Xuan, D.X. Effects of mineral admixtures on the thermal expansion properties of hardened cement paste. *Constr. Build. Mater.* **2010**, *24*, 1761–1767. [CrossRef]
124. Shimasaki, I.; Rokugo, K.; Morimoto, H. On thermal expansion coefficient of concrete at very early age. In *Proceedings of International, Workshop on Control of Cracking in Early-Age Concrete*; Tohoku University: Sendai, Japan, 1999.
125. Ghabezloo, S.; Sulem, J.; Saint-Marc, J. The effect of undrained heating on a fluid-saturated hardened cement paste. *Cem. Concr. Res.* **2009**, *39*, 54–64. [CrossRef]
126. Abbasnia, R.; Shekarchi, M.; Ahmadi, J. Evaluation of concrete drying shrinkage related to moisture loss. *ACI Mater. J.* **2013**, *110*, 269–277. [CrossRef]
127. Parveen, S.; Rana, S.; Fangueiro, R. Macro- and nanodimensional plant fiber reinforcements for cementitious composites. In *Sustainable and Nonconventional Construction Materials Using Inorganic Bonded Fiber Composites*; Savastano Junior, H., Fiorelli, J., dos Santos, S.F., Eds.; Woodhead Publishing: Sawston, UK, 2017; pp. 343–382. [CrossRef]
128. Larosche, C.J. Types and causes of cracking in concrete structures. *Fail. Distress Repair Concr. Struct.* **2009**, 57–83. [CrossRef]
129. Jianxia, S. Durability Design of Concrete Hydropower Structures. *Compr. Renew. Energy* **2012**, *6*, 377–403. [CrossRef]
130. Demirboga, R.; Farhan, K.Z. *Palm oil fuel ash (POFA). Sustainable Concrete Made with Ashes and Dust from Different Sources*; Springer: Berlin/Heidelberg, Germany, 2022; pp. 279–330. [CrossRef]
131. Muthukrishnan, S.; Gupta, S.; Kua, H.W. Application of rice husk biochar and thermally treated low silica rice husk ash to improve physical properties of cement mortar. *Theor. Appl. Fract. Mech.* **2019**, *104*, 102376. [CrossRef]
132. Bagheri, A.R.; Alibabaie, M.; Babaie, M. Reduction in the permeability of plastic concrete for cut-off walls through utilization of silica fume. *Constr. Build. Mater.* **2008**, *22*, 1247–1252. [CrossRef]
133. Bentz, D.P.; Jensen, O.M.; Coats, A.M.; Glasser, F.P. Influence of silica fume on diffusivity in cement-based materials: I. Experimental and computer modeling studies on cement pastes. *Cem. Concr. Res.* **2000**, *30*, 953–962. [CrossRef]

134. Japanese Standards Association. *(JSA). Japanese Industrial Standards (JIS) R 5201—Physical Testing Methods for Cement;* Japanese Standards Association: Tokyo, Japan, 2019; p. 107.
135. Dhanoa, M.S.; Barnes, R.J.; Lister, S.J. Standard Normal Variate Transformation and De-trending of Near-Infrared Diffuse Reflectance Spectra. *Appl. Spectrosc.* **1989**, *43*, 772–777.

molecules

MDPI

Article

Correction of Temperature Variation with Independent Water Samples to Predict Soluble Solids Content of Kiwifruit Juice Using NIR Spectroscopy

Harpreet Kaur [1,2,*], Rainer Künnemeyer [3] and Andrew McGlone [2]

1 The Dodd Walls Centre for Photonic and Quantum Technologies, School of Engineering, The University of Waikato, Hamilton 3216, New Zealand
2 The New Zealand Institute for Plant and Food Research Limited, Ruakura, Hamilton 3214, New Zealand; Andrew.McGlone@plantandfood.co.nz
3 The Dodd Walls Centre for Photonic and Quantum Technologies, The University of Otago, Dunedin 9054, New Zealand; r.kunnemeyer@gmail.com
* Correspondence: harpreet.kaur@plantandfood.co.nz

Abstract: Using the framework of aquaphotomics, we have sought to understand the changes within the water structure of kiwifruit juice occurring with changes in temperature. The study focuses on the first (1300–1600 nm) and second (870–1100 nm) overtone regions of the OH stretch of water and examines temperature differences between 20, 25, and 30 °C. Spectral data were collected using a Fourier transform–near-infrared spectrometer with 1 mm and 10 mm transmission cells for measurements in the first and second overtone region, respectively. Water wavelengths affected by temperature variation were identified. Aquagrams (water spectral patterns) highlight slightly different responses in the first and second overtone regions. The influence of increasing temperature on the peak absorbance of the juice was largely a lateral wavelength shift in the first overtone region and a vertical amplitude shift in the second overtone region of water. With the same data set, we investigated the use of external parameter orthogonalisation (EPO) and extended multiple scatter correction (EMSC) pre-processing to assist in building temperature-independent partial least square regression models for predicting soluble solids concentration (SSC) of kiwifruit juice. The interference component selected for correction was the first principal component loading measured using pure water samples taken at the same three temperatures (20, 25, and 30 °C). The results show that the EMSC method reduced SSC prediction bias from 0.77 to 0.1 °Brix in the first overtone region of water. Using the EPO method significantly reduced the prediction bias from 0.51 to 0.04 °Brix, when applying a model made at one temperature (30 °C) to measurements made at another temperature (20 °C) in the second overtone region of water.

Keywords: soluble solids content; Brix; kiwifruit juice; aquaphotomics; near infrared spectroscopy; extended multiplicative scatter correction (EMSC); external parameter orthogonalisation (EPO)

Citation: Kaur, H.; Künnemeyer, R.; McGlone, A. Correction of Temperature Variation with Independent Water Samples to Predict Soluble Solids Content of Kiwifruit Juice Using NIR Spectroscopy. *Molecules* **2022**, *27*, 504. https://doi.org/10.3390/molecules27020504

Academic Editors: Roumiana Tsenkova and Jelena Muncan

Received: 15 December 2021
Accepted: 10 January 2022
Published: 14 January 2022

1. Introduction

Water is the major constituent of fruits, typically more than 80% [1,2], and absorbs near-infrared (NIR) radiation [3,4]. The NIR spectrum of fruit shows a strong absorption peak around 970 nm, which corresponds to the second overtone of the OH stretch in water [5,6]. NIR spectroscopy (NIRS) models for predicting dry matter (DM) and soluble solids content (SSC) of fruit (apples) have been developed using the narrow spectral range from 800 to 1100 nm around this absorption peak [5].

NIRS models are called robust when their prediction accuracy is relatively insensitive to unknown changes in external factors [7]. A factor that can strongly affect NIR model performance is temperature [8]. Shifts in the water absorbance bands with temperature can reduce model performance [9–12]. Acharya et al. [12] have studied the effect of temperature on prediction models of fruit quality, observing that a calibration equation developed at one fixed temperature could not reliably predict on samples measured at a different temperature. Roger et al. [10] found a model offset bias of 8 °Brix for a temperature variation of 20 °C (range 5–25 °C) for SSC prediction in apples. Several techniques have been previously investigated to compensate fruit model predictions for fluctuations in sample temperature. Kawano et al. [9] developed calibration equations for peaches using samples at different temperatures. Peirs et al. [13] similarly developed robust calibration models for a wide range of apple cultivars, incorporating samples at all temperature ranges expected in future measurements. Roger et al. [10] removed the temperature-induced bias in SSC predictions on apples by applying the external parameter orthogonalisation (EPO) algorithm, as a pre-processing step, to remove the part of the spectral data matrix most affected by temperature. Several new techniques have been reported recently in the literature, indicating the problem is far from solved for all circumstances [14].

The framework of aquaphotomics appears suitable for examining the temperature sensitivity of fruit spectra. Aquaphotomics is an NIR spectral analysis methodology that focuses on changes in the pattern of water absorbance bands due to perturbations by extraneous factors. The field has aided the understanding of the role of water in biological systems [15–18]. The effect of perturbations on water binding structures has been observed due to variation in solute concentration, temperature, and other environmental factors [16,18,19]. The aquaphotomics methodology defines 12 water absorption bands in the first overtone region of water, called the water matrix coordinates (WAMACS), which describe the water states in an aqueous system. The methodology has been applied to the study of apple juice when the sample temperature is increased from 20 to 30 °C, revealing an increase in free water molecule states that raises the spectral absorbance at 1414 nm [20].

In this paper, we use the aquaphotomics approach to study the changes in the water structure of kiwifruit juice caused by variation of temperature in the vicinity of the 1450 nm (first overtone of OH stretch of water) and 970 nm (second overtone of OH stretch of water) absorbances. The second overtone region has had very little research attention from an aquaphotomics perspective, which is surprising given the importance of that region for intact fruit quality prediction by NIR, including on kiwifruit [21,22]. Physically filtered fruit juices, removing most particulate matter, minimize light scattering variation between samples and thus provide an ideal medium for fundamental aquaphotomics studies involving controlled temperature perturbations of the sample water chemistry. The results from such studies, if clarifying the fundamental mechanisms involved, may help in understanding and/or overcoming the temperature sensitivities associated with NIRS whole fruit measurements.

We also evaluate the pre-processing modeling methods, extended multiplicative scatter correction (EMSC), and EPO, using pure water spectra as interferent, to minimize the temperature sensitivity of NIRS models for the SSC of kiwifruit juice. Previous aquaphotomics analysis showed the effective use of EMSC for minimizing the temperature sensitivity of apple juice models for SSC prediction, where the spectral measurements were over the 1300–1600 nm first overtone region, and the required interferent spectra were derived from pure water measurements [20]. The EPO technique is somewhat similar in requiring the specification of an interferent spectrum. It has been previously explored for the development of temperature-insensitive NIR models of intact apple SSC across the second overtone region using common fruit samples, measured at different temperatures to derive the required interferent spectra [10].

2. Materials and Methods

2.1. Sample Preparation

A total of 100 fully ripe Zespri® SunGold Kiwifruit (*Actinidia chinensis* var. *chinensis* 'Zesy002') were purchased from New Zealand retail stores. Juice was expressed from about 2 cm thick endcaps, removed from the stem and calyx ends of each fruit, and was collected in Eppendorf tubes. The samples were centrifuged at 13,400 rpm for 3 min

(MiniSpin, Eppendorf, Hamburg, Germany) and then filtered through a 0.2 μm syringe filter to produce a clear juice (Figure 1). The samples were stored in a refrigerator at 4 °C. Fourier transform–near-infrared (FT-NIR) spectra and reference SSC measurements were performed the next day after the samples were equilibrated to room temperature (20 °C). Milli-Q water with a resistivity of 18.2 MΩ cm was produced using a water purification system (Millipore, Thermofisher Scientific, Knox, Australia).

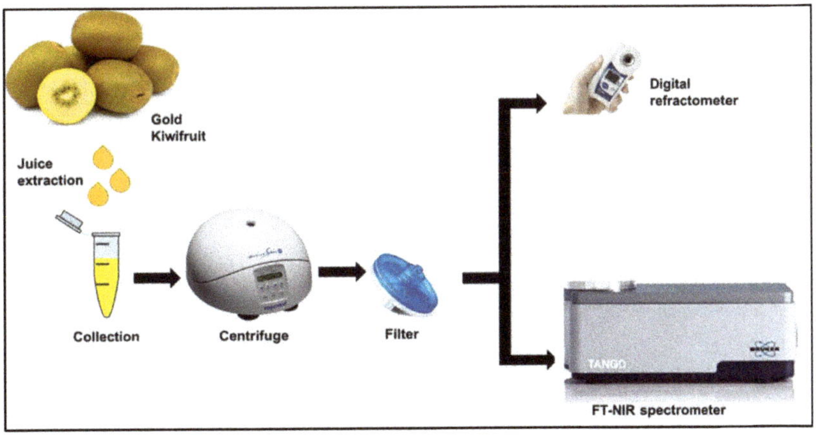

Figure 1. Experimental procedure for kiwifruit soluble solids content (SSC) measurement.

2.2. *Reference SSC (°Brix) Measurement*

The SSC value of the kiwifruit juice samples was measured at room temperature using a digital refractometer (PAL-1, Atago Co., Ltd., Tokyo, Japan), calibrated with Milli-Q water. The Brix value was recorded after placing approximately 0.5 mL of juice into the measurement chamber of the refractometer; this was enough to fully cover the optical interface.

2.3. *FT-NIR Spectral Measurements*

Transmittance spectra of the juice samples were measured at 20, 25, and 30 °C (±1 °C) with an FT-NIR spectrometer (Tango, Bruker Corporation, Bremen, Germany) equipped with a temperature-controlled holder. Two measurements were acquired for each juice sample, using quartz cuvettes of 1 mm and 10 mm optical path length for the 1300–1600 nm and 870–1100 nm wavelength ranges, respectively [23]. For each measurement, one spectrum was the average of 32 successive scans and was recorded with a resolution of 16 cm^{-1}. The total number of juice spectra was 600 (100 samples × 1 consecutive scan × 3 temperatures × 2 cuvettes). The samples were divided into two sets, one for the 1300–1600 nm and one for the 870–1100 nm wavelength ranges. After the removal of five outliers, anomalous readings speculated to be laboratory blunders, the final data set consisted of 95 juice samples (285 spectra for three temperatures) in each wavelength set. The spectral region above 1800 nm was discarded because of the high absorption in aqueous samples. To monitor interfering signals, a reference spectrum of Milli-Q water was taken at the beginning, middle, and end of the experiment, which resulted in a total of 18 water spectra (3 samples × 1 consecutive scan × 3 temperatures × 2 cuvettes).

2.4. *Aquaphotomics Analysis*

Aquaphotomics water matrix coordinates (WAMACS) were created using the peak wavelengths identified in a principal component analysis (PCA) of the full data set of fruit juice spectra over the three temperatures in the first and second overtone regions of the OH stretch of water. An anharmonic oscillator model was used to establish 12 water bands in the second overtone region that corresponded to the previously established wavelengths in the first overtone region of water [24]. Aquagrams displaying the resulting water spectral pattern (WASP) in each overtone region were studied to observe the effect of temperature variation.

2.5. *Multivariate Analysis*

Predictive models were developed using MATLAB version R2018b (MathWorks Inc., Natick, MA, USA) and the PLS toolbox version 8.6.2 (Eigenvector Research Inc., Wenatchee, WA, USA). The analysis involved the development of predictive models using spectra pre-processed by:

2.5.1. SNV + 2D

This is the standard normal variate transformation of the raw spectra followed by second derivative processing (Savitzky–Golay second-order derivative with smoothing parameters: width 15, order 2).

2.5.2. EMSC

This is the extended multiplicative scatter correction of the raw spectra. The concept of EMSC pre-treatment was introduced by Martens et al. [25,26]. EMSC was designed to remove chemical variabilities by using a model framework that segregates the spectral response of the analyte of interest from that of a known interference.

Equation (1) describes the theory of EMSC:

$$X = b_0 + b_1\overline{X} + b_2 I + e \quad (1)$$

where X is the raw observed spectra, $\overline{X}$ is the mean spectrum (the mean of all calibration spectra), I is an interferent spectrum (to be determined), b_0, b_1, and b_2 are fitting constants, and e is the residual [18]. Rearranging Equation (1) leads to:

$$\frac{X - b_0}{b_1} - \frac{b_2 I}{b_1} = \overline{X} + \frac{e}{b1} \quad (2)$$

The left-hand side of Equation (2) defines the corrected spectra,

$$\hat{X} = \frac{X - b_0}{b_1} - \frac{b_2 I}{b_1} \quad (3)$$

where the constant terms can be estimated by multiple linear regression (MLR).

2.5.3. EPO

This is the external parameter orthogonalisation of the raw spectral matrix **X**. The concept of EPO was introduced by Roger et al. [10]. It is a pre-processing method that aims at removing the part of the **X** matrix space most influenced by the external parameter variations. The method identifies the parasitic subspace for removal by computing a PCA on a small set of spectra measured on the same objects, while the external parameter is varying.

The theory of the EPO algorithm is outlined below [27].

The spectra matrix **X** (size n × m) can be written as:

$$\mathbf{X} = \mathbf{XP} + \mathbf{XQ} + \mathbf{R} \quad (4)$$

where **P** is the projection matrix (size m × m) of the useful part of the spectra: **X*** = **XP**; **Q** is the projection matrix (size m × m) of the not useful part (e.g., influenced by temperature) of the spectra: **X#** = **XQ**; **R** is the residual matrix (size n × m); n is the number of samples, and m is the number of wavelengths.

The aim of EPO is to obtain the useful spectra $\mathbf{X^*} = \mathbf{X}(\mathbf{I} - \mathbf{Q})$, while matrix $\mathbf{Q}$ can be written as $\mathbf{Q} = \mathbf{GG^T}$ where $\mathbf{G^T}$ is the transpose of $\mathbf{G}$. The transformed spectra for both the calibration and validation sets are then calculated as $\mathbf{X^*} = \mathbf{XP}$ where $\mathbf{P} = \mathbf{I} - \mathbf{GG^T}$, and $\mathbf{I}$ is the identity matrix. To estimate $\mathbf{G}$, the uninformative part of the spectra that is orthogonal to the useful part of the spectra, the principal component of the difference spectra $\mathbf{D}$ is calculated. $\mathbf{D}$ is the difference matrix generated by subtracting the average spectra for the samples at the lowest temperature (in our case) from the samples at all temperatures.

2.5.4. All Temperature Method

This involved combining samples from all three temperatures and applying a standard pre-treatment on all spectra, both calibration and validation, of SNV transformation followed by 2nd derivative processing.

2.6. Statistical Analysis

The main data set in the long-wavelength region (1300–1600 nm) and the short wavelength region (870–1100 nm) was split into three subsets for 20, 25, and 30 °C temperature, respectively. The samples were first rank ordered by SSC value and then systematically split into ten different groups, using a Venetian blind selection approach, delivering SSC equivalence between the groups. This arrangement enabled a 10-way leave-each-group-out approach to calibration-validation set modeling and analysis. Each of the ten calibration–validation sets were created by holding out a single group in turn, as an independent validation data set, and leaving the remaining nine groups to be combined as the calibration data set. Consequently, the total number of samples in each calibration set was 71, and in each validation set was 24. A separate 10-way Venetian blind cross-validation process was also undertaken with the calibration modeling on each calibration data set.

3. Results and Discussion

The SSC of kiwifruit juice ranged from 11.9 to 19.2 °Brix, with a mean of 16.54 °Brix and a standard deviation of 1.26 °Brix. Figure 2 shows the distribution of SSC for all fruit juice samples in the experiment. There was a very small number of relatively low SSC samples, below 14 °Brix, which may be population outliers.

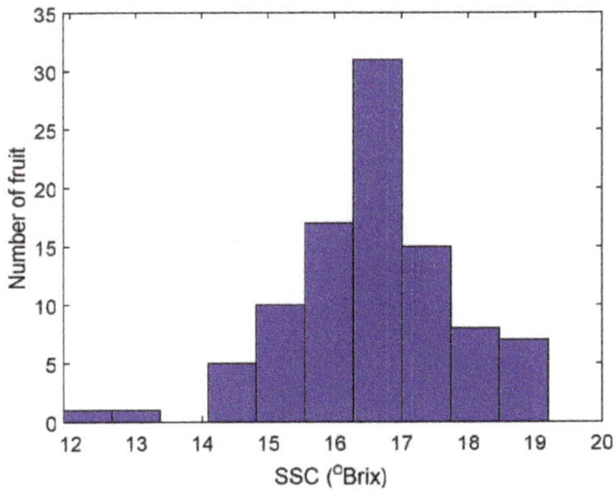

Figure 2. Number of fruit vs SSC for the kiwifruit juice samples.

3.1. The Raw Spectra

The absorbance plot in Figure 3 illustrates that as the temperature increased in kiwifruit juice, the absorbance curve in the first overtone region shifted to shorter wavelengths with a broadening of the peak and a decrease in intensity (Figure 3a). However, in the second overtone region, there was a slight upward shift in intensity towards the shorter wavelengths with increasing temperature (Figure 3b). The isosbestic points were 1444 nm (before the water peak wavelength) and 994 nm (after the water peak wavelength), each approximately 4 nm away from reported pure water isosbestic points at 1440 nm and 990 nm, respectively [28].

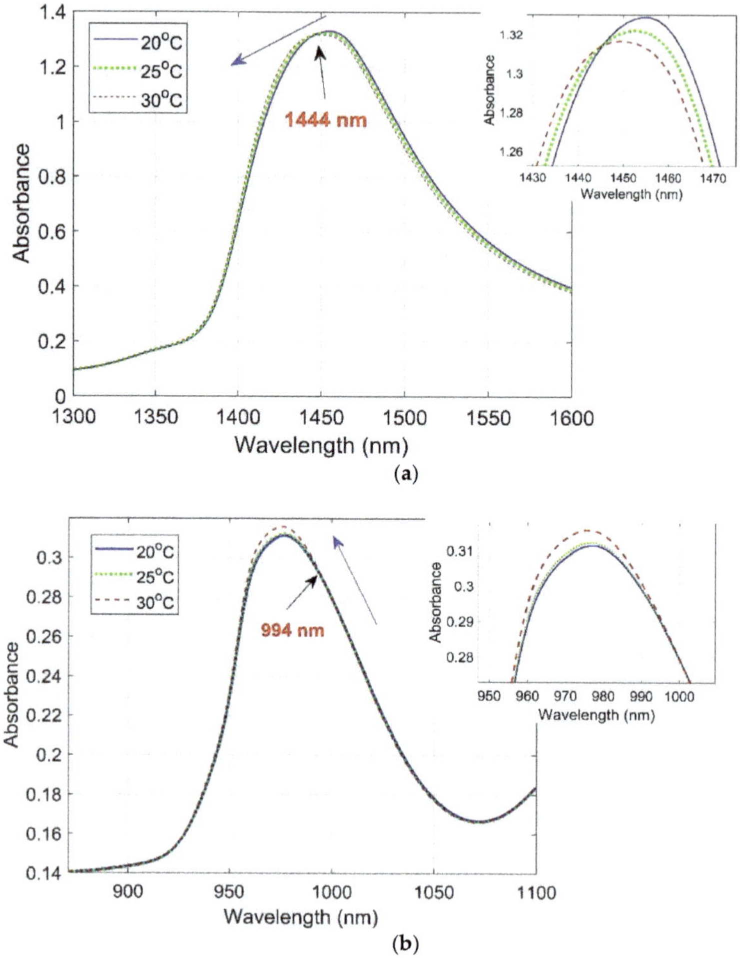

Figure 3. Average raw absorbance spectra of kiwifruit juice at three temperatures 20, 25, and 30 °C in (**a**) the first overtone and (**b**) the second overtone region of the OH stretch of water. Labels indicate wavelengths of the isosbestic points.

3.2. Aquaphotomics Analysis

The wavelengths of the peak and trough in the PC1 spectrum (from PCA on all juice samples and temperatures) were at 1414 nm and 1494 nm (the first overtone), and 963 nm and 1027 nm (the second overtone), as shown in Figure 4a,b. These wavelength pairs correspond to C5 (S_0: free water) and C11 (S_4: species with four hydrogen bonds) activation for the first overtone, and C6 (water hydration) and C12 (strongly bonded water) activation for the second overtone region. The remaining WAMACS assignments, not directly identified from the PCA, were selected as the midpoints of each known water band in Table 1. As expected, the zero-crossing points for the two PC1 plots were identical to the isosbestic points observed in Figure 3.

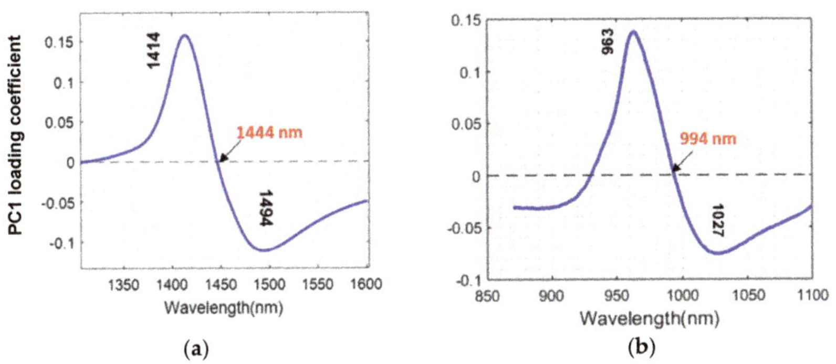

Figure 4. PC1 loading of kiwifruit juice in (**a**) the first overtone and (**b**) the second overtone region of the OH stretch of water. Labels indicate peak wavelengths (black) and zero-crossing points (red).

Table 1. Temperature-perturbed water wavelengths of kiwifruit juice in the first [16,29] and the second overtone regions of OH stretch of water [30].

WAMACS	Assignment	Wavelengths in Overtone Region		Activated Wavelengths, nm	
		First (1300–1600 nm)	Second (800–1100 nm)	First Overtone	Second Overtone
C1	ν_3—asymmetric stretching vibration	1336–1348	900–908		
C2	OH stretch—water solvation shell)	1360–1366	916–920		
C3	$\nu_1 + \nu_3$—H_2O symmetric stretching and asymmetric stretching vibration	1370–1376	923–927		
C4	OH stretch (water solvation shell)	1380–1388	930–935		
C5	S_0 (free water)	1398–1418	942–955	1414	
C6	Water hydration, H_5O_2	1421–1430	957–963		963
C7	S_1—water molecules with 1 hydrogen bond	1432–1444	965–973		
C8	$\nu_2 + \nu_3$—H_2O bending and asymmetric stretching vibration	1448–1454	975–979		
C9	S_2—water molecules with 2 hydrogen bonds	1458–1468	982–989		
C10	S_3—water molecules with 3 hydrogen bonds	1472–1482	992–998		
C11	S_4—water molecules with 4 hydrogen bonds	1482–1495	998–1007	1494	
C12	Strongly bonded water or ν_1, ν_2	1506–1516	1014–1021		1027

3.3. *Aquagrams*

The aquagrams of average spectra of the juice at three temperatures are illustrated in Figure 5a,b for the two overtone regions. There are strong similarities in the two overtone regions, free water species increasing with temperature as the water structure becomes less organized as a result of increased molecular motion and less stable H-bonds. However, there is a difference with the asymmetric stretching and bending ($\nu_2 + \nu_3$) only observed to increase with temperature for the second overtone region. We might have expected that the same water coordinates to be similarly highlighted in the first and second overtone region. However, this is not quite the case here.

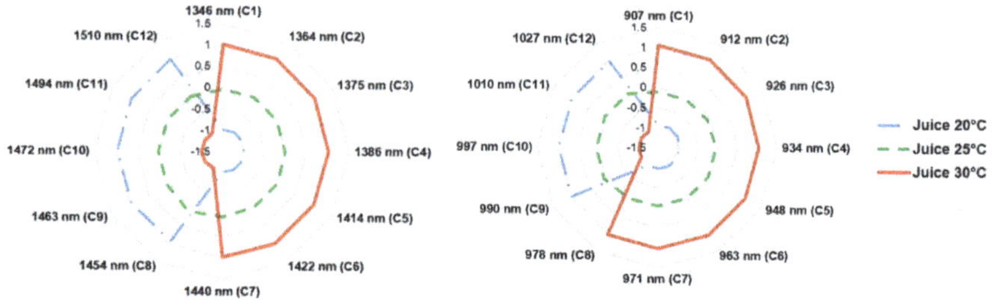

(a) (b)

Figure 5. Aquagrams at three temperatures in (**a**) the first overtone (1300–1600 nm) (**b**) the second overtone (870–1100 nm) region of the OH stretch of water in kiwifruit juice.

3.4. EMSC Correction

Pure Water Analysis

When applying PCA to the water spectra, the shape of the PC1 loading in the first overtone region (Figure 6) is very similar to that reported by Segtnan et al. [8] and Maeda et al. [31], indicating a change in water structure due to a change in temperature. The shape of the PC1 loading of water in the second overtone region (Figure 6) is similar to the PC1 loading in the first overtone region. Hence, the respective PC1 loadings, for the first overtone and second overtone regions were used as the interferent spectra in the EMSC correction method (Equation (3)).

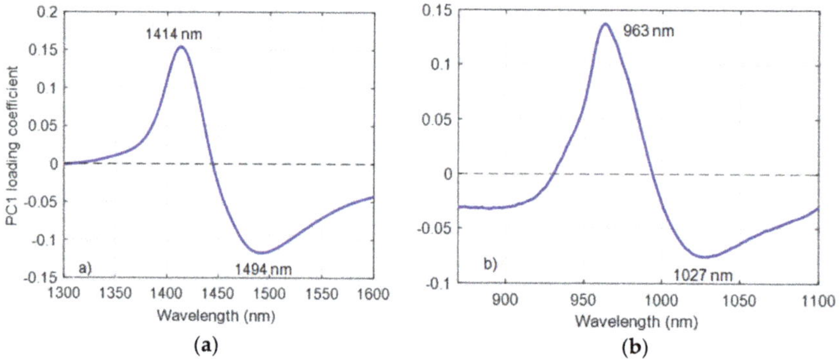

(a) (b)

Figure 6. PC1 loading of water in (**a**) the first overtone and (**b**) the second overtone region of the OH stretch of water. Labels indicate peak and trough wavelengths.

3.5. EPO Correction

PCA of the Difference Matrix D for EPO Correction

There was a variation in the temperature around the peak wavelength region of the juice spectra (Figure 3). When applying PCA to the difference matrix, D, of water and juice spectra (Figure 7), the shape of the PC1 loadings (Figure 8a,b) were nearly identical, and the peak and trough positions were identical to those determined in the PCA of the raw juice and water spectra (Figures 4 and 6). Therefore, the PC1 loadings of the difference matrix, D, of water were used in the EPO correction (Figure 6) as the interferent spectra to correct juice spectra against temperature variation.

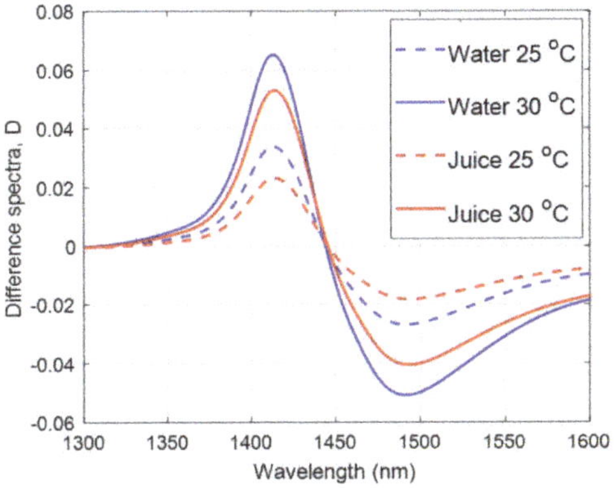

Figure 7. Average raw absorbance difference spectra of water and kiwifruit juice after subtracting average raw absorbance spectrum of water and juice at 20 °C, respectively.

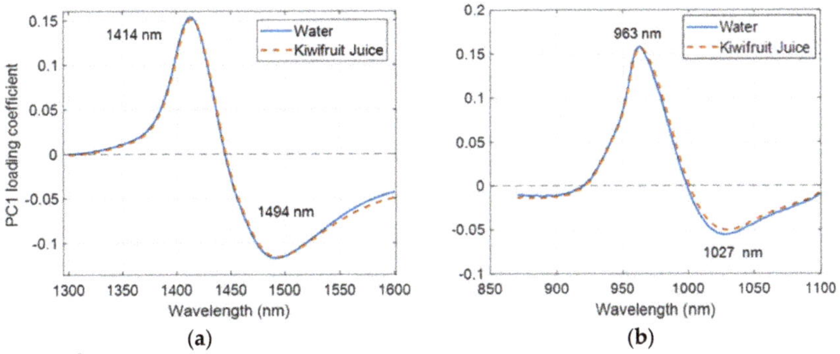

Figure 8. PC1 loading of water and juice difference matrix in the (**a**) 1300–1600 nm region with a 1 mm cuvette; and (**b**) 870–1100 nm region with a 10 mm cuvette. Labels indicate the peak and trough wavelengths.

3.6. Prediction of SSC

Application of both the EMSC and EPO pre-processing techniques generally reduced the SSC prediction bias by a large margin in both the first (Figure 9) and second (Figure 10) overtone regions, especially compared with SNV + 2D pre-processing. Beyond that, and particularly comparing EMSC and EPO, it is difficult to see any consistent trends or patterns in the results. For instance, in the first overtone region, the EMSC method seems advantageous (lower bias) compared with the EPO method when applying a model calibrated at 30 °C to a validation set at 20 or 25 °C (Figure 9c). However, that does not apply in reverse, a model calibrated at 20 °C is perhaps slightly better under the EPO method when applied to validation sets at 25 and 30 °C. In the second overtone region, the EPO method seems to have the advantage, although oddly it fails badly, even compared with the SNV + 2D method, when using a model calibrated at 25 °C on a validation set at 30 °C (Figure 10b). The variation in results of any particular method is relatively large, represented by standard deviation error bars in the graphs, and suggests a large amount of modeling noise between the various combinations of calibration and validation data sets.

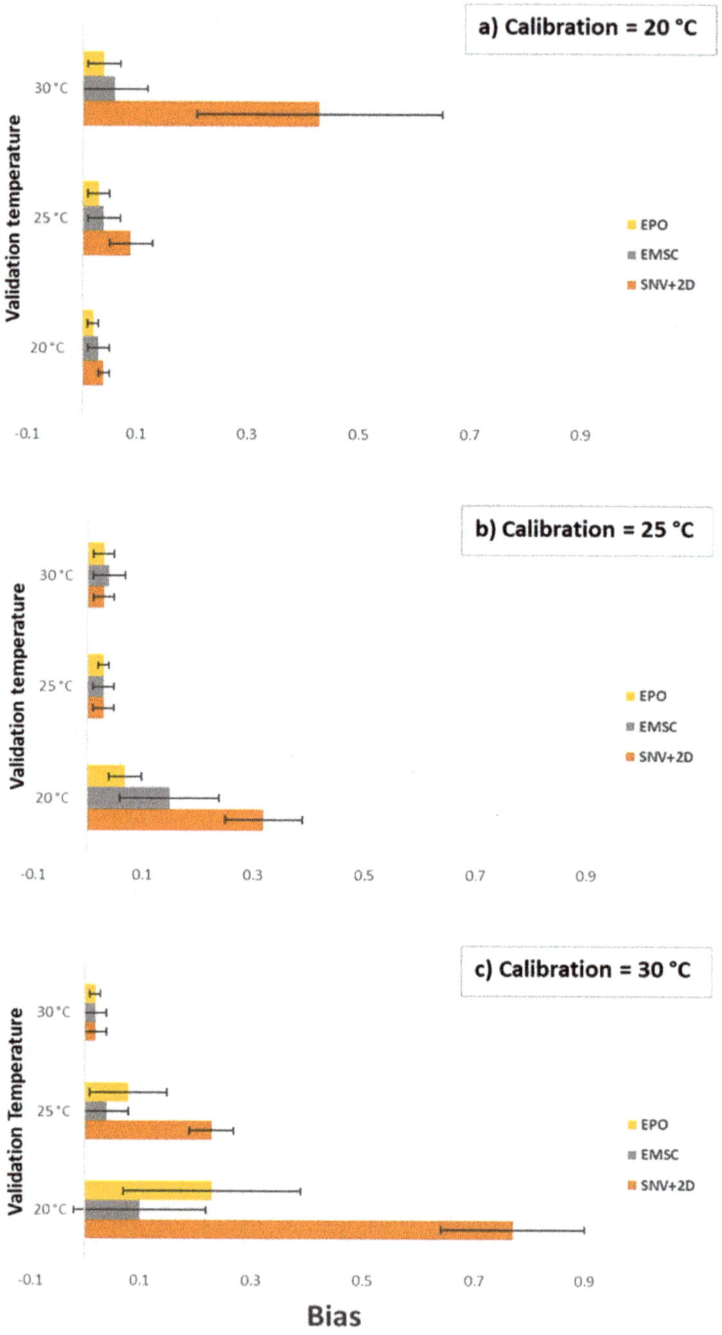

Figure 9. Validation temperature vs. bias at for SSC prediction of kiwifruit juice in the first overtone (1300–1600 nm) region of the OH stretch of water at calibration temperature (**a**) 20 °C, (**b**) 25 °C, and (**c**) 30 °C. Error bars show standard deviation.

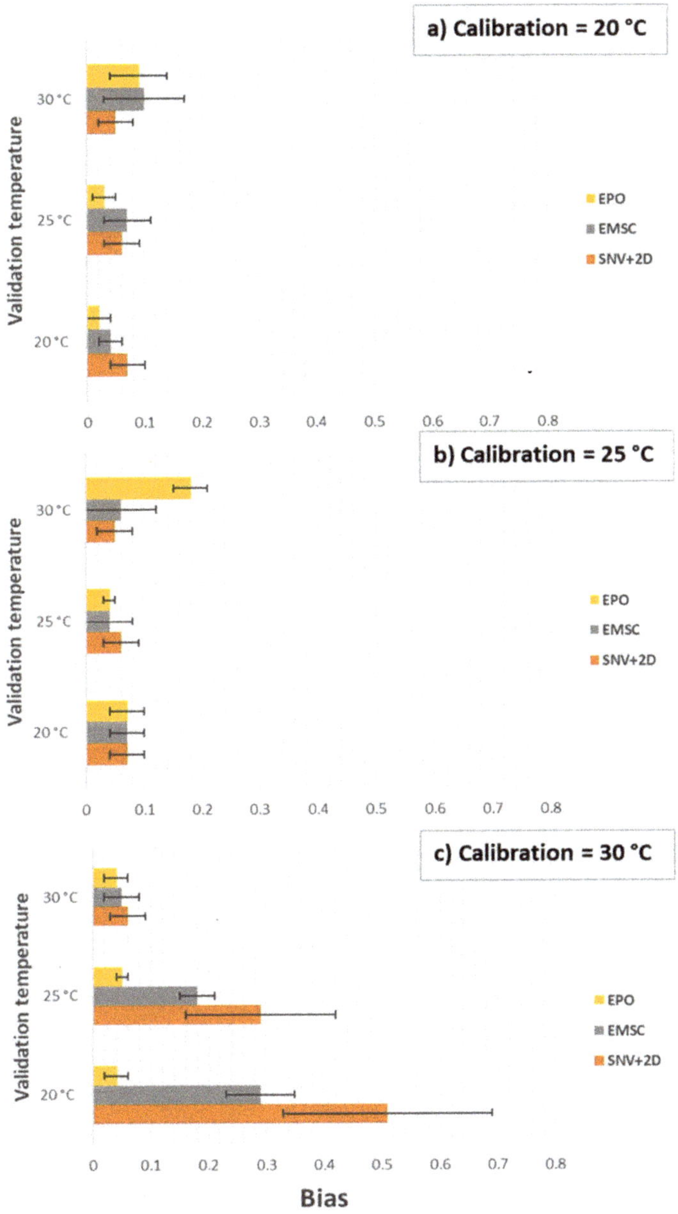

Figure 10. Validation temperature vs. bias for SSC prediction of kiwifruit juice in the second overtone (870–1100 nm) region of the OH stretch of water at calibration temperature (**a**) 20 °C, (**b**) 25 °C, and (**c**) 30 °C. Error bars show standard deviation.

The performance of each method is shown in detail in Tables 2 and 3. The result for the All-Temperature method is listed for comparison. The all-temperature method resulted in the lowest overall biases of 0.03 in the first overtone region and less than 0.06 in the second overtone region of water. However, the EPO method consistently produced the lowest SEP and RMSECV for the first and second overtone regions of water. The RMSECV errors in the first and second overtone regions were fairly consistent, approximately 0.09 and 0.12 respectively when using the EPO method for calibration models at 20, 25, and 30 °C. However, the bias results were not consistent. For example, the calibration model at 30 °C predicting at 20 °C, produced a bias of 0.23 in the first overtone region whereas a bias of 0.04 was generated in the second overtone region. The best choice of wavelength region may depend on other matters, such as sample thickness—analysis of thicker samples, as in thicker than the 1 mm pathlength, may demand the use of the second overtone region of water to achieve sufficient light transmission.

Table 2. Performance comparison for soluble solids content (SSC) prediction of kiwifruit juice in the first overtone (1300–1600 nm) region of the OH stretch of water at different temperatures.

With 1 mm Cuvette in the First Overtone Region (1300–1600 nm)								
N_{cal} = 72, N_{val} = 23								
Calibration				Validation				
T_{cal} [°C]	Method	r^2_{cv}	RMSECV	T_{val} [°C]	r^2_p	RMSEP	BIAS	SEP
All	SNV + 2D	0.99	0.12 (±0.00)	20	0.99	0.12 (±0.01)	0.03 (±0.02)	0.12 (±0.01)
				25	0.99	0.12 (±0.02)	0.03 (±0.01)	0.12 (±0.02)
				30	0.99	0.13 (±0.02)	0.03 (±0.01)	0.12 (±0.02)
20	SNV + 2D	0.99	0.14 (±0.01)	20	0.98	0.16 (±0.01)	0.04 (±0.01)	0.15 (±0.01)
				25	0.96	0.24 (±0.05)	0.09 (±0.04)	0.22 (±0.05)
				30	0.98	0.48 (±0.21)	0.43 (±0.22)	0.19 (±0.02)
	EMSC	0.99	0.14 (±0.01)	20	0.99	0.13 (±0.02)	0.03 (±0.02)	0.13 (±0.01)
				25	0.98	0.15 (±0.02)	0.04 (±0.03)	0.14 (±0.02)
				30	0.99	0.15 (±0.04)	0.06 (±0.06)	0.13 (±0.02)
	EPO	0.99	0.10 (±0.01)	20	0.99	0.09 (±0.02)	0.02 (±0.01)	0.09 (±0.02)
				25	0.99	0.09 (±0.01)	0.03 (±0.02)	0.09 (±0.01)
				30	0.99	0.10 (±0.02)	0.04 (±0.03)	0.09 (±0.01)
25	SNV+2D	0.99	0.13 (±0.02)	20	0.98	0.37 (±0.05)	0.32 (±0.07)	0.18 (±0.04)
				25	0.98	0.15 (±0.03)	0.03 (±0.02)	0.14 (±0.03)
				30	0.99	0.14 (±0.01)	0.03 (±0.02)	0.14 (±0.02)
	EMSC	0.99	0.12 (±0.01)	20	0.99	0.21 (±0.07)	0.15 (±0.09)	0.13 (±0.01)
				25	0.98	0.15 (±0.04)	0.03 (±0.02)	0.15 (±0.04)
				30	0.99	0.14 (±0.02)	0.04 (±0.03)	0.13 (±0.02)
	EPO	0.99	0.09 (±0.00)	20	0.99	0.11 (±0.03)	0.07 (±0.03)	0.09 (±0.02)
				25	0.99	0.09 (±0.01)	0.03 (±0.01)	0.08 (±0.01)
				30	0.99	0.09 (±0.02)	0.03 (±0.02)	0.09 (±0.01)
30	SNV+2D	0.99	0.14 (±0.00)	20	0.97	0.80 (±0.13)	0.77 (±0.13)	0.21 (±0.04)
				25	0.98	0.28 (±0.04)	0.23 (±0.04)	0.15 (±0.03)
				30	0.99	0.14 (±0.01)	0.02 (±0.02)	0.14 (±0.01)
	EMSC	0.99	0.13 (±0.00)	20	0.99	0.18 (±0.10)	0.10 (±0.12)	0.13 (±0.03)
				25	0.99	0.14 (±0.01)	0.04 (±0.04)	0.12 (±0.01)
				30	0.99	0.13 (±0.01)	0.02 (±0.02)	0.12 (±0.01)
	EPO	0.99	0.09 (±0.00)	20	0.99	0.26 (±0.15)	0.23 (±0.16)	0.10 (±0.03)
				25	0.99	0.13 (±0.06)	0.08 (±0.07)	0.09 (±0.02)
				30	0.99	0.09 (±0.01)	0.02 (±0.01)	0.09 (±0.01)

Table 3. Performance comparison for SSC prediction of kiwifruit juice in the first overtone (870–1100 nm) region of the OH stretch of water at different temperatures.

With 10 mm Cuvette in the Second Overtone Region (870–1100 nm)								
N_{cal} = 72, N_{val} = 23								
Calibration				Validation				
T_{cal} [°C]	Method	r^2_{cv}	RMSECV	T_{val} [°C]	r^2_p	RMSEP	BIAS	SEP
All	SNV + 2D	0.98	0.17 (±0.01)	20	0.98	0.18 (±0.04)	0.06 (±0.05)	0.16 (±0.03)
				25	0.98	0.17 (±0.02)	0.05 (±0.02)	0.16 (±0.03)
				30	0.98	0.18 (±0.02)	0.04 (±0.02)	0.17 (±0.02)
20	SNV + 2D	0.98	0.20 (±0.01)	20	0.97	0.21 (±0.03)	0.07 (±0.03)	0.21 (±0.04)
				25	0.97	0.20 (±0.04)	0.06 (±0.03)	0.20 (±0.03)
				30	0.97	0.19 (±0.03)	0.05 (±0.03)	0.20 (±0.03)
	EMSC	0.99	0.14 (±0.01)	20	0.98	0.15 (±0.03)	0.04 (±0.02)	0.14 (±0.03)
				25	0.98	0.18 (±0.02)	0.07 (±0.04)	0.16 (±0.02)
				30	0.98	0.20 (±0.05)	0.10 (±0.07)	0.17 (±0.03)
	EPO	0.99	0.12 (±0.01)	20	0.99	0.13 (±0.01)	0.02 (±0.02)	0.13 (±0.01)
				25	0.98	0.14 (±0.02)	0.03 (±0.02)	0.14 (±0.02)
				30	0.98	0.17 (±0.03)	0.09 (±0.05)	0.15 (±0.02)
25	SNV+2D	0.98	0.20 (±0.01)	20	0.97	0.21 (±0.03)	0.07 (±0.03)	0.21 (±0.04)
				25	0.97	0.20 (±0.04)	0.06 (±0.03)	0.20 (±0.03)
				30	0.97	0.19 (±0.03)	0.05 (±0.03)	0.20 (±0.03)
	EMSC	0.99	0.15 (±0.01)	20	0.97	0.19 (±0.01)	0.07 (±0.03)	0.18 (±0.02)
				25	0.99	0.14 (±0.03)	0.04 (±0.04)	0.12 (±0.03)
				30	0.98	0.17 (±0.03)	0.06 (±0.06)	0.14 (±0.02)
	EPO	0.99	0.12 (±0.01)	20	0.97	0.21 (±0.02)	0.07 (±0.04)	0.19 (±0.03)
				25	0.99	0.13 (±0.02)	0.04 (±0.02)	0.12 (±0.01)
				30	0.98	0.24 (±0.05)	0.18 (±0.06)	0.15 (±0.03)
30	SNV+2D	0.98	0.19 (±0.01)	20	0.97	0.55 (±0.18)	0.51 (±0.18)	0.21 (±0.04)
				25	0.98	0.35 (±0.12)	0.29 (±0.13)	0.18 (±0.01)
				30	0.97	0.19 (±0.03)	0.06 (±0.03)	0.18 (±0.03)
	EMSC	0.98	0.17 (±0.02)	20	0.98	0.34 (±0.06)	0.29 (±0.06)	0.16 (±0.03)
				25	0.98	0.25 (±0.01)	0.18 (±0.03)	0.16 (±0.03)
				30	0.98	0.17 (±0.05)	0.05 (±0.03)	0.15 (±0.05)
	EPO	0.99	0.13 (±0.00)	20	0.98	0.14 (±0.02)	0.04 (±0.02)	0.14 (±0.02)
				25	0.99	0.14 (±0.01)	0.05 (±0.01)	0.13 (±0.01)
				30	0.99	0.12 (±0.01)	0.04 (±0.02)	0.12 (±0.01)

4. Conclusions

The aquaphotomics study here has revealed that the free water components of kiwifruit juice increase and the bound water components decrease as the temperature rises from 20 to 30 °C. The key aquaphotomics wavebands in the first and second overtone regions were identified. The influence of increasing temperature on the peak absorbance of kiwifruit juice spectra was a lateral (wavelength) shift in the first overtone region and a vertical shift in the second overtone region of water. In the second overtone region, the C8 asymmetric stretching and bending component ($\nu_2 + \nu_3$) became more prominent in the aquagram with increasing temperature, which was not the case in the first overtone region.

Predictive modeling of the SSC of kiwifruit juice over the temperature range 20 to 30 °C was more robust (lower offset bias) when using EPO and EMSC pre-processing with an interference term generated from PCA of a simple and independent pure water-temperature spectral matrix experimentally generated over the same temperature range. The water-temperature matrix only needs to be created once and, in being independent of the kiwifruit juice samples, considerably simplifies the generation of temperature-independent predictions. The consequence of this is that model calibration data on actual juice samples need only be measured at one temperature, the EPO and/or EMSC pre-processing enables application at any other temperature within the measured temperature range. This approach may apply to other applications, such as other fruit juices or intact fruit modeling problems, where robustness against temperature changes is desirable.

Author Contributions: Conceptualization, H.K., R.K. and A.M.; methodology, H.K., R.K. and A.M.; resources, A.M.; writing—original draft preparation, H.K.; writing—review and editing, R.K. and A.M.; supervision, R.K. and A.M. All authors have read and agreed to the published version of the manuscript.

Funding: Harpreet Kaur acknowledges the financial support of a PhD scholarship from The University of Waikato, the Ministry of Business, Innovation and Employment (MBIE), The New Zealand Institute for Plant & Food Research Limited, The New Zealand.

Institutional Review Board Statement: Not applicable.

Informed Consent Statement: Not applicable.

Conflicts of Interest: The authors declare no conflict of interest.

Sample Availability: Samples of the compounds are not available from the authors.

References

1. Popkin, B.M.; D'Anci, K.E.; Rosenberg, I.H. Water, hydration, and health. *Nutr. Rev.* **2010**, *68*, 439–458. [CrossRef] [PubMed]
2. DeMan, J.M. Water. In *Principles of Food Chemistry*; Springer: Boston, MA, USA, 1999; pp. 1–32.
3. Pegau, W.S.; Gray, D.; Zaneveld, J.R.V. Absorption and attenuation of visible and near-infrared light in water: Dependence on temperature and salinity. *Appl. Opt.* **1997**, *36*, 6035–6046. [CrossRef]
4. Tsenkova, R. Aquaphotomics: Water in the biological and aqueous world scrutinised with invisible light. *Spectrosc. Eur.* **2010**, *22*, 6–10.
5. McGlone, V.A.; Jordan, R.B.; Seelye, R.; Clark, C.J. Dry-matter—a better predictor of the post-storage soluble solids in apples? *Postharvest Biol. Technol.* **2003**, *28*, 431–435. [CrossRef]
6. Nicolaï, B.M.; Beullens, K.; Bobelyn, E.; Peirs, A.; Saeys, W.; Theron, K.I.; Lammertyn, J. Nondestructive measurement of fruit and vegetable quality by means of NIR spectroscopy: A review. *Postharvest Biol. Technol.* **2007**, *46*, 99–118. [CrossRef]
7. Wang, Y.; Veltkamp, D.J.; Kowalski, B.R. Multivariate instrument standardization. *Anal. Chem.* **1991**, *63*, 2750–2756. [CrossRef]
8. Segtnan, V.H.; Šašić, Š.; Isaksson, T.; Ozaki, Y. Studies on the Structure of Water Using Two-Dimensional Near-Infrared Correlation Spectroscopy and Principal Component Analysis. *Anal. Chem.* **2001**, *73*, 3153–3161. [CrossRef] [PubMed]
9. Kawano, S.; Abe, H.; Iwamoto, M. Development of a Calibration Equation with Temperature Compensation for Determining the Brix Value in Intact Peaches. *J. Near Infrared Spectrosc.* **1995**, *3*, 211–218. [CrossRef]
10. Roger, J.M.; Chauchard, F.; Bellon-Maurel, V. EPO–PLS external parameter orthogonalisation of PLS application to temperature-independent measurement of sugar content of intact fruits. *Chemometr. Intell. Lab. Syst.* **2003**, *66*, 191–204. [CrossRef]
11. Golic, M.; Walsh, K.B. Robustness of calibration models based on near infrared spectroscopy for the in-line grading of stonefruit for total soluble solids content. *Anal. Chim. Acta* **2006**, *555*, 286–291. [CrossRef]
12. Acharya, U.K.; Walsh, K.B.; Subedi, P. Effect of temperature on SWNIRS based models of fruit DM and colour. In Proceedings of the NIR 2013—16th International Conference on Near Infrared Spectroscopy, Montpellier, France, 2–7 June 2013; pp. 674–676. Available online: http://hdl.cqu.edu.au/10018/1017629 (accessed on 16 July 2019).
13. Peirs, A.; Scheerlinck, N.; Nicolaï, B. Temperature compensation for near infrared reflectance measurement of apple fruit soluble solids contents. *Postharvest Biol. Technol.* **2003**, *30*, 233–248. [CrossRef]
14. Mishra, P.; Roger, J.M.; Rutledge, D.N.; Woltering, E. Two standard-free approaches to correct for external influences on near-infrared spectra to make models widely applicable. *Postharvest Biol. Technol.* **2020**, *170*, 111326. [CrossRef]
15. Tsenkova, R. Aquaphotomics: Exploring water-light interactions for a better understanding of the biological world. Part 2: Japanese food, language and why NIR for diagnosis? *NIR News* **2006**, *17*, 814. [CrossRef]
16. Tsenkova, R.; Kovacs, Z.; Kubota, Y. Aquaphotomics: Near Infrared Spectroscopy and Water States in Biological Systems. In *Membrane Hydration: The Role of Water in the Structure and Function of Biological Membranes*; Disalvo, E.A., Ed.; Springer International: New York, NY, USA, 2015; pp. 189–211.
17. Tsenkova, R.; Munćan, J.; Pollner, B.; Kovacs, Z. Essentials of Aquaphotomics and Its Chemometrics Approaches. *Front. Chem.* **2018**, *6*, 363. [CrossRef] [PubMed]

18. Gowen, A.; Stark, E.; Tsuchisaka, T.; Tsenkova, R. Extended multiplicative signal correction as a tool for aquaphotomics. *NIR News* **2011**, *22*, 9–13. [CrossRef]
19. Gowen, A.A.; Amigo, J.M.; Tsenkova, R. Characterisation of hydrogen bond perturbations in aqueous systems using aquaphotomics and multivariate curve resolution-alternating least squares. *Anal. Chim. Acta* **2013**, *759*, 8–20. [CrossRef] [PubMed]
20. Kaur, H.; Künnemeyer, R.; McGlone, A. Investigating aquaphotomics for temperature-independent prediction of soluble solids content of pure apple juice. *J. Near Infrared Spectrosc.* **2020**, *28*, 103–112. [CrossRef]
21. McGlone, V.A.; Kawano, S. Firmness, dry-matter and soluble-solids assessment of postharvest kiwifruit by NIR spectroscopy. *Postharvest Biol. Technol.* **1998**, *13*, 131–141. [CrossRef]
22. Kaur, H.; Künnemeyer, R.; McGlone, A. Comparison of hand-held near infrared spectrophotometers for fruit dry matter assessment. *J. Near Infrared Spectrosc.* **2017**, *25*, 267–277. [CrossRef]
23. Kaur, H.; Künnemeyer, R.; McGlone, A. Investigating Aquaphotomics for Fruit Quality Assessment. In Proceedings of the 3rd Aquaphotomics International Symposium Exploring Water Molecular Systems in Nature, Awaji, Japan, 2–6 December 2018.
24. Osborne, B.G.; Fearn, T.; Hindle, P.H. *Practical NIR Spectroscopy with Applications in Food and Beverage Analysis*; Longman Food Technology, No; Longman Scientific & Technical: Harlow, UK, 1993. Available online: https://nla.gov.au/nla.cat-vn2895403 (accessed on 5 August 2019).
25. Martens, H.; Stark, E. Extended multiplicative signal correction and spectral interference subtraction: New preprocessing methods for near infrared spectroscopy. *J. Pharm. Biomed. Anal.* **1991**, *9*, 625–635. [CrossRef]
26. Martens, H.; Bruun, S.W.; Adt, I.; Sockalingum, G.D.; Kohler, A. Pre-processing in biochemometrics: Correction for path-length and temperature effects of water in FTIR bio-spectroscopy by EMSC. *J. Chemom.* **2006**, *20*, 402–417. [CrossRef]
27. Minasny, B.; McBratney, A.B.; Bellon-Maurel, V.; Roger, J.-M.; Gobrecht, A.; Ferrand, L.; Joalland, S. Removing the effect of soil moisture from NIR diffuse reflectance spectra for the prediction of soil organic carbon. *Geoderma* **2011**, *167*, 118–124. [CrossRef]
28. Workman, J.J.; Weyer, L. *Practical Guide to Interpretive Near-Infrared Spectroscopy*; CRC Press: Boca Raton, FL, USA, 2007.
29. Muncan, J.; Tsenkova, R. Aquaphotomics—From Innovative Knowledge to Integrative Platform in Science and Technology. *Molecules* **2019**, *24*, 2742. Available online: https://www.mdpi.com/1420-3049/24/15/2742 (accessed on 28 July 2019). [CrossRef] [PubMed]
30. Kaur, H. Investigating Aquaphotomics for Fruit Quality Assessment. Ph.D. Thesis, The University of Waikato, Hamilton, New Zealand, 2020. Available online: https://hdl.handle.net/10289/13693 (accessed on 17 August 2020).
31. Maeda, H.; Ozaki, Y.; Tanaka, M.; Hayashi, N.; Kojima, T. Near Infrared Spectroscopy and Chemometrics Studies of Temperature-Dependent Spectral Variations of Water: Relationship between Spectral Changes and Hydrogen Bonds. *J. Near Infrared Spectrosc.* **1995**, *3*, 191–201. [CrossRef]

molecules

MDPI

Article

Interactions of Linearly Polarized and Unpolarized Light on Kiwifruit Using Aquaphotomics

Damenraj Rajkumar [1,2,3,*], Rainer Künnemeyer [2,3], Harpreet Kaur [2], Jevon Longdell [1,3] and Andrew McGlone [2]

1 Department of Physics, University of Otago, Dunedin 9016, New Zealand; jevon.longdell@otago.ac.nz
2 The New Zealand Institute for Plant and Food Research Limited, Ruakura 3216, New Zealand; Rainer.Kunnemeyer@plantandfood.co.nz (R.K.); harpreet.kaur@plantandfood.co.nz (H.K.); Andrew.McGlone@plantandfood.co.nz (A.M.)
3 The Dodd Walls Centre for Photonic and Quantum Technologies, University of Otago, Dunedin 9054, New Zealand
* Correspondence: damen.rajkumar@plantandfood.co.nz

Abstract: Near infrared (NIR) spectroscopy is an important tool for predicting the internal qualities of fruits. Using aquaphotomics, spectral changes between linearly polarized and unpolarized light were assessed on 200 commercially grown yellow-fleshed kiwifruit (*Actinidia chinensis* var. *chinensis* 'Zesy002'). Measurements were performed on different configurations of unpeeled (intact) and peeled (cut) kiwifruit using a commercial handheld NIR instrument. Absorbance after applying standard normal variate (SNV) and second derivative Savitzky–Golay filters produced different spectral features for all configurations. An aquagram depicting all configurations suggests that linearly polarized light activated more free water states and unpolarized light activated more bound water states. At depth ($\geq$1 mm), after several scattering events, all radiation is expected to be fully depolarized and interactions for incident polarized or unpolarized light will be similar, so any observed differences are attributable to the surface layers of the fruit. Aquagrams generated in terms of the fruit soluble solids content (SSC) were similar for all configurations, suggesting the SSC in fruit is not a contributing factor here.

Keywords: aquaphotomics; water; spectra; band assignment; functionality; polarization; kiwifruit; near infrared spectroscopy

Citation: Rajkumar, D.; Künnemeyer, R.; Kaur, H.; Longdell, J.; McGlone, A. Interactions of Linearly Polarized and Unpolarized Light on Kiwifruit Using Aquaphotomics. *Molecules* **2022**, *27*, 494. https://doi.org/10.3390/molecules27020494

Academic Editors: Roumiana Tsenkova and Jelena Muncan

Received: 15 December 2021
Accepted: 10 January 2022
Published: 13 January 2022

1. Introduction

Preference for high-quality fruit has propelled the development of non-destructive techniques for postharvest fruit grading. Although the final decision before purchasing fruit depends upon consumers, the development of instruments used to mimic human judgement is important [1]. One such technique uses near-infrared spectroscopy (NIRS), which has seen success in predicting fruit internal qualities such as soluble solids content (SSC) and dry matter content (DMC) by utilizing multivariate and statistical analyses such as principal components analysis (PCA) and partial least squares regression (PLSR) to create prediction models [2]. Nevertheless, there is still a requirement for improvement of the technique in several areas such as calibration robustness for fruits harvested from different seasons and calibration model transfer between instruments [3,4].

Usually, unpolarized light is used in NIRS. Crossed polarizers in the incident and detection light path are sometimes applied to reduce the amount of specular reflection received [5]. However, polarized light may offer advantages as suggested by some recent studies on pears and apples [6,7].

Implementing polarized light in NIR spectroscopy is simple but, nonetheless, there are few reported studies using polarized light to assess internal quality of fruits, probably because of multiple scattering in the biological tissue, which quickly depolarizes any initially polarized radiation [8]. The degree of polarization for circularly and linearly polarized light has been observed to decrease as green 'Conference' pears mature and has been attributed to starch, a polarization sensitive structure, hydrolyzing into smaller sugar molecules, resulting in a decrease in reduced scattering [6]. Advancements in polarized light interactions with tissue such as polarization gating spectroscopy have suggested that polarized light can be utilized to probe shallow penetration depths in biological material and that by varying the polarization state between circular and linear polarized light, specific sampling depths can be achieved [8–10]. Structural color in *Pollia condensata* has been determined to be caused by Bragg reflection of helicoidally stacked cellulose microfibrils, reflecting either left or right circularly polarized light [11]. This suggests that utilizing polarized light may be able to infer physical structures in fruits.

Aquaphotomics is a recent scientific discipline conceptualized by Professor Dr Roumiana Tsenkova that utilizes water as a 'detector' for scientifically investigating changes associated with water structures and improving NIRS predictions [12]. For example, using the aquaphotomics approach, temperature changes in water have been identified leading to improved NIRS apple juice SSC predictions, by correcting for temperature using the method of extended multiplicative scatter correction (EMSC) [13]. Water is the major constituent of fruits but other compounds, with active OH functional groups, such as sugars, starch, and cellulose, contribute to the overall pattern of water absorption peaks in the NIR range. The second overtone region of the OH stretch, which gives rise to the strong water peak around 970 nm, is of major interest to the use of NIRS for non-destructive measurement of fruit properties [14,15].

The objective of this study was to investigate the effects of polarized and unpolarized light on unpeeled (intact) and peeled (sliced) yellow-fleshed kiwifruit (*Actinidia chinensis* var. *chinensis* 'Zesy002') in the second overtone region of the OH stretch of water, using aquaphotomics. Previous studies involving the removal of apple skin resulted in an improvement of prediction models for SSC and firmness, probably because of removal of the highly scattering skin [16]. By removing kiwifruit skin, it is assumed that scattering effects will reduce considerably. Sugar molecules such as sucrose are optically active and rotate the plane of linearly polarized light, which is why the effects of SSC measured on kiwifruits are investigated using linearly polarized and unpolarized light [17].

2. Materials and Methods

Unpeeled (intact) and peeled (cut) kiwifruit (Figure 1) were placed directly on top of the ring adapter, enabling an interactance mode NIRS measurement to be made.The measurement setup (Figure 2) consisted of a bespoke ring adapter that ensured only diffuse transmitted light was collected, a linear polarizer (LPNIRE100-B, Thorlabs Inc., Newton, NJ, USA) and a handheld NIR instrument (F-750, Felix Instruments Oregon, Camas, WA, USA).

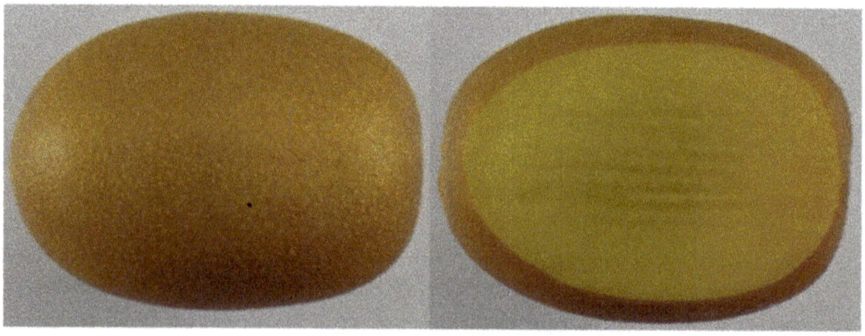

Figure 1. Example of unpeeled (**Left**) and peeled (**Right**) kiwifruit.

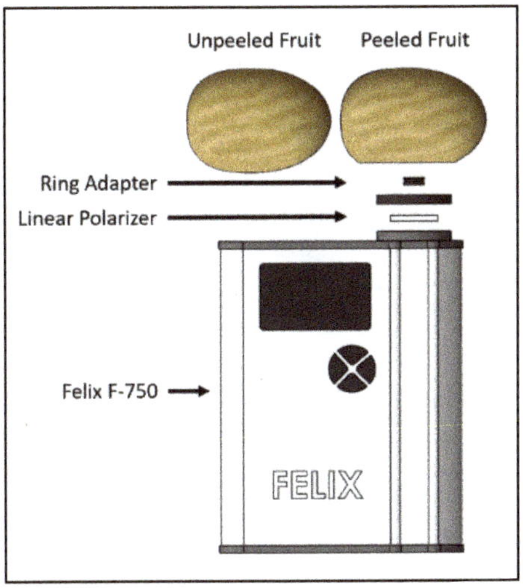

Figure 2. An illustration of the measurement of set up depicting peeled and unpeeled kiwifruit, a ring adapter, a linear polarizer and a Felix F-750.

2.1. Sample Preparation

Two hundred yellow-fleshed kiwifruit, sourced from a local kiwifruit packhouse (Te Puke, New Zealand), were stored at room temperature (22 ± 1 °C). Forty fruits were measured each day for five days and all fruit, except Day 1 fruit, were subjected to 100 ppm ethylene for 24 h to accelerate ripening. Using the F-750 instrument (Oregon, Camas, WA, USA), fruit was measured under four different configurations: Unpeeled Unpolarized (UU), Unpeeled Polarized (UP), Peeled Unpolarized (PU) and Peeled Polarized (PP). Unpeeled and peeled refer to intact and sliced fruit, respectively, where sliced fruit had two 2 mm slices sectioned off using a commercial meat slicer (WFS30MGB3, Wedderburn, New Zealand) to expose internal fruit tissue. After slicing, the sections of each fruit were re-placed onto the cut surface, with the whole fruit then being wrapped in cling wrap (Gladwrap®, Plant Based Cling Wrap, Sydney, Australia) to reduce moisture loss.

2.2. Spectra Collection

The linear polarizer selectively transmits an electromagnetic wave that oscillates along a defined plane and absorbs the rest. Light scattered back towards the detector consists of two components: light having undergone few scattering events and multiply scattered light [18]. The polarizer in this configuration measures light of the same input polarization state and half of the depolarized light. Only co-polarized light was measured in the polarized light configurations,

$$I_{co-pol}(\lambda) = I_{||}(\lambda) + I_{\perp}(\lambda), \quad (1)$$

where $I_{||}(\lambda)$ refers to light having undergone a few scattering events and $I_{\perp}(\lambda)$ refers to depolarized light that has undergone multiple scattering events.

All measurements were made at room temperature (22 ± 1 °C) with the F-750 recording the average of five scans on one side of a kiwifruit. This process was repeated four times at the same location, once for each configuration. Each fruit was orientated with its stem end along the transmission axis of the linear polarizer. A separate scan was recorded for each configuration using a reflectance standard (Spectralon SRS-99-020, Labsphere, North Sutton, NH, USA) and a custom reference holder.

2.3. Destructive Measurements

After measurements were complete, DMC (% FW) and SSC (°Brix) were destructively measured. For DMC, an approximately 3 mm thick kiwifruit cross-sectional slice was sectioned off from the equatorial middle of each fruit. The kiwifruit slice was weighed, then dried for 24 h at 65 °C to remove moisture. The weight of the dried kiwifruit slice was then measured and the DMC was calculated as the ratio of the dry to wet weight.

For SSC, a refractometer (PAL-1, Atago Co. Ltd., Tokyo, Japan) was referenced to 0°Brix using Milli-Q water. Stem and blossom endcaps were sectioned off, about 5 mm in from the ends, and approximately 0.5 mL of juice was squeezed into the digital refractometer. The final SSC (°Brix) value was obtained by averaging the measurements from both ends of the kiwifruit.

2.4. Multivariate and Aquaphotomics Analysis

The fruit interactance measurements, normalized using the reference scans, were transformed to absorbance data (i.e., base 10 logarithm). The subsequent analysis used pre-processing techniques to identify key differences in measurements made in the different configurations. Pre-processing methods used on the absorbance data were:

- Mean centering;
- Standard Normal Variate (SNV);
- SNV followed by second derivative processing (SNV + 2D). The second derivative was calculated using the Savitzky–Golay method with a filter window width of 7 nm and second order polynomial smoothing. A filter width of seven was chosen as higher widths may 'wash' out any interesting features, and to improve the resolution.

Principal Components Analysis (PCA) analysis was carried out using PLS toolbox version 8.6.2 (Eigenvector Research Inc., Manson, WA, USA) operating under MATLAB version 2021a (MathWorks Inc., Natick, MA, USA). PCA is a useful tool that can reduce dimensionality and simplify interpretation of all kiwifruit absorbance for each configuration [19]. PCA is also useful for identifying wavelengths of interest between configurations. Loading and score plots of the first three principal components were used to explain variances for all configurations.

Aquaphotomics analysis utilizes 12 wavebands, called the water matrix coordinates (WAMACS), which are sensitive to perturbations of the water structure. The WAMACS in the range of 800–1100 nm, corresponding to the second overtone of water, were calculated using the anharmonic oscillator model and the WAMACS wavebands known in the first overtone region around 1450 nm [20]. Each WAMACS waveband represents a combination of water vibrational states and different water species, namely S0, S1, S2, S3 and S4, where the number refers to the number of hydrogen bonds. Owing to the limited optical bandwidth of the F-750 instrument, exact wavelengths provide only an indication of wavebands that are important when differentiating between configurations. Specific wavelengths were determined using:

- SNV + 2D absorbance spectra of all configurations, noting any features.
- Average SSC difference spectra (SNV + 2D absorbance) between the Low, Medium and High SSC groups.
- Principal components analysis (PCA) of different configurations, including loading and score plots.

Once selected, WAMACS wavelengths used for aquagrams were generated to visualize water perturbations using a relative standard normal variate transformation:

$$A'_\lambda = \frac{(A_\lambda - \mu_\lambda)}{\sigma_\lambda}, \quad (2)$$

where A_λ is the pre-processed absorbance value for a sample at wavelength λ, and μ and σ are the mean and standard deviation of the pre-processed absorbance values across all configurations at that specific wavelength. Aquagrams were then generated using a spider plot function available in MATLAB [21].

3. Results and Discussion

Table 1 shows the variation in SSC for all 200 kiwifruit. Fruits were assigned to Low (7–11.9°Brix), Medium (12.1–14.9°Brix) or High (15–20.5°Brix) SSC groups to compare results across all configurations at different average SSC. Total SSC varied from 7 to 20.5°Brix, with a standard deviation of 2.9°Brix.

Table 1. Variation of SSC by different SSC level grouping (Low, Medium, High).

SSC Group	SSC (°Brix)	Average (°Brix)
Low SSC (N = 61)	7–11.9	10.4
Medium SSC (N = 69)	12.1–14.9	13.5
High SSC (N = 70)	15–20.5	16.9
All SSC (N = 200)	7–20.5	13.7

3.1. Raw and SNV Spectra

Raw absorbance spectra of all kiwifruit are shown in Figure 3 in the range 800–1050 nm, where the filled areas for each configuration represent mean ± standard deviation at each wavelength. For the peeled fruit (skin removed), the absorbance increased, relative to the unpeeled fruit, for both the linearly polarized and unpolarized light and there was a substantial increase in absorbance (decreased light intensity) when using the linear polarizer (Figure 3). This demonstrates that removal of skin increases absorbance for linearly polarized and unpolarized light and that a substantial intensity, reduction is observed when using a linear polarizer. The increase in absorbance after peeling was similar to that previously observed on peeled apples [16]. The SNV transformation of the spectra also revealed clear separation between the linearly polarized and unpolarized configurations, with the former exhibiting slight broadening of the water peak compared with the latter. This can be related to the lower penetration depth of polarized light compared with unpolarized light, because of fewer interactions within the fruit tissue [22].

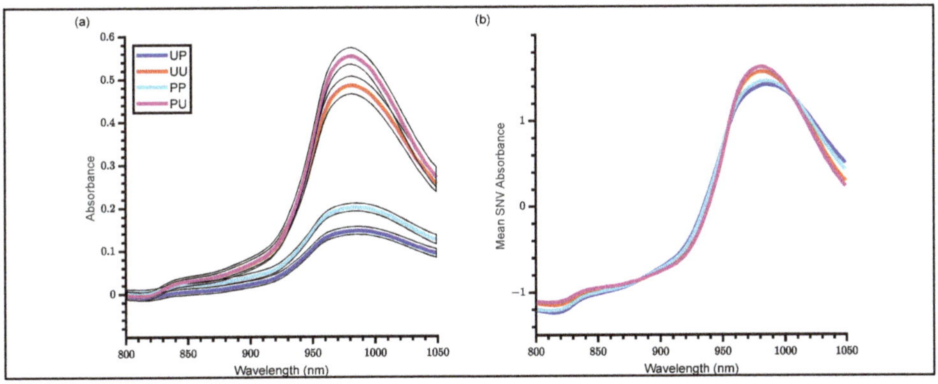

Figure 3. Absorbance spectra (800–1050 nm) of kiwifruit for unpeeled polarized (blue), unpeeled unpolarized (red), peeled polarized (cyan) and peeled unpolarized (magenta) for (**a**) Raw absorbance with filled areas representing mean ± std and (**b**) Mean SNV absorbance for each configuration.

3.2. WAMACS Wavelength Selection

Taking a second derivative of the SNV absorbance (SNV + 2D) revealed further differences between co-polarized and unpolarized light measurements (Figure 4). One feature included a prominent reduction in the second derivative absorbance from unpolarized to polarized light at 942 nm. Another was an apparent flattening of the linearly polarized light compared with unpolarized light from 970 to 1000 nm.

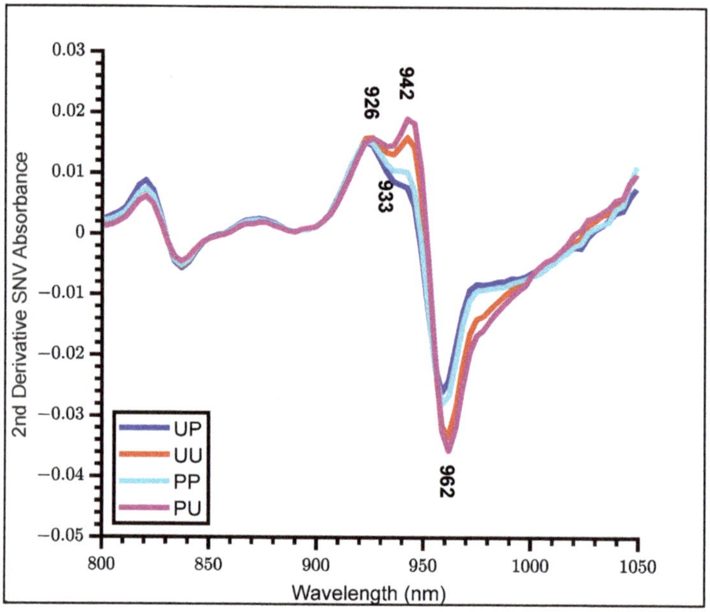

Figure 4. Standard Normal Variate (SNV) + 2D absorbance for each configuration (Blue—Unpeeled Polarized, Red—Unpeeled Unpolarized, Cyan—Peeled Polarized and Magenta—Peeled Unpolarized kiwifruit) in the range of 800–1050 nm.

In general, the peeled configurations exhibited higher second derivative absorbance at 942 nm and lower absorbance from 960 to 1000 nm than unpeeled configurations. Kiwifruit skins are complex structures, made of largely dry dead fruit cells that will be highly scattering and result in light losses that contribute to relatively higher absorbance measurements on the unpeeled fruit compared to on the peeled fruit [23].

PCA loading and score plots for SNV and second derivatives are shown in Figure 5, where just over 95% of the variance was captured by the first three principal components (PC1—82.91%, PC2—10.80% and PC3—1.61%). Each score plot is arranged in order of Unpeeled Polarized, Unpeeled Unpolarized, Peeled Polarized, and Peeled Unpolarized (Blue, Red, Cyan and Magenta, respectively) with every 200 sample numbers indicating a new configuration.

For each principal component plot, maxima and minima wavelengths in the range of 900 to 1020 nm were identified for use with the aquaphotomics analysis. There was a clear separation between the polarized and unpolarized configurations in PC1, where there was a slight tendency for peeled configurations to shift negatively. This appears to be due to a negative correlation at 946 nm, a wavelength corresponding to a free water state (S_0), described as water molecules with a free OH^- functional groups. Separation between polarization states shifted positively at 965 nm, a wavelength corresponding to water molecules bonded with one hydrogen bond. Trends with the higher PCs were not so obvious.

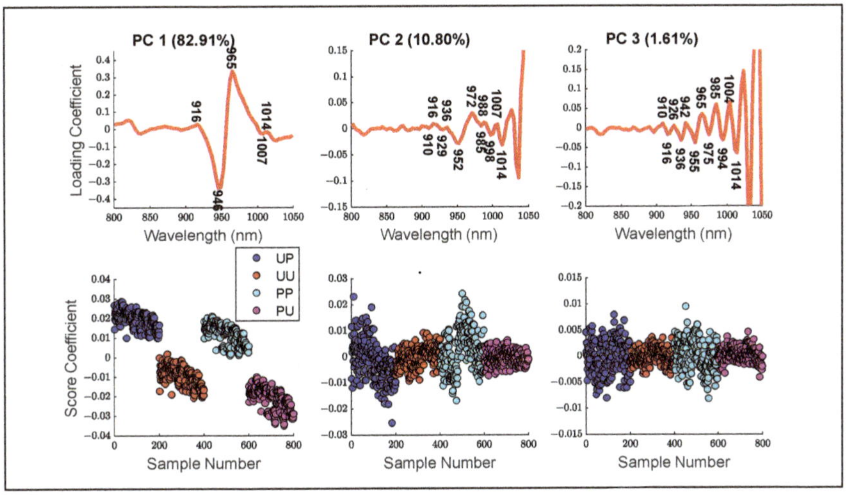

Figure 5. Principal Component Analysis (PCA) loading and score plots with variance explained at the top of each loading plot. For score plots, Blue (Unpeeled Polarized, 1–200), Red (Unpeeled Unpolarized, 201–400), Cyan (Peeled Polarized, 401–600) and Magenta (Peeled Unpolarized, 601–800 kiwifruit) are shown.

Average SSC difference spectra (SNV + 2D absorbance) were calculated for each configuration (Figure 6) by subtracting the average spectra for all groups from the average spectra of the Low SSC group. The changes for the polarized light configurations were at 946 and 965 nm, an increase and decrease in SNV + 2D absorbance, respectively, as SSC increased. The unpolarized light configurations had similar changes occurring at 949 nm and 968 nm with the unpeeled configurations having extra features at 975 nm and 978 nm, possibly caused by the presence of the skin. All minor maxima and minima in each configuration were considered in the subsequent aquaphotomics analysis.

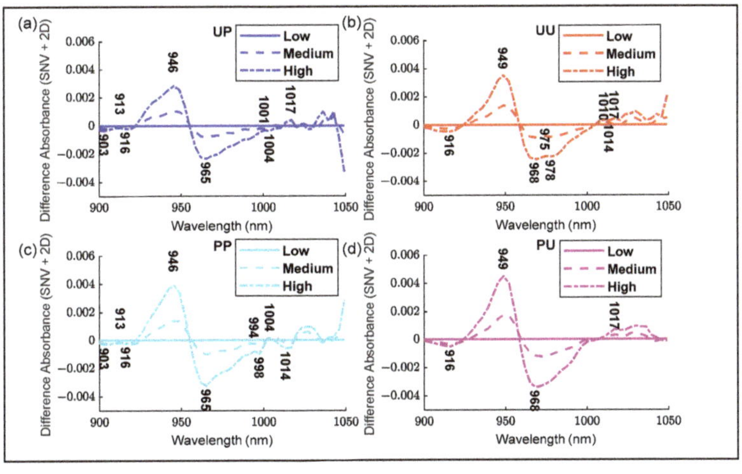

Figure 6. Standard Normal Variate (SNV) + 2D Soluble Solids Content (SSC) Difference Spectra for each configuration. (**a**) Unpeeled Polarized, (**b**) Unpeeled Unpolarized, (**c**) Peeled Polarized and (**d**) Peeled Unpolarized kiwifruit. Low, medium and high designations are represented by solid, dashed and dashed-dot lines, respectively.

3.3. Aquaphotomics Analysis

A summary of the important WAMACS coordinates is shown in Table 2, the water bands based on calculations using the anharmonic oscillator model for the second overtone of water [20]. C1 to C5 are related to free water species and C6 to C12 are related to bound water species. Using PCA results (Figure 5), activated wavelengths, from within each band, were identified at 916 nm (C2) from PC1, PC2 and PC3; 946 nm (C5) from PC1; 965 nm (C7) from PC1; 988 nm (C9) from PC2; 1007 nm (C11) and 1014 nm (C12) from PC1 and PC2. Using the SNV + 2D spectra (Figure 4), activated wavelengths were identified at 926 nm (C3), 933 nm (C4) and 962 nm (C6). From the average SSC difference spectra (Figure 6), activated wavelengths were identified at 903 nm (C1), 975 nm (C8) and 994 nm (C10).

Table 2. Assignment of water absorbance bands for second overtone of water using the anharmonic oscillator model [20].

WAMACS	Assignment	Water Bands (nm)	Activated Wavelengths (nm)
C1	v3—asymmetric stretching vibration	900–908	903
C2	OH stretch—(water solvation shell)	916–920	916
C3	v1 + v3H_2O symmetric stretching and asymmetric stretching vibration	923–927	926
C4	OH stretch (water solvation shell)	930–935	933
C5	S0 (free water)	942–955	946
C6	Water hydration, H_5O_2	957–963	962
C7	S1—Water molecules with one hydrogen bond	965–973	965
C8	v2 + v3H_2O bending andasymmetric stretching vibration	975–979	975
C9	S2—Water molecules with 2 hydrogen bonds	982–989	988
C10	S3—Water molecules with 3 hydrogen bonds	992–998	994
C11	S4—Water molecules with 4 hydrogen bonds	998–1007	1007
C12	Strongly bonded water (v1, v2)	1014–1021	1014

3.4. Aquagrams

3.4.1. Aquagram for Polarized and Unpolarized Light

The overall aquagram of all configurations (Figure 7) suggests that polarized light has relatively greater absorbance at free water states (C1 to C5) than unpolarized light, which relatively favors bound water states (C6 to C10). The exception is the bound water states at C11 and C12, where polarized light configurations exhibited relatively greater absorbance than unpolarized light. C11 and C12 are closely related to strongly bonded hydrogen water molecules so it is possible that these water structures could be polarization dependent but, as such, there is no explanation on why absorbance of C12 for unpeeled polarized is higher than peeled polarized configuration and vice versa for C11 [19]. Peeled configurations exhibited relatively greater absorbance for bound water states than the unpeeled configurations.

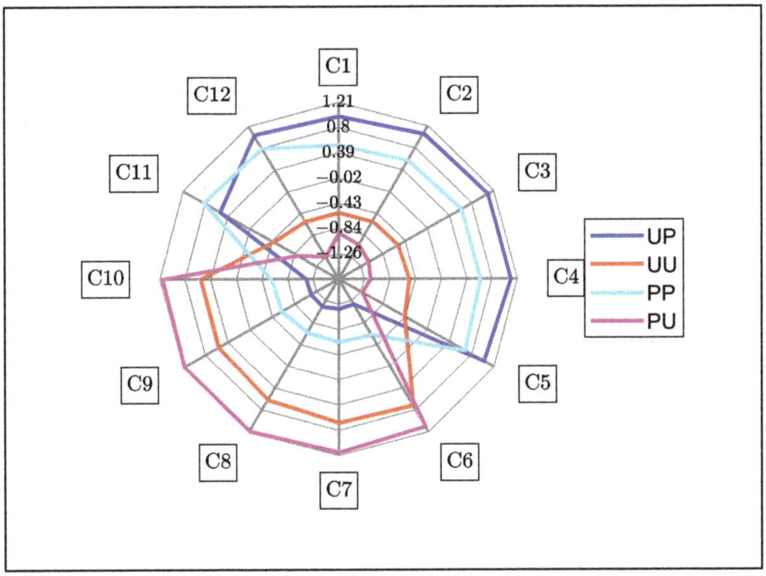

Figure 7. Aquagram for all configurations. Blue—Unpeeled Polarized, Red—Unpeeled Unpolarized, Cyan—Peeled Polarized and Magenta—Peeled Unpolarized kiwifruit.

Polarized light is quickly depolarized in biological material such as fruit tissues, due to multiple scattering [8]. Light undergoes multiple scattering events to become entirely diffuse and depolarized (isotropically scattered) in a distance of the order of 1 mm in fruit tissue [24]. Hence, water structure interactions of polarized light are expected to be similar to unpolarized light after a penetration depth of approximately 1 mm due to such depolarization. Differences observed between polarized and unpolarized are, thus, attributable to the near-surface region of fruit and the relatively shorter pathlength of polarized light [22]. There is also potential for polarization-sensitive structures such as cellulose and starch causing differences between unpolarized and linearly polarized light. Starch granules in particular produce Maltese cross patterns when placed between crossed polarizers, a common phenomenon with birefringent material [25]. The second overtone of water contains mixed absorbance from all these structures, meaning that it may be difficult to differentiate differences between polarized and unpolarized through conventional means [14].

3.4.2. Aquagram for Soluble Solids Content

Similar aquagrams patterns are produced for all configurations irrespective of the SSC grouping (Figure 8). Alignment with the free water species (C1 to C5) decreased, with the bound water species (C6 to C11) alignment increasing, as the average SSC increased. This is similar to previous work involving SSC grouping [20]. The aquagram suggests that differences between polarized and unpolarized responses were not related to the SSC. There is no explanation why, but it is worth noting that at C6, from the Low to High SSC group, the relative absorbance decreased for unpolarized light whereas it stayed the same for polarized configurations.

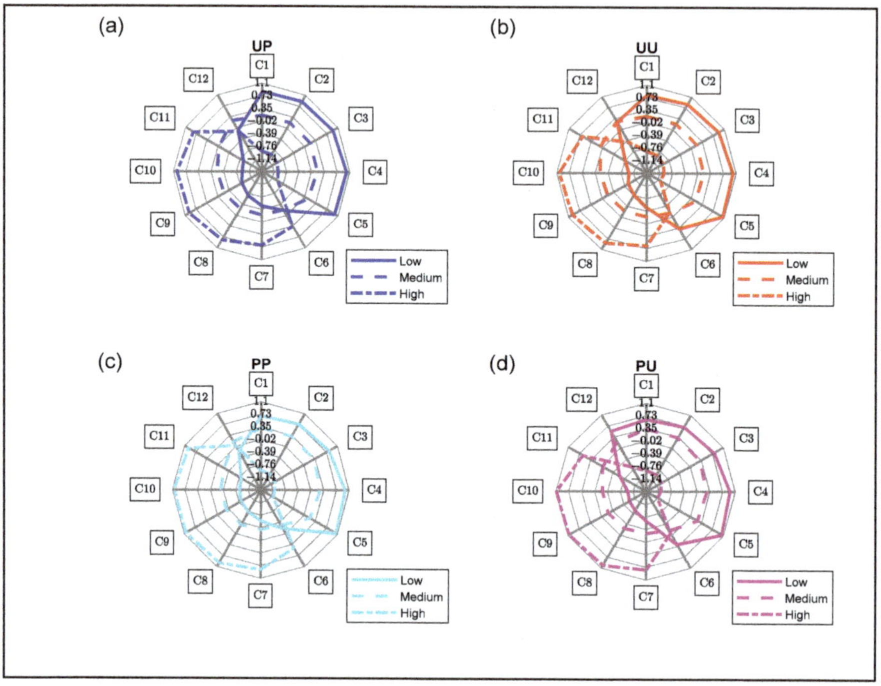

Figure 8. Aquagram for all configurations with different kiwifruit SSC (low, medium and high) for (**a**) Unpeeled Polarized, (**b**) Unpeeled Unpolarized, (**c**) Peeled Polarized and (**d**) Peeled Unpolarized. Solid Line—Low SSC, Dashed Line—Medium SSC and Dashed-Dot Line—High SSC.

4. Conclusions

Two hundred yellow-fleshed kiwifruit were spectrally measured, in the NIR range from 800 to 1050 nm, under four different combinations of unpeeled and peeled fruit, and linearly polarized and unpolarized light. Clear differences in the absorbance patterns were observed between the polarized and unpolarized light, but less so between the unpeeled and peeled fruit. Differences in fruit SSC did not appear to be a significant factor associated with these differences. Under an aquaphotomics framework, there was the suggestion that bound water states absorbed more unpolarized light than polarized light. It is speculated that differences are due to polarization sensitive structures, particularly in the near surface layers, and further work is needed to investigate and explain these differences in response due to the polarization state of light.

Author Contributions: Conceptualization, D.R., R.K. and H.K.; methodology, D.R., H.K. and A.M.; resources, A.M.; writing—original draft preparation, D.R.; writing—review and editing, R.K., H.K., J.L. and A.M.; supervision, R.K., H.K., J.L. and A.M. All authors have read and agreed to the published version of the manuscript.

Funding: Damenraj Rajkumar acknowledges financial support of a PhD scholarship from The New Zealand Institute for Plant and Food Research Limited, New Zealand. This research was funded by The New Zealand Ministry of Business Innovation and Employment Endeavour Fund Contract #33780.

Institutional Review Board Statement: Not applicable.

Informed Consent Statement: Not applicable.

Data Availability Statement: The data presented in this study are available on request from the corresponding author.

Conflicts of Interest: The authors declare no conflict of interest.

Sample Availability: Samples of the compounds are not available from the authors.

References

1. Abbott, J.A. Quality measurement of fruits and vegetables. *Postharvest Biol. Technol.* **1999**, *15*, 207–225. [CrossRef]
2. Schaare, P.; Fraser, D. Comparison of reflectance, interactance and transmission modes of visible-near infrared spectroscopy for measuring internal properties of kiwifruit (*Actinidia chinensis*). *Postharvest Biol. Technol.* **2000**, *20*, 175–184. [CrossRef]
3. Nicolaï, B.M.; Beullens, K.; Bobelyn, E.; Peirs, A.; Saeys, W.; Theron, K.I.; Lammertyn, J. Nondestructive measurement of fruit and vegetable quality by means of NIR spectroscopy: A review. *Postharvest Biol. Technol.* **2007**, *46*, 99–118. [CrossRef]
4. Xie, L.; Wang, A.; Xu, H.; Fu, X.; Ying, Y. Applications of near-infrared systems for quality evaluation of fruits: A review. *Trans. ASABE* **2016**, *59*, 399–419.
5. Nguyen-Do-Trong, N.; Dusabumuremyi, J.C.; Saeys, W. Cross-polarized VNIR hyperspectral reflectance imaging for non-destructive quality evaluation of dried banana slices, drying process monitoring and control. *J. Food Eng.* **2018**, *238*, 85–94. [CrossRef]
6. Nassif, R.; Pellen, F.; Magné, C.; Le Jeune, B.; Le Brun, G.; Abboud, M. Scattering through fruits during ripening: Laser speckle technique correlated to biochemical and fluorescence measurements. *Opt. Express* **2012**, *20*, 23887–23897. [CrossRef]
7. Sarkar, M.; Gupta, N.; Assaad, M. Monitoring of fruit freshness using phase information in polarization reflectance spectroscopy. *Appl. Opt.* **2019**, *58*, 6396–6405. [CrossRef]
8. Tuchin, V.V. Polarized light interaction with tissues. *J. Biomed. Opt.* **2016**, *21*, 071114. [CrossRef]
9. Gomes, A.J.; Turzhitsky, V.; Ruderman, S.; Backman, V. Monte Carlo model of the penetration depth for polarization gating spectroscopy: Influence of illumination-collection geometry and sample optical properties. *Appl. Opt.* **2012**, *51*, 4627–4637. [CrossRef]
10. Da Silva, A.; Deumie, C.; Vanzetta, I. Elliptically polarized light for depth resolved optical imaging. *Biomed. Opt. Express* **2012**, *3*, 2907–2915. [CrossRef]
11. Vignolini, S.; Rudall, P.J.; Rowland, A.V.; Reed, A.; Moyroud, E.; Faden, R.B.; Baumberg, J.J.; Glover, B.J.; Steiner, U. Pointillist structural color in Pollia fruit. *Proc. Natl. Acad. Sci. USA* **2012**, *109*, 15712–15715. [CrossRef]
12. Muncan, J.; Tsenkova, R. Aquaphotomics—From Innovative Knowledge to Integrative Platform in Science and Technology. *Molecules* **2019**, *24*, 2742. [CrossRef] [PubMed]
13. Kaur, H.; Künnemeyer, R.; McGlone, A. Investigating aquaphotomics for temperature-independent prediction of soluble solids content of pure apple juice. *J. Near Infrared Spectrosc.* **2020**, *28*, 103–112. [CrossRef]
14. Osborne, B.G.; Fearn, T.; Hindle, P.H. *Practical NIR Spectroscopy with Applications in Food and Beverage Analysis*; Longman Scientific and Technical: Essex, England, 1993.
15. McGlone, V.A.; Jordan, R.B.; Seelye, R.; Martinsen, P.J. Comparing density and NIR methods for measurement of kiwifruit dry matter and soluble solids content. *Postharvest Biol. Technol.* **2002**, *26*, 191–198. [CrossRef]
16. Lu, R.; Guyer, D.E.; Beaudry, R.M. Determination of firmness and sugar content of apples using near-infrared diffuse reflectance. *J. Texture Stud.* **2000**, *31*, 615–630. [CrossRef]
17. Compton, R.; Mahurin, S.; Zare, R.N. Demonstration of optical rotatory dispersion of sucrose. *J. Chem. Educ.* **1999**, *76*, 1234. [CrossRef]
18. Gobrecht, A.; Bendoula, R.; Roger, J.-M.; Bellon-Maurel, V. Combining linear polarization spectroscopy and the Representative Layer Theory to measure the Beer–Lambert law absorbance of highly scattering materials. *Anal. Chim. Acta* **2015**, *853*, 486–494. [CrossRef]
19. Tsenkova, R.; Munćan, J.; Pollner, B.; Kovacs, Z. Essentials of aquaphotomics and its chemometrics approaches. *Front. Chem.* **2018**, *6*, 363. [CrossRef]
20. Kaur, H. Investigating Aquaphotomics for Fruit Quality Assessment. Ph.D. Thesis, The University of Waikato, Hamilton, New Zealand, 2020.
21. Moses. Spider_Plot. Moses. GitHub. 2021. Available online: https://github.com/NewGuy012/spider_plot/releases/tag/16.6 (accessed on 24 November 2021).
22. Liu, Y.; Kim, Y.L.; Li, X.; Backman, V. Investigation of depth selectivity of polarization gating for tissue characterization. *Opt. Express* **2005**, *13*, 601–611. [CrossRef]
23. Redgwell, R.J.; MacRae, E.; Hallett, I.; Fischer, M.; Perry, J.; Harker, R. In vivo and in vitro swelling of cell walls during fruit ripening. *Planta* **1997**, *203*, 162–173. [CrossRef]
24. Fang, Z.-h.; Fu, X.-p.; He, X.-m. Investigation of absorption and scattering characteristics of kiwifruit tissue using a single integrating sphere system. *J. Zhejiang Univ.-Sci. B* **2016**, *17*, 484–492. [CrossRef] [PubMed]
25. Tongdang, T. Some properties of starch extracted from three Thai aromatic fruit seeds. *Starch-Stärke* **2008**, *60*, 199–207. [CrossRef]

molecules

MDPI

Article

NIRS and Aquaphotomics Trace Robusta-to-Arabica Ratio in Liquid Coffee Blends

Balkis Aouadi [1], Flora Vitalis [1], Zsanett Bodor [1,2], John-Lewis Zinia Zaukuu [3], Istvan Kertesz [1] and Zoltan Kovacs [1,*]

1 Department of Measurements and Process Control, Institute of Food Science and Technology, Hungarian University of Agriculture and Life Sciences, 14-16. Somlói Street, H-1118 Budapest, Hungary; aouadi.balkis@phd.uni-mate.hu (B.A.); vitalis.flora@phd.uni-mate.hu (F.V.); zsanett.bodor93@gmail.com (Z.B.); kertesz.istvan@uni-mate.hu (I.K.)

2 Department of Dietetics and Nutrition Faculty of Health Sciences, Semmelweis University, 17. Vas Street, H-1088 Budapest, Hungary

3 Department of Food Science and Technology, Kwame Nkrumah University of Science and Technology (KNUST), Kumasi 00233, Ghana; zaukuu.jz@knust.edu.gh

* Correspondence: kovacs.zoltan.food@uni-mate.hu

Abstract: Coffee is both a vastly consumed beverage and a chemically complex matrix. For a long time, an arduous chemical analysis was necessary to resolve coffee authentication issues. Despite their demonstrated efficacy, such techniques tend to rely on reference methods or resort to elaborate extraction steps. Near infrared spectroscopy (NIRS) and the aquaphotomics approach, on the other hand, reportedly offer a rapid, reliable, and holistic compositional overview of varying analytes but with little focus on low concentration mixtures of Robusta-to-Arabica coffee. Our study aimed for a comparative assessment of ground coffee adulteration using NIRS and liquid coffee adulteration using the aquaphotomics approach. The aim was to demonstrate the potential of monitoring ground and liquid coffee quality as they are commercially the most available coffee forms. Chemometrics spectra analysis proved capable of distinguishing between the studied samples and efficiently estimating the added Robusta concentrations. An accuracy of 100% was obtained for the varietal discrimination of pure Arabica and Robusta, both in ground and liquid form. Robusta-to-Arabica ratio was predicted with R^2CV values of 0.99 and 0.9 in ground and liquid form respectively. Aquagrams results accentuated the peculiarities of the two coffee varieties and their respective blends by designating different water conformations depending on the coffee variety and assigning a particular water absorption spectral pattern (WASP) depending on the blending ratio. Marked spectral features attributed to high hydrogen bonded water characterized Arabica-rich coffee, while those with the higher Robusta content showed an abundance of free water structures. Collectively, the obtained results ascertain the adequacy of NIRS and aquaphotomics as promising alternative tools for the authentication of liquid coffee that can correlate the water-related fingerprint to the Robusta-to-Arabica ratio.

Keywords: coffee; NIRS; aquagrams; chemometrics; authentication; PCA; PCA-LDA; PLSR

Citation: Aouadi, B.; Vitalis, F.; Bodor, Z.; Zinia Zaukuu, J.-L.; Kertesz, I.; Kovacs, Z. NIRS and Aquaphotomics Trace Robusta-to-Arabica Ratio in Liquid Coffee Blends. *Molecules* **2022**, 27, 388. https://doi.org/10.3390/molecules27020388

Academic Editor: Stefano Materazzi

Received: 17 December 2021
Accepted: 5 January 2022
Published: 8 January 2022

1. Introduction

The worldwide appeal of coffee, consumed not only as a functional beverage, but also as a provider of unique cultural experiences, stems from its distinct organoleptic features. These criteria are mostly defined by the respective geographic and varietal origin as well as the brewing processes.

While genus *Coffea* exists under numerous varieties, *Coffea arabica* and *Coffea canephora* are the two commonly consumed ones [1]. Arabica, the priciest of the two and marketed as having the higher quality grade, has been a prime target for fraud, propelled by the potential economic gains [2].

On the consumer front, rising demands for safe products that impart the desired nutritional and sensory values and authentically state the actual ingredients present are driving a palpable sense of responsibility shared by the food industry operators and academia alike. With regulations stipulating no more than 1% of foreign materials in coffee [3], this challenge becomes even more daunting.

Upon adulteration, affecting the flavor profile of coffee is not the sole repercussion on coffee quality. Other reported aspects comprise alterations of the antioxidant capacity and reduction of the levels of bioactive compounds [4].

Although a common practice, mixing the two coffee varieties, unless otherwise stated, can be considered as a milder type of coffee forgery. Innumerable studies investigated the efficiency of detecting such occurrences. Wermelinger et al. [5], for instance, attempted the quantification of the Robusta fraction in a coffee blend via Raman spectroscopy. Mixtures with Robusta contents of 5, 10, 25, 33, 50, and 75% *w*/*w* were classified. Kahweol, exclusively present in Arabica beans, enabled the discrimination of the two extracted lipid fractions of Arabica and Robusta with a detection limit ranging from 4.9 to 7.5% *w*/*w*. The higher the content of Robusta, naturally richer in unsaturated fatty acids, the greater the shift of the peak once situated at 1665 cm^{-1} (6006 nm).

For Schievano et al. [6], nuclear magnetic resonance (NMR) was the method of choice for authenticating coffee blends by quantifying 16-O-methylcafestol (16-OMC). The study accurately detected Robusta, at concentrations below 0.9%, with detection and quantitation limits of 5 and 20 mg per kg, respectively. Pure Arabica was equally 100% distinguished from Robusta-Arabica mixtures. Other suggested discriminators consisted of fatty acids, tocopherols, or sterols. These, however, necessitate additional extraction and separation operations as suggested by Schievano et al. [6].

Similarly, Milani et al. [3] used NMR to authenticate coffee adulterated with barley, corn, coffee husks, soybean, rice, and wheat added in 50% *w*/*w* proportion to pure coffee. Soft independent modelling by class analogy (SIMCA) provided 100% correct classification for both training and prediction sets and limits of detection of 0.31–0.86% in medium as well as in dark roasted coffee were obtained.

The differential electronic nose was employed by Brudzewski et al. [7] in analyzing Arabica coffee adulterated with 10, 20, 30, 40, 50, 60, 70, 80, and 90% Robusta. With an average error of 0.21%, the adopted 30-fold cross-validation model permitted the recognition of all mixtures.

For Pizarro et al., the approach differed, where calibration models developed from near-infrared spectra produced prediction models with root mean square error of prediction (RMSEP) of 0.79%. The added Robusta ranged from 0 to 60% *w*/*w* [8]. The methodology followed by Spaniolas et al. [9], consisted in differentiating the two varieties based on a lab-on-a-chip system and a limit of detection of 5% was achievable.

Other forms of adulteration involve the addition of both corn and soybean. Such cases were studied by Arrieta et al. and Daniel et al. [10,11], who deployed the voltametric electronic tongue and capillary electrophoresis-tandem mass spectrometry, respectively. Although efficient (R^2 of 0.973 and 0.941 for the prediction of corn and soybean in case of e-tongue), these techniques demand high levels of technicity and relatively lengthy processing.

Combined with multivariate curve resolution (MCR), near infrared hyperspectral imaging was utilized to determine coffee husks, soil, wood sticks, and roasted corn kernel powders added in quantities of 1–40% [12]. Quantitative models with absolute errors not exceeding 4% were obtained.

Roasted barley, rice, and wheat powders are also some of the low-cost additions made to pure Arabica for increased profit margins. Song et al. [13] applied high performance liquid chromatography (HPLC) to quantitatively analyze coffee blends containing 1, 2, 3, 4, 5, 10, and 20% *w*/*w* of these powders. For the purpose of the study, monosaccharides, nicotinic acid, and trigonelline served as chemical indicators of the authenticity of coffee. Of all studied indices, glucose aided the most in the discrimination of pure and adulterated

Arabica. The corresponding discrimination limit was 1% *w*/*w* with significant difference in ANOVA ($p < 0.05$).

Coffee quality analysis has mainly focused on beans and powders and only a few studies used aqueous coffee solutions. Amongst those who attempted to do so, Suhandy and Yulia intentionally added 10–60% of Robusta to Arabica and collected the UV-visible spectra of the aqueous solutions in the 200–400 nm range. They proved that the selection of specific intervals as a basis for building the partial least squares (PLS) models enhances the performance of the model, resulting in a ratio prediction to deviation (RPD) of 2.15 [14].

By conducting the present study, one of our objectives was to assess the applicability of aquaphotomics, as an innovative NIR-based approach in pinpointing potential blending of the two coffee varieties.

With demonstrated efficiency in a panoply of applications, aquaphotomics offers a holistic approach to the study of biosystems and the analysis of food matrices [15]. Aquaphotomics-related studies have substantiated that placing an emphasis on the water molecular system can in fact be an alternative to other more laborious techniques. In a sense, by applying various perturbations, structural changes of water species are induced and thus can be reflective, by comparison to control samples, of the state of the studied matrix. Most importantly, it brings about a new perspective regarding one of the commonly encountered limitations of conventional analysis: water.

This feature has been already used to track changes induced by cheese ripening [16], to screen water's quality in the presence of certain contaminants [17], to elucidate yoghurt fermentation mechanisms [18], to authenticate honey [19], and many more applications [20–23]. With regards to coffee analysis, this approach could prove particularly beneficial in case of the shortage of beans, the absence of technically qualified coffee quality assessors as well as the insufficiency of the chemicals used for other sophisticated methods. The practical implications of the study could be particularly promising in cases where the authentication and detection of the adulteration is not possible in powder form namely with the expansion of the ready-to-drink (RTD) coffee market.

The aim of our research was to authenticate coffee both in its ground and liquid states using conventional NIRS and aquaphotomics. To do so, a comparative assessment of the quantification accuracy of Robusta-to-Arabica ratio in mixtures containing 0.5–35% of Robusta was conducted. Determining the impact such blending has on the respective water spectral pattern of the studied samples was also one of the prime objectives of our study. The obtained performances were evaluated by the inclusion of marketed blends of different varietal composition and geographical origin throughout the analysis steps.

2. Results and discussion

2.1. Varietal Discrimination of Pure Ground Coffee

A primary step consisted in assessing whether or not the applied method could discriminate between the pure varieties of ARA1, ARA2, ARA3, ROB1, ROB2, and ROB3 in the form of ground coffee.

Analysis of pure ground coffee samples of differing varieties by means of principal component analysis, as showcased in Figure 1, demonstrates a pattern of separation along the axis of PC1, which together with PC2 accounts for 99% of the data variability. The efficacy of NIRS in terms of separating the samples was not only based on their respective varieties, but also on their provenance as the different samples came from different sources: Brazil (ARA1), Columbia (ARA2), Ethiopia (ARA3), Vietnam (ROB1), Uganda (ROB2), and India (ROB3). This trend suggests the compositional variability within each of the evaluated varieties. Indeed, studies have shown the role of geographical origin in conferring a specific chemical composition to coffee. This is in accordance with the findings reported by Giraudo et al. [24], who proved that intra-varietal differences of coffee beans originating from different countries and continents can be traced by their respective NIR spectral patterns. According to the corresponding loadings vector (Figure 1c), the wavebands 1390, 1408,

1438, 1452, and 1512 nm contributed the most to this separation. The PCA-LDA model scores yielded 100% recognition and prediction of the pure Arabica and Robusta varieties.

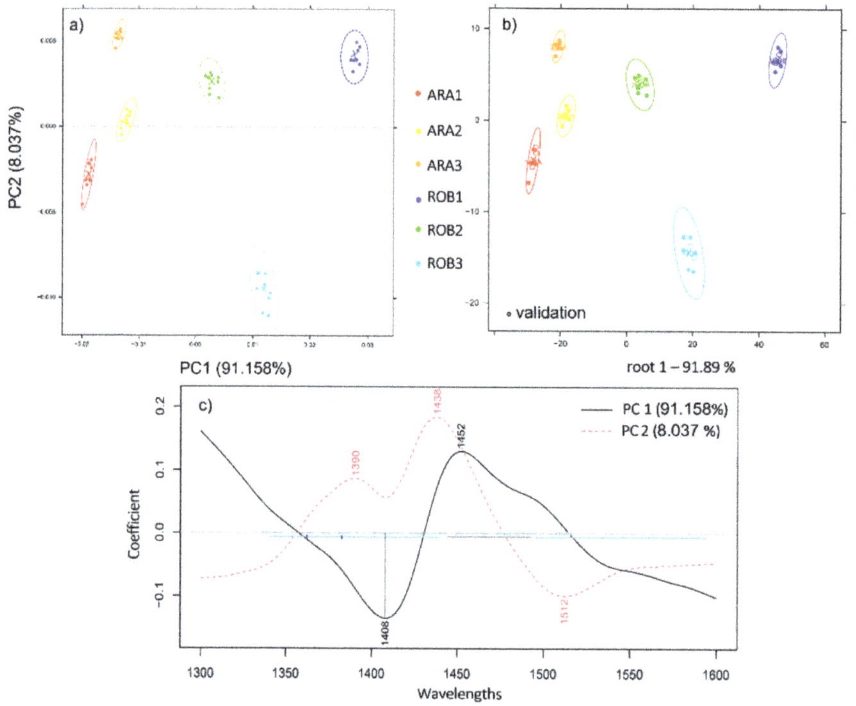

Figure 1. (**a**) Principal component analysis (PCA) on pure arabica (ARA1, ARA2, ARA3) and Robusta (ROB1, ROB2, ROB3) ground coffee samples in the wavelength range of 1300–1600 nm, N = 54, Savitzky-Golay smoothing (window size 19) and MSC; (**b**) PCA-LDA classification plot of pure Arabica (ARA1, ARA2, ARA3) and Robusta (ROB1, ROB2, ROB3) ground coffee samples, N = 54; (**c**) The respective PCA loading plot.

2.2. Near Infrared Analysis of Ground Coffee Mixtures

For the remainder of our study, we focused on the mixtures prepared by mixing the pair (ARA3, ROB3). To determine if a recognizable pattern is ascribable to the adulterated Arabica depending on the added Robusta, principal component analysis was performed in the 1st overtone (1300–1600 nm), 2nd overtone (800–1100 nm), as well as in the truncated spectral range of the instrument, 800–1670 nm. The model illustrating the most distinctive pattern was obtained in the range 800–1670 nm using the smoothed and MSC pretreated spectra (Figure 2a). According to the loadings plot (Figure 2c), the wavelengths responsible for the variance in the data are mostly those located at 970, 1106, 1126, 1266, 1298, 1318, and 1464 nm. Previous studies have attributed bond vibrations at 1126 nm of the 2 × C-H stretching and 2 × C-H deformation and (CH2)n C-H stretching second overtone to coffee fatty acids and chlorogenic acid (CGA) [25]. Indeed, these constituents have already proven to be good discriminators of the varietal origin of coffee [26].

Relying solely on the visual inspection of the separated samples, the truncated range 800–1670 nm served better for the pattern recognition of the mixtures with PCA. The analysis of the samples by means of linear discriminant analysis, however, proved better when performed at the first overtone 1300–1600 nm. An accurate recognition and prediction of 95.87% and 94.45% were obtained, respectively, using the raw spectra. The misclassifications occurred mainly between sample pairs (1% and 3%; 3% and 5%) whereas those comprising at least 10% Robusta were 100% accurately classified.

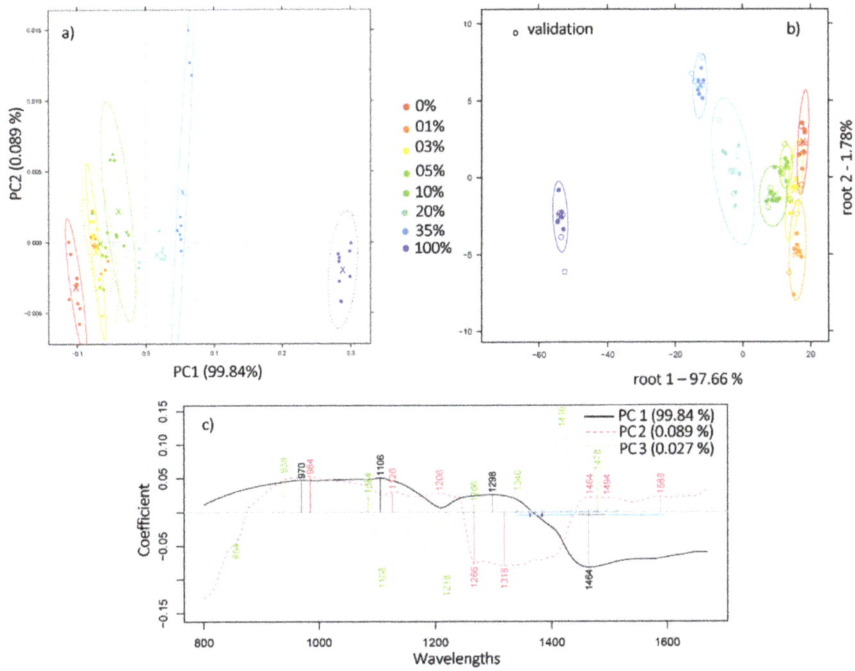

Figure 2. (**a**) PCA scores plot reveals separation along PC1 axis of the mixtures containing Robusta concentration in the range 1%–35%, N = 72, wavelength range 800–1670 nm, Savitzky-Golay smoothing (window size 19) and MSC; (**b**) PCA-LDA classification plot of the robusta adulterated ground coffee in the concentration range 1%–35%, wavelength range 1300-1600 nm, N = 72; (**c**) PCA loadings plot.

Once the mixtures were correctly classified, PLSR models were built in order to assess the feasibility of near infrared spectroscopy in predicting the Robusta to Arabica ratio. By leaving one group out (three consecutive scans of the same replicate) cross-validation, the model built on the smoothed first derivative of the spectra enabled a coefficient of determination (R^2CV) of 0.99 and an error (RMSECV) of 2.4% (Figure 3a). Similar results ($R^2 > 0.99$ and RMSE below 1.2% *w*/*w*) were found when evaluating Arabica-Robusta mixtures in the range of 0–60% [8].

The corresponding regression vector showcases the most significant wavelengths in terms of accurately determining the added Robusta. These peaks are located at 1324, 1374, 1402, 1422, 1444, 1470, 1498, 1518, 1540, and 1556 nm (Figure 3b). Prior studies have assigned wavelengths in the 1400–1600 nm range to some typical components of coffee, such as caffeine, sugar, and chlorogenic acids [27]. The addition of Robusta, naturally richer in chlorogenic acid and caffeine content [28], could explain the prominence of these particular wavebands when predicting the added Robusta.

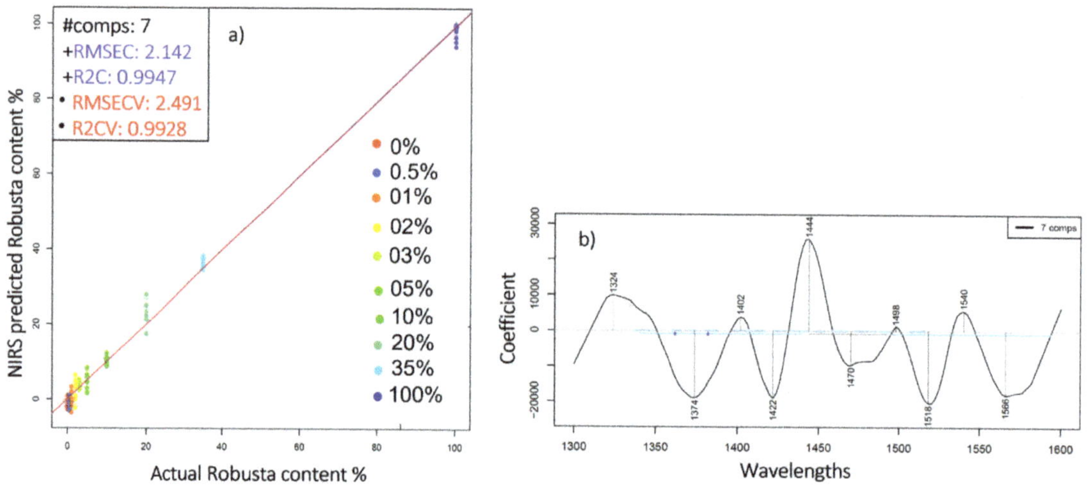

Figure 3. (**a**) PLSR analysis of the ground coffee mixtures derived from the smoothed (Savitzky-Golay smoothing (window size 19)) first derivative spectra for the prediction of added Robusta (% *w*/*w*); (**b**) The respective regression vector in the range 1300–1600 nm.

The PCA-LDA classification and PLSR prediction of the Robusta-to-Arabica ratio were also performed on the marketed blends B10% and B30%. Figure 4a illustrates the obtained results where B10% and B30% were discriminated from the pure Arabica and Robusta ground coffee samples with 100% accuracies of recognition and prediction. The regression model built to predict the Robusta content and cross-validated by leaving three consecutive scans of each replicate at a time enabled an estimation of added Robusta with R^2CV and RMSECV values of 0.97 and 3.93% *w*/*w*, respectively (Figure 4b). This slight difference compared to the model constructed only on the mixtures could be due to the different composition of the marketed blends B10% and B30%, obtained by combining other Arabica and Robusta varieties, from a geographical origin other than that of ARA3 and ROB3.

2.3. Near Infrared Analysis of Pure Liquid Coffee Extracts

Performing principal component analysis on the pure Arabica (ARA3) and Robusta (ROB3) liquid extracts in the short wavelength range of 800–1100 nm revealed a pattern of separation into two respective clusters depending on the coffee variety (Figure 5). Combined, PC1 and PC2 accounted for more than 99% of the data variance and the bands contributing the most to this separation were positioned at 950, 982, and 1034 nm.

Next, absorbances of ARA3 and ROB3 aqueous samples as projected on the aquagram were investigated in 12 characteristic wavelength ranges in the 2nd water overtone in NIR region. What the aquagram accentuated is that Robusta coffee extracts, contrarily to Arabica, were majorly characterized by water molecules that are structured into water shells (908 nm), V1 and V2 bonded water while Arabica has high hydrogen bonded water structures (1060 nm) and is rich in water clusters with two, three, and four hydrogen bonds (1018, 1036, and 1044 nm) (Figure 6a). Wu et al. [29] are among those who investigated the compositional analysis of milk in the short NIR wavelength range (800–1050 nm) and reported the potential assignment of the 1018 and 1042 nm to the interaction of fat–water. The fact that Arabica is naturally richer in fat content can explain the high absorbance observed at these bands [30].

The incorporation of marketed blends B10% and B30% into the aquagram calculation is presented in (Figure 6b). Notably, the resulting water spectral pattern followed a logical sequence. Out of the two studied blends, the one with the highest Arabica content (B10%) had a similar pattern to pure Arabica, with slightly lower absorbance values. When the percentage of Robusta increased, as is the case of B30% blend, higher absorbances in the wavelength range of 890–954 nm were emphasized.

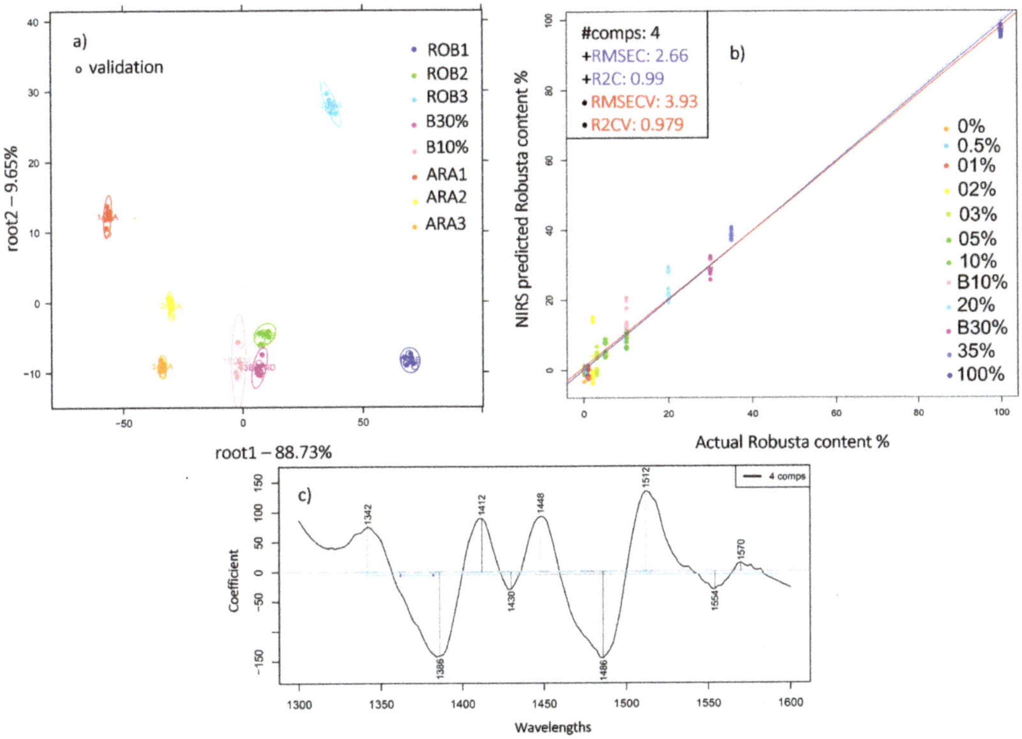

Figure 4. (**a**) PCA-LDA Classification of pure ground Arabica (ARA1, ARA2, ARA3), Robusta (ROB1, ROB2, ROB3) and marketed blends B10%, B30% in the range 1300–1600 nm, N = 72, spectral pretreatment: Savitzky-Golay smoothing (window size 19) and 1st derivative; (**b**) PLSR analysis of the ground coffee mixtures and B10% and B30%, spectral pretreatment: Savitzky-Golay smoothing (window size 17) and SNV; (**c**) The respective regression vector in the 1300–1600 nm.

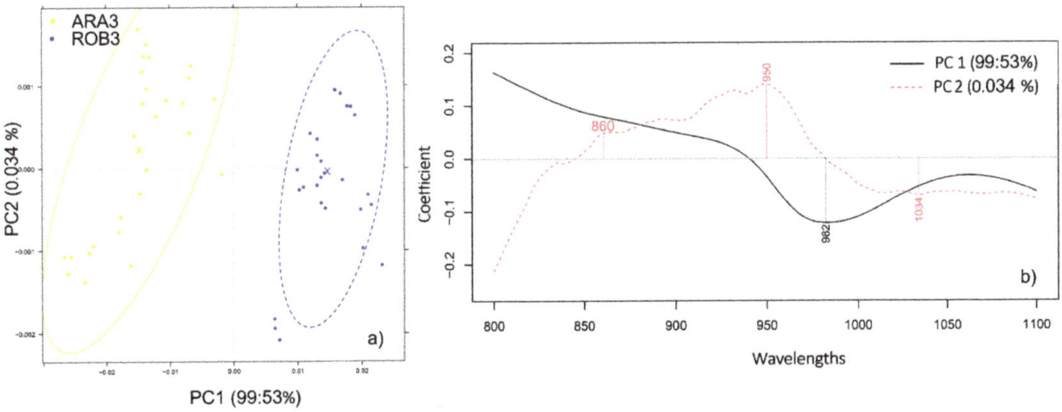

Figure 5. (**a**) PCA analysis applied to the spectra of pure Arabica (ARA3) and Robusta (ROB3) liquid extracts in the 800–1100 nm range, N = 54, spectral pretreatment: Savitzky-Golay smoothing (window size 19) and MSC; (**b**) The respective PCA loadings plot.

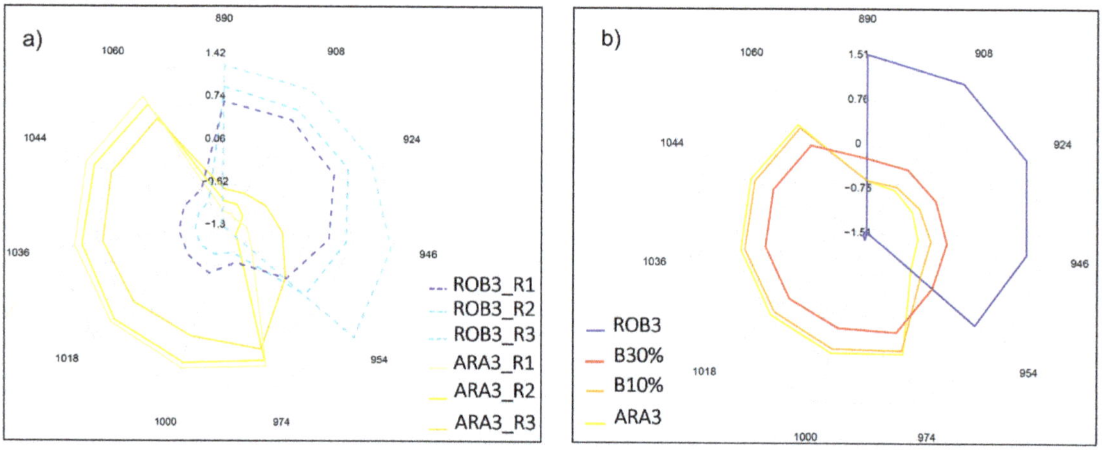

Figure 6. (**a**) Aquagram representation of the spectral pattern of pure Arabica and Robusta liquid extracts at the second overtone region (800–1100 nm), R1, R2, R3 denote replicates, N = 9 each; (**b**) Water spectral pattern of marketed blends B10% and B30%, pure Arabica (ARA3) and pure Robusta (ROB3), N = 27 each.

Likewise, PCA-LDA was proven performant when assigning the samples ARA3, B10%, B30%, and ROB3 to their specific classes, with an accurate recognition of 91.26% of the samples while at the prediction level 83.39% were correctly categorized. The separation is most apparent along the axis of the first discriminant factor (Figure 7). The misclassifications occurred mostly between samples with proximate composition. Thus, B10% was primarily misclassified in 14.78% of the cases to the group 0% (ARA3) while B30% was identified as B10% in 11.11% of cases.

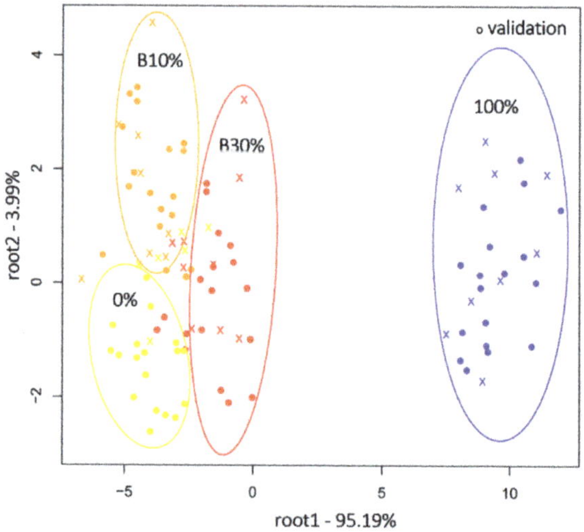

Figure 7. PCA-LDA classification of marketed blends B10% and B30%, pure Arabica (0%) and pure Robusta (100%) at the second overtone region (800–1100 nm), N = 108, NrPCs = 18.

2.4. Near Infrared Analysis of Liquid Coffee Mixtures

When all adulteration levels were considered, LDA models destined at regrouping the samples into their corresponding groups enabled a 100% recognition of the different mixtures, and the prediction rate amounted to 71.32%. The following table recaps where misclassification occurred presumably due to the low Robusta concentrations or to the proximity of certain levels (Table 1). The classification was even less efficient when the model blends (B10%; B30%) were included into the construction of the predictive model (55.58% prediction rate). The blend B10% was misidentified as belonging to the group containing 5% Robusta in 11.14% of the studied cases and misclassified with 3.67% to the following groups: B30%, 35%, 20%, 10%. B30%, on the other hand, was wrongly categorized as belonging to the groups B10%, 35%, and 3% in 7.44% of the cases. While the blending ratio of these model blends fits into the range covered by our study, their heterogenous composition could have an effect on the classification accuracy. Indeed, the effect of the blend composition on the accuracy of the classification model has already been proven by Tavares et al. [31], who, basing their study on the analysis of the lipid extracts by HPLC, proved that proportions as high as 10% of maize and 20% of coffee by-products are required to identify the adulteration of coffee by means of PCA and LDA.

Table 1. PCA-LDA classification model on the NIRS data of pure and adulterated mixtures after three-fold cross-validation (N = 268).

		Validation Accuracy %									
		Robusta-to-Arabica Ratio									
		0%	0.5%	1%	2%	3%	5%	10%	20%	35%	100%
Robusta-to-Arabica ratio	0%	**66.74**	8.03	0	7.44	0	11.11	11.11	0	0	0
	0.5%	14.79	**51.92**	7.45	7.44	14.78	7.44	7.44	0	3.67	0
	1%	0	3.96	**70.41**	0	7.44	0	0	11.11	0	0
	2%	0	8.03	0	**81.44**	7.44	0	0	0	0	0
	3%	3.67	20.02	3.67	0	**55.56**	7.44	3.67	0	0	0
	5%	3.67	0	3.67	3.67	11.11	**66.67**	3.67	7.44	3.67	0
	10 %	7.45	8.03	0	0	3.67	3.67	**66.67**	7.44	3.67	0
	20%	3.67	0	14.79	0	0	3.67	7.44	**70.33**	3.67	0
	35%	0	0	0	0	0	0	0	3.67	**85.32**	0
	100%	0	0	0	0	0	0	0	0	0	**100**

Averaging the consecutive scans and the parallel spectra of each of the studied mixtures and those of the controls (pure Arabica and pure Robusta) was proven effective when it comes to improving the accuracy of the predictive PLSR model. The optimal cross-validated model was the one built in the second overtone region, 800–1100 nm, and was characterized by R^2CV and RMSECV values of 0.95 and 6.35% w/w, respectively (Figure 8a). Again, the blends lowered the accuracy of the regression model ($R^2CV = 0.9$). The most prominent wavelengths corresponded to 840, 870, 954, and 990 nm (Figure 8c). Interestingly, the band situated at 954nm was already proven relevant when differentiating pure Arabica and Robusta based on their water spectral patterns (Figure 6). Similar results ($R^2 = 0.95$) were obtained by Núñez et al. [32] when examining the HPLC-UV fingerprints of brewed Arabica coffee containing Robusta in proportions ranging from 15% to 85%.

The complexity of differentiating between the mixtures with the lowest adulteration levels was evidenced primarily by their respective water spectral pattern where an overlapping of blends containing Robusta fractions as low as 0.5%, 1%, and 2% occurred. Notably, above these concentration levels, the higher the ratio Robusta to Arabica was, the higher the absorbance in the wavelengths that are characteristic of pure Robusta. Inversely, the lower the added Robusta, the higher the absorbance in the wavelengths characteristic of pure Arabica (Figure 9a).

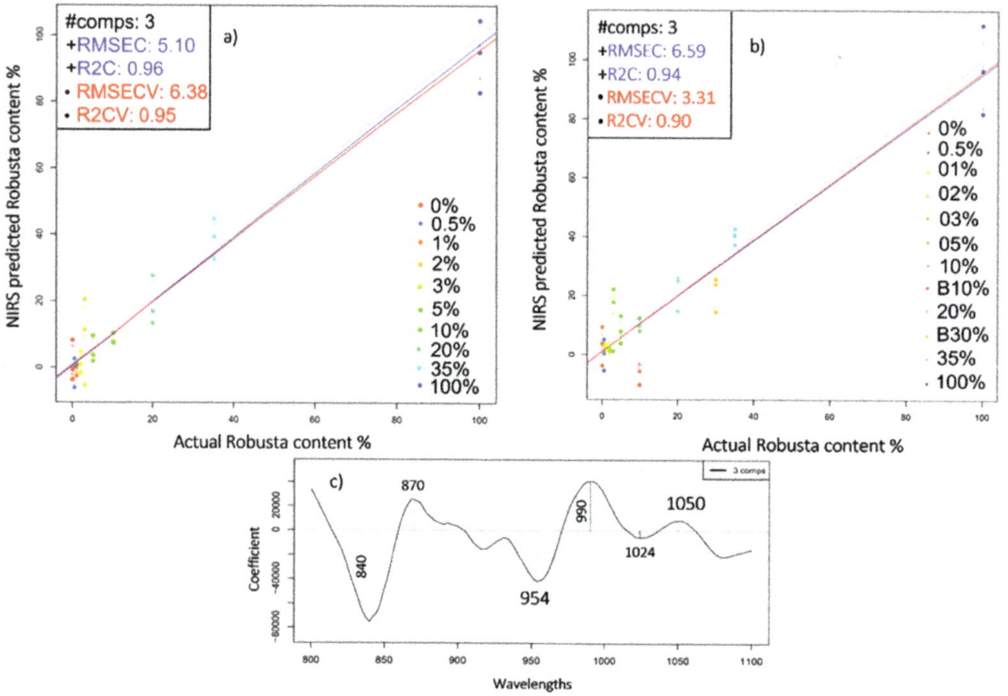

Figure 8. (**a**) Y-fit graph of the prediction of Robusta concentration in liquid mixtures N = 30; (**b**) PLSR analysis on the dataset containing marketed blends B10% and B30% and the mixtures, N = 36; (**c**) Regression vector of the predictive model (**b**) in the 800–1100 nm range. Spectral pre-processing: Averaging consecutive scans, Savitzky-Golay smoothing (window size 19), 1st derivative.

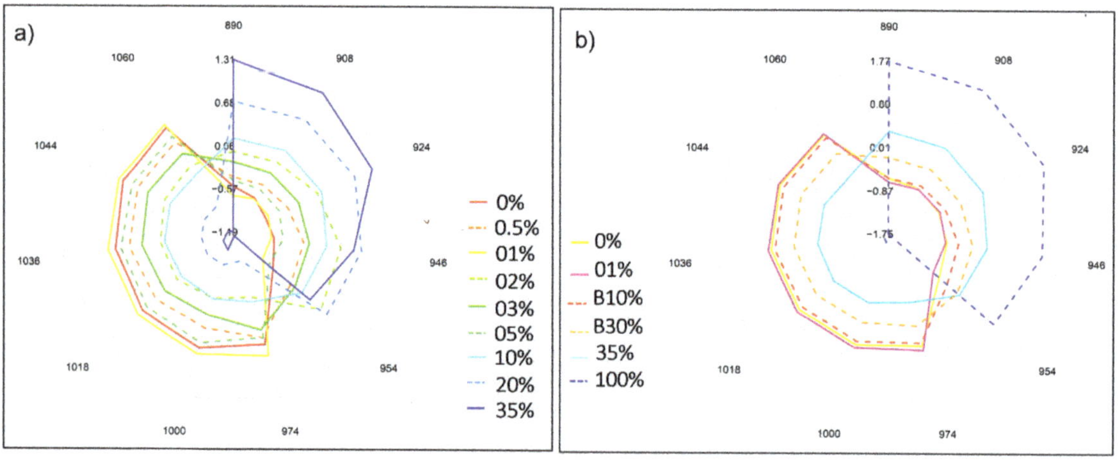

Figure 9. (**a**) Aquagrams of aqueous solutions of Robusta-Arabica blends in the concentration range of 0.5–35% and pure Arabica (0%) in the second overtone region; (**b**) Aquagram of the dataset comprising pure Arabica (0%), pure Robusta (100%), Robusta-Arabica blends (01% and 35%) and marketed blends (B10% and B30%).

Assessing whether or not the inclusion of marketed blends B10% and B30% can still be translated into distinctive water spectral patterns, in the presence of lab generated mixtures covering both low (1%) and high blending ratios (35%), was also attempted and confirmed the adequacy of the analysis from an aquaphotomics standpoint in terms of highlighting the respective composition of the studied samples. Once again, the intricacy of detecting the lowest blending ratio was reflected by a slight overlapping with pure Arabica extract (Figure 9b).

3. Materials and Methods

3.1. Samples Preparation

For the purpose of our study, Arabica beans originating from Brazil (ARA1), Columbia (ARA2), and Ethiopia (ARA3) and Robusta beans sourced from Vietnam (ROB1), Uganda (ROB2), and India (ROB3) were French-roasted, ground, and procured by Bourbon café (Tahitótfalu, Hungary). Mixtures comprising 0.5, 1, 2, 3, 5, 10, 20, 35% *w*/*w* Robusta were prepared by pairing ARA3 and ROB3. The threshold above which the addition of Robusta can have a palpable effect on coffee aroma is 35% [31]. Alongside these mixtures, marketed blends of different provenance and serving as test samples were considered. The 1st blend B10% consisted of 90% Arabica (South American) and 10% Robusta (South-east Asian), whereas the 2nd blend B30% comprised 70% Arabica (Central and South American) and 30% Robusta (Southeast Asian). Triplicate samples were prepared for each of the mixture concentration levels.

After formulating the mixtures, water extracts of the pure coffee varieties, the mixtures, as well as the marketed blends were prepared by pouring 100 mL Milli-Q water, heated at boiling point, onto 8 g of coffee. After five minutes, the samples were filtered using a 25 µm pore-sized quantitative filter Whatman paper. The obtained extracts were cooled to room temperature (25 °C) prior to analysis.

3.2. Instrumental Analysis

A benchtop MetriNIR Spectrometer (MetriNIR Research, Development and Service Co., Budapest, Hungary) was used to collect the spectral data in the wavelength range of 740–1700 nm. For a more representative spectra of each of the ground coffee mixtures, the cuvette was rotated between the three consecutive scans of each sample type during scanning.

In the case of the aqueous samples, a thermoregulated cuvette with a sample layer thickness of 0.5 mm was used to maintain the temperature of the samples at 25 °C. The cuvette was thoroughly washed with Milli-Q water between measurements and dried for the next sample. A total of 324 spectra, made up of three consecutive scans of the three refills of the triplicates of each mixture, were acquired. For reference data, Milli-Q water spectra were taken after every 5th sample measurement.

Two modes of spectra acquisition were adopted, diffuse reflectance mode in the case of powders and transflectance mode for liquids.

3.3. Data Processing

The selected spectral ranges were the truncated 800–1670 nm region, used to reduce spectral noise, as well as the first (1300–1600 nm) and second (800–1100 nm) overtone regions of water (more specifically OH bond), necessary for the aquaphotomics based analysis [17,32].

A set of spectral preprocessing methods were tested in terms of their effect on the obtained results. Initially, an essential step was to conduct spectral smoothing using Savitzky Golay filter by fitting the spectral points into a 2nd polynomial within the selected window width (11, 17, or 19 points). The smoothing was also jointly applied with one of the following pretreatments: multiplicative scatter correction (MSC), detrend (DeTr), standard normal variate (SNV), 1st or 2nd derivative.

The chemometric tools used for the statistical analysis of the multivariate data consisted mostly of principal component analysis (PCA), used as a pattern recognition and dimensionality reduction tool. In addition, hybrid principal component analysis-linear discriminant analysis (PCA-LDA) models served as multi-class classifiers. Ensuring that the number of PCs was optimal for further modeling was essential. In doing so, the PCs guaranteeing a combination of the best validation accuracy and the minimal difference between training and validation accuracies were selected. The dataset was split into a calibration set (two thirds) and a validation set (one third) and the three-fold cross validation (CV) method was used to assess the predictive accuracy of the PCA-LDA model in classifying pure Arabica and Robusta, their resulting mixtures at different blending ratios, as well as the marketed blends.

Subsequently, to relate the NIR spectrum to the added Robusta, partial least squares regression modelling (PLSR) was performed. Different validation methods were considered before deciding upon the model that ensures the most accurate prediction of the Robusta-to-Arabica ratio. The evaluation of the PLS models was done by computing the coefficient of determination (R^2) and the root mean square error (RMSE) of both the calibration and cross-validation. These metrics assess the fit of the tested data to the regression line while estimating the difference between predicted and actual values. The closer R^2 is to 1 and the lower RMSEC is, the more accurate the model [33]. As per the validation methods, they ranged from the least robust leave one sample out validation to more robust cross-validation based on the grouping defined by specific class variables (by repeats, by sample type, etc.). Testing the accuracy of the predictive models was performed using the two commercialized blends B10% and B30%. Only the best models were displayed in the present manuscript.

Aquagrams, representative tools of the water spectral pattern, were investigated both at the 1st and 2nd overtone regions at selected water matrix coordinates (WAMACs). These WAMACs consisted of the following wavelengths: 890, 908, 924, 946, 954, 975, 1001, 1019, 1036, 1044, and 1060 nm in case of the 2nd overtone and involved 1342, 1364, 1374, 1384, 1412, 1426, 1440, 1452, 1462, 1476, 1488, and 1512 nm when plotted in the 1st overtone range [34]. Based on literature, these wavelengths have been assigned to specific water molecular structures and have demonstrated their practicality with regard to highlighting the effect of certain perturbations on the studied system [17,19,22]. While both of the overtone ranges (1st and 2nd) were considered, the one portraying the most water spectral pattern differences between the studied samples corresponded to the 2nd overtone region and was the one presented in the manuscript.

In order to minimize sources of variations within each sample type, averaging of the repeats, refills, and consecutives was also attempted throughout the analysis.

4. Conclusions

To date, coffee adulteration issues have been addressed extensively, however; few are the studies that were not based on complex coffee extraction methods. Even fewer studies did not resort to chemical markers for the differentiation of the two coffee varieties (Arabica and Robusta) in liquid state.

Our study sought to extend the research done on coffee quality analysis through the application of both conventional NIR spectroscopy and its novel approach, aquaphotomics.

Conventional spectroscopy provided satisfactory results in terms of distinguishing pure Arabica and Robusta ground coffee from different geographical origins with 100% correct classification accuracy. When mixtures of these varieties were prepared by varying the blending ratios, accurate classification and quantification models were achieved depending on the Robusta to Arabica content. Only 5.55% of the ground coffee mixtures were misidentified by means of LDA analysis. As per the prediction of the Robusta-to-Arabica ratio, it was estimated with R^2CV of 0.99 and an error (RMSECV) of 2.4% *w*/*w*.

On the other hand, implementing aquaphotomics-based research was found to give typical spectral fingerprints to the aqueous blends. As the added Robusta increased, the corresponding mixtures had higher absorbances in the wavelengths associated with pure Robusta. A prominence of bonds attributed to water shells, as well as V1 and V2 bonded water was featured in their respective aquagrams. Conversely, those with higher Arabica fraction presented characteristic spectral patterns at the WAMACS linked to pure Arabica. The marked spectral features, in the latter case, were mainly attributed to an abundance of high hydrogen bonded water structures and water clusters with two, three, and four hydrogen bonds. The efficacy of the implemented approach was further corroborated when marketed blends were examined, correctly discriminated, and their Robusta contents accurately estimated (R^2CV of 97% and 90% by NIRS and aquaphotomics respectively).

What the findings of this study pinpoint is that aquaphotomics could be a suitable, cost-effective alternative to other technically demanding authentication tools. Most importantly, it offers novel insights regarding the changes of the water spectral pattern induced by the increased amount of Robusta. If implemented, this approach could reveal undeclared blending of coffee and contribute to the detection of potential adulteration. Nevertheless, it is worth pointing out that the applied method requires further refining with the inclusion of other coffee mixtures prepared under different roasting and brewing processes.

Author Contributions: Conceptualization, B.A. and Z.K.; Data curation, B.A., Z.B. and J.-L.Z.Z.; Formal analysis, B.A., F.V., Z.B., J.-L.Z.Z. and Z.K.; Funding acquisition, Z.K.; Investigation, B.A., F.V. and I.K.; Methodology, I.K. and Z.K.; Project administration, Z.K.; Resources, Z.K.; Software, B.A., F.V., Z.B., J.-L.Z.Z. and Z.K.; Supervision, Z.K.; Validation, Z.K.; Visualization, B.A.; Writing—original draft, B.A.; Writing—review & editing, B.A., F.V., Z.B., J.-L.Z.Z., I.K. and Z.K. All authors have read and agreed to the published version of the manuscript.

Funding: This research was supported by the European Union and co-financed by the European Social Fund (grant agreement no. EFOP-3.6.3-VEKOP-16-2017-00005); by the European Union and co-financed by the European Regional Development Fund and the Hungarian Government (grant agreement no. GINOP-2.2.1-18-2020-00025); and by the Thematic Excellence Program awarded by the Ministry for Innovation and Technology (grant agreement no. NKFIH-831-10/2019). This project was supported by the Doctoral School of Food Science of the Hungarian University of Agriculture and Life Sciences (B.A., Z.B., F.V.), and the ÚNKP-21-3-I-MATE/44 (F.V.) New National Excellence Program of the Ministry for Innovation and Technology from the source of the National Research, Development and Innovation Fund.

Institutional Review Board Statement: Not applicable.

Informed Consent Statement: Not applicable.

Data Availability Statement: The data presented in this study are available on request from the corresponding author. The data are not publicly available, due to privacy reasons.

Conflicts of Interest: The authors declare no conflict of interest.

References

1. Toci, A.T.; Farah, A.; Pezza, H.R. Critical Reviews in Analytical Chemistry Coffee Adulteration : More than Two Decades of Coffee Adulteration : More than Two Decades of Research. *Crit. Rev. Anal. Chem.* **2016**, *46*, 83–92. [CrossRef] [PubMed]
2. Sezer, B.; Apaydin, H.; Bilge, G.; Boyaci, I.H. Coffee Arabica Adulteration: Detection of Wheat, Corn and Chickpea. *Food Chem.* **2018**, *264*, 142–148. [CrossRef] [PubMed]
3. Milani, M.I.; Rossini, E.L.; Catelani, T.A.; Pezza, L.; Toci, A.T.; Pezza, H.R. Authentication of Roasted and Ground Coffee Samples Containing Multiple Adulterants Using NMR and a Chemometric Approach. *Food Control* **2020**, *112*, 107104. [CrossRef]
4. Paola de Pádua Gandra, F.; Ribeiro Lima, A.; Batista Ferreira, E.; Cardoso De Angelis Pereira, M.; Gualberto Fonseca Alvarenga Pereira, R. Adding Adulterants to Coffee Reduces Bioactive Compound Levels and Antioxidant Activity. *J. Food Nutr. Res.* **2017**, *5*, 313–319. [CrossRef]
5. Wermelinger, T.; D'Ambrosio, L.; Klopprogge, B.; Yeretzian, C. Quantification of the Robusta Fraction in a Coffee Blend via Raman Spectroscopy: Proof of Principle. *J. Agric. Food Chem.* **2011**, *59*, 9074–9079. [CrossRef] [PubMed]
6. Schievano, E.; Finotello, C.; De Angelis, E.; Mammi, S.; Navarini, L. Rapid Authentication of Coffee Blends and Quantification of 16-O-Methylcafestol in Roasted Coffee Beans by Nuclear Magnetic Resonance. *J. Agric. Food Chem.* **2014**, *62*, 12309–12314. [CrossRef]
7. Brudzewski, K.; Osowski, S.; Member, S.; Dwulit, A. Recognition of Coffee Using Differential Electronic Nose. *IEEE Trans. Instrum. Meas.* **2012**, *61*, 1803–1810. [CrossRef]

8. Pizarro, C.; Esteban-Díez, I.; González-Sáiz, J.M. Mixture Resolution According to the Percentage of Robusta Variety in Order to Detect Adulteration in Roasted Coffee by near Infrared Spectroscopy. *Anal. Chim. Acta* **2007**, *585*, 266–276. [CrossRef] [PubMed]
9. Spaniolas, S.; May, S.T.; Bennett, M.J.; Tucker, G.A. Authentication of Coffee by Means of PCR-RFLP Analysis and Lab-on-a-Chip Capillary Electrophoresis. *J. Agric. Food Chem.* **2006**, *54*, 7466–7470. [CrossRef]
10. Arrieta, A.A.; Arrieta, P.L.; Mendoza, J.M. Analysis of Coffee Adulterated with Roasted Corn and Roasted Soybean Using Voltammetric Electronic Tongue. *Acta Sci. Pol. Technol. Aliment.* **2019**, *18*, 35–41. [PubMed]
11. Daniel, D.; Lopes, F.S.; dos Santos, V.B.; do Lago, C.L. Detection of Coffee Adulteration with Soybean and Corn by Capillary Electrophoresis-Tandem Mass Spectrometry. *Food Chem.* **2018**, *243*, 305–310. [CrossRef]
12. Forchetti, D.A.P.; Poppi, R.J. Detection and Quantification of Adulterants in Roasted and Ground Coffee by NIR Hyperspectral Imaging and Multivariate Curve Resolution. *Food Anal. Methods* **2020**, *13*, 44–49. [CrossRef]
13. Song, H.Y.; Jang, H.W.; Debnath, T.; Lee, K.G. Analytical Method to Detect Adulteration of Ground Roasted Coffee. *Int. J. Food Sci. Technol.* **2019**, *54*, 256–262. [CrossRef]
14. Suhandy, D.; Yulia, M. The Quantification of Adulteration in Arabica Coffee Using UV-Visible Spectroscopy in Combination with Two Different PLS Regressions. *Aceh Int. J. Sci. Technol.* **2017**, *6*, 59–67. [CrossRef]
15. Muncan, J.; Tsenkova, R. Aquaphotomics-From Innovative Knowledge to Integrative Platform in Science and Technology. *Molecules* **2019**, *24*, 2742. [CrossRef]
16. Atanassova, S.; Naydenova, N.; Kolev, T.; Iliev, T.; Mihaylova, G. Near Infrared Spectroscopy and Aquaphotomics for Monitoring Changes during Yellow Cheese Ripening. *Agric. Sci. Technol.* **2016**, *3*, 390.
17. Kovacs, Z.; Bázár, G.; Oshima, M.; Shigeoka, S.; Tanaka, M.; Furukawa, A.; Nagai, A.; Osawa, M.; Itakura, Y.; Tsenkova, R. Water Spectral Pattern as Holistic Marker for Water Quality Monitoring. *Talanta* **2015**, *147*, 598–608. [CrossRef] [PubMed]
18. Muncan, J.; Tei, K.; Tsenkova, R. Real-Time Monitoring of Yogurt Fermentation Process by Aquaphotomics near-Infrared Spectroscopy. *Sensors* **2021**, *21*, 177. [CrossRef] [PubMed]
19. Bázár, G.; Romvári, R.; Szabó, A.; Somogyi, T.; Éles, V.; Tsenkova, R. NIR Detection of Honey Adulteration Reveals Differences in Water Spectral Pattern. *Food Chem.* **2016**, *194*, 873–880. [CrossRef]
20. Cui, X.; Liu, X.; Yu, X.; Cai, W.; Shao, X. Water Can Be a Probe for Sensing Glucose in Aqueous Solutions by Temperature Dependent near Infrared Spectra. *Anal. Chim. Acta* **2017**, *957*, 47–54. [CrossRef] [PubMed]
21. Mura, S.; Cappai, C.; Franco, G.; Barzaghi, S.; Stellari, A.; Maria, T.; Cattaneo, P. Vibrational Spectroscopy and Aquaphotomics Holistic Approach to Determine Chemical Compounds Related to Sustainability in Soil pro Fi Les. *Comput. Electron. Agric.* **2019**, *159*, 92–96. [CrossRef]
22. Mcglone, A.; Kaur, H.; Ku, R. Investigating Aquaphotomics for Temperature-Independent Prediction of Soluble Solids Content of Pure Apple Juice. *J. Near Infrared Spectrosc.* **2020**, *28*, 103–112.
23. Matija, L.R.; Tsenkova, R.N.; Miyazaki, M.; Banba, K.; Muncan, J.S. Aquagrams: Water Spectral Pattern as Characterization of Hydrogenated Nanomaterial. *FME Trans.* **2012**, *40*, 51–56.
24. Giraudo, A.; Grassi, S.; Savorani, F.; Gavoci, G.; Casiraghi, E.; Geobaldo, F. Determination of the Geographical Origin of Green Coffee Beans Using NIR Spectroscopy and Multivariate Data Analysis. *Food Control* **2019**, *99*, 137–145. [CrossRef]
25. Esteban-Díez, I.; González-Sáiz, J.M.; Pizarro, C. Prediction of Sensory Properties of Espresso from Roasted Coffee Samples by Near-Infrared Spectroscopy. *Anal. Chim. Acta* **2004**, *525*, 171–182. [CrossRef]
26. Kamiloglu, S. Authenticity and Traceability in Beverages. *Food Chem.* **2019**, *277*, 12–24. [CrossRef]
27. Ribeiro, J.S.; Ferreira, M.M.C.; Salva, T.J.G. Chemometric Models for the Quantitative Descriptive Sensory Analysis of Arabica Coffee Beverages Using near Infrared Spectroscopy. *Talanta* **2011**, *83*, 1352–1358. [CrossRef] [PubMed]
28. Adnan, A.; Naumann, M.; Morlein, D.; Pawelzik, E. Reliable Discrimination of Green Coffee Beans Species: A Comparison of UV-Vis-Based Determination of Caffeine and Chlorogenic Acid with Non-Targeted near-Infrared Spectroscopy. *Foods* **2020**, *9*, 788. [CrossRef]
29. Wu, D.; He, Y.; Feng, S. Short-Wave near-Infrared Spectroscopy Analysis of Major Compounds in Milk Powder and Wavelength Assignment. *Anal. Chim. Acta* **2008**, *610*, 232–242. [CrossRef]
30. Speer, K.; Kölling-Speer, I. The Lipid Fraction of the Coffee Bean. *Braz. J. Plant Physiol.* **2006**, *18*, 201–216. [CrossRef]
31. Assis, C.; Oliveira, L.S.; Sena, M.M. Variable Selection Applied to the Development of a Robust Method for the Quantification of Coffee Blends Using Mid Infrared Spectroscopy. *Food Anal. Methods* **2018**, *11*, 578–588. [CrossRef]
32. Tsenkova, R.; Muncan, J.; Pollner, B.; Kovacs, Z. Essentials of Aquaphotomics and Its Chemometrics Approaches. *Front. Chem.* **2018**, *6*, 363. [CrossRef] [PubMed]
33. Næs, T.; Isaksson, T.; Fearn, T.; Davies, T. *A User-Friendly Guide to Multivariate Calibration and Classification*; NIR Publications: Chichester, UK, 2002; Volume 6.
34. Kovacs, Z.; Pollner, B.; Bazar, G.; Muncan, J.; Tsenkova, R. A Novel Tool for Visualization of Water Molecular Structure and Its Changes, Expressed on the Scale of Temperature Influence. *Molecules* **2020**, *25*, 2234. [CrossRef] [PubMed]

molecules

MDPI

Article

Identification of Stingless Bee Honey Adulteration Using Visible-Near Infrared Spectroscopy Combined with Aquaphotomics

Muna E. Raypah [1], Ahmad Fairuz Omar [1,*], Jelena Muncan [2], Musfirah Zulkurnain [3] and Abdul Rahman Abdul Najib [1]

[1] School of Physics, Universiti Sains Malaysia, Pulau Pinang 11800, Malaysia; muna_ezzi@usm.my (M.E.R.); abdulrahmannajib95@gmail.com (A.R.A.N.)
[2] Aquaphotomics Research Department, Faculty of Agriculture, Kobe University, Kobe 658-8501, Japan; jmuncan@people.kobe-u.ac.jp
[3] Food Technology Division, School of Industrial Technology, Universiti Sains Malaysia, Pulau Pinang 11800, Malaysia; musfirah.z@usm.my
* Correspondence: fairuz_omar@usm.my

Abstract: Honey is a natural product that is considered globally one of the most widely important foods. Various studies on authenticity detection of honey have been fulfilled using visible and near-infrared (Vis-NIR) spectroscopy techniques. However, there are limited studies on stingless bee honey (SBH) despite the increase of market demand for this food product. The objective of this work was to present the potential of Vis-NIR absorbance spectroscopy for profiling, classifying, and quantifying the adulterated SBH. The SBH sample was mixed with various percentages (10–90%) of adulterants, including distilled water, apple cider vinegar, and high fructose syrup. The results showed that the region at 400–1100 nm that is related to the color and water properties of the samples was effective to discriminate and quantify the adulterated SBH. By applying the principal component analysis (PCA) on adulterants and honey samples, the PCA score plot revealed the classification of the adulterants and adulterated SBHs. A partial least squares regression (PLSR) model was developed to quantify the contamination level in the SBH samples. The general PLSR model with the highest coefficient of determination and lowest root means square error of cross-validation ($R^2_{CV} = 0.96$ and $RMSE_{CV} = 5.88\ \%$) was acquired. The aquaphotomics analysis of adulteration in SBH with the three adulterants utilizing the short-wavelength NIR region (800–1100 nm) was presented. The structural changes of SBH due to adulteration were described in terms of the changes in the water molecular matrix, and the aquagrams were used to visualize the results. It was revealed that the integration of NIR spectroscopy with aquaphotomics could be used to detect the water molecular structures in the adulterated SBH.

Keywords: adulteration; stingless bee honey; visible and near-infrared spectroscopy; PCA; PLSR; aquaphotomics

Citation: Raypah, M.E.; Omar, A.F.; Muncan, J.; Zulkurnain, M.; Abdul Najib, A.R. Identification of Stingless Bee Honey Adulteration Using Visible-Near Infrared Spectroscopy Combined with Aquaphotomics. *Molecules* **2022**, *27*, 2324. https://doi.org/10.3390/molecules27072324

Academic Editor: Maged Henary

Received: 22 February 2022
Accepted: 1 April 2022
Published: 3 April 2022

1. Introduction

Honey is a natural food that may be used not only as a sweetener but also as a medication because of its therapeutic effects on human health. Flower honey is the most prevalent kind of honey, and it is made by honeybees (*Apis Mellifera* L.) from the nectar of various types of flowers, depending on the geographical region and season, while stingless bee honey is made from the nectar of trees and is a naturally higher moisture content [1]. Other compounds are often added to commercially sold honey for nutrition and medical purposes, and some are added to spoof the pure honey. Honey is often threatened by cheaper, commercially accessible sugar syrups with similar chemical compositions [2]. Even if these standards are followed to maintain high levels of quality, contaminations and/or adulterations might occur during manufacture, compromising the product's quality and safety [3]. Adulterants in honey are any substances that are mixed with pure honey. Adulteration raises glucose levels, which can lead to diabetes, belly weight gain, and obesity. It also elevates blood lipid levels, which can lead to high blood pressure. Various adulteration activities of honey have been reported in the market, with the most common being the addition of edible syrups such as high-fructose corn syrup and corn syrup [4]. Many approaches, both traditional and modern, have been used and developed to distinguish pure honey from contaminated or non-honeys [5].

Spectroscopy has been more popular in the detection of honey adulteration in recent years due to its speed, simplicity, environmental friendliness, and nondestructive nature. It's worth noting that strategies for proving the authenticity of products are always evolving in response to these increasingly widespread behaviors [3]. Recently, several spectroscopy methods, such as Raman spectroscopy [6], NIR spectroscopy on *Apis mellifera* [7–9], and stingless bee honey [1,9] were conducted to determine the adulteration. The combination of NIR spectroscopy application and chemometric methods [10,11] shows a simple, rapid, and nondestructive method on adulterated honey. Moreover, honey consistency is possibly fluid, viscous, or partially to completely crystalline [12]. Because hydrogen bonds, which are associated with water, are present in most natural samples, this method can be used in a variety of domains [9]. In the research of adulteration detection in honey, spectroscopic techniques such as near- and mid-infrared spectroscopy were used [4]. Researchers are constantly developing efficient and sensitive detection methods using NIR spectroscopic approaches to detect adulterants in honey [13]. At present, honey adulteration is generally detected on the bees' honey. Stingless bee honey has a high-water content, slight sweetness, acidic flavor, fluid texture, and slow crystallization [14]. Compared to bees' honey, stingless bee honey contains a higher amount of water, ranging between 25 to 56 g/100 g, and higher acidity, which influences its shelf-life and keeping quality. Honey produced by stingless bees (Melipona sp. and Trigona sp.) is recognized for its unique sour taste and odor [15]. Based on the local beekeepers' report, the adulteration of SBH involves dilution with water to increase the yield volume of the honey to fraudulently increase income. In addition, in certain cases, cheaper honey is blended with a sour-tasting liquid such as vinegar to create a sour taste that resembles that of SBH, and then market it at a high price commensurate with the authentic SBH [16]. However, due to the complexity of food matrices, most standard approaches can only detect a small number of adulterants in stingless bee honey without a thorough examination of all of its attributes. Hence, less research is available on the adulterated stingless bee honey.

After carbohydrates, water is the second-largest component of honey and is considered as one of the most important features that affect several characteristics of honey, such as viscosity, flavor, specific weight, shelf-life, and crystallization [17,18]. In the case of stingless bee honeys, the water content $\sim$ 20% is generally higher compared to the genus Apis and can be even higher than 40% depending on the bee species [19]. As a result, water is a very significant component that should be considered during the analysis of SBHs. It is well-known that different water molecular structures can be identified based on their respective absorbance bands in the NIR region, providing the NIR spectroscopy with the ability to detect subtle changes associated with water molecular structure changes. This is especially utilized in aquaphotomics [20,21], a spectroscopy-based science that employs the structure of water in bio-aqueous systems to interpret their functionality, and the results can be visualized using simple and quick tools called aquagrams [22,23]. Recent studies applied aquaphotomics for the detection of honey adulteration in which the structural changes of honey upon adulteration were explained in the terms of the changes in the water molecular matrix [9,13].

Apart from the common type of honey that is produced by bees of the genus Apis, demand for the honey produced from the stingless bee genus has increased recently and carries commercial value higher than the one of the genus Apis. However, despite holding increasing market demand, there are fewer studies and literature available regarding stingless bee honey's (SBH) physicochemical properties, particularly its optical visible and near-infrared (Vis-NIR) properties. SBH has limited industrial production, lower shelf life, and lack of an institutional quality standard, due to the scant knowledge about the product and the distribution limitation of SBHs in the world market compared with honey from the genus Apis [24]. This deficiency of information weighs down the definition of quality attributes and standards concerning SBHs. Most of the physicochemical characteristics of honey available are related to beehive products directed to Apis products [25]. As a result, SBH is not controlled by food control authorities, since it is not included in the international standards for honey [26]. For that reason, consumers have no quality assurance on SBH products [25,27]. In other words, the lack of comprehensive physicochemical data allows the recognition of possible adulteration activities to become even harder to implement for SBH. Hence, this research is designed to quantify the alteration in the Vis-NIR spectra of the SBH concerning adulteration by different percentages of added water, apple cider vinegar, and high fructose syrup. In addition, multivariate analysis including principal component analysis (PCA) and partial least squares regression (PLSR) is performed on the Vis-NIR spectroscopy in the region of 400–1100 nm. What is more, the analysis of the adulterated SBH using aquaphotomics is presented. To the best of the authors' knowledge, this is the first time to evaluate the adulterated SBH using the combination of aquaphotomics and NIR spectroscopy in the region 800–1100 nm.

2. Results and Discussion

2.1. *Vis-NIR Spectra of Pure and Adulterated SBH Samples*

The raw spectra of the samples (n = 31) are presented in Figure 1, and the adulterated samples are labeled by the type and percentage of adulteration. The spectral profiles in the Vis-NIR region showed three distinctive groups, where fructose-syrup (FS)-adulterated honey samples are particularly different compared to the water (W)- and apple-cider (AC)-adulterated honey. Depending on the adulterant type, there is a vastly different baseline offset, an effect that can be attributed to light scattering due to the sugar crystals present in the honey samples [28,29]. Alternatively, an increase in the baseline could be explained by increased bulk and hydration water content, that causes an increase in the scattering [23,30,31]. Most probably, the two phenomena are inter-connected, suggesting an altered water–sugar interaction by adding apple cider and water that results in changes in the crystallization degree.

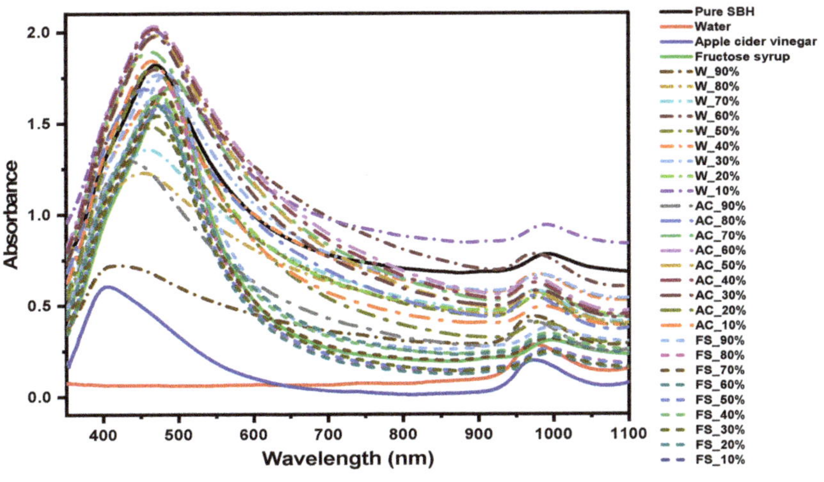

Figure 1. Spectra for pure SBH, adulterants, and adulterated SBH samples (n = 31).

The Vis-NIR spectra (400–1100 nm) of pure SBH and the adulterants together with SBH adulterated with various percentages of each adulterant are shown in Figure 2. It is apparent from Figure 2 that the baseline offset shows the largest differences depending on the percentage of added adulterant in the spectra of water-adulterated honey, followed by apple cider and the smallest variations can be observed in the fructose-syrup-adulterated honey samples. Interestingly, the spectrum of pure honey is furthest away from the fructose-syrup-adulterated honey spectra. While the changes in the color of the honey may be subtle, as can be seen in the visible part of the spectrum, the observed spectral characteristics in the NIR region of the spectra suggest a change in other optical properties that may be connected to the scattering of light, for example, the refractive index [32], or the optical rotation, as was shown to be the case in other honey adulteration studies [33–35].

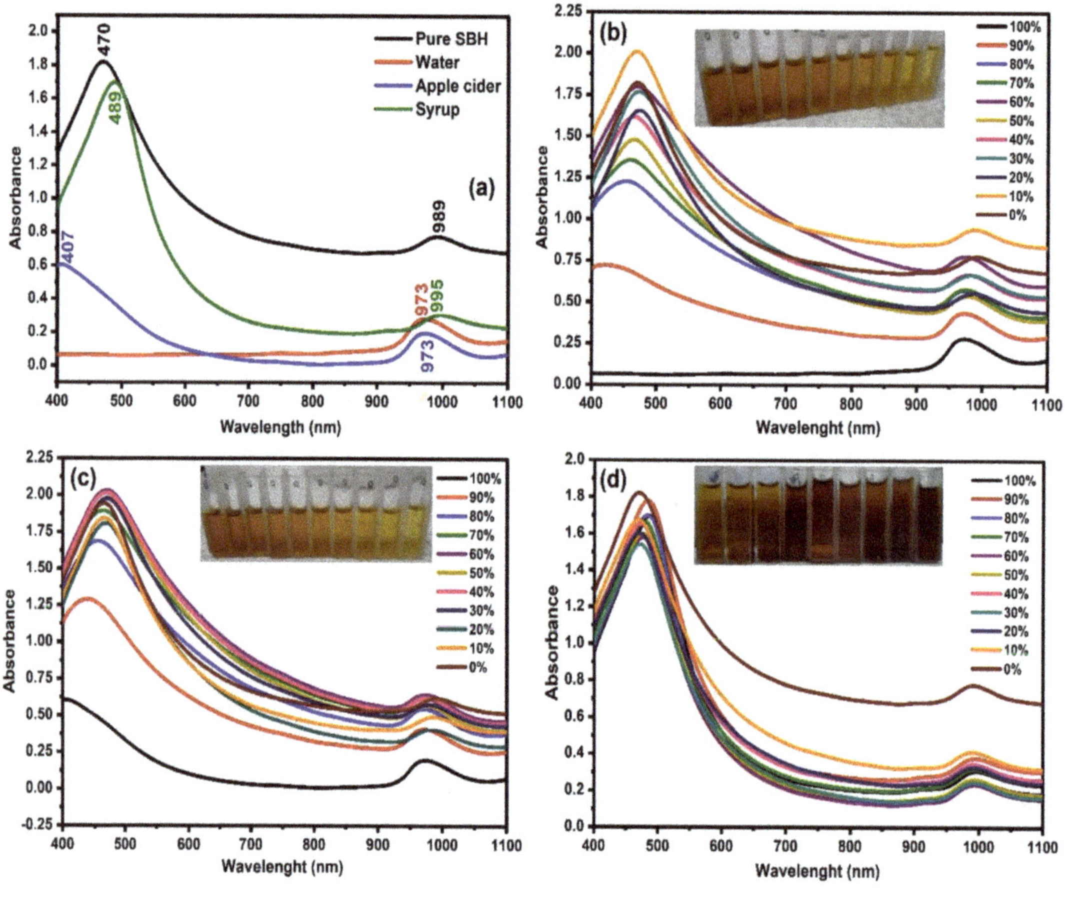

Figure 2. Vis-NIR spectra of (**a**) Pure SBH and adulterants and adulterated SBH by different percentages of water (**b**), apple cider (**c**), and fructose syrup (**d**).

As can be seen in Figure 2a, there are differences in intensity and wavelength peak between samples in the visible region. The peaks at a visible region for the pure SBH, apple cider, and fructose syrup are located at 470 nm, 407 nm, and 489 nm, respectively. The color of honey is the first quality aspect that affects consumer predilection. The color of honey is related to the floral origin or the plant source, minerals, phenolic contents, storage time, and temperature [36]. The absorbance at 400–500 nm is related to the honey compounds that absorb the light, such as the blue–violet light range at 400 nm, that resulted in the characteristic orange-amber color of honey [37]. On the other hand, some intensity differences can be observed in the visible region at 400–700 nm. The higher absorbance intensity designates the dark color of the sample [38]. The pure SBH spectrum presented the highest intensity in this range, followed by apple cider vinegar and fructose syrup. Pure honey remained in the middle range, with its orange-amber color, followed by the apple cider and fructose syrup, that exhibited different colors. The band around the region between 550 nm and 600 nm characterizes the maximum emission of riboflavin (vitamin B2) presented in the samples [39].

Likewise, the raw spectra in Figure 2a demonstrated that the absorption peaks of the samples are mainly located in the NIR region. The peak of absorbance within the NIR region for water and apple cider is located at 973 nm, which is associated with the second overtone of the symmetric and asymmetric OH-stretching bands [40–42]. The apple cider generally contains up to 94% of water content [43]. The NIR absorbance for fructose syrup is further shifted to a higher wavelength with a peak of 995 nm, while the NIR peak for pure SBH was recorded at 989 nm. The determination of the original Vis-NIR properties of the samples is important in setting the potential benchmarking on the authenticity of the SBH, thus allowing the detection—and, preferably, the quantification—of the adulterant through the alteration on the spectral attributes of the sample. Figure 2b–d shows the Vis-NIR spectra of SBH adulterated by different percentages of water, apple cider, and fructose syrup, respectively. The adulteration is shown at an increasing percentage from 10 to 90%, while 0% refers to the spectrum of pure SBH and 100% to the spectrum of the adulterant. The color of pure SBH can range from white to dark amber [44,45]. From the images of the samples, the SBH adulterated with water and apple cider exhibits visible color changes from light amber to water white (based on the Pfund scale) [46,47]. However, the SBH sample adulterated with fructose syrup does not show significant changes from the visual perception.

Spectroscopic and colorimetric techniques can provide a more exact evaluation of honey color and are used to identify the small differences between the color of honeys [47]. A further possible practice for the determination of honey color is using the colorimetric parameters based on spectral information. This can be achieved in a chromaticity diagram (or a color space) developed for the perception of the human eye, such as the CIELAB/CIE XYZ/CIELUV color space. In the case of honey analysis, the CIELAB color space is the most widely applied [2,36,48,49], used in this study concerning illuminant D65 and a visual angle of 10° [48,49]. The absorbance spectra of the samples were transformed to transmission spectra using the Unscrambler Software and transferred to a Chromaticity Diagram template developed in the OriginPro 2021 Software. It must be highlighted that colorimeters apply continuous filters and provide the X, Y, and Z tristimulus values as output, while spectrometers measured the transmission/reflection/emission spectra. Since color parameters values are derived from the spectral data, the results may carry the error caused by the spectral resolution of the spectrometer.

Within the approximately uniform CIELAB color space, two-color coordinates, a^* and b^*, as well as lightness L^* are defined. L^* is an approximate measurement of the degree of lightness within the range of 0–100 (0 for black till 100 for white). The a^* coordinate determines the greenness/redness of the sample. The greenish color is in the negative range, while the reddish color is in the positive range. The b^* coordinate indicates the blue or yellow color, where blueness is in the negative range and yellowness in the positive range. It was found that water and apple cider were the lightest by visual comparison and have the highest values of the parameter L^*, that indicates the lightness—94.55 and 84.12, respectively. The L^* value decreased further in pure SBH (30.08) and fructose syrup (46.35). The SBH in this study can be considered as dark honey, since $L^* \leq 50$ [36]. This could be attributed to the floral source, the species of bee, and the location of honey production. It was shown that the honey with the highest levels of total minerals exhibit quite low values of L^*, coinciding with a dark color [49]. Furthermore, these results were in close relationship with the absorbance spectra shown in Figure 2a and confirm that the absorbance increased with the decreasing lightness value, as reported by Bertoncelj et al. [36]. What is more, the CIE XYZ (or CIE 1931) chromaticity diagram is displayed in Supplementary Figures S1 and S2. In these figures, the adulterated samples were labeled as H_W9 to H_W1, H_C9 to H_C1, and H_S9 to H_S1, which means the honey is adulterated with water, apple cider vinegar, and fructose syrup from 90% to 10%, respectively. The chromaticity diagram (Figure S1) and its zoom-in view (Figure S2) proved the variation in the value of L^* due to the addition of adulterants, which is related to the interpretation in Figure 2.

The plot of parameters a^* and b^* of the samples is shown in Figure 3. From the diagram, it is apparent that, depending on L^*, the samples were clearly distinguished from each other, as it was more obvious in adulterants and pure SBH. Additionally, the adulterated honey with fructose syrup is clearly distinguished from the other adulterated samples. Likewise, at a specific level of adulteration, the adulterated honey samples due to water and apple cider vinegar at a specific range of a^* and b^* are overlapped in the (a^*, b^*) scheme, resulting from their similar color characteristics.

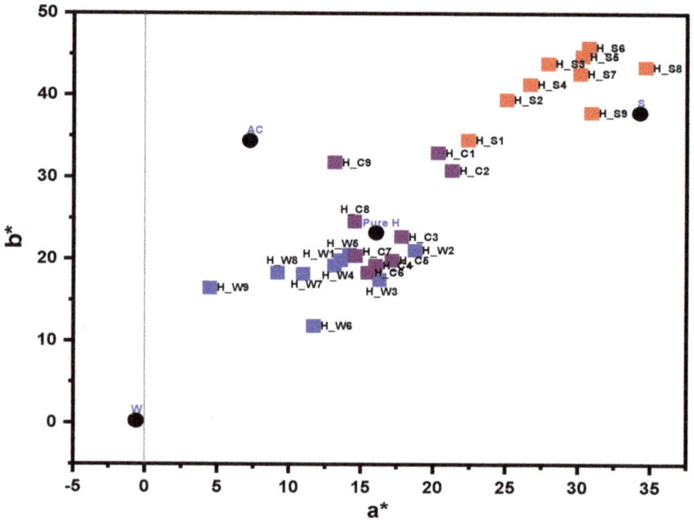

Figure 3. Location zone of adulterants and honey samples in the (a^*, b^*) diagram.

The Vis-NIR spectra can be characterized with two main peaks, at 470 nm and 980 nm, for the SBH as reported earlier [50]. The high fructose syrup showed a similar peak characterization, at 500 nm and 980 nm. On the other hand, apple cider also showed two main peaks at 400 nm and 970 nm, while water only exhibited a peak at 970 nm. In order to be able to quantify the spectral alteration due to the added adulterant in the pure SBH sample, the relationship between the absorbance at 470 nm and 970 nm with the percentage of adulterant was plotted and is shown in Figure 4a and b, respectively. In general, there is no substantial degradation in the value of absorbance for SBH adulterated with 10 to 60% of water and apple cider. The spectral degradation begins to take place when the quantity of adulterant is raised to 70% onwards. This observation was found for both 470 and 970 nm. As presented in Figure 4, the relationship between the concentration of adulterant and absorbance can be quantified by a linear correlation coefficient (R), where the R values of 0.8456 and 0.6653 were generated between the absorbance at 470 nm with the percentage of water and apple cider, respectively. In addition, the R of 0.7295 was generated between the absorbance at 970 nm with the percentage of water, but a very low R, of 0.3716, was produced for the apple cider. Nevertheless, at 470 nm, the SBH adulterated with fructose syrup showed no notable correlation with the spectral absorbance, with data fluctuating between 1.548 and 1.822 with a standard deviation of 0.073. For a similar dataset, the absorbance at 970 nm dropped 0.353 points from 0.743 when the pure SHB sample was added with 10% of syrup. However, the continuous addition of fructose syrup did not cause further reduction in the value of absorbance, where the data only fluctuated between 0.202 and 0.39 with a standard deviation of 0.058.

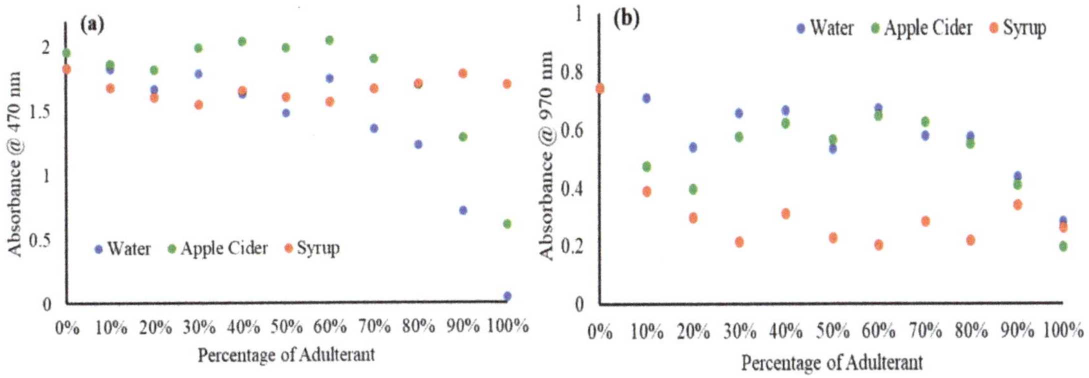

Figure 4. Relationship between the percentage of added adulterant and absorbance at (**a**) 470 nm and (**b**) 970 nm.

The peak shift in the Vis and NIR spectra towards the percentage of added adulterant was also investigated. From Figure 5a, for the visible region, a hypochromic shift occurs from 469 nm to 386 nm for water and from 466 nm to 405 nm for apple cider. SBH adulterated with fructose syrup, on the other hand, causes a consistent bathochromic shift from 469 nm to 489 nm, with the increment of added adulterant. The shift in the wavelength is predominantly from 50% of added adulterants. The pattern of the response curve is almost similar to Figure 4a due to the transformation in the SBH color caused by the adulteration. Water and apple cider cause the SBH samples to lose their yellow-red property, while the addition of fructose syrup enriched the yellow-red properties of the SBH due to the original color properties of the fructose syrup (as can be seen in Figure 2).

The relationship between the wavelength of the NIR peak and the amount of the adulterants in SBH samples is depicted in Figure 5b. Generally, the NIR region exhibits a broad peak where multiple wavelengths share similar maximum values compared to visible absorbance. This is more significant for SBH samples adulterated with apple cider and fructose syrup. The NIR peak absorbance for pure SBH is located between 987 and 992 nm. The NIR peak shifted significantly to a lower NIR wavelength until it reached the centralized water peak at 970 nm with the increase in water and apple cider. A previous study reported that the combination of NIR wavelengths between 960 and 965 nm within C-H and O-H bands can reliably quantify sugars including fructose, glucose, and sucrose [51].

Generally, the addition of water and apple cider (predominantly composed of water) reduced the values of the soluble solids content 'SSC' comparably, while the addition of high fructose syrup increased the SSC further, especially at concentrations beyond 60%, as shown in Figure 5c. Pure SBH has an average SSC of 74.5 °Brix. According to a review written by [44], the SSC for SBH ranges from 64.5 to 75.8 °Brix and is lower than the one for Apis mellifera honey due to its higher water content and lower sugar content. The sugar composition of SBH was recently discovered to be predominantly trehalulose, which explains its lower total fructose and glucose contents [52]. The pure apple cider recorded 4.1 °Brix contributed by sugar and organic acids. Pure high fructose syrup, on the other hand, recorded a much higher SSC, at 17.8 °Brix.

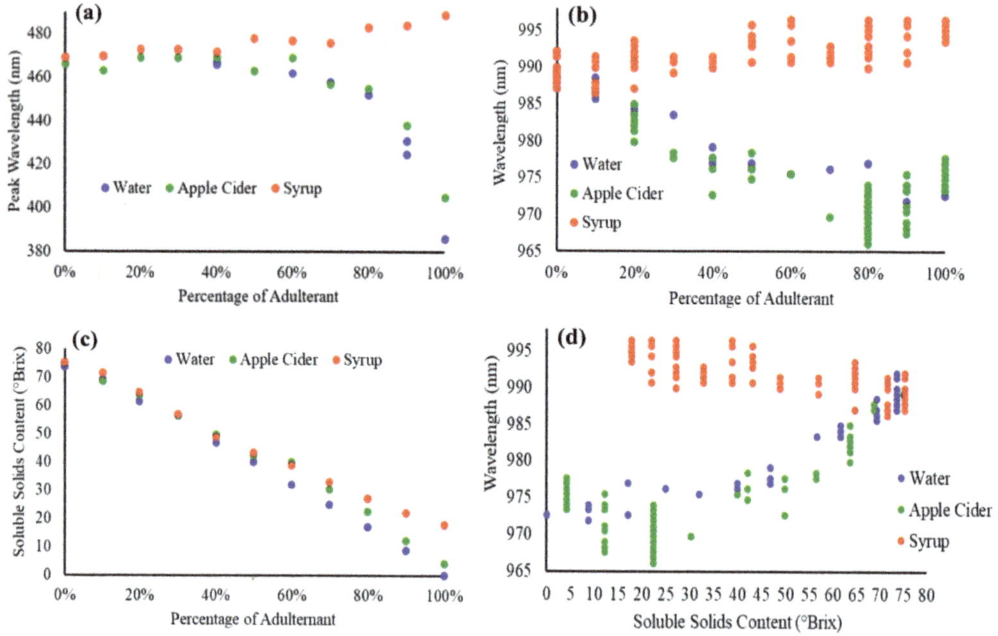

Figure 5. (**a**) Visible and (**b**) near-infrared peak absorbance of the samples against the percentage of added adulterant, (**c**) relationship between soluble solids content (in °Brix) and the percentage of added adulterant, and (**d**) absorbance at near-infrared peak and the soluble solids content of the samples.

The wavelength of the NIR peak was plotted against the soluble solids content of the samples, as shown in Figure 5d. The increase in °Brix value showed a gradual increment of the NIR wavelength beyond 970 nm for both samples adulterated with water and apple cider. These results are in agreement with some studies in which the experiment was conducted to analyze the NIR properties of water-sugar solutions [51,53,54]. In these studies, raising sugar concentration in water (i.e., high SSC) causes the water band to be more symmetric and, as a result, shifts the peak absorbance towards the longer wavelength. Omar et al. [50] also reported that the addition of water to both SBH and Apis mellifera honey resulted in a shift of the NIR absorbance peak towards a lower wavelength. However, the increase in °Brix value of the SBH that was adulterated with syrup exhibits a very minimal shift towards a lower wavelength for the higher SSC of the adulterated samples.

2.2. PCA Analysis and PLSR Modeling

Room temperature Vis-NIR spectra of pure and adulterated honey were exported from the spectral software system and introduced directly into the Unscrambler software to generate the chemometric models. A PCA was performed on the Vis-NIR spectra (400–1100 nm) due to its ability to decrease dimensionality. To enhance the spectral quality and attain a good clustering for samples, the raw data were first pre-processed using moving average smoothing (within a 25-segment size) and baseline transformations. The 3D score plot for all the samples according to the first three principal components (PCs) is shown in Figure 6a. 2D PCA score plots of PC1 vs. PC2, PC1 vs. PC3, and PC2 vs. PC3 are presented in Supplementary Figure S3–S5, respectively. As presented in Figure 6a, the samples were clustered into seven groups, that corresponded to the three adulterants (water 'W', apple cider 'AC', and fructose syrup 'FS') and four groups of SBHs (pure and adulterated honey). The honey samples were clustered into different groups and zones based on the presence of adulterants, suggesting that these samples have distinctive properties concerning the adulteration type. In addition, the cumulative explained variance of the first three PCs was 99.11% of the total variance of spectral data, which indicates that these PCs can reflect most of the basic characteristics of the raw data.

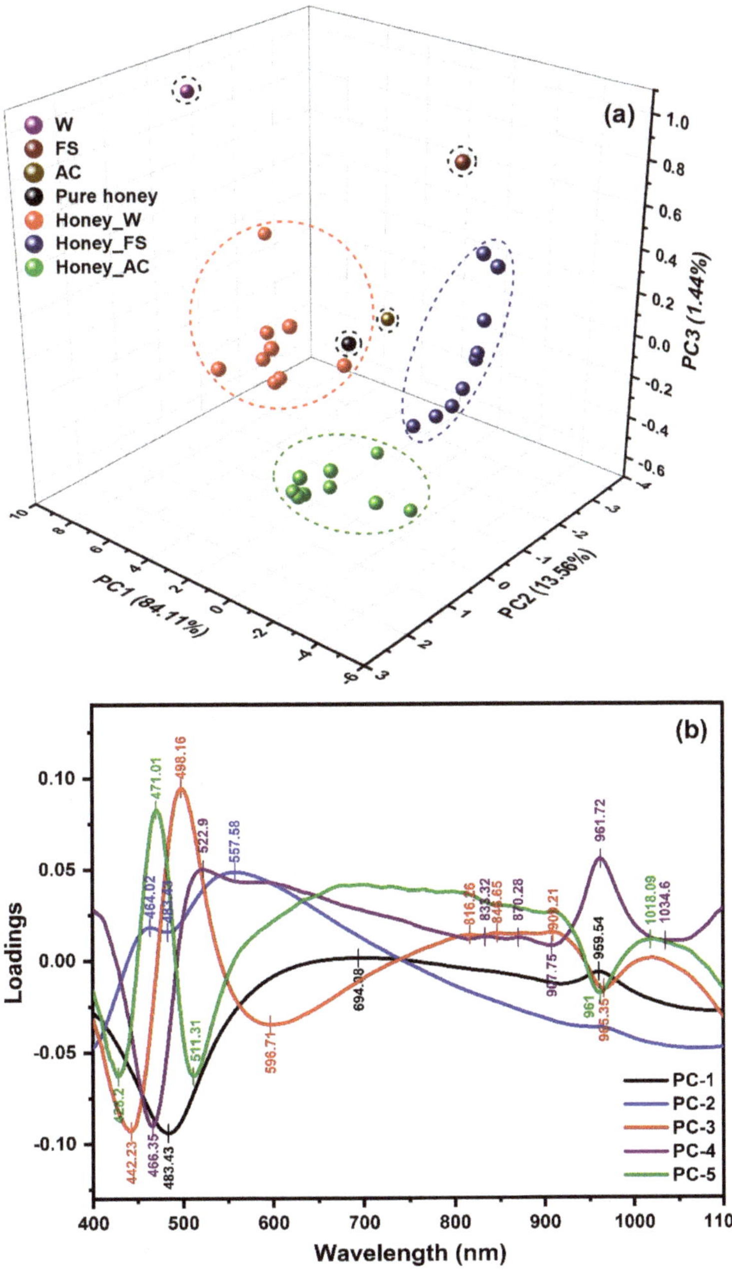

Figure 6. PCA analysis: (**a**) 3D score plot of the first three PCs and (**b**) x-loadings of PC1-PC5 of Vis-NIR spectra (400–1100 nm).

The PCA loadings reveal the wavelengths that show the maximum difference at the individual PCs [55]. The loadings of each wavelength to differentiate the SBHs were evaluated and displayed in Figure 6b for the first five components (PC1 to PC5). Several contributive wavelengths with high x-loadings are recognized at Vis and NIR regions. These wavelengths including 442, 466, 471, 483, 498, 511, 558, and 597 nm in the Vis region, and 816, 833, 847, 870, 908, 909, 960, 961, 965, 1018, and 1035 nm in the NIR region. The peaks at the visible region are related to the color of the honey and the effect of the adulterations' type and level on the color of honey samples, while the peaks in the NIR region are located within the areas of the third overtone of the C-H stretching band [56,57], the second overtone of the OH stretching band of water [9,58,59], and the second overtone of the N-H stretching band. These spectral features arise from the major components of honey, including carbohydrates, water, proteins, and amino acids [60]. The findings demonstrated that the potential adulteration of SBH by common adulterants such as water, apple cider, and high fructose syrup can be discriminated with a clear separation. Despite the complexity of detection involving the influences of the adulterants on the color changes of the SBH honey, distinct trends can be discriminated by considering both visible and NIR regions.

Table 1 summarizes the results of various pre-treatments that were applied to optimize the calibration performance of the global PLSR model utilized to quantify the level of the adulteration in the SHB samples. It is shown that R_C^2 and R_{CV}^2 are approximately similar for all the models examined, and therefore the model with the lowest $RMSE_{CV}$ was chosen. As displayed in Table 1, the most accurate model that produces the lowest $RMSE_{CV}$ corresponds to the moving average smoothing and the first polynomial detrending transformations using seven factors (LVs). The PLSR modeling results are presented in Figure 7. Figure 7a shows the loading plot of the regression vectors of the best PLSR model (Factor 7). The regression vectors with higher loading values displayed a high compatibility with the spectral bands presented in the PCA analysis. The positions of the spectral peaks in the regression coefficient plot of the model were marked to determine the bands that have the biggest weights in the calibration on adulterated honey. These bands characterize the diverse water structures and carbohydrates. Figure 7b demonstrated the linear regression of actual and predicted adulteration levels in the SBH samples. The value of R_C^2, R_{CV}^2, $RMSE_C$, and $RMSE_{CV}$ were 0.98, 0.96, 3.93%, and 5.88%, respectively. The obtained values of $RMSE_C$ and $RMSE_{CV}$ of the global PLSR model suggested its good predictive capacity and the appropriateness of the selected spectral region, 400–1100 nm.

Table 1. Calibration and cross-validation results of the PLSR model performed on pre-processed spectral data at the range 400–1100 nm.

Pre-Processing Methods	LVs	$RMSE_C$ (%)	$RMSE_{CV}$ (%)	R_C^2	R_{CV}^2
Raw absorbance	7	3.65	6.43	0.98	0.95
Smoothing	7	4.20	6.49	0.97	0.95
Detrend 1st polynomial	7	2.34	6.33	0.99	0.95
1st derivative SG	6	3.85	6.29	0.98	0.95
Smoothing, Detrend 1st Polynomial	**7**	**3.93**	**5.88**	**0.98**	**0.96**
Smoothing, detrend 1st polynomial, 1st derivative SG	6	4.08	6.58	0.98	0.94

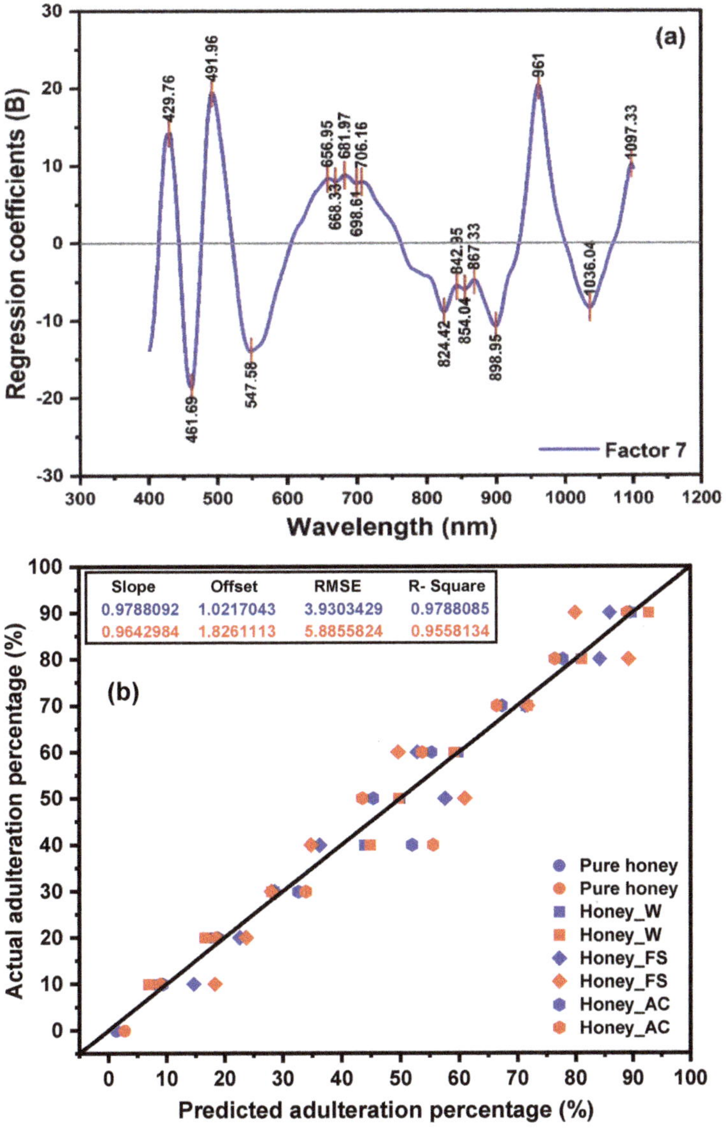

Figure 7. PLSR model results: (**a**) regression coefficients plot of Factor 7 and (**b**) calibration (in blue) and cross-validation (in red) at the 400–1100 nm spectral interval for SBH samples.

2.3. Evaluation of the Structural Changes of Adulterated SBH Based on Aquaphotomics

The aquagrams in Figures 8–10 presented the structural changes in stingless bee honey after adulteration by water, apple cider, and fructose syrup, respectively. The radial axes of aquagrams are defined by 16 absorbance bands that can be considered as WAMACs. The aquagrams show WASPs of adulterated honey compared to the WASP of pure honey (the black line on Figures 8–10). Clearly, the aquagrams of honey adulterated by water and apple cider (Figures 8 and 9) showed similar WASPs. The first common characteristic is the decrease of the absorbance of adulterated SBH samples in the region 980–1035 nm. In this region, the higher the adulteration percentage the lower the absorbance, and this behavior can be noticed in regular steps of absorbance reduction. The lowest aquagram line in this region corresponds to pure adulterants (water and apple cider, which is a highly aqueous sample). The second common characteristic is the increase of absorbance in the region 939–970 nm, and a gradual shift towards the lower wavelengths with the increase in the percentage of adulteration. These observations are in agreement with the previous findings by Omar et al. [50] on the NIR spectral behavior of SBH adulterated with water. Particularly, it was noticed that the main NIR absorbance peak was related to water absorbance located around 950–1050 nm and that as the honey was diluted with the addition of water, the peak shifted towards lower wavelengths. Therefore, it can be concluded that the observed characteristics showed that the honey is becoming more liquid as it is more diluted by adulterants. In aquagrams, this process is represented by the restructuring of water that contains more weakly hydrogen-bonded water and free water as the percentage of adulterant is increased.

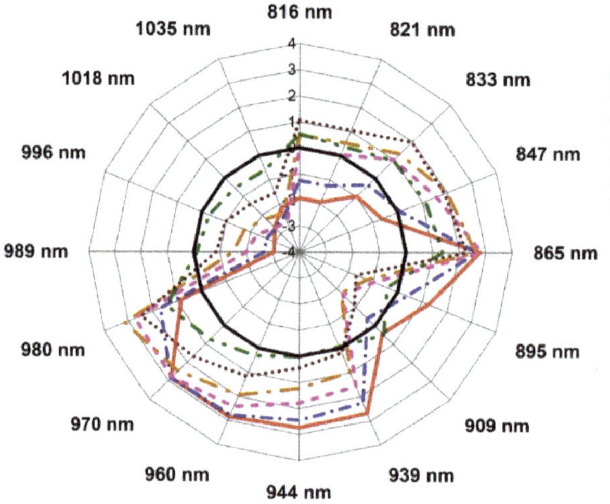

Figure 8. Aquagrams of pure SBH, water, and adulterated SBH with various percentages of water.

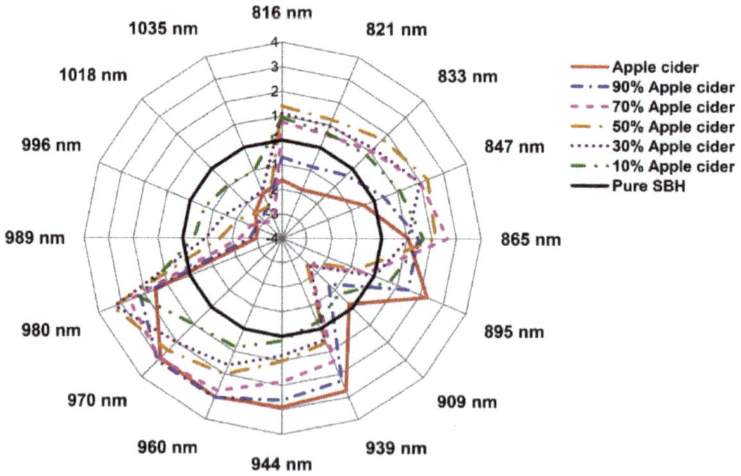

Figure 9. Aquagrams of pure SBH, apple cider vinegar, and adulterated SBH with various percentages of apple cider vinegar.

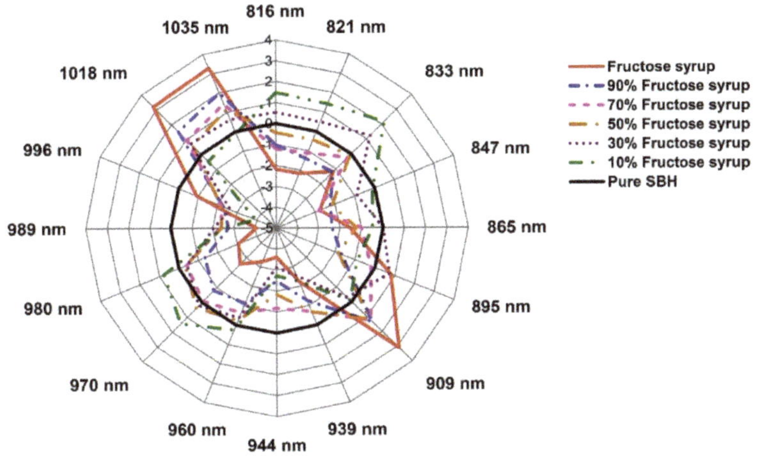

Figure 10. Aquagrams of pure SBH, fructose syrup, and adulterated SBH with various percentages of fructose syrup.

The bands 939 nm, 944 nm, 960 nm, 970 nm, and 980 nm correspond to overtones of the WAMACs located respectively at 1408.5 nm and 1416 nm (both bands can be assigned to free water molecules), 1440 nm (water dimer), 1455 nm (water hydration shell OH-$(H_2O)_{4,5}$ and bulk water), and 1470 nm (can be attributed to water molecules with 2 or 3 hydrogen bonds) [21]. In the region 980–1035 nm, the bands 989 nm and 996 nm can be ascribed to overtones of the WAMACs located at 1483.5 nm and 1494 nm (both bands corresponding to water molecules with 4 hydrogen bonds) [21]. The bands 1018 and 1035 nm are very close to the bands which are identified as NIR absorbance bands for water (1010 and 1030 nm) [61], while the band at 1020 nm is attributed to OH with possible H-bonding in water at 1–2 °C [62]. If it is assumed that both 1018 nm and 1035 nm bands are overtones of water bands in the first overtone of the water region, the recalculation would produce the wavelengths 1527 and 1552.5 nm, respectively. In the aquaphotomics application on honey adulteration by Bazar et al. [13], the bands 1528–1532 nm and 1564–1572 nm have high absorbance in pure honey and a decrease in a regular trend with the addition of adulterant, similar to the performance in this study. They attributed the bands above 1500 nm (in our case this would correspond to the bands above 1000 nm) to ice-like clusters of liquid water, formed by a very small amount of monomeric water species, a major part of it bound by one hydrogen bond at the periphery and two hydrogen bonds in the center. These structures represent highly organized water structures with strong H-bonds. The ice-like structures of liquid water are stable clusters with less free -OH and typically generated around macromolecules such as sugars [53]. It was shown that the addition of sugar decreases the amount of weakly H-bonded molecules, while it increases the number of H-bonded water molecules, resulting in highly organized water structures [63]. This means that these water structures include the main sugars in honey. In view of that, the bands 1018 nm and 1035 nm can be assigned to strongly hydrogen-bonded water in a crystallized form that is presented in pure honey due to the high sugar content; this water can also be thought of in terms of sugar–water interaction. The addition of water or apple cider acts on these structures as a heater, melting them and creating more weakly hydrogen-bonded water. These findings are in agreement with what was observed during the initial inspection of the raw spectra in Figure 1 and confirm that the origin of the scattering and changes in the baseline, that was so prominent in the case of adulteration by water and apple cider, are indeed due to the altered water–sugar interaction, with the increase of bulk and hydration water and changes in the crystallization of sugars in honey.

A similar decrease in absorbance at aquagrams for honey adulteration by both water and apple cider happens at the 909 nm band. This band was found to be strongly related to the sugar C-H group [51,64–67], and so it can be assigned to the sugar–water interaction. The entire 870–890 nm region can be attributed to carbohydrates [68], and the band at 895 nm may be related to some specific type in apple cider. The band at 895 nm clearly makes the difference in spectral patterns of honey adulterated by water and apple cider and is highly characteristic and presented with high absorbance in the case of apple cider. Alternatively, it may also be ascribed to the absorbance of protonated water clusters $H^+.(H_2O)_3$ [69]. The region 816–865 nm incorporates several overlapped spectroscopic features of compounds with C-H and O-H groups, including proteins, carbohydrates, hydrocarbons, alcohols, and water [62], with water being a stronger absorber around 830–840 nm [68,70].

The aquagram of SBH adulterated with fructose syrup in Figure 10 shows a spectral pattern quite different from those of Figures 8 and 9. With an increase in the percentage of fructose syrup, there is an increase in absorbance at 1018–1035 nm and 909 nm. The fructose syrup is a highly concentrated solution of sugars, and this agrees well with the assignments of these bands to the sugar–water interaction. These two features are the most prominent characteristic of honey adulterated with fructose syrup, while the absorbance shows a marked decrease at other bands. Adulteration with fructose syrup seems to obliterate the features of honey, resulting in a significant decline in absorbance at all bands, even when the adulteration is at the lowest level of 10%. Hence, it can be deduced that the adulteration of honey with fructose syrup is the most serious case compromising the honey's structure and functionality.

From the above discussion, our findings agree with the earlier reports about the effects of the adulteration of honey. A fast and simple method for the detection of SBH adulteration was presented using aquagrams for the region 800–1100 nm, where the most common photodetectors available in the market offer the best sensitivity [51]. For the development of a simple multispectral sensor, the results suggested that the bands at 865 nm and 980 nm have the highest specificity for the detection of the adulteration of SBH by water. In the case of apple cider vinegar, the highest specificity for adulteration detection was found at the bands 865 nm, 970 nm, and 980 nm, and lastly, for adulteration by fructose syrup, the bands at 847 nm, 939 nm, 944 nm, 989 nm, and 996 nm. Therefore, using eight wavelengths (847 nm, 865 nm, 939 nm, 944 nm, 970 nm, 980 nm, 989 nm, and 996 nm), a simple and multispectral portable measurement system for detecting SBH adulteration can be developed based on the method presented in this work, that allows for the detection of adulteration and the type of adulterant.

3. Materials and Methods

3.1. Honey Samples

The pure stingless bee honey (SBH) sample was purchased from MUKAS Stingless Bee Farm, which is located in Kedah, Malaysia. All samples were harvested in the year 2018, stored in airtight jars, and refrigerated until analysis.

3.2. Adulterants

The three types of adulterants used in this study were distilled water, apple cider vinegar, and high fructose syrup, which are common SBH adulterants used in the market. Both apple cider and fructose syrup were purchased from Sinaran Saintifik Enterprise, Penang, Malaysia.

3.3. Honey Adulteration Sample Preparation

The pure SBH samples were adulterated by three different types of adulterants, which were distilled water, apple cider vinegar, and high fructose syrup. The SBH samples were adulterated with various degrees of adulteration (10%, 20%, 30%, 40%, 50%, 60%, 70%, 80% and 90%). The mixture was classified as adulterated honey, and the sample was thoroughly shaken until a homogenous mixture was formed. Prior to analysis, the honey samples were stored in glass jars, in a dark place, at room temperature. The overall number of samples was 31, comprising 1 pure SBH sample (0%), 3 adulterants (100%), and 27 adulterated honey samples (10–90%). The adulterated SBH samples consisted of 3 groups of 9 samples each, adulterated with water, apple cider vinegar, and high fructose syrup, accordingly. The adulteration level was from 10 to 90% with an interval of 10%.

3.4. Vis-NIR Spectroscopy

The visible and near-infrared (Vis-NIR) absorbance spectroscopy measurement of the samples was conducted using the QE65000 spectroscopic system (Ocean Optics, Inc., Dunedin, FL, USA) with a spectral range between 400 and 1100 nm. Pure and adulterated honey samples in glass holders (1 cm × 1 cm) were scanned at room temperature (∼25 °C) using the QE65000 spectrometer. The absorbance measurement of the sample is relative to an empty cuvette and was calculated using Equation (1):

$$A_\lambda = -\log_{10}\left(\frac{S_\lambda - D_\lambda}{R_\lambda - S_\lambda}\right) \quad (1)$$

where:

A_λ is the absorbance at wavelength λ

S_λ is the intensity of light transmitted through the sample at wavelength λ

D_λ is the dark intensity at wavelength λ

R_λ is the intensity of light transmitted through the reference (empty cuvette)

3.5. Color Analysis

Color characteristics were determined using a Chromaticity Diagram template developed in the OriginPro 2021 Software Package (version 9.8, Origin Lab Corporation, Northampton, MA, USA). The template was designed to calculate the color parameters from the spectra according to the equations from the CIE Technical Committee [71]. The CIELAB color space was utilized [2,36,48,49], with reference to illuminant D65 and a visual angle of 10° (CIE 1964 Supplementary Standard Observer) [48,49]. The wavelength range used in the calculation was 380–780 nm [47].

3.6. Total Soluble Solids

The soluble solids content (SSC: °Brix) of the prepared samples was measured using a PAL-3 refractometer from Atago, Co. (Tokyo, Japan) with a range of measurements from 0 to 93 °Brix and a resolution of 0.1 °Brix.

3.7. Multivariate Analysis

First, the Vis-NIR spectral data were preprocessed with some transformations to minimize unwanted effects, that include baseline variation, light scattering, and path length variances [72]. A moving average smoothing with a segment size of 25 was performed to eliminate random variations of the data set and correct the scatter effect. Baseline correction was used to adjust the spectral offset. The first-order detrending transformation was used to remove the baseline of the signals in the spectral data [73] and detach the particular absorption features [74]. The first derivative order of Savitzky–Golay (SG) with 25 smoothing points was utilized to reduce the baseline variation and augment the spectral features [75].

A principal component analysis (PCA) was applied to study the clustering of the samples. The three-dimensional (3D) score plot and the corresponding loadings of the principal components (PCs) were presented for the pre-processed spectra. In addition, the partial least squares regression (PLSR) model was developed to quantify the adulteration level in honey samples. The regression model was validated by the full cross-validation method. The precision and accuracy of the PLSR model was evaluated by the determination coefficient (R^2) and the root mean square error (RMSE) of calibration and cross-validation

(R_C^2, R_{CV}^2, $RMSE_C$, $RMSE_{CV}$). A good model should have a high R^2 and a low RMSE. The PLSR models with 1–10 factors (latent variables 'LVs') were examined, and the optimal number of LVs was selected based on the lowest value of the $RMSE_{CV}$. Both PCA and PLSR were performed using the Unscrambler Software (version 10.4, CAMO Software AS, Oslo, Norway).

3.8. Aquagrams

An aquaphotomics analysis was applied to examine the influence of each adulterant depending on the concentration. The raw spectra were pre-processed using Savitzky–Golay's second-order polynomial smoothing with 21 points to remove noise, linear baseline correction to correct the baseline slope, and normal variate transformation (SNV) to remove the baseline offset. These pre-processing methods were applied on datasets split according to the adulterant type, because of the specific effects of each adulterant on the baseline. First, the loadings of PCA and regression coefficients of PLSR were inspected for consistently appearing and highly influential variables, that can be considered as Water Matrix Coordinates (WAMACs). Based on this evaluation, the wavelength region from 800 to 1100 nm was opted for aquaphotomics analysis, where 16 important absorbance bands were selected to be presented on the aquagrams. Afterwards, the absorbance values were normalized following the procedure for calculation of classic aquagrams [23], and the spectrum of pure honey was subtracted to allow for the comparison with the adulterated honey samples. The water absorbance spectral patterns (WASPs) of honey with each additive (water, apple cider, and syrup) were presented on aquagram plots featuring normalized absorbance and displayed on radar axes defined by selected WAMACs. Pre-processing was performed using the commercially available software Pirouette 4.0 (Infometrix Inc., Bothell, WA, USA), and the aquagrams were prepared in Microsoft Office Excel 2016 (Microsoft Co., Redmond, WA, USA) and depicted using the OriginPro 2021 Software Package (version 9.8, Origin Lab Corporation, Northampton, MA, USA).

4. Conclusions

The characteristics of pure and adulterated SBH were studied using visible (Vis) and near-infrared (NIR) spectroscopy. The SBH was adulterated with various adulterants, including distilled water, apple cider vinegar, and high fructose syrup, with a percentage ranging from 10% to 90%. The visible peak of the SBH was altered, but the shift in the visible peak was apparent only for the level of adulterants beyond 50%. On the other hand, the shift in NIR is only significant for SBH adulterated with water and apple cider, contributed by the change in the water structure of the samples. The classification of the adulterants and both pure and adulterated SBHs was attained using a principal component analysis (PCA). A partial least squares regression (PLSR) global model was developed to quantify the adulteration level in the honey samples. An optimum PLSR prediction model with $R_{CV}^2 = 0.96$ and $RMSE_{CV} = 5.88$ % was acquired. In conclusion, Vis-NIR absorbance spectroscopy at the region 400–1100 nm has proven a promising method in identifying the adulterated SBH. The alteration in the spectral attribute, however, is highly dependent on the nature of the liquid added to the pure SBH. Furthermore, the results showed that the region at 400–1100 nm that is related to the color and water properties of the samples is effective to discriminate and quantify the adulterated SBHs.

For the first time, the adulteration of SBH has been investigated using the combination of the spectroscopy technique and the aquaphotomics approach at the short-wavelength NIR region (800–1100 nm). The adulteration level in SBH including 10% was identified, irrespectively of the adulterant type. It was found that each adulterant resulted in a change in the spectral pattern of honey in a unique way that can be explained by the interaction of the adulterant with the chemical structure of honey. This method can be applied for developing highly sensitive and portable measurement systems for detecting adulterated SBH.

Supplementary Materials: The following supporting information can be downloaded at: https://www.mdpi.com/article/10.3390/molecules27072324/s1, Figure S1. CIE x, y chromaticity diagram showing the variation of color of the samples ($n = 31$). Figure S2. Zoom-in view of CIE x, y chromaticity diagram of the samples ($n = 31$). Figure S3. 2D scores plot of PC1 vs. PC2 of the samples ($n = 31$). Figure S4. 2D scores plot of PC1 vs. PC3 of the samples ($n = 31$). Figure S5. 2D scores plot of PC2 vs. PC3 of the samples ($n = 31$).

Author Contributions: Conceptualization, A.F.O.; methodology, A.F.O.; software, M.E.R. and J.M.; formal analysis, A.F.O., M.E.R. and J.M.; investigation, A.R.A.N.; resources, A.F.O.; data curation, A.R.A.N.; writing-original draft preparation, A.F.O.; writing-review and editing, M.E.R., M.Z. and J.M.; visualization and; supervision, A.F.O.; project administration and funding acquisition, A.F.O. All authors have read and agreed to the published version of the manuscript.

Funding: This research was funded by Tsuki no Shizuku Foundation, Japan of a research grant for aquaphotomics.

Institutional Review Board Statement: Not avalilable.

Informed Consent Statement: Not avalilable.

Data Availability Statement: Not avalilable.

Acknowledgments: The authors would like to thank and acknowledge the financial support of a research grant for aquaphotomics from Tsuki no Shizuku Foundation, Japan.

Conflicts of Interest: The authors declare no conflict of interest.

Sample Availability: Samples of the compounds are not available from the authors.

References

1. Ávila, S.; Hornung, P.S.; Teixeira, G.L.; Beux, M.R.; Lazzarotto, M.; Ribani, R.H. A chemometric spproach for moisture control in stingless bee honey using near infrared spectroscopy. *J. Near Infrared Spectrosc.* **2018**, *26*, 379–388. [CrossRef]
2. Valinger, D.; Longin, L.; Grbeš, F.; Benković, M.; Jurina, T.; Kljusurić, J.G.; Tušek, A.J. Detection of honey adulteration-The potential of UV-VIS and NIR spectroscopy coupled with multivariate analysis. *LWT Food Sci. Technol.* **2021**, *145*, 111316. [CrossRef]
3. Lastra-Mejías, M.; Izquierdo, M.; González-Flores, E.; Cancilla, J.C.; Izquierdo, J.G.; Torrecilla, J.S. Honey Exposed to laser-induced breakdown spectroscopy for chaos-based botanical classification and fraud assessment. *Chemom. Intell. Lab. Syst.* **2020**, *199*, 103939. [CrossRef]
4. Huang, F.; Song, H.; Guo, L.; Guang, P.; Yang, X.; Li, L.; Zhao, H.; Yang, M. Detection of adulteration in Chinese honey using NIR and ATR-FTIR spectral data fusion. *Spectrochim. Acta Part A Mol. Biomol. Spectrosc.* **2020**, *235*, 118297. [CrossRef] [PubMed]
5. Shiddiq, M.; Asyana, V.; Aliyah, H. Identification of Pure and Adulterated Honey Using Two Spectroscopic Methods. *J. Physic Conf. Ser.* **2019**, *1531*, 012022. [CrossRef]
6. Salvador, L.; Guijarro, M.; Rubio, D.; Aucatoma, B.; Guillén, T.; Vargas Jentzsch, P.; Ciobotă, V.; Stolker, L.; Ulic, S.; Vásquez, L.; et al. Exploratory Monitoring of the Quality and Authenticity of Commercial Honey in Ecuador. *Foods* **2019**, *8*, 105. [CrossRef]
7. Guelpa, A.; Marini, F.; du Plessis, A.; Slabbert, R.; Manley, M. Verification of authenticity and fraud detection in South African honey using NIR spectroscopy. *Food Control* **2017**, *73*, 1388–1396. [CrossRef]
8. Li, S.; Zhang, X.; Shan, Y.; Su, D.; Ma, Q.; Wen, R.; Li, J. Qualitative and quantitative detection of honey adulterated with high-fructose corn syrup and maltose syrup by using near-infrared spectroscopy. *Food Chem.* **2017**, *218*, 231–236. [CrossRef]
9. Yang, X.; Guang, P.; Xu, G.; Zhu, S.; Chen, Z.; Huang, F. Manuka honey adulteration detection based on near-infrared spectroscopy combined with aquaphotomics. *LWT* **2020**, *132*, 109837. [CrossRef]
10. Peng, J.; Xie, W.; Jiang, J.; Zhao, Z.; Zhou, F.; Liu, F. Fast Quantification of Honey Adulteration with Laser-Induced Breakdown Spectroscopy and Chemmometric Methods. *Foods* **2020**, *9*, 341. [CrossRef]
11. Elhamdaoui, O.; El Orche, A.; Cheikh, A.; Mojemmi, B.; Nejjari, R.; Bouatia, M. Development of Fast Analytical Methods for the Detection and Quantification of Honey Adulteration Using Vibrational Spectroscopy and Chemometrics Tools. *J. Anal. Methods Chem.* **2020**, *2020*, 8816249. [CrossRef] [PubMed]
12. Molnar, C.M.; Berghian-Grosan, C.; Magdas, D.A. An optimized green preparation method for the successful application of Raman spectroscopy in honey studies. *Talanta* **2020**, *208*, 120432. [CrossRef] [PubMed]
13. Bázár, G.; Romvári, R.; Szabó, A.; Somogyi, T.; Éles, V.; Tsenkova, R. NIR detection of honey adulteration reveals differences in water spectral pattern. *Food Chem.* **2016**, *194*, 873–880. [CrossRef] [PubMed]
14. Pimentel, T.C.; Rosset, M.; de Sousa, J.M.B.; de Oliveira, L.I.G.; Mafaldo, I.M.; Pintado, M.M.E.; de Souza, E.L.; Magnani, M. Stingless bee honey: An overview of health benefits and main market challenges. *J. Food Biochem.* **2021**, *46*, e13883. [CrossRef]
15. Chan, B.K.; Haron, H.; Talib, R.A.; Subramaniam, P. Physical properties, antioxidant content and anti-oxidative activities of Malaysian stingless kelulut (*Trigona* spp.) honey. *J. Agric. Sci.* **2017**, *9*, 32–40.

16. Mail, M.H.; Rahim, N.A.; Amanah, A.; Khawory, M.H.; Shahudin, M.A.; Seeni, A. FTIR and elementary analysis of Trigona honey, Apis honey and adulterated honey mixtures. *Biomed. Pharmacol. J.* **2019**, *12*, 2011–2017. [CrossRef]
17. Do Nascimento, A.S.; Marchini, L.C.; de Carvalho, C.A.L.; Araújo, D.F.D.; de Olinda, R.A.; da Silveira, T.A. Physical-chemical parameters of honey of stingless bee (Hymenoptera: Apidae). *Am. Chem. Sci. J.* **2015**, *7*, 139–149. [CrossRef]
18. Ramón-Sierra, J.M.; Ruiz-Ruiz, J.C.; de la Luz Ortiz-Vázquez, E. Electrophoresis characterisation of protein as a method to establish the entomological origin of stingless bee honeys. *Food Chem.* **2015**, *183*, 43–48. [CrossRef]
19. Bijlsma, L.; de Bruijn, L.L.; Martens, E.P.; Sommeijer, M.J. Water content of stingless bee honeys (Apidae, Meliponini): Interspecific variation and comparison with honey of Apis mellifera. *Apidologie* **2006**, *37*, 480–486. [CrossRef]
20. Muncan, J.; Tsenkova, R. Aquaphotomics—From innovative knowledge to integrative platform in science and technology. *Molecules* **2019**, *24*, 2742. [CrossRef]
21. Tsenkova, R. Aquaphotomics: Dynamic spectroscopy of aqueous and biological systems describes peculiarities of water. *J. Near Infrared Spectrosc.* **2009**, *17*, 303–313. [CrossRef]
22. Tsenkova, R. Aquaphotomics: Water in the biological and aqueous world scrutinised with invisible light. *Spectrosc. Eur.* **2010**, *22*, 6.
23. Tsenkova, R.; Munćan, J.; Pollner, B.; Kovacs, Z. Essentials of aquaphotomics and its chemometrics approaches. *Front. Chem.* **2018**, *6*, 363. [CrossRef] [PubMed]
24. Guerrini, A.; Bruni, R.; Maietti, S.; Poli, F.; Rossi, D.; Paganetto, G.; Muzzoli, M.; Scalvenzi, L.; Sacchetti, G. Ecuadorian stingless bee (Meliponinae) honey: A chemical and functional profile of an ancient health product. *Food Chem.* **2009**, *114*, 1413–1420. [CrossRef]
25. De Almeida-Muradian, L.B.; Stramm, K.M.; Estevinho, L.M. Efficiency of the FT-IR ATR spectrometry for the prediction of the physicochemical characteristics of M elipona subnitida honey and study of the temperature's effect on those properties. *Int. J. Food Sci. Technol.* **2014**, *49*, 188–195. [CrossRef]
26. Alimentarius, C. Revised codex standard for honey. *Codex Stan* **2001**, *12*, 1982.
27. Souza, B.A.; Roubik, D.W.; Barth, O.M.; Heard, T.A.; Enríquez, E.; Carvalho, C.; Villas-Bôas, J.; Marchini, L.; Locatelli, J.; Persano-Oddo, L.; et al. Composition of stingless bee honey: Setting quality standards. *Interciencia* **2006**, *31*, 867–875.
28. Shenk, J.S.; Workman, J.J., Jr.; Westerhaus, M.O. Application of NIR spectroscopy to agricultural products. In *Handbook of Near-Infrared Analysis*; CRC Press: Boca Raton, FL, USA, 2007; pp. 365–404.
29. Rust, A.; Marini, F.; Allsopp, M.; Williams, P.J.; Manley, M. Application of ANOVA-simultaneous component analysis to quantify and characterise effects of age, temperature, syrup adulteration and irradiation on near-infrared (NIR) spectral data of honey. *Spectrochim. Acta Part A Mol. Biomol. Spectrosc.* **2021**, *253*, 119546. [CrossRef]
30. Tsenkova, R.N.; Iordanova, I.K.; Toyoda, K.; Brown, D.R. Prion protein fate governed by metal binding. *Biochem. Biophys. Res. Commun.* **2004**, *325*, 1005–1012. [CrossRef]
31. Chatani, E.; Tsuchisaka, Y.; Masuda, Y.; Tsenkova, R. Water molecular system dynamics associated with amyloidogenic nucleation as revealed by real time near infrared spectroscopy and aquaphotomics. *PLoS ONE* **2014**, *9*, e101997. [CrossRef]
32. Martin, K. In vivo measurements of water in skin by near-infrared reflectance. *Appl. Spectrosc.* **1998**, *52*, 1001–1007. [CrossRef]
33. Abdel-Aal, E.M.; Ziena, H.; Youssef, M. Adulteration of honey with high-fructose corn syrup: Detection by different methods. *Food Chem.* **1993**, *48*, 209–212. [CrossRef]
34. Bidin, N.; Zainuddin, N.H.; Islam, S.; Abdullah, M.; Marsin, F.M.; Yasin, M. Sugar detection in adulterated honey via fiber optic displacement sensor for food industrial applications. *IEEE Sens. J.* **2015**, *16*, 299–305. [CrossRef]
35. Nikolova, K.; Panchev, I.; Sainov, S.; Gentscheva, G.; Ivanova, E. Selected physical properties of lime bee honey in order to discriminate between pure honey and honey adulterated with glucose. *Int. J. Food Prop.* **2012**, *15*, 1358–1368. [CrossRef]
36. Bertoncelj, J.; Doberšek, U.; Jamnik, M.; Golob, T. Evaluation of the phenolic content, antioxidant activity and colour of Slovenian honey. *Food Chem.* **2007**, *105*, 822–828. [CrossRef]
37. Lanza, E.; Li, B. Application for near infrared spectroscopy for predicting the sugar content of fruit juices. *J. Food Sci.* **1984**, *49*, 995–998. [CrossRef]
38. Aliaño-González, M.J.; Ferreiro-González, M.; Espada-Bellido, E.; Palma, M.; Barbero, G.F. A screening method based on Visible-NIR spectroscopy for the identification and quantification of different adulterants in high-quality honey. *Talanta* **2019**, *203*, 235–241. [CrossRef]
39. Lenhardt, L.; Bro, R.; Zeković, I.; Dramićanin, T.; Dramićanin, M.D. Fluorescence spectroscopy coupled with PARAFAC and PLS DA for characterization and classification of honey. *Food Chem.* **2015**, *175*, 284–291. [CrossRef]
40. Peters, R.D.; Noble, S.D. Using near infrared measurements to evaluate NaCl and KCl in water. *J. Near Infrared Spectrosc.* **2019**, *27*, 147–155. [CrossRef]
41. Li, H.; Yang, W.; Lei, J.; She, J.; Zhou, X. Estimation of leaf water content from hyperspectral data of different plant species by using three new spectral absorption indices. *PLoS ONE* **2021**, *16*, e0249351. [CrossRef]
42. Das, B.; Sahoo, R.N.; Pargal, S.; Krishna, G.; Verma, R.; Viswanathan, C.; Sehgal, V.K.; Gupta, V.K. Evaluation of different water absorption bands, indices and multivariate models for water-deficit stress monitoring in rice using visible-near infrared spectroscopy. *Spectrochim. Acta Part A Mol. Biomol. Spectrosc.* **2021**, *247*, 119104. [CrossRef] [PubMed]
43. Vembadi, A.; Menachery, A.; Qasaimeh, M.A. Cell cytometry: Review and perspective on biotechnological advances. *Front. Bioeng. Biotechnol.* **2019**, *7*, 147. [CrossRef] [PubMed]

44. Nordin, A.; Sainik, N.Q.A.V.; Chowdhury, S.R.; Saim, A.B.; Idrus, R.B.H. Physicochemical properties of stingless bee honey from around the globe: A comprehensive review. *J. Food Compos. Anal.* **2018**, *73*, 91–102. [CrossRef]
45. Pontis, J.A.; Costa, L.A.M.A.D.; Silva, S.J.R.D.; Flach, A. Color, phenolic and flavonoid content, and antioxidant activity of honey from Roraima, Brazil. *Food Sci. Technol.* **2014**, *34*, 69–73. [CrossRef]
46. Belay, A.; Solomon, W.K.; Bultossa, G.; Adgaba, N.; Melaku, S. Botanical origin, colour, granulation, and sensory properties of the Harenna forest honey, Bale, Ethiopia. *Food Chem.* **2015**, *167*, 213–219. [CrossRef]
47. Bodor, Z.; Benedek, C.; Urbin, Á.; Szabó, D.; Sipos, L. Colour of honey: Can we trust the Pfund scale?–An alternative graphical tool covering the whole visible spectra. *LWT* **2021**, *149*, 111859. [CrossRef]
48. Shamsudin, S.; Selamat, J.; Sanny, M.; Abd Razak, S.B.; Jambari, N.N.; Mian, Z.; Khatib, A. Influence of origins and bee species on physicochemical, antioxidant properties and botanical discrimination of stingless bee honey. *Int. J. Food Prop.* **2019**, *22*, 239–264. [CrossRef]
49. González-Miret, M.L.; Terrab, A.; Hernanz, D.; Fernández-Recamales, M.Á.; Heredia, F.J. Multivariate correlation between color and mineral composition of honeys and by their botanical origin. *J. Agric. Food Chem.* **2005**, *53*, 2574–2580. [CrossRef]
50. Omar, A.F.; Yahaya, O.K.M.; Tan, K.C.; Mail, M.H.; Seeni, A. The influence of additional water content towards the spectroscopy and physicochemical properties of genus Apis and stingless bee honey. In *Optical Sensing and Detection IV*; International Society for Optics and Photonics: Bellingham, WA, USA, 2016.
51. Omar, A.F.; Atan, H.; MatJafri, M.Z. Peak response identification through near-infrared spectroscopy analysis on aqueous sucrose, glucose, and fructose solution. *Spectrosc. Lett.* **2012**, *45*, 190–201. [CrossRef]
52. Fletcher, M.T.; Hungerford, N.L.; Webber, D.; Carpinelli de Jesus, M.; Zhang, J.; Stone, I.S.; Blanchfield, J.T.; Zawawi, N. Stingless bee honey, a novel source of trehalulose: A biologically active disaccharide with health benefits. *Sci. Rep.* **2020**, *10*, 1–8. [CrossRef]
53. Giangiacomo, R. Study of water–sugar interactions at increasing sugar concentration by NIR spectroscopy. *Food Chem.* **2006**, *96*, 371–379. [CrossRef]
54. Bakier, S. Application of NIR spectroscopy for the analysis of water-carbohydrate interactions in water solutions. *Acta Agrophys* **2008**, *11*, 7–21.
55. Kovacs, Z.; Bázár, G.; Oshima, M.; Shigeoka, S.; Tanaka, M.; Furukawa, A.; Nagai, A.; Osawa, M.; Itakura, Y.; Tsenkova, R. Water spectral pattern as holistic marker for water quality monitoring. *Talanta* **2016**, *147*, 598–608. [CrossRef]
56. Šašić, S.; Ozaki, Y. Short-wave near-infrared spectroscopy of biological fluids. 1. Quantitative analysis of fat, protein, and lactose in raw milk by partial least-squares regression and band assignment. *Anal. Chem.* **2001**, *73*, 64–71. [CrossRef] [PubMed]
57. Tsenkova, R.; Muncan, J. *Aquaphotomics for Bio-Diagnostics in Dairy: Applications of Near-Infrared Spectroscopy*; Springer: Singapore, 2021.
58. Bakhsheshi, M.F.; Lee, T.-Y. *Non-Invasive Monitoring of Brain Temperature by Near-Infrared Spectroscopy*; Taylor & Francis: Milton Park, UK, 2015; Volume 2, pp. 31–32.
59. Osborne, B.G. Near-infrared spectroscopy in food analysis. *Encycl. Anal. Chem. Appl. Theory Instrum.* **2006**, *2*, 31–32.
60. Da Silva, P.M.; Gauche, C.; Gonzaga, L.V.; Costa, A.C.O.; Fett, R. Honey: Chemical composition, stability and authenticity. *Food Chem.* **2016**, *196*, 309–323. [CrossRef] [PubMed]
61. Murray, I.; Williams, P.; Norris, K. *Near-Infrared Technology in the Agricultural and Food Industries*; American Association of Cereal Chemists: St. Paul, MN, USA, 1987.
62. Williams, P.; Manley, M.; Antoniszyn, J. *Near Infrared Technology: Getting the Best out of Light*; African Sun Media: Stellenbosch, South Africa, 2019.
63. Bázár, G.; Kovacs, Z.; Tanaka, M.; Furukawa, A.; Nagai, A.; Osawa, M.; Itakura, Y.; Sugiyama, H.; Tsenkova, R. Water revealed as molecular mirror when measuring low concentrations of sugar with near infrared light. *Anal. Chim. Acta* **2015**, *896*, 52–62. [CrossRef]
64. Golic, M.; Walsh, K.; Lawson, P. Short-wavelength near-infrared spectra of sucrose, glucose, and fructose with respect to sugar concentration and temperature. *Appl. Spectrosc.* **2003**, *57*, 139–145. [CrossRef]
65. Miyamoto, K.; Kitano, Y. Non-destructive determination of sugar content in satsuma mandarin fruit by near infrared transmittance spectroscopy. *J. Near Infrared Spectrosc.* **1995**, *3*, 227–237. [CrossRef]
66. Guthrie, J.; Reid, D.; Walsh, K.B. Assessment of internal quality attributes of mandarin fruit. 2. NIR calibration model robustness. *Aust. J. Agric. Res.* **2005**, *56*, 417–426. [CrossRef]
67. Mekonnen, B.K.; Yang, W.; Hsieh, T.H.; Liaw, S.K.; Yang, F.L. Accurate prediction of glucose concentration and identification of major contributing features from hardly distinguishable near-infrared spectroscopy. *Biomed. Signal Processing Control* **2020**, *59*, 101923. [CrossRef]
68. McGlone, V.A.; Kawano, S. Firmness, dry-matter and soluble-solids assessment of postharvest kiwifruit by NIR spectroscopy. *Postharvest Biol. Technol.* **1998**, *13*, 131–141. [CrossRef]
69. Headrick, J.M.; Diken, E.G.; Walters, R.S.; Hammer, N.I.; Christie, R.A.; Cui, J.; Myshakin, E.M.; Duncan, M.A.; Johnson, M.A.; Jordan, K.D. Spectral signatures of hydrated proton vibrations in water clusters. *Science* **2005**, *308*, 1765–1769. [CrossRef] [PubMed]
70. Workman, J., Jr. *The Handbook of Organic Compounds, Three-Volume Set: Nir, ir, r, and Uv-Vis Spectra Featuring Polymers and Surfactants*; Elsevier: Amsterdam, The Netherlands, 2000.
71. Illumination, I.C.o. *CIE 15: Technical Report: Colorimetry*; CIE Technical Committee: Vienna, Austria, 2004.

72. Tigabu, M.; Odén, P.C. Multivariate classification of sound and insect-infested seeds of a tropical multipurpose tree, Cordia africana, with near infrared reflectance spectroscopy. *J. Near Infrared Spectrosc.* **2002**, *10*, 45–51. [CrossRef]
73. Barnes, R.; Dhanoa, M.S.; Lister, S.J. Standard normal variate transformation and de-trending of near-infrared diffuse reflectance spectra. *Appl. Spectrosc.* **1989**, *43*, 772–777. [CrossRef]
74. Dotto, A.C.; Dalmolin, R.S.D.; Grunwald, S.; ten Caten, A.; Pereira Filho, W. Two preprocessing techniques to reduce model covariables in soil property predictions by Vis-NIR spectroscopy. *Soil Tillage Res.* **2017**, *172*, 59–68. [CrossRef]
75. Wang, L.; Lee, F.S.; Wang, X.; He, Y. Feasibility study of quantifying and discriminating soybean oil adulteration in camellia oils by attenuated total reflectance MIR and fiber optic diffuse reflectance NIR. *Food Chem.* **2006**, *95*, 529–536. [CrossRef]

molecules

MDPI

Article

Revealing the Effect of Heat Treatment on the Spectral Pattern of Unifloral Honeys Using Aquaphotomics

Zsanett Bodor [1,2], Csilla Benedek [2], Balkis Aouadi [1], Viktoria Zsom-Muha [1] and Zoltan Kovacs [1,*]

1 Department of Measurements and Process Control, Institute of Food Science and Technology, Hungarian University of Agriculture and Life Sciences, 14-16 Somlói Street, H-1118 Budapest, Hungary; bodor.zsanett@phd.uni-mate.hu (Z.B.); aouadi.balkis@phd.uni-mate.hu (B.A.); zsomne.muha.viktoria@uni-mate.hu (V.Z.-M.)

2 Department of Dietetics and Nutrition, Faculty of Health Sciences, Semmelweis University, 17 Vas Street, H-1088 Budapest, Hungary; benedek.csilla@se-etk.hu

* Correspondence: kovacs.zoltan.food@uni-mate.hu

Abstract: In this study we aimed to investigate the effect of heat treatment on the spectral pattern of honey using near infrared spectroscopy (NIRS). For the research, sunflower, bastard indigo, and acacia honeys were collected from entrusted beekeepers. The honeys were not subject to any treatment before. Samples were treated at 40 °C, 60 °C, 80 °C, and 100 °C for 60, 120, 180, and 240 min. This resulted in 17 levels, including the untreated control samples. The 5-hydroxymethylfurfural (HMF) content of the honeys was determined using the Winkler method. NIRS spectra were recorded using a handheld instrument. Data analysis was performed using ANOVA for the HMF content and multivariate analysis for the NIRS data. For the latter, PCA, PCA-LDA, and PLSR models were built (using the 1300–1600 nm spectral range) and the wavelengths presenting the greatest change induced by the perturbations of temperature and time intervals were collected systematically, based on the difference spectra and the weights of the models. The most contributing wavelengths were used to visualize the spectral pattern changes on the aquagrams in the specific water matrix coordinates. Our results showed that the heat treatment highly contributed to the formation of free or less bonded water, however, the changes in the spectral pattern highly depended on the crystallization phase and the honey type.

Keywords: honey; heat treatment; NIRS; chemometrics; aquagram; PCA; PCA-LDA; PLRS; WAMACs; HMF

Citation: Bodor, Z.; Benedek, C.; Aouadi, B.; Zsom-Muha, V.; Kovacs, Z. Revealing the Effect of Heat Treatment on the Spectral Pattern of Unifloral Honeys Using Aquaphotomics. *Molecules* **2022**, *27*, 780. https://doi.org/10.3390/molecules27030780

Academic Editor: Stefano Materazzi

Received: 11 December 2021
Accepted: 21 January 2022
Published: 25 January 2022

1. Introduction

Honey, as a natural sweetener used since ancient times [1], is a perfect candidate for the increasing demand for unprocessed, natural, and "healthy" products. According to the literature, honey is produced by honeybees (*Apis mellifera*) from the nectar and sap of living plants or honeydew [2,3]. Owing to its valuable nutritional composition and relatively high price on the market, it represents an important value for the consumers. Honey is composed of sugars (95% of the dry matter content [4]), water (<20%) and numerous nutritious compounds, such as minerals, amino acids, vitamins, and phytochemicals [5,6]. The composition of honey is highly influenced by both botanical and geographical origin [6]. However, there are other factors—for example storage conditions or processing—that can have an impact on the composition and sensory characteristics (e.g., aroma, color) of honey [7,8]. The processing of honey includes heat treatment, which is often applied for the elimination of the crystals or to delay crystallization.

Honey crystallization is a naturally occurring process, depending mainly on the ratio of fructose and glucose and the water/glucose fraction. Other factors, such as the presence of pollen and other particles can also influence the crystallization process. Honeys with a higher glucose content (28–30 g/100 g), fructose/glucose ratio < 1.14 and/or glucose/moisture ratio ≥ 2.1 crystallize faster. The crystals are usually not preferred by the consumers due to the unpleasant organoleptic properties of the (rough) crystals [9,10]. Moreover, the crystallized state makes the handling of honey more difficult for the producers and beekeepers. Therefore, heat treatment can be applied for the liquefaction of honey, for which numerous methods are available [11]. The most common techniques are the treatment in chambers by hot air or water bath. Nowadays, different types of honey heater equipments are also available [12,13]. According to Hungarian regulations, the core temperature of honey cannot exceed 40 °C during the processing of honey [14], because at higher temperature levels the composition of honey changes significantly [15]. Other adverse aspects are also noticeable, including, but not limited to, changes of taste/aroma [16–18], decay of vitamins [19], changes of the color [9,10,20,21], Maillard-reaction-induced decrease or increase of antioxidants [9,22,23], decrease of enzyme activity (diastase, invertase), and formation of hydroxymethylfurfural (HMF) [7,10,13,18,19,24]. These attributes also change during long-term normal storage, but heating, especially above 50 °C, highly accelerates these processes. One of the most important indicators of heat treatment is the HMF content, which cannot be higher than 40 mg/kg in honeys (except honeys from tropical regions, where the limit is 80 mg/kg) [2,3,25]. Nevertheless, even at temperatures lower than 60 °C, significant changes can occur in terms of the composition and sensory properties of honey. However, based on the literature, the detection of heat treatment below 60 °C can be challenging when based on HMF content as the sole indicator [16,18,26–28].

Currently, multivariate, correlative techniques can offer fingerprint-like information on the analytes, thus representing powerful alternatives to conventional methods. As one of these techniques, near infrared spectroscopy (NIRS) has already been applied to detect the changes deriving from heat treatment [18,29,30]. A new application field of NIRS, called aquaphotomics, aims to check the changes in the water structure of the samples as a result of different perturbations [31]. As honey is a supersaturated solution of sugars in water, the aquaphotomics approach could be a perfect choice for the detection of overheating or other mishandling of honey. Previously, aquaphotomics has been applied to detect changes in honey resulting from adulteration with sugar syrups [32–35]. However, to the best of the authors knowledge, the aquaphotomics approach has never been applied to evaluate the effect of heat treatment on the compositional changes of honey.

Therefore, this study intends to investigate the effect of heat treatment on the spectral pattern of unifloral honeys using aquaphotomics.

2. Results

2.1. HMF Content of the Honeys

The initial HMF contents of the three investigated honey types were different: sunflower honeys had an average HMF content of 18.55 ± 0.28 mg/kg, bastard indigo honeys presented 14.68 ± 1.61 mg/kg, and acacia honeys contained 6.96 ± 0.38 mg/kg (Table 1.). These all fulfill the requirements of the legislation (maximum 40 mg/kg) [2,3]. Based on the two-way ANOVA test, the effect of time interval, temperature, and their interaction was found to significantly affect the HMF content of all of the studied honey samples.

No significant difference was found among time intervals within the 40 °C group in sunflower, bastard indigo, and acacia honeys. In the case of the 60 °C group, no clear trend was observed. However, in the case of the honeys heated to 80 °C and 100 °C, the samples heat treated for 60 min had significantly lower HMF content compared to honeys heat treated for 120, 180, and 240 min. Moreover, an increasing trend can be observed in the 80 °C and 100 °C groups with the increase of the treatment time.

In the case of the honeys heat treated for 60 min, the sunflower and acacia honeys treated at 100 °C had higher HMF contents compared to the lower temperatures when the effect of temperature within time intervals was evaluated. Honey samples heat treated for 120 min showed different results in the case of the three honey types. The HMF values of the sunflower honey (120 min group) showed that all the samples were significantly different from each other and the HMF value increased with the increase of the temperature. Results of the bastard indigo honey showed that only the honeys heat treated at 100 °C showed significantly higher HMF contents compared to the lower temperature groups. Acacia honey showed no significant differences between 40 °C and 60 °C, while the 80 °C group had significantly higher HMF contents than the honeys heated at lower temperature levels; the same applied for the 100 °C treated group. The same trend was found in the case of acacia honey for 180 min and 240 min treated honeys. The groups of the 180 min and 240 min treatment of sunflower honey showed that only the 80 °C and 100 °C treated honeys differed significantly from the other temperature levels. In the case of the bastard indigo honey samples heated for 180 min, only the honeys heated at 100 °C showed a significantly higher HMF compared to the honeys heated at lower temperatures. The sunflower honeys heated for 240 min showed the same trend as the bastard indigo and acacia honeys.

Table 1. Results of the HMF content of the honey samples from the heat treatment experiment.

		Hydroxymethylfurfural Content, mg/kg				
		Control	**40 °C**	**60 °C**	**80 °C**	**100 °C**
Sunflower	**Control**	18.5 ± 0.3				
	60 min		20.2 ± 1.5 ^{aA}	16.2 ± 1 ^{aA}	17.6 ± 0.2 ^{aA}	40.3 ± 0.8 ^{aB*}
	120 min		17.3 ± 1.3 ^{aA}	20.5 ± 0.7 ^{bB}	31.8 ± 1.3 ^{bC*}	155.1 ± 2.7 ^{bD*}
	180 min		18.4 ± 1.6 ^{aA}	19.9 ± 1.8 ^{bA}	37.2 ± 0.6 ^{cB*}	241.5 ± 7.4 ^{cC*}
	240 min		17.5 ± 1.4 ^{aA}	19.5 ± 2 ^{abA}	52 ± 2.7 ^{dB*}	463.6 ± 28.3 ^{dC*}
Bastard indigo **	**Control**	14.7 ± 1.6				
	60 min		14.1 ± 2.8 ^{aAB}	18 ± 2.3 ^{abB}	11.9 ± 1.1 ^{aA}	16.7 ± 0.9 ^{aAB}
	120 min		15.1 ± 3.5 ^{aA}	15.8 ± 0.6 ^{abA}	14.3 ± 1 ^{bA}	81.4 ± 4 ^{bB*}
	180 min		15.7 ± 1.1 ^{aA}	21.1 ± 3.5 ^{bA}	19.8 ± 0.6 ^{cA}	146.4 ± 2.3 ^{cB*}
	240 min		12.9 ± 1.4 ^{aA}	13.7 ± 1.3 ^{aA}	28.2 ± 1.1 ^{dB}	306 ± 17.8 ^{dC*}
Acacia	**Control**	7.0 ± 0.4				
	60 min		9.1 ± 1.3 ^{aA}	7.7 ± 0.3 ^{aA}	8 ± 0.4 ^{aA}	16.1 ± 1.7 ^{aB*}
	120 min		8 ± 0.6 ^{aA}	8.8 ± 1.4 ^{aA}	13.3 ± 0.9 ^{bB*}	44.7 ± 4.3 ^{bC*}
	180 min		8.6 ± 1 ^{aA}	9.6 ± 0.3 ^{aA}	12.2 ± 0.8 ^{bB*}	89.1 ± 2.8 ^{cC*}
	240 min		10 ± 1.1 ^{aA}	9.6 ± 0.9 ^{aA}	18.8 ± 2.4 ^{cB*}	211.6 ± 5 ^{dC*}

Letters represent the significant differences between the samples based on the results of an ANOVA test and pairwise comparisons at $p < 0.05$: lowercase letters (a,b,c,d) stand for the differences between time intervals (columns) within a temperature level; capital letters (A,B,C,D) are for the differences between temperature levels within time intervals (rows); * are for a significantly different level compared to the control sample. ** Results of bastard indigo were previously presented at a conference [29].

Sunflower and acacia honey samples heat treated at 80 °C for 120 min or longer, and the samples heated at 100 °C (all time intervals) showed significantly higher HMF contents compared to control. In the case of the bastard indigo honey, only the samples heated at 100 °C for 120, 180, 240 min had a significantly higher HMF than that of the control. Moreover, it should be highlighted that the limit (40 mg/kg) was reached only in the case of the 100 °C treatment of the bastard indigo and acacia honeys, whereas for sunflower honey, the temperature level of 80 °C and duration of 240 min induced a higher value than the limit. This shows that longer low-level heat treatments and even higher temperatures are not detected by this conventional method, however, even at these lower temperatures (from 60 °C) irreversible changes occur in honeys. Our results are in line with the work of Romanian researchers who also found that more intense HMF formation occurred at higher temperatures, such as 100 °C [24]. Bogdanov [36] also showed that the HMF limit of 40 mg/kg could be reached after one or two days at 60 °C or after a month at 40 °C. However, in a Hungarian study it has been shown that the sensory properties of honey such as the flavor, color, consistency, and odor changed at lower temperatures [37]; the global taste was already affected at 40 °C and 60 °C, based on the results obtained by the potentiometric electronic tongue. Moreover, the group also found that the color changed significantly at 50 °C and 60 °C [18].

The differences in the formation of HMF and the trends observed could originate from the fact that the initial pH, free acidity, amino acid, and sugar composition (especially fructose ratio) of the three honey types are different, which could have a significant impact on the formation of HMF [38].

The obtained results demonstrate the poor ability of HMF to indicate heat treatments of honey samples and thus the need for additional or alternative methods that can provide a higher sensitivity in the detection of such processes that may be misleading to consumers. As such, NIRS and specifically aquaphotomics may be involved in the quality authentication of honeys.

2.2. *Models of the Botanical Origin of Honey Types*

The NIRS-based models built for the discrimination of the three types of honey (acacia, sunflower, and bastard indigo) not subjected to any heat treatment (control samples) showed that all the three groups can be separated from each other with 100% accuracy using principal-component-analysis-based linear discriminant analysis (PCA-LDA) (Figure 1a). The aquagram of the honeys also showed completely different spectral patterns for the three honey types. While sunflower honey was mainly characterized by high absorbances at the wavelengths attributed to highly hydrogen-bonded water (1511 nm and 1489 nm), the most abundant water molecular structures for acacia honey consisted of water shells (1363 nm), combinations of antisymmetric and symmetric stretching modes of water and V1- and V2-bonded water [39]. Similar to sunflower honey, bastard indigo honey also presented peaks located at the water matrix coordinates (WAMACs), associated with strongly hydrogen-bounded water molecules, but also at regions attributed to free water (1412 nm), thus attesting the complexity of the physicochemical composition and the crystallization phase of each of the studied honeys (Figure 1b).

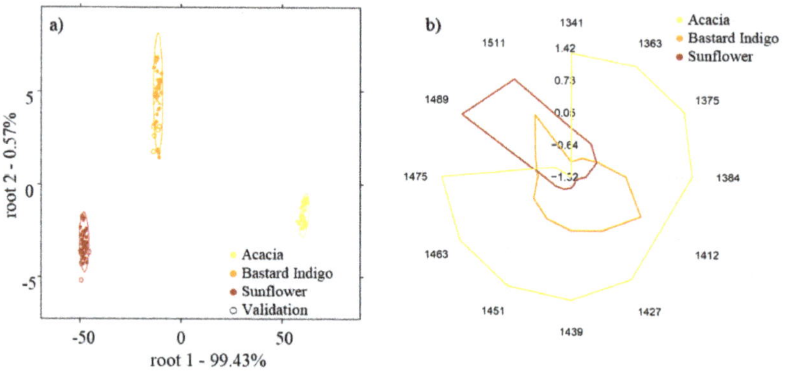

Figure 1. Differentiation of the botanical origin of the three control honeys: (**a**) PCA-LDA score plot for the discrimination of the botanical origin and (**b**) aquagrams of the honey samples of different botanical origins.

2.3. *Results of the Principal Component Analysis*

Principal component analysis calculated separately for the three honey (acacia, sunflower, bastard indigo) types showed similar results. In the case of the sunflower honey (Figure 2), there was a discrimination pattern through PC1 that described 99.40% of the variance. The group of control samples was completely separated from the scores of honey samples treated at different temperatures (40, 60, 80, 100 °C) and showed a slight overlapping with the honey samples treated at 40 °C. The higher treatment levels overlapped with each other. In this case the 1347 nm, 1446 nm, 1527 nm, and 1576 nm values contributed to the formation of PC1. The PCA model of heating time separation also showed a discrimination tendency through PC1 that described 97.57% of the variance. Values obtained at 1316 nm, 1405 nm, 1446 nm, 1489 nm, 1524 nm, 1553 nm, and 1585 nm contributed to the formation of PC1. In this case, the control slightly overlapped with the honeys treated for 60 min. However, it can also be seen that there are separated subgroups in each time treatment group, which shows the higher effect of the temperature on the spectra of honey.

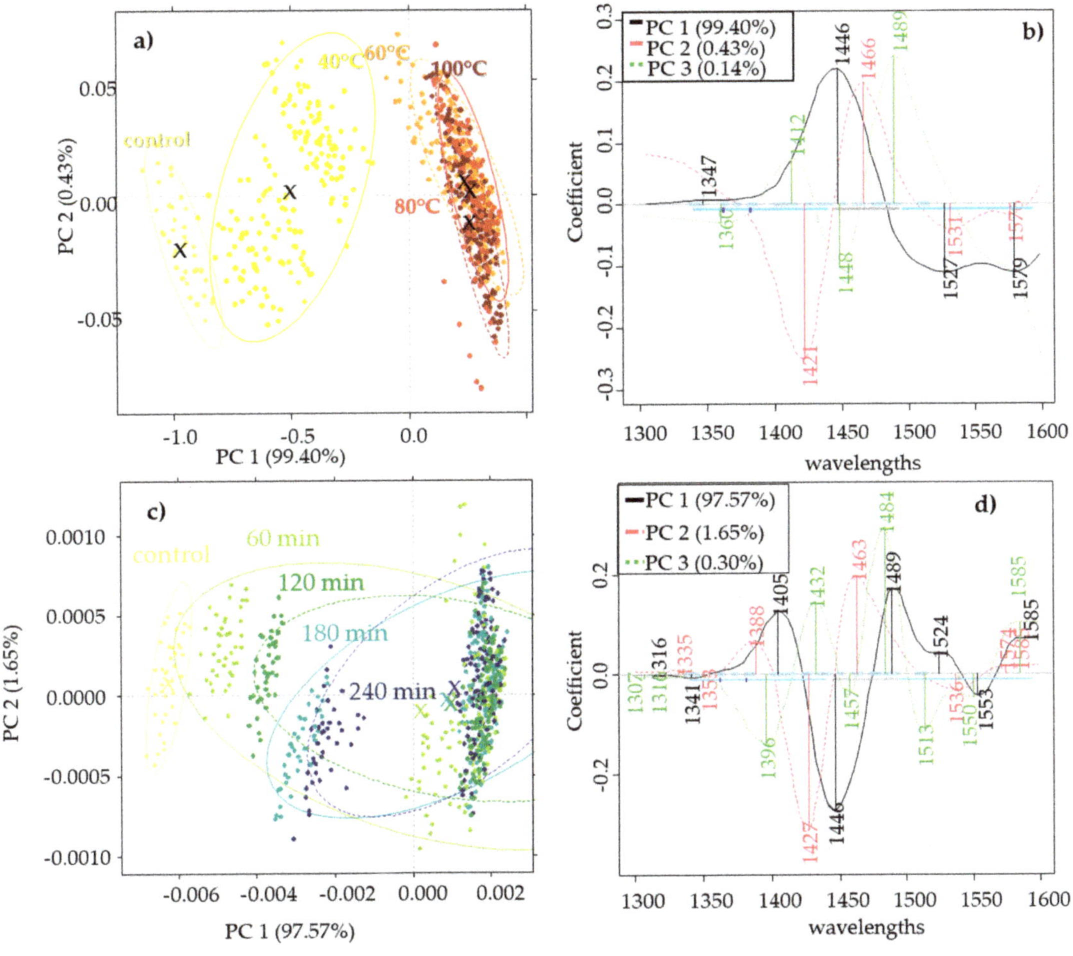

Figure 2. Principal component analysis of the control and heat-treated sunflower honeys: (**a**) PCA score plot for temperature pattern visualization with a Savitzky–Golay smoothing (window size 13) and SNV pretreatment; (**b**) the respective PCA loading plot; (**c**) PCA score plot for the time pattern visualization with a Savitzky–Golay smoothing (window size 13) and Savitzky–Golay 2nd derivative (window size 13, 2nd order derivative) pretreatment; (**d**) the respective PCA loading plot.

In the case of the bastard indigo honey, the trends were similar to the sunflower honeys, where the 1534 nm and 1582 nm values contributed to PC1 with the highest weight. The model built to visualize the effect of time intervals showed that the values obtained at 1335 nm, 1448 nm, 1531 nm, and 1579 nm had the highest contribution to PC1, however, in this case, there was no obvious separation trend based on the time intervals.

In the case of acacia honey, the trends were not as obvious as in the case of the other two honey types. The PCA model presenting the temperature pattern showed only a slight separation tendency through the first two principal components. PC1 was mainly obtained by the wavelengths at 1405 nm, 1454 nm, 1524, and 1565 nm. The model depicting the time pattern did not show any clear trend for the separation of the time intervals.

The wavelengths contributing to the model illustrating the temperature level patterns showed that in the case of all the honey types, the regions at 1524–1534 nm and 1582–1585 nm were the most affected ones. The region at 1524–1553 nm can be assigned to the ionic hydrogen bonding vibration in $OH-(H_2O)_{2-4}$ [40], while the 1582–1585 nm region is characteristic of fructose, sucrose, and glucose [32].

The models showing the pattern of time interval discrimination were also similar where 1316 nm and 1335 nm could be assigned to the weakly H-bonded water. The domination of the free -OH is related to this region. The peaks at 1405 nm, and 1432 nm and 1446 nm are related to the free water and water molecules with one hydrogen bond, respectively, while the region at 1448–1454 nm can be assigned to the $OH-(H_2O)_{4,5}$ water solvation shell. The assigned wavelengths also revealed that water molecules with four hydrogen bonds were also formed by the heat treatment (1489 nm) [32,41].

Similar results were obtained in a Hungarian study investigating low-level heat treatment of honeys (at 40, 50, and 60 °C for 30, 60, and 120 min) using near-infrared spectroscopy in the range of 950–1630 nm. In this research, the sunflower honeys showed a similar trend based on the PCA, the separation of the control sample was clear and a slight overlapping was found with the 40 °C treated samples, however, the 60 °C treated honeys separated completely from the control honey [18]. However, no clear separation tendency was observed for the acacia honeys.

2.4. Results of the PCA-LDA Analysis

The general (including all the sublevels of time and temperature treatments) PCA-LDA models, built separately for each honey type, did not provide strong classification accuracies in the case of the different honey types. The general model built for the classification of the different temperature levels showed average training (recognition) and cross-validation (prediction) accuracies of 80.18% and 68.79%, 82.24% and 75.95%, and 64.82% and 48.44% for the sunflower, bastard indigo, and acacia honeys, respectively. The models of the time interval classifications weren't effective with 52.70% and 35.29%, 63.78% and 41.33%, 47.38% and 25.93% accuracies for the sunflower, bastard indigo and acacia honeys, respectively. However, the detailed (i.e., built for the classification of time intervals within temperature levels, or built for the classification of temperature levels within time intervals) models provided better classification accuracies.

In Figure 3a,b, an example of the PCA-LDA score plot for the discrimination of the temperature or time interval of the applied heat treatment within the time or temperature groups, respectively, is showcased (detailed models). Loadings on the plot show the 20 wavelengths that contributed the most to the separation of the groups.

In each of the models, the presented results were chosen from 41 pretreatment combinations after a leave-one-sample-out cross-validation, based on the best validation accuracy.

Detailed temperature-level PCA-LDA models (Table 2 upper part) provided the best results in the case of the sunflower honey. Honeys heated for 240 min showed a 100% classification accuracy of the temperature levels. The models of the honeys heated for 60 min showed a slightly lower accuracy (97.47%) after validation. The temperature groups 60 °C and 80 °C also provided worse results; however, in the case of all the models, the control was classified correctly. The classification models of bastard indigo weren´t accurate, but similarly, the honeys heated for four hours showed the best classification of temperature. In this case, all the models provided 100% correct classification of the control. Models of the acacia honey weren´t as performant as those of the other two groups, where the control classification accuracy was higher in the honeys heated for longer time intervals.

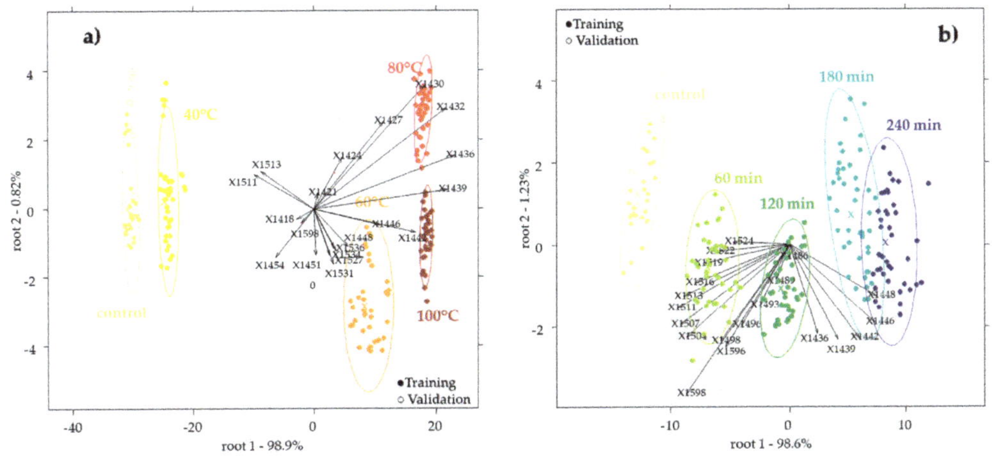

Figure 3. PCA-LDA score plot of the sunflower honey with the 20 most important loadings: (**a**) temperature classification model of honeys treated for 60 min with a Savitzky–Golay smoothing (window size 21) and SNV pretreatment; (**b**) time classification model of honey heated at 40 °C with Savitzky–Golay smoothing (window size 13), MSC and detrending pretreatment.

Table 2. PCA-LDA classification accuracies of the detailed temperature level and time interval classification models.

Honey	Subgroup	Pretreatment	Training %	Validation %	Control %
		Temperature Classification within Time Group			
Sunflower	within 60 min	sgol@2-21-0_snv	99.93	97.47	100
	within 120 min	sgol@2-13-0_sgol@2-13-2	97.74	87.55	100
	within 180 min	sgol@2-17-0	99.82	91.37	100
	within 240 min	sgol@2-13-0_sgol@2-17-2	100	100	100
Bastard indigo	within 60 min	sgol@2-17-0_deTr	81.11	62.38	100
	within 120 min	sgol@2-17-0_deTr	88.99	78.56	100
	within 180 min	sgol@2-17-0_deTr	92.74	83.71	100
	within 240 min	sgol@2-13-0_sgol@2-21-1	97.92	93.22	100
Acacia	within 60 min	sgol@2-21-0_deTr_msc	85.74	66.30	51.28
	within 120 min	sgol@2-13-0_sgol@2-17-1	91.11	59.94	69.23
	within 180 min	sgol@2-13-0_msc	91.56	72.17	76.92
	within 240 min	sgol@2-13-0_sgol@2-17-1	84.69	66.10	76.92
		Time Classification within Temperature Group			
Honey	**Subgroup**	**Pretreatment**	**Training %**	**Validation %**	**Control %**
Sunflower	within 40 °C	sgol@2-13-0_deTr_msc	98.63	96.36	100
	within 60 °C	sgol@2-17-0_sgol@2-21-1	90.58	72.47	100
	within 80 °C	sgol@2-21-0_sgol@2-13-1	84.80	57.27	100
	within 100 °C	sgol@2-13-0_sgol@2-13-2	89.95	72.21	100
Bastard indigo	within 40 °C	sgol@2-17-0_deTr	97.05	95.16	100
	within 60 °C	sgol@2-17-0	76.15	47.94	100
	within 80 °C	sgol@2-13-0_sgol@2-13-2	82.80	55.40	100
	within 100 °C	sgol@2-17-0	89.52	61.66	100
Acacia	within 40 °C	sgol@2-21-0_sgol@2-13-1	71.19	42.99	56.41
	within 60 °C	sgol@2-21-0_deTr_msc	62.21	31.96	71.79
	within 80 °C	sgol@2-17-0_msc	82.77	58.66	82.05
	within 100 °C	sgol@2-13-0_sgol@2-17-2	94.79	72.64	79.49

Each row represents the best model chosen from the 41 pretreatment combinations, the average classification accuracies for the training, validation, and the control correct classification are computed from the leave-one-sample-out cross validation confusion tables. sgol@x-y-z means Savitzky–Golay smoothing, where x denotes the polynomial order, y the window size and z the order of derivation; msc denotes multiplicative scatter correction; snv denotes standard normal variate; detr denotes detrending.

The detailed models for the classification of the time levels within temperature groups (Table 2 lower part) provided the best training and validation accuracies in the case of the sunflower honey, followed by bastard indigo, and acacia samples. In general, these models were worse than the models of the temperature classification within time intervals. The validation accuracies of the sunflower and bastard indigo honeys showed similar trends, where the best models were obtained for the time interval classification within 40 °C, followed by the model at 100 °C, while the models of the other two temperatures were weaker. In the case of acacia honey, the best model was achieved for the time interval classification within 80 °C, while similarly to bastard indigo, the worst model was obtained for the 60 °C treated group. The control was classified correctly in all the models of sunflower and bastard indigo. The models of the acacia honey provided the best results for the control: a correct classification for the models with 80 °C, followed by 100 °C, 60 °C, and 40 °C.

Poor results were also obtained for acacia samples in a Hungarian study [18]. This could be due to the lower nutritional content and the different crystallization phases of the honey samples. These results support the findings of Segato et al., 2019, who also found that the changes in NIR spectra as a result of heat treatment are highly phase-related, which could come from the fact that the scattering of the crystals is different in the different crystallization phases [42].

2.5. Results of the Partial Least Square Regression of Honeys

The results presented here were chosen from 41 pretreatment combinations after leave-one-sample-out cross-validation, based on the best R^2CV.

Results of the general (including all the temperature levels or time intervals) PLSR models of the three honey types provided the best results in the case of the sunflower honeys, followed by bastard indigo, and acacia honeys. The prediction of temperature provided a R^2CV of 0.81 and RMSECV of 10.70 °C, R^2CV of 0.76 and RMSECV of 11.82 °C, R^2CV of 0.36 and RMSECV of 19.00 °C for the sunflower, bastard indigo, and acacia honeys, respectively.

The prediction model of time intervals was much worse where in all the honey types, the R^2CV was lower than 0.26 and the error RMSECV was higher than 60 min. Therefore, more detailed models were calculated, their corresponding parameters are shown in Supplementary Table S1.

The detailed temperature level PLSR models built for the prediction of the applied temperature within the four studied time intervals (Supplementary Table S1 upper part) provided the best results in the case of sunflower honey. The residual prediction deviation (RPD) values were between 2.35 and 3.96 while the R^2CV was higher than 0.80 in all four models. The best prediction accuracy was obtained for the 240 min group. The model parameters of the bastard indigo honey were worse than in the case of the sunflower honey, however, the RPDCV values were >2.0 in all cases and the R^2CV values were between 0.76 and 0.88. Similarly, the 240 min group provided the best results. The prediction models of the acacia honey were worse than the results of the two other honey types. The RPD values were below 2.0 and the R^2CV values ranged between 0.29 and0.68. The best models were obtained in the case of the 60 min group, while those built for the 180 min group were less effective.

The detailed time interval PLSR models (Supplementary Table S1 lower part) also provided better results in the case of the sunflower honey compared to the bastard indigo and acacia honeys. The best results were obtained for the 40 °C group with an R^2CV value of 0.97 and RPDCV > 5.0. Lower prediction accuracies were obtained for the 80 °C group with an R^2CV of 0.83 and RPDCV of 2.45. In the case of the bastard indigo honey, the model of the 40 °C group provided the best results (R2CV = 4.13 and RPDCV = 4.13). The 60 °C and 80 °C groups models weren´t as accurate with R2CV < 0.5. For acacia honey, the most accurate prediction was achieved in the case of the 100 °C group with R2CV and RPDCV values of 0.83 and 2.45, respectively.

Summarizing, similar to the results of PCA-LDA, the best results were achieved in the case of the sunflower followed by the bastard indigo and acacia honeys.

2.6. Results of the Aquagrams Visualizing the Effect of Temperature and Time Intervals

The aquagrams plotted at the water matrix coordinates for each honey type as predefined based on the subtraction spectra, the PCA loadings of the temperature (Figure 2a) and time visualization models (Figure 2b), as well as the most contributing wavelengths of the previously presented PCA-LDA models (Figure 3a,b) and PLSR regression models (Supplementary Figure S1b,d), are presented in Figure 4 (sunflower honey), Figure 5 (bastard indigo honey), and Figure 6 (acacia honey).

To better understand the effect of the heat treatment parameters (time and temperature) on the water spectral pattern of each honey type, their respective aquagrams were inspected while fixating one parameter and changing the other.

As portrayed in Figure 4, across the different temperature levels (Figure 4 upper part) and time intervals (Figure 4 lower part), the control group for sunflower honey is markedly distinguished from the heat-treated samples.

Within each time interval, and as the applied temperature increases, lower absorbances at the highly hydrogen-bonded bands (1489 nm to 1513 nm) and higher ones at the free water conformations are observed. This pattern is particularly pronounced at the 60 min time frame (Figure 4e), where exceeding the temperature of 40 °C (maximum allowed) to reach 60 °C translates into a larger scale change of the spectral pattern.

As can be seen from the aquagrams, at the lowest applied temperature of 40 °C, the heating period can have a significant influence on the water structure (Figure 4a). This influence can still be noticed at 60 °C (Figure 4b), but this change towards the less hydrogen-bounded water structure is not that prominent anymore when higher temperatures are considered (Figure 4c,d).

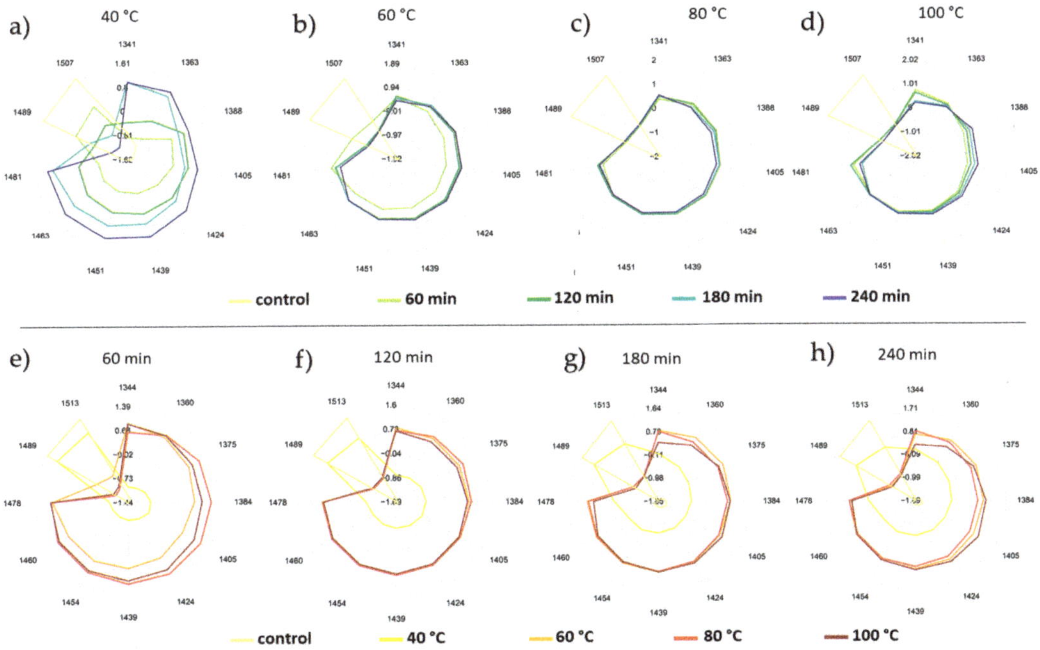

Figure 4. Aquagrams of the sunflower honey: (**a**–**d**) aquagrams showing pattern of time intervals; (**e**–**h**) aquagrams showing the pattern of temperature levels.

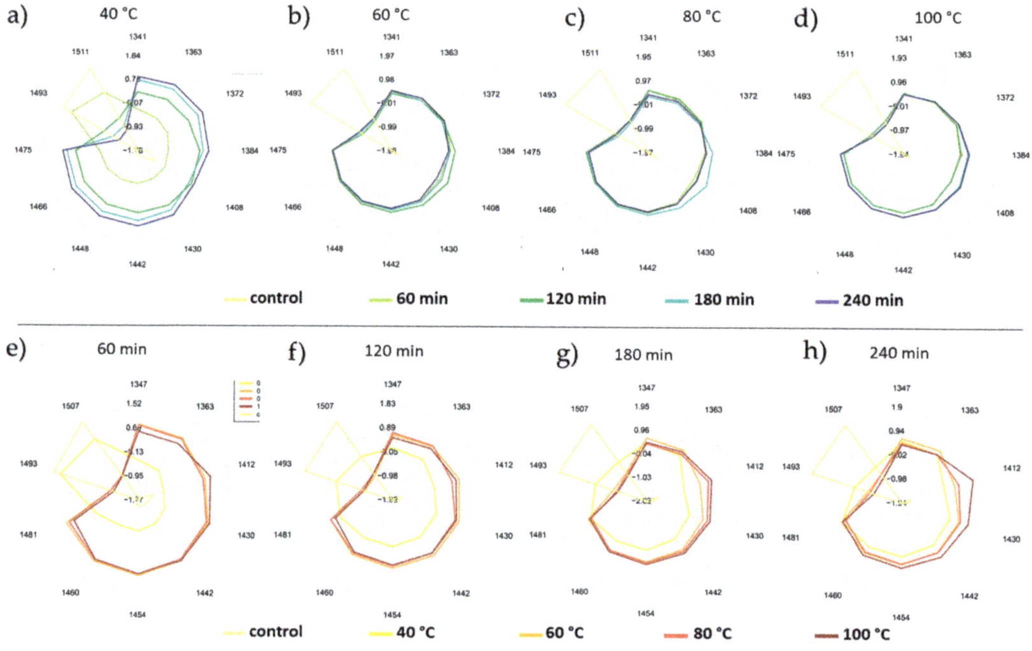

Figure 5. Aquagrams of the bastard indigo honey: (**a**–**d**) aquagrams showing pattern of time intervals; (**e**–**h**) aquagrams showing the pattern of temperature levels.

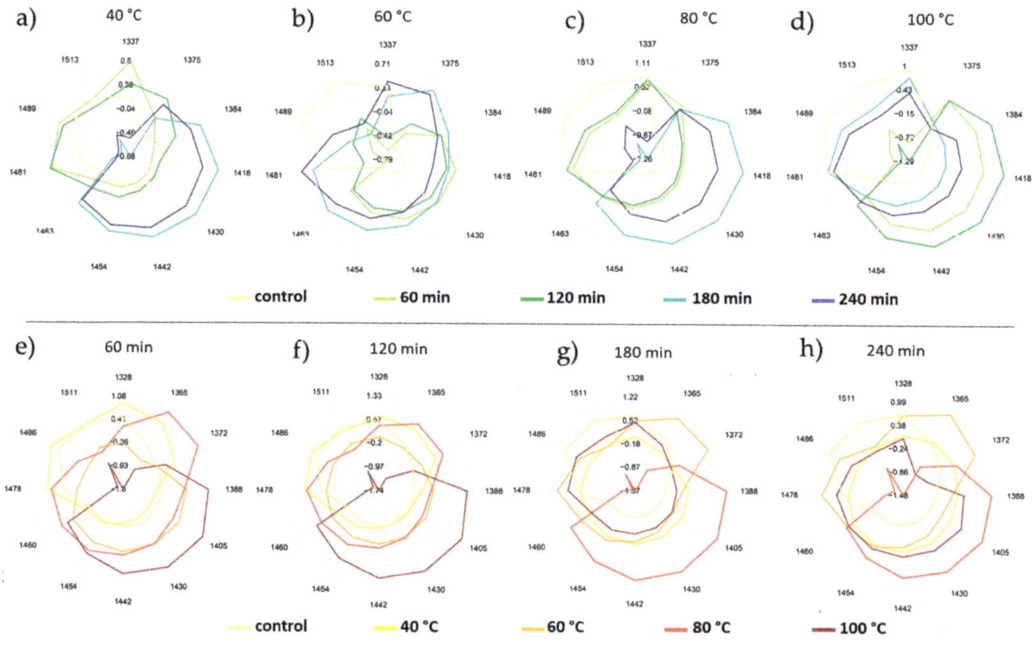

Figure 6. Aquagrams of the acacia honey: (**a**–**d**) aquagrams showing pattern of time intervals; (**e**–**h**) aquagrams showing the pattern of temperature level.

Following the same rationale when analyzing the bastard indigo honey samples (Figure 5), the impact of the temperature (Figure 5 upper part) and time interval (Figure 5 lower part) of the heat treatment is reflected in the aquagram through the liquefaction of the initially bonded water into more free water structures (Figure 5). Again, the time interval can be considerably impactful when it comes to affecting the existing water structures at 40 °C (Figure 5a), but not as much when the honey was heated up to 60 °C, 80 °C, and 100 °C (Figure 5b–d).

Explanation of the heat treatment effect on acacia honey (Figure 6), on the other hand, was less manageable. While the alteration of the water conformation is clearly reflected in the corresponding aquagram (Figure 6), these changes do not follow a logical pattern either along the varying time intervals (Figure 6 upper part), nor on the basis of the applied temperatures levels (Figure 6 lower part).

Such a behavior can be justified by the inherent differences in terms of the crystallization state and the physicochemical features of acacia honey compared to sunflower and bastard indigo honey samples [43]. This peculiar state has already been proven when the water spectral patterns of the three studied honey types were investigated in the absence of heat treatment (control group), where acacia, unlike the other two honey types, had abundant free water and less hydrogen-bonded water molecules. Segato et al. [42] also found that the changes of the spectral pattern in honeys are phase-related, and he also found that honey that was initially in liquid state (such as acacia in this study) showed less changes compared to the completely crystallized (like sunflower in our case) and less crystallized samples (like bastard indigo honey in our case). The HMF content of the honeys also showed similar trends: the HMF formation was the most intense in the sunflower honey, followed by bastard indigo and acacia honeys (Table 1). However, it should be noted that the NIRS seemed to be more sensitive to the changes from the effect of heat treatment, as the aquagrams, PCA-LDA, and PCA models showed the changes even at lower levels, while in the case of the HMF, only honeys heated at 80 °C for at least 120 min and 100 °C showed significant changes compared to the control honeys.

These findings do illustrate that the potential adulteration of honey by means of heat processing can be reflected in the respective aquagrams. Not only can this approach indicate—to some extent—the differences induced by the temperature levels at different time periods but it can also confirm the complexity of detecting such instances that are not only dictated by the thermal treatment parameters but can highly depend on the initial crystallization state of the honey.

3. Materials and Methods

3.1. Honey Samples

Three types of unifloral honey were collected from reliable beekeepers. The honeys were not processed or heat treated after the collection from the beehive. Sunflower (*Helianthus annuus)*, bastard indigo (*Amorpha fruticosa*), and acacia (*Robinia pesudoacacia*) honeys were used in the study. Three bottles per honey type, each of 1 kg, were collected from the three honeys (nine bottles in total). The three individual bottles were used as replicates (R) in the experiments.

The samples were portioned out to 100 mL glass sample holders with a closing polyethylene cap; 50 g of honey was weighed into the glasses. After portioning, the samples were processed by heat treatment. The samples were heated to 40 °C, 60 °C, 80 °C, or 100 °C and kept at temperature for 60, 120, 180, or 240 min each. This resulted in 17 heat treatment levels (including the untreated control), where 3 samples were created for each treatment level (the three replicates originated from the three bottles), resulting in 51 samples per type and 153 samples in total. The heat treatment was performed in a drying chamber.

3.2. Hydroxymethylfurfural Measurements of Honey

HMF determination of honey was performed according to the guideline of the International Honey Commission [44], using the spectrophotometric Winkler method. A Thermo Helios Alpha (Thermo Fischer Scientific Inc., Waltham, MA, USA) UV–VIS spectrophotometer (±0.001 units of absorbance, 1 cm light path) at 550 nm, using quartz cuvettes, was applied for the HMF quantifications.

3.3. Near-Infrared Spectroscopy Measurements

The NIRS measurements were performed using a handheld NIR-S-G1 Spectrometer (InnoSpectra Co., Hsinchu, Taiwan). Spectra were recorded in the range of 900–1700 nm, with 3 nm wavelength step in a transflectance setup. The layer thickness of the sample in the cuvette was 0.4 mm, which ensured that the maximum absorbance values did not exceed two absorbance unit. Each sample was measured three times applying three different fills with five consecutive scans, each resulting in 15 spectra per sample, and a total of 45 spectra per heat treatment level (per unifloral honey). Samples were measured in randomized order. After each five samples, a reference water sample was measured.

3.4. Statistical Analyis

3.4.1. ANOVA Analysis of the HMF Content

The HMF results of the honey samples were analyzed using ANOVA. Before the building of the ANOVA models, assumptions such as the normality (using Shapiro–Wilk test) and homogeneity of the variances (using Levene's test) were checked. To calculate which heat treatment levels differed significantly from the control, a one-way ANOVA test was performed. Additionally, a two-way ANOVA was used to check if the temperature level, time interval, and their interaction (time interval*temperature level) have a significant effect on the HMF formation in honeys. In case of a significant interaction, the significant differences within temperature and within time intervals were analyzed at the $p < 0.05$ significance level. Moreover, in the case of a significant ANOVA model, a post hoc test was applied the following way: when the homogeneity of the variances was assumed, Tukey's test was used and if it was not assumed, then Games–Howell's test was used for the pairwise comparison [45].

3.4.2. Spectral Range and Spectral Pretreatments

The spectral range of 1300–1600 nm was applied throughout the analysis. The evaluations were performed according to the protocol of aquaphotomics described by Tsenkova et al., 2018 [39]. The three honey types were evaluated separately. Prior to the data analysis, an outlier detection was applied on the dataset using the built-in outlier detection function of the aquap2 package [46].

After the inspection of the raw spectra, spectral pretreatment optimization was performed using 41 pretreatment combinations. A Savitzky–Golay (Sgol) smoothing (2nd order polynomial) with different window sizes (21, 17, or 13) and derivation varieties (no derivation, 1st, and 2nd derivative) was applied to reduce the noise in the spectra and to reveal overlapping peaks. Standard normal variate or multiplicative scatter correction was applied to reduce the baseline shift. Detrending and the aforementioned techniques were tested in single, double, or triple variations.

3.4.3. Modellings of the NIR Dataset

Principal Component Analysis—PCA

Principal component analysis was performed on the three honey types separately to reveal the patterns of time interval and temperature level. The PCA plots were colored according to the temperature level and the time interval. The models of the PCA were built using the best pretreatment obtained during the PCA-LDA of the general models (including all the temperature or time intervals) built for the temperature and time discrimination. This resulted in two models per honey type—one model for the presentation of the temperature pattern, and one for the time interval pattern.

PCA-Linear Discriminant Analysis—PCA-LDA

The hybrid PCA-LDA analysis was used to build the classification models. All the models were built using the 41 pretreatment combinations. As a first step, a classification model was built for the discrimination of the botanical types, then general models were built for the classification of the temperature groups (general temperature model) and for the classification of time groups (general time interval model), including all the sublevels of time or temperature treatments. However, due to the high interaction of temperature and time interval, models were also built for the classification of time intervals within each of the temperature groups (detailed time interval models) and for the temperature levels within each time interval (detailed temperature models). It resulted in a total of eight models per honey type (four models for the time interval discrimination within the temperature groups and four models for the temperature-level discrimination within the time intervals), and 24 models in total after choosing the models with the highest validation accuracy. A PC number optimization was also performed where the models with the highest validation accuracy and at the same time lowest difference between training and validation accuracy were chosen. The final models were validated using a leave-one-sample-out validation (LOSO), where all scans of one replicate of the samples were left out in each iteration step of the cross-validation.

Partial Least Square Regression (PLSR)

A partial least square regression was first performed on the three honey types separately for the prediction of time intervals and temperatures. A PLSR was also performed to regress on the time interval within each temperature level (detailed time interval models) and temperature level within each time interval (detailed temperature-level models). This also resulted in 8 models per honey type, and a total of 24 models, similarly to the PCA-LDA analysis. The correlation between the actual and predicted values was reported by the R2C and R2CV values. The error of the prediction was calculated using the root mean square error of the training (RMSEC) and validation (RMSECV). Besides the RMSE values, the residual prediction deviation (RPD) was also calculated for the training (RPDC) and validation (RPDCV). All the models were validated with a leave-one-sample-out (LOSO) cross-validation, where the spectra of one replicate of the samples were left out. In the case of the PLRS models, the pretreatment optimization was also performed, where the models with the best model parameters (based on the RMSECV, R2CV, and RPDCV) were chosen.

Subtraction Spectra

Subtraction spectra were calculated for the time interval subsets (detailed time interval models) and temperature level subsets (detailed temperature level models), where the control sample was subtracted from the others to reveal the wavelengths showing the greatest changes occurring upon the heat treatment temperature or time, respectively. The subtraction was performed on spectra that were pretreated with MSC and Savitzky–Golay smoothing (2nd order polynomial, window size of 21) with a 2nd derivation separately.

3.4.4. Determination of the Water Matrix Coordinates for the Aquagrams

The wavelengths belonging to the water matrix coordinates were chosen from the PCA loadings, PCA-LDA weights, PLRS regression vectors, and subtraction spectra. The wavelengths presenting the highest change due to the temperature or the time interval perturbation were collected. The assigned wavelengths were collected and grouped to the 12 water matrix coordinates (WAMACs) defined by Tsenkova [47] and the wavelengths presented the most frequently (within one WAMAC) were chosen for the calculation of the classic aquagrams.

Calculation of the aquagrams was performed in such a way as to illustrate the spectral pattern changes as a result of time intervals within one temperature level (detailed time interval models) and also to illustrate the effect of temperature level within one time interval (detailed temperature models). In total, 24 aquagrams were calculated, eight for each of the three honey types.

4. Conclusions

In this study, three different honey types were analyzed in terms of the effect of the heat treatment at different temperatures and different time intervals. The impact of the applied processing was measured by determining the HMF content and by NIRS. The temperatures and their interaction highly influenced the HMF formation of honey; however, the temperature level had a higher effect than the time interval. The dynamics of HMF formation differed for the three honey types, which underlines the importance of the initial physicochemical composition, defined by the origin of the honey, in the HMF production. However, only honeys heated at 80 °C and 100 °C provided significant changes in HMF content, which shows the limited ability of HMF as a sole indicator of honey heat treatment.

The PCA-LDA models provided better results for the temperature-level classifications than for the time interval. In general, sunflower honey provided better results on the classification and prediction accuracies than the other two honey types. In all cases, the worst model parameters were obtained for the acacia honeys. It can be concluded that the NIRS was more sensitive than HMF in detecting the effect of heat treatment. Nevertheless, these results indicate that the changes generated byheat treatment are related to the initial crystallization phase (as the sunflower was completely crystallized, bastard indigo was mid-crystallized and the acacia was in liquid form) and the composition of the samples; therefore, it is not possible to set up general principles for the detection of heat processing in honeys. On the other hand, our results prove that even at a low temperature treatment (40 °C), measurable changes occur in the spectra of the honey, and that these spectral changes are mainly related to the transformation of the highly bonded water to less H-bonded water or free water. Besides the water structure, the sugar composition was also modified, which could be concluded from the changes in the wavelength range of 1580–1590 nm.

Our research reveals the potential of NIRS and specifically aquaphotomics in the detection of the changes induced in the water structure of honey by heat treatment. In the future, it would also be important to see how the spectral pattern is affected as a result of heat treatment after recrystallization and storage.

Supplementary Materials: The following are available online, Table S1: Results of the partial least square regression models built for the prediction of time interval within temperature group and temperature within time intervals. Figure S1: Partial least square regression plot of the sunflower honeys: (a) regression plot of honeys heated for 60 min regressed on the temperature levels with Savitzky–Golay smoothing (window size: 17) and detrending; (b) the respective regression vector; (c) regression plot of honeys heated at 40 °C regressed on the time intervals with Savitzky–Golay smoothing (window size: 17), detrending, and MSC; (d) the respective regression vector.

Author Contributions: Conceptualization, Z.B., C.B. and Z.K.; formal analysis, Z.B.; funding acquisition, V.Z.-M. and Z.K.; investigation, Z.B.; methodology, Z.B., C.B. and Z.K.; project administration, Z.B. and Z.K.; resources, Z.B., C.B., B.A. and Z.K.; supervision, C.B. and Z.K.; validation, Z.K.; visualization, Z.B. and B.A.; writing—original draft, Z.B.; writing—review and editing, Z.B., C.B., B.A., V.Z.-M. and Z.K. All authors have read and agreed to the published version of the manuscript.

Funding: This research was supported by the European Union and cofinanced by the European Social Fund (grant agreement no. EFOP-3.6.3-VEKOP-16-2017-00005); by the European Union and cofinanced by the European Regional Development Fund and the Hungarian Government (grant agreement no. GINOP-2.2.1-18-2020-00025); and by the Thematic Excellence Programme awarded by the Ministry for Innovation and Technology (grant agreement no. NKFIH-831-10/2019).

Institutional Review Board Statement: Not applicable.

Informed Consent Statement: Not applicable.

Data Availability Statement: The data presented in this study are available on request from the corresponding author. The data are not publicly available, due to privacy reasons.

Acknowledgments: This project was supported by the Doctoral School of Food Science of the Hungarian University of Agriculture and Life Sciences. Authors owe thanks to the beekeepers who provided the honey samples and to Chiraz Ghdir for their assistance in laboratory work.

Conflicts of Interest: The authors declare no conflict of interest.

Sample Availability: Not available.

References

1. Crane, E. The Past and Present Importance of Bee Products to Man. In *Bee Products Properties, Applications, and Apitherapy*; Mizrahi, A., Lensky, Y., Eds.; Springer: Boston, MA, USA, 1997; pp. 1–13.
2. Codex Alimentarius Commission. *Codex Standard for Honey, CODEX STAN 12-1981*; 2001; Volume 11, p. 7. Available online: https://www.fao.org/fao-who-codexalimentarius/sh-proxy/es/?lnk=1&url=https%253A%252F%252Fworkspace.fao.org%252Fsites%252Fcodex%252FStandards%252FCXS%2B12-1981%252FCXS_012e.pdf (accessed on 10 December 2021).
3. The European Council Council Directive 2001/110/EC of 20 December 2001 Relating to Honey. *Official J. Eur. Union* **2001**, 47–52. Available online: https://eur-lex.europa.eu/LexUriServ/LexUriServ.do?uri=OJ:L:2002:010:0047:0052:EN:PDF (accessed on 10 December 2021).
4. Bogdanov, S. Honey Composition. In *Book of Honey*; Bee Hexagon Knowledge Network, 2014; pp. 27–36. Available online: https://www.researchgate.net/publication/304011775_Honey_Composition (accessed on 10 December 2021).
5. Bodor, Z.; Benedek, C.; Kovacs, Z.; Zinia Zaukuu, J.-L. Identification of Botanical and Geographical Origins of Honey-Based on Polyphenols. In *Plant-Based Functional Foods and Phytochemicals*; Apple Academic Press: Palm Bay, FL, USA, 2021; pp. 125–161.
6. Da Silva, P.M.; Gauche, C.; Gonzaga, L.V.; Costa, A.C.O.; Fett, R. Honey: Chemical Composition, Stability and Authenticity. *Food Chem.* **2016**, *196*, 309–323. [CrossRef] [PubMed]
7. Al-Diab, D.; Jarkas, B. Effect of Storage and Thermal Treatment on the Quality of Some Local Brands of Honey from Latakia Markets. *J. Entomol. Zool. Stud.* **2015**, *3*, 328–334.
8. Visquert, M.; Vargas, M.; Escriche, I. Effect of Postharvest Storage Conditions on the Colour and Freshness Parameters of Raw Honey. *Int. J. Food Sci. Technol.* **2014**, *49*, 181–187. [CrossRef]
9. Turkmen, N.; Sari, F.; Poyrazoglu, E.S.; Velioglu, Y.S. Effects of Prolonged Heating on Antioxidant Activity and Colour of Honey. *Food Chem.* **2006**, *95*, 653–657. [CrossRef]
10. Samira, N. The Effect of Heat Treatment on the Quality of Algerian Honey. *Researcher* **2016**, *8*, 1–6.
11. Bogdanov, S. Liquefaction of Honey. *Apiacta* **1993**, *28*, 4–10.
12. Tosi, E.A.; Ré, E.; Lucero, H.; Bulacio, L. Effect of Honey High-Temperature Short-Time Heating on Parameters Related to Quality, Crystallisation Phenomena and Fungal Inhibition. *LWT—Food Sci. Technol.* **2004**, *37*, 669–678. [CrossRef]
13. Tosi, E.; Martinet, R.; Ortega, M.; Lucero, H.; Ré, E. Honey Diastase Activity Modified by Heating. *Food Chem.* **2008**, *106*, 883–887. [CrossRef]
14. Codex Alimentarius Hungaricus 2-100 számú Irányelv megkülönböztető jelöléssel ellátott mézfélék (2-100 Honey with distinctive quality indication). In *Codex Alimentarius Hungaricus*; Codex Alimentarius Hungaricus (Ed.) Magyar Élelmiszerkönyv Bizottság, 2009; pp. 3–6. Available online: https://elelmiszerlanc.kormany.hu/download/1/3b/a2000/2-100.pdf (accessed on 21 October 2017).
15. Zábrodská, B.; Vorlová, L. Adulteration of Honey and Available Methods for Detection—A Review. *Acta Vet. Brno* **2014**, *83*, S85–S102. [CrossRef]
16. Visser, F.R.; Allen, J.M.; Shaw, G.J. The Effect of Heat on the Volatile Flavour Fraction from a Unifloral Honey. *J. Apic. Res.* **1988**, *27*, 175–181. [CrossRef]
17. Inan, Ö.; Özcan, M.M.; Arslan, D.; Ünver, A. Some Physico-Chemical and Sensory Properties of Heat Treated Commercial Pine and Blossom Honey. *J. Apic. Res.* **2012**, *51*, 347–352. [CrossRef]
18. Bodor, Z.; Koncz, F.; Zinia Zaukuu, J.-L.; Kertész, I.; Gillay, Z.; Kaszab, T.; Kovács, Z.; Benedek, C. Effect of Heat Treatment on Chemical and Sensory Properties of Honeys. *Animal Welfare* **2017**, *13*, 39–48.
19. Chua, L.S.; Adnan, N.A.; Abdul-Rahaman, N.L.; Sarmidi, M.R. Effect of Thermal Treatment on the Biochemical Composition of Tropical Honey Samples. *Int. Food Res. J.* **2014**, *21*, 773–778.
20. Csóka, M.; Tolnay, P.; Szabó, S.A. Hársméz színjellemzőinek változása hőkezelés hatására, illetve a tárolás során—Alteration in Linden Honey Colour Properties by Storage and Heat Treatment. *Élelmiszervizsgálati Közlemények* **2014**, *60*, 44–49.
21. Zhao, H.; Cheng, N.; Zhang, Y.; Sun, Z.; Zhou, W.; Wang, Y.; Cao, W. The Effects of Different Thermal Treatments on Amino Acid Contents and Chemometric-Based Identification of Overheated Honey. *LWT* **2018**, *96*, 133–139. [CrossRef]
22. Singh, I.; Singh, S. Honey Moisture Reduction and Its Quality. *J. Food Sci. Technol.* **2018**, *55*, 3861–3871. [CrossRef]
23. Nicoli, M.; Anese, M.; Parpinel, M. Influence of Processing on the Antioxidant Properties of Fruit and Vegetables. *Trends Food Sci. Technol.* **1999**, *10*, 94–100. [CrossRef]

24. Cozmuta, A.M.; Cozmuta, L.M.; Varga, C.; Marian, M.; Peter, A. Effect of Thermal Processing on Quality of Polyfloral Honey. *Rom. J. Food Sci.* **2011**, *1*, 45–52.
25. Codex Alimentarius Hungaricus 1-3-2001/110 számú Előírás Méz (1-3-2001/110 Regulation Honey). In *Codex Alimentarius Hungaricus*; Codex Alimentarius Hungaricus (Ed.) Magyar Élelmiszerkönyv Bizottság, 2002; pp. 1–7. Available online: http://www.hermanottointezet.hu/sites/default/files/dokumentumok/mez.pdf (accessed on 16 October 2017).
26. Dimins, F.; Kuka, P.; Kuka, M.; Cakste, I. The Criteria of Honey Quality and Its Changes during Storage and Thermal Treatment. *Proc. Latvia Univ. Agric.* **2006**, *16*, 73–78.
27. Oroian, M. Physicochemical and Rheological Properties of Romanian Honeys. *Food Biophys.* **2012**, *7*, 296–307. [CrossRef]
28. Turhan, I.; Tetik, N.; Karhan, M.; Gurel, F.; Reyhan Tavukcuoglu, H. Quality of Honeys Influenced by Thermal Treatment. *LWT—Food Sci. Technol.* **2008**, *41*, 1396–1399. [CrossRef]
29. Bodor, Z.; Ghdir, C.; Zaukuu, J.; Benedek, C.; Kovacs, Z. Detection of Heat Treatment of Honey with near Infrared Spectroscopy. *Hungarian Agric. Engin.* **2019**, *36*, 57–62. [CrossRef]
30. Verdú, S.; Ivorra, E.; Sánchez, A.J.; Barat, J.M.; Grau, R. Spectral Study of Heat Treatment Process of Wheat Flour by VIS/SW-NIR Image System. *J. Cereal Sci.* **2016**, *71*, 99–107. [CrossRef]
31. Muncan, J.; Kuroki, S.; Moyankova, D.; Morita, H.; Atanassova, S.; Djilianov, D.; Tsenkova, R. Protocol for Aquaphotomics Monitoring of Water Molecular Structure in Leaves of Resurrection Plants during Desiccation and Recovery. *Protocol. Exch.* **2019**. [CrossRef]
32. Bázár, G.; Romvári, R.; Szabó, A.; Somogyi, T.; Éles, V.; Tsenkova, R. NIR Detection of Honey Adulteration Reveals Differences in Water Spectral Pattern. *Food Chem.* **2016**, *194*, 873–880. [CrossRef]
33. Bodor, Z.; Zaukuu, J.Z.; Aouadi, B.; Benedek, C.; Kovacs, Z. Application of NIRS and Aquaphotomics for the Detection of Adulteration of Honey, Paprika and Tomato Paste. In *Proceedings of the SZIEntific Meeting for Young Researchers—Ifjú Tehetségek Találkozója*; University, S.I., Ed.; Szent Itsván University: Budapest, Hungary, 2019; pp. 76–91.
34. Yang, X.; Guang, P.; Xu, G.; Zhu, S.; Chen, Z.; Huang, F. Manuka Honey Adulteration Detection Based on Near-Infrared Spectroscopy Combined with Aquaphotomics. *LWT* **2020**, *132*, 109837. [CrossRef]
35. Ferreiro-González, M.; Espada-Bellido, E.; Guillén-Cueto, L.; Palma, M.; Barroso, C.G.; Barbero, G.F. Rapid Quantification of Honey Adulteration by Visible-near Infrared Spectroscopy Combined with Chemometrics. *Talanta* **2018**, *188*, 288–292. [CrossRef]
36. Bogdanov, S. Wiederverflüssigung Des Honigs; Bern. 1992. Available online: https://www.agroscope.admin.ch/dam/agroscope/de/dokumente/themen/nutztiere/bienen/honverfl_d.pdf.download.pdf/honverfl_d.pdf (accessed on 15 April 2020).
37. Bodor, Z.; Zaukuu, J.-L.Z.; Benedek, C.; Kovacs, Z. Detection of Heat Treatment of Honey by Rapid Correlative Techniques. Available online: http://www.ihc-platform.net/bodoretaloralpresentationmalta.pdf (accessed on 9 September 2019).
38. Shapla, U.M.; Solayman, M.; Alam, N.; Khalil, M.I.; Gan, S.H. 5-Hydroxymethylfurfural (HMF) Levels in Honey and Other Food Products: Effects on Bees and Human Health. *Chem. Cent. J.* **2018**, *12*, 1–18. [CrossRef] [PubMed]
39. Tsenkova, R.; Munćan, J.; Pollner, B.; Kovacs, Z. Essentials of Aquaphotomics and Its Chemometrics Approaches. *Front. Chem.* **2018**, *6*, 1–25. [CrossRef]
40. Xantheas, S.S. Ab Initio Studies of Cyclic Water Clusters $(H_2O)_n$, N=1–6. III. Comparison of Density Functional with MP2 Results. *J. Chem. Phys.* **1995**, *102*, 4505. [CrossRef]
41. Muncan, J.; Tsenkova, R. Aquaphotomics—From Innovative Knowledge to Integrative Platform in Science and Technology. *Molecules* **2019**, *24*, 2742. [CrossRef] [PubMed]
42. Segato, S.; Merlanti, R.; Bisutti, V.; Montanucci, L.; Serva, L., Lucatello, L.; Mirisola, M.; Contiero, B.; Conficoni, D.; Balzan, S.; et al. Multivariate and Machine Learning Models to Assess the Heat Effects on Honey Physicochemical, Colour and NIR Data. *Eur. Food Res. Technol.* **2019**, *245*, 2269–2278. [CrossRef]
43. Oddo, L.P.; Piro, R. Main European Unifloral Honeys: Descriptive Sheets. *Eur. Food Res. Technol.* **2018**, *244*, 118–126.
44. Bogdanov, S. Harmonised Methods of the International Honey Commission. *Int. Honey Comm. (IHC)* **2009**, *5*, 1–62.
45. Tabachnick, B.G.; Fidell, L.S. *Using Multivariate Statistics*, 6th ed.; Pearson Education: Harlow, Essex, UK, 2013.
46. Pollner, B.; Kovacs, Z. R-Package Aquap2–Multivariate Data Analysis Tools for R Including Aquaphotomics Methods. Available online: https://www.aquaphotomics.com/aquap2/ (accessed on 28 July 2021).
47. Tsenkova, R. Introduction Aquaphotomics: Dynamic Spectroscopy of Aqueous and Biological Systems Describes Peculiarities of Water. *J. Near Infrared Spectrosc.* **2009**, *17*, 303–314. [CrossRef]

molecules

MDPI

Article

Aquaphotomic, E-Nose and Electrolyte Leakage to Monitor Quality Changes during the Storage of Ready-to-Eat Rocket

Laura Marinoni [1,*], Marina Buccheri [1], Giulia Bianchi [1] and Tiziana M. P. Cattaneo [1,2]

1 Research Centre for Engineering and Agro-Food Processing, Council for Agricultural Research and Economics, 20133 Milano, Italy; marina.buccheri@crea.gov.it (M.B.); giulia.bianchi@crea.gov.it (G.B.); tiziana.cattaneo@crea.gov.it (T.M.P.C.)
2 Department of Agricultural and Forestry Sciences (DAFNE), Tuscia University, 01100 Viterbo, Italy
* Correspondence: laura.marinoni@crea.gov.it

Abstract: The consumption of ready-to-eat (RTE) leafy vegetables has increased rapidly due to changes in consumer diet. RTE products are perceived as fresh, high-quality, and health-promoting. The monitoring of the RTE quality is crucial in relation to safety issues. This study aimed to evaluate the maintenance of RTE rocket salad freshness packed under modified atmospheres. A portable E-nose, the electrolyte leakage test (which measures the index of leaf damage—I_{LD}), and NIR spectroscopy and Aquaphotomics were employed. Two trials were carried out, using the following gas mixtures: (A) atmospheric air (21% O_2, 78% N_2); (B) 30% O_2, 70% N_2; (C) 10% CO_2, 5% O_2, 85% N_2. Samples were stored at 4 °C and analyzed at 0, 1, 4, 7, 11, and 13 days. ANOVA, PCA, PLS were applied for data processing. E-nose and I_{LD} results identified the B atmosphere as the best for maintaining product freshness. NIR spectroscopy was able to group the samples according to the storage time. Aquaphotomics proved to be able to detect changes in the water structure during storage. These preliminary data showed a good agreement NIR/I_{LD} suggesting the use of NIR for non-destructive monitoring of the damage to the plant membranes of RTE rocket salad.

Keywords: storage; ready-to-eat rocket; water; NIR; E-nose; electrolyte leakage; Aquaphotomics

Citation: Marinoni, L.; Buccheri, M.; Bianchi, G.; Cattaneo, T.M.P. Aquaphotomic, E-Nose and Electrolyte Leakage to Monitor Quality Changes during the Storage of Ready-to-Eat Rocket. *Molecules* **2022**, *27*, 2252. https://doi.org/10.3390/molecules27072252

Academic Editors: Roumiana Tsenkova, Jelena Muncan and Stefano Materazzi

Received: 11 February 2022
Accepted: 28 March 2022
Published: 30 March 2022

1. Introduction

The consumption of ready-to-eat (RTE) leafy vegetables has increased rapidly due to changes that have occurred in the dietary pattern of the consumer. RTE products are perceived as natural, fresh, convenient, high-quality, and health-promoting [1,2]. Rocket (*Eruca sativa* Mill.) salad is principally consumed as an RTE product, either alone or mixed with other vegetables [3]. It shows different characteristics from other types of salad, as it belongs to the Brassicaceae family. For this reason, it is a source of compounds with biological activity beneficial for human health, such as glucosinolates. Glucosinolates are then hydrolyzed by the enzyme myrosinase with the release of isothiocyanates, which are compounds with antimicrobial activity [4]. Because of its high content of bioactive compounds, different health-promoting functions are attributed to rocket plants [5], but, as with most leafy vegetables, rocket leaves have very high metabolic activity [6], which limits their shelf-life. During storage, the high respiration rate and ethylene production lead to leaf yellowing due to chlorophyll degradation, loss of turgidity, off-flavor development, and general deterioration [7].

Many postharvest technologies, such as refrigeration and modified atmosphere packaging (MAP), are successfully employed to delay the senescence of packed vegetables [8]. These techniques are determinants in preserving visual quality and microbial safety of minimally processed fruit and vegetables during the supply chain [9]. MAP is effective in prolonging the shelf-life of fresh-cut produce by modifying the ratios between gases within the packaging. Successful applications of MAP (with low O_2 and high CO_2 levels) to minimally processed fruits and vegetables have been extensively reported in the literature [2], since low O_2 concentration causes a decrease in respiration, this inhibits the growth of postharvest pathogens, and slows down the deterioration rate. However, very low levels of O_2 may induce anaerobic fermentation with the corresponding accumulation of unpleasant odors, undesirable tastes, and tissue damage [2,8,10]. Moreover, the presence of a very high CO_2 concentration (25%) in the storage atmosphere has been found to be deleterious for fresh-cut artichokes, while only slight beneficial effects were observed at lower concentrations (5 and 15%) [11].

The monitoring of the quality of RTE vegetables is crucial, especially in relation to safety issues [12]. It is essential to evaluate the product quality both during storage and at the end of its shelf-life.

Several techniques are used to monitor the quality of fresh-cut fruit and vegetables during shelf-life, such as the evaluation of texture, respiration rate, pH, microbiological and sensory quality, nutritional and antioxidants status [13]. Among them, the electrolyte leakage test measures the cell membrane permeability, resulting in an index of leaf damage. This method is widely used in the investigation of various stress conditions, such as quality changes during shelf-life in different ready-to-eat products [14–16], including rocket salad [3,17]. However, all these methods are generally expensive and time-consuming, require the destruction of the sample, and are not suited to automation.

Among the non-destructive techniques, the electronic nose (E-nose) is a fast and reliable method to evaluate the volatile fingerprint in the headspace of food. According to Gardner and Bartlett [18], the electronic nose is "an instrument which comprises an array of electronic chemical sensors with partial specificity and an appropriate pattern-recognition system, capable of recognizing simple or complex odors". The sensors respond to the whole set of headspace volatiles, giving an idea of the metabolic changes that take place in the headspace of food [19]. More than 70 volatiles have been identified in the headspace of fresh rucola, 20 of which contribute to the leaf aroma [20]. Some typical volatile compounds found in RTE rocket salad are dimethyl sulfide, dimethyl disulfide, dimethyl sulfoxide, and furans derivatives [20,21].

Near-infrared (NIR) spectroscopy, in combination with chemometrics and Aquaphotomics, represents a powerful, rapid, and non-destructive analytical tool to monitor the quality of packaged foods by evaluating the changes occurring during the storage [22].

Aquaphotomics is a recent scientific discipline based on NIR measurements and multivariate spectral analysis that investigates the water–light interactions in biological systems. This approach exploits the fact that changes in the water matrix reflect, as would a mirror, the molecules the water surrounds [23,24]. Aquaphotomics is based on the high sensitivity of water's hydrogen bonds that reflect any change in the aqueous system highlighting perturbations that can be observed, measured, analyzed, and interpreted [24]. According to this approach, the NIR spectra acquired in living systems under various perturbations (temperature, ion concentrations, oxidative stress, illumination, disease, and damage) are characterized by 12 water absorption ranges (6–20 nm width each) in the spectral region of the first overtone of water (1300–1600 nm). Such spectral ranges have been called Water Matrix Coordinates (WAMACs) and labelled Ci, i = 1–12. Within the WAMACs, specific water absorbance bands are related to specific water molecular conformations (water species and water molecular structures) [24]. When a perturbation produces changes at specific water absorbance bands, and when this is determined consistently and repeatedly throughout the Aquaphotomics analysis, these water absorbance bands (WABs) are considered 'activated' by the respective perturbation. The selected WABs are plotted in spider charts, named 'aquagrams', which depict the Water Absorbance Spectral Patterns (WASPs) [24].

This work aimed to evaluate and monitor the changes occurring during the storage of ready-to-eat rocket salad packed under modified atmospheres. The electrolyte leakage test and rapid and non-destructive techniques, such as NIR spectroscopy coupled to Aquaphotomics and a Portable Electronic Nose, were employed.

2. Results and Discussion

2.1. E-Nose Analyses

In a previous preliminary work [25], the evaluation of the storage of the fresh-cut spring rocket (Trial 1) was carried out only through two non-destructive techniques, electronic nose and NIR spectroscopy.

The E-nose was applied in order to evaluate the evolution of the volatile compounds profile of rocket salad during storage. Preliminary results of Trial 1, only summarized here, highlighted the great influence of three broad-range sensors, W5S, W1S, and W2S, on the characterization of the samples. Such sensors are indicated as sensitive towards a wide range of compounds; however, they possess some selectivity towards specific compounds; respectively, methane, and alcohols for W1S and W2S. These compounds, indeed, indicate anaerobic conditions or fermentation reactions likely characterizing the late storage stages, and the related signals mainly characterized the last checkpoints of all the samples. In particular, C samples showed a peculiar pattern, with an important impact of the three sensors at all sampling points. The E-nose profile of treatment C underwent major changes during the storage, while treatments A and B showed more constant sensor values. Profile B reflected minimal variations occurring inside the rocket bag, suggesting that the B atmosphere was the best in maintaining the product's initial conditions [25].

In the second experiment carried out on second-cut autumn rocket (Trial 2) and fully reported here, the three broad-range sensors were confirmed as the predominant ones in the characterization of the samples. Figure 1 shows the biplot of PCA illustrating the mutual relationships between samples and sensors.

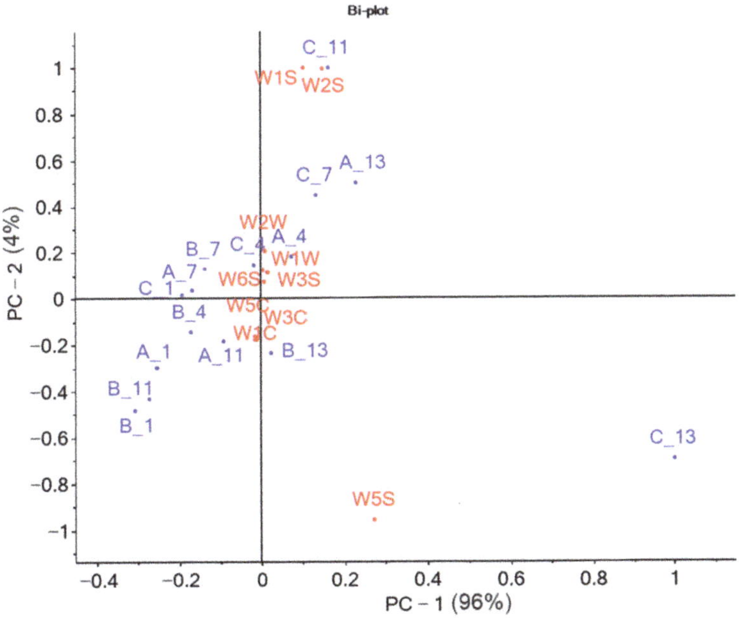

Figure 1. Biplot of E-nose sensor responses and samples scores (average values) during the storage of rocket salad.

The three broad-range sensors were responsible for the positioning in the multivariate space of the longer-stored samples. W1S and W2S greatly described the sample C11 and, to a lesser extent, C7 and A13. W5S mainly characterized the C13 sample. The other sensors, sensitive to aromatic compounds, alkanes, terpenes, and organic sulfur compounds, were located close to the axes intersection and described the short-term stored samples. These findings are in accordance with Mastrandrea et al. [26], who studied the changes in volatile compounds responsible for flavor in wild rocket stored in MAP conditions. They found volatile and aromatic compounds, including sulfur, C6, and C5 compounds, acetaldehyde, isothiocyanate, and thiocyanate derivatives. These compounds are responsible for the typical odor and flavor notes of fresh rocket [26]. Interestingly, A11, B11, and B13 samples clustered close to the fresher samples, indicating that these two active atmospheres played a crucial role in limiting metabolic changes inside the bags during the storage.

In Trial 2, E-nose profiles differed among the treatments (Figure 2a). Samples A and B showed lower sensor values compared to treatment C, which was characterized, in particular, by very high W5S sensor values.

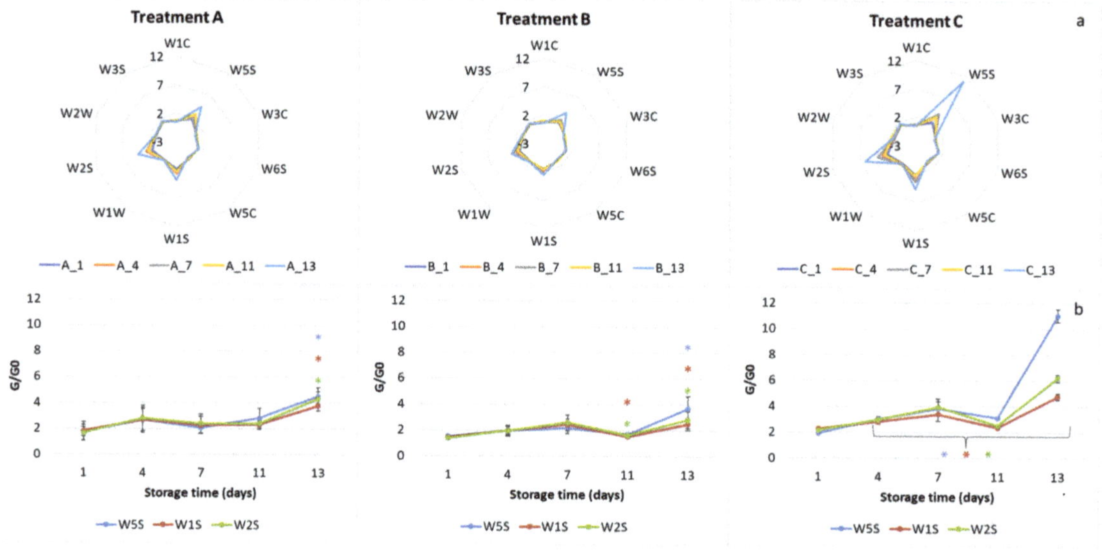

Figure 2. E- nose profiles (**a**) and trend curves of W5S, W1S and W2S sensors (**b**) of the three treatments during the storage: Trial 2. Data are reported as mean values ± standard deviation. Colored asterisks indicate significant differences in the corresponding sensor signals according to ANOVA and Tukey's post hoc test ($p < 0.05$).

Figure 2b reports in detail the trend of the three broad-range sensors. Treatment A showed constant values until t = 11 and then a marked significant increase at t = 13 of all sensors. Treatment B showed significant differences on days 11 and 13 for the W1S and W2S sensors and only at time t = 13 for the W5S. Sample C showed significant differences for all sampling points with maximum values at the last checkpoint, indicating a possible accumulation of a wide range of compounds, such as methane and alcohols, in the package atmosphere. The fact that the three sensors mainly described the samples of treatment C, which is characterized by low oxygen, agrees with the literature data [10,27–29]. Indeed, alcohols, such as ethanol and methanol, have been reported to be released under restricted O_2 conditions [10,27]. Ethanol, for example, is considered a major fermentative metabolite, while methanol is reported to come from enzymatic degradation of pectin by pectin methyl esterase [28]. It can be assumed that in the C treatment, the lack of O_2 for aerobic respiration led to a switch to anaerobic respiration, with a release of alcohols. Increases in fermentative volatiles such as ethanol are reported to negatively affect the sensory properties of the product [30–32]. Indeed, Allende et al. [29] reported that products with high respiration rates require high levels of O_2 in the package to maintain their quality.

2.2. Electrolyte Leakage Analyses

The present work also shows the results, of both trials, of the electrolyte leakage test.

The index of leaf damage (I_{LD}), measured by an electrolyte leakage test, can be considered a good indicator of the product's freshness [33]. In the first trial (spring mowing, Figure 3a), I_{LD} remained more or less constant in all treatments until day 4. On day 7, it increased significantly only in C treatment (LSD > 0.61). In treatments A and B, the increase in I_{LD} took place only after 10 days. In any case, treatments A and B showed lower I_{LD} values than treatment C until the end of the storage (13 days).

In the second trial (autumn mowing, Figure 3b), the leaves' behavior was slightly different. All the treatments showed an I_{LD} value far higher than in the first trial. I_{LD} values were constant until day 7, after which all the values increased almost exponentially. Moreover, in this case, the C treatment showed the worst performance reaching, at the end of the storage, the highest I_{LD} value (LSD > 2.2).

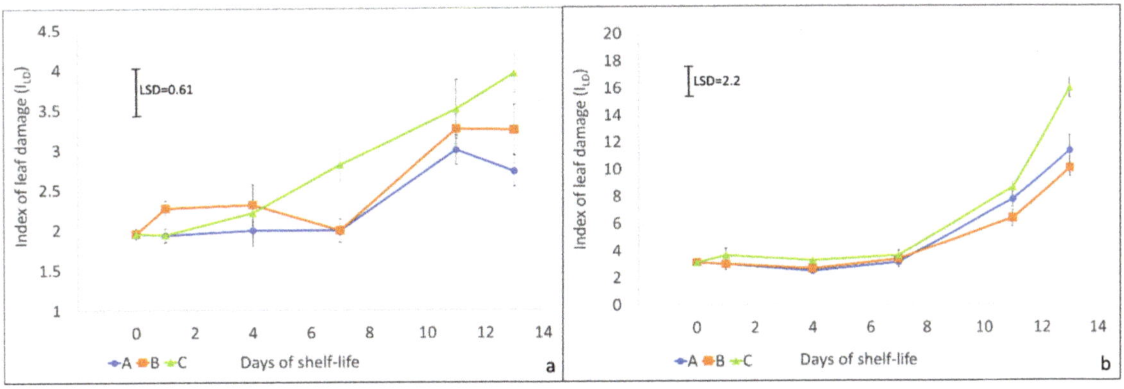

Figure 3. Index of leaf damage (I_{LD}) of rocket salad samples of trial 1 (**a**) and 2 (**b**) ± standard error. The result of the LSD post-hoc test is reported in each graph ($p < 0.05$).

Considering both trials, the low I_{LD} values of the samples in the first days agree with the findings of Luca et al. [16], who reported a low index of leaf damage until day 8 of shelf-life in wild rocket leaves. The higher value of treatment C at the end of the storage period indicates that a modified atmosphere enriched with CO_2 can negatively affect rocket leaves, inducing faster deterioration of the samples. Mastrandrea et al. [34] obtained similar results on rocket leaves under passive modified atmosphere conditions: high CO_2 and low oxygen concentration increased off-odors production and decreased shelf-life.

The different behavior of rocket leaves (higher deterioration in the second trial) can be due to the two different seasons when the mowing took place. Environmental conditions, including temperature, solar radiation, and rainfall, have an important influence on the quality of brassica leafy species [35,36]. Furthermore, rocket is capable of regrowing after mowing, giving under optimal pedo-climatic conditions up to 5–6 cropping in a season [37]. Hall et al. [38] reported that the harvest season and the mowing number affect the leaf water content, with late cuttings and summer cuttings having higher dry weight (lower water content). In the two experiments, two rocket harvests were analyzed— the first cut in the early spring and the last cut in the early autumn. The different harvest season and the cutting number could have affected the leaves' composition, and especially their water content [36,38,39]. For this reason, leaves from plants of the first trial (April) were probably more resistant to deterioration than those of the second trial (October).

2.3. NIR Spectroscopy and Aquaphotomics

NIR data of Trial 1, as well as those of E-nose, have recently been presented as a poster [25]. In the present paper, these are reported in more detail and compared with those of Trial 2 and with the electrolyte leakage data.

Figure 4 shows the averaged raw NIR spectra of the packed rocket salad samples of Trial 1 (a) and 2 (b). The raw spectra showed broad and overlapped bands related to water absorptions at 960–990 (second overtone -OH stretching), 1150–1170 (combination of the first overtone -OH stretching and OH bending), and 1430–1440 nm (first overtone -OH stretching) [24]. The spectra of leafy vegetables originate from the interaction of the electromagnetic radiation with the compounds that absorb it (chlorophyll, carotenoids, water, cellulose and hemicelluloses, starch, lignin, proteins) and from reflection and internal scattering phenomena of the non-absorbed radiation [40]. The leaf can be modeled as a stack of four layers, each of which owns different physical characteristics and optical properties. The light interacting with the leaf can be subjected to phenomena of specular reflection, absorption, transmission, and scattering [40–42]. The difference in vegetable surface, thickness, and structure, as occurs for leaves and petioles, determines a different reflection of the electromagnetic radiation [40]. Furthermore, the growing season is recognized to have an influence on the chemical-physical characteristics of the leaves, such as the amount of dry matter, the leaf area surface, and the thickness [43]. Bonasia et al. [44] reported higher dry matter concentration, higher specific leaf area, and more thickened leaves for rocket salad grown in winter-spring compared to the autumn-winter product. The differences in the sample composition caused by the growing season could have affected the raw spectra of Trial 2, which were more heterogeneous and dispersed than in the first trial. Furthermore, rocket leaves from Trial 2 (October mowing) were more variable in shape and dimensions, while the petioles were thicker than those from Trial 1 (April mowing). This distinct leaf morphology probably caused a change in the arrangement of the layers of leaves and petioles inside the package that gave rise to differences in the optical phenomena in the two systems, resulting in different spectra.

The application of pre-treatments made the peaks narrower and more defined, allowing their easier identification. Figure 4c,d show the detail of the second derivative spectra truncated to 1300–1600 nm in order to examine the first overtone of the water. The presence of wavelength shifts in the analyzed range supported the hypothesis that Aquaphotomics could be helpful to discriminate between the different treatments.

2.3.1. Trial 1

To highlight and enhance the small differences found in the second derivative of the spectra, the normalization was performed on Trial 1 spectra according to Tsenkova et al. [24] (Figure 5).

The graph allowed the identification of the wavelengths most involved in the characterization of the different samples. In order to identify further characterizing wavelengths, the PCA and PLS models were calculated on the pre-treated spectra.

The explorative PCA explained 98% of the total variance showing samples grouped according to the storage time (Figure 6): (i) $t = 0$; (ii) $t = 1$ samples; (iii) $t = 4$ samples; (iv) $t = 7$ to $t = 13$ samples. Interestingly, sample B at 7 days located together with $t = 4$ samples. This suggested that the characteristics of the biosystem of the 4 days samples were also maintained for 7 days rocket samples stored in atmosphere B.

According to the loadings plot (Figure 6b), the separation along PC1 between fresh and longer-stored samples was mainly based on a wavelength of 1373 nm, while the separation along PC2 was due to 1453 nm. According to Tsenkova et al. [24], these wavelengths correspond to the absorbance of the free OH stretch and of strongly hydrogen-bonded water, respectively.

A preliminary PLS model was built up with pre-treated spectra and the I_{LD} index. Figure 7 shows the scatter plot of the model (Figure 7a) together with the factor loadings (Figure 7b).

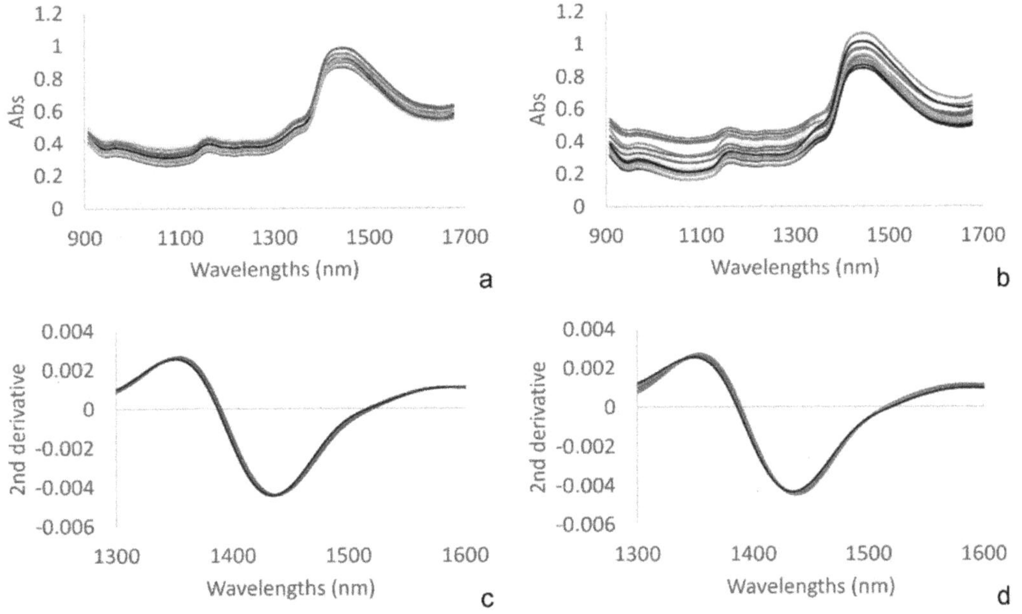

Figure 4. Averaged raw NIR spectra of the packed rocket salad samples of Trial 1 (**a**) and 2 (**b**) and detail of the second derivative spectra truncated to 1300–1600 nm of Trial 1(**c**) and 2 (**d**).

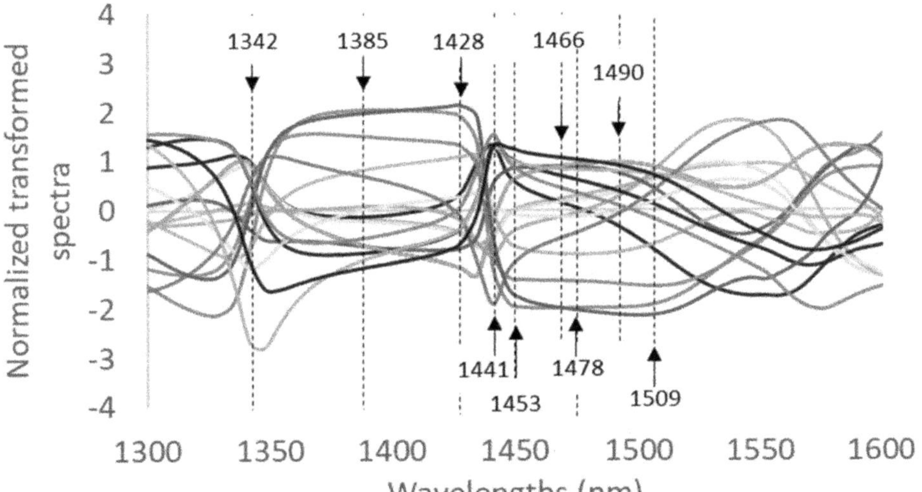

Figure 5. Normalized spectra of the packed rocket salad samples of Trial 1.

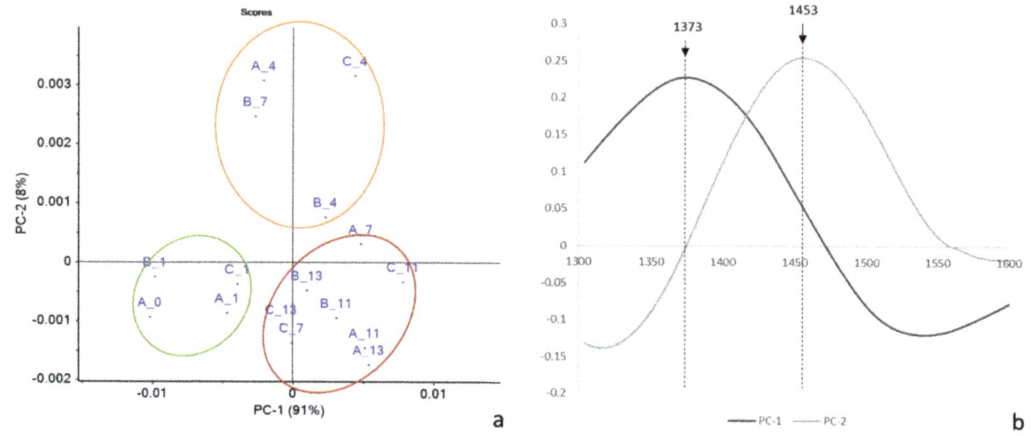

Figure 6. PCA score (**a**) and loading (**b**) plots of pre-treated NIR spectra of rocket salads of Trial 1 (each point corresponded to the mean spectra for each checkpoint).

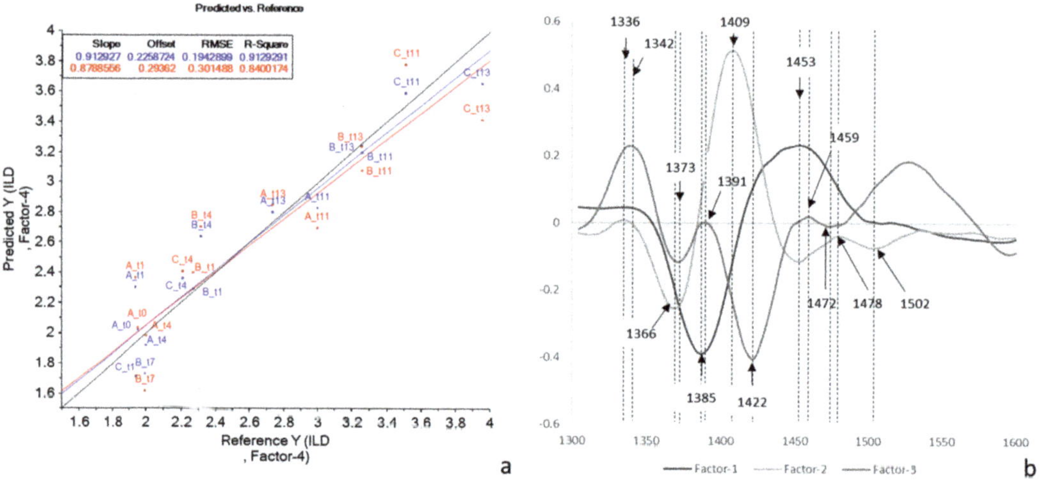

Figure 7. Scatter plot of calibration (blue) and cross validation (red)performance of predictive models built with pretreated NIR spectra and I_{LD} values (**a**); PLS Factor Loadings (**b**).

The model showed an R-value in calibration of 0.92 and an R-value in cross-validation of 0.83, with a standard error in cross-validation of 0.30%. The good performance of the preliminary predictive model indicated some relationship between the NIR spectra and the plant membrane damage index. The NIR spectrum of a leaf is indeed strongly influenced by its structure, thickness, and state of hydration, which in turn is an index of plant stress [45]. Aday [46] also found agreement between FT-NIR spectroscopy and electrolyte leakage data on mushrooms treated with electrolyzed water in combination with passive atmosphere packaging.

Based on the common WABs found in normalized spectra and in the PCA and PLS loadings plots, 12 wavelengths inside the WAMACs ranges were selected for the construction of aquagrams. Each wavelength corresponds to the absorption of specific water molecular species. The wavelengths are listed and described in Table 1.

Table 1. Selected wavelengths.

Selected Wavelengths	WAMACs [22]
1342	C1—ν3
1366	C2—water solvation shell, OH-(H_2O) n, n = 1, 2, 4
1373	C3—ν1 + ν3
1385	C4—water solvation shell, OH-(H_2O)1,4 and superoxide, O2-(H_2O)4
1416	C5—free water molecules (S0)
1428	C6—water hydration, H-OH bend and O . . . O
1441	C7—water molecules with 1 hydrogen bond (S1)
1453	C8—ν2 + ν3, Water solvation shell, OH-(H_2O)4,5
1466	C9—water molecules with 2 hydrogen bonds (S2)
1478	C10—water molecules with 3 hydrogen bonds (S3)
1490	C11—water molecules with 4 hydrogen bonds (S4)
1509	C12—ν1, ν2, strongly bound water

The aquagrams of Trial 1 highlighted differences among the samples, giving rise to different WASPs for each sampling time and for each treatment (Figure 8).

Treatments A and C of the Trial 1 showed a shift from left to right up to the fourth day; then, the graph went back to the left. For treatment B, the inversion occurred on the seventh day. This behavior indicates a prevalence of hydrogen-bonded water species and strongly-bound water [47] in the freshly cut rocket. With the progress of the storage, a situation is reached in which free water or weakly hydrogen-bonded water prevails [47]. This point could indicate the loss of freshness of the product. From these premises, it can be assumed that Aquaphotomics estimated the first loss of freshness after 4 days from packaging for the A and C treatments, and after 7 days for the B treatment. This suggested that treatment B was the best at preserving the freshness of rocket salad, in agreement with the E-nose findings.

2.3.2. Trial 2

Based on the characteristics of the second sampling (autumn rocket, October mowing, presence of larger leaves and long petioles), the adequacy of the Aquaphotomics model was verified. The data processing procedure was repeated as for the first trial.

PCA is reported in Figure 9.

Again, there was a good separation of the samples according to the days of storage along PC1, which accounted for 98% of the variance (Figure 9a). The group of samples from day 4 was separated from the others along PC2. Interestingly, the B11 sample ranked alongside the first checkpoints, while the C7 sample was superimposed on t = 11/13 samples.

According to the loadings plot (Figure 9b), the separation along PC1 between fresh and longer-stored samples was mainly based on a wavelength at 1366 nm, while the separation along PC2 was due to 1385 and 1521 nm. According to Tsenkova et al. [24], the wavelengths at 1366 and 1385 nm correspond to the absorbance of water solvation shells.

The PLS regression between NIR spectra and I_{LD} data was also tentatively applied to the data from Trial 2. However, in this case, the results were not satisfactory. Better results were achieved after the application of Moving Average smoothing and the first derivative Norris Gap, obtaining R = 0.86 in calibration. However, the results in cross-validation were not as encouraging (R cross-val = 0.54), not making the model useful for practical use. It should be noted that the NIR spectra were acquired on both the sides of intact and sealed salad bags and, therefore, on the whole salad, including both leaves and petioles. Conversely, the I_{LD} data resulted from a destructive analysis carried out exclusively on the leaves. Furthermore, it can be observed from Figure 3b that the samples up to day 7 were characterized by a very low variability of I_{LD} (2.5–3.7), with a detrimental effect on quantitative calibrations [48]. These two aspects could explain the low performance obtained for this model.

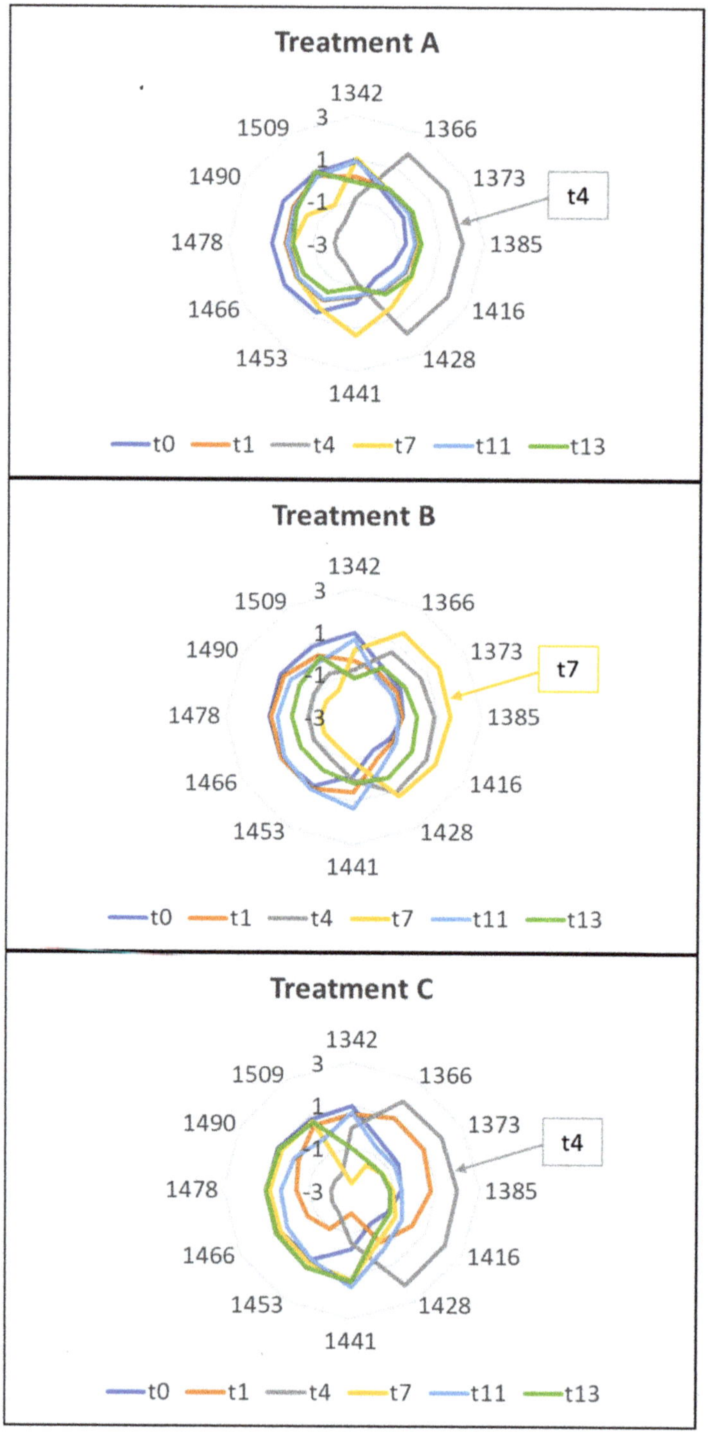

Figure 8. Aquagrams of the rocket samples belonging to the three treatments during the storage: Trial 1.

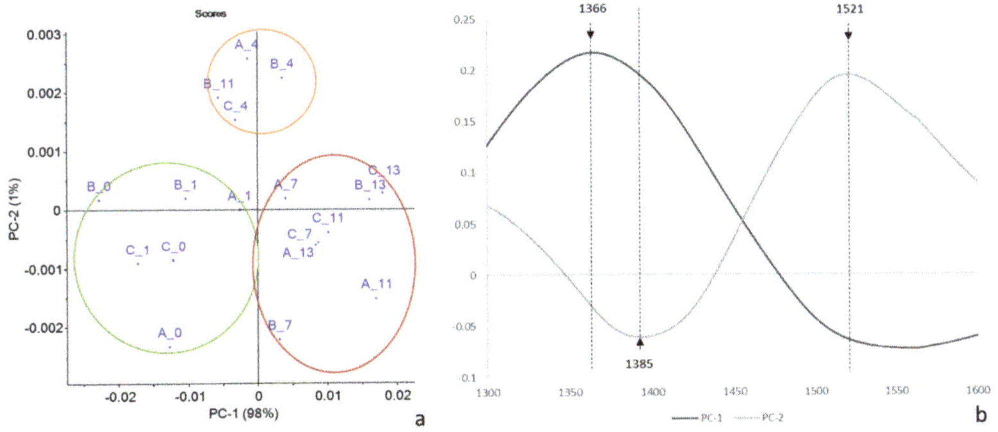

Figure 9. PCA score (**a**) and loading (**b**) plots of pre-treated NIR spectra of rocket salads of Trial 2 (each point corresponded to the mean spectra for each checkpoint).

The aquagrams were built using the same WABS as in Trial 1 (Figure 10).

The aquagrams of Trial 2 showed a different and opposite profile compared to Trial 1. As previously reported, the presence of plant material with different physiological and metabolic characteristics, due to the different growing and harvesting season [38,39,43,44], might have affected the hydration state of the stored product. Furthermore, morphological variability could have influenced the aquagram trends.

Treatments A and B showed similar profiles, with the fresh product (t0) profile very different from all the others. Consequently, it was difficult to identify a trend as a function of storage time. Fresh samples located on the right side of the chart, showed a prevalence of free water, while the stored samples were more characterized by bound water. The profiles of checkpoints 1–13, on the other hand, looked very similar, and almost overlapped in the region of 1441–1478 nm. This could indicate that the major changes in water occurred immediately after packaging. Major variations occurred at 1416–1428 nm and between 1490–1509 nm. Conversely, treatment C showed different profiles for the various sampling days.

These results suggested building a dedicated series of aquagrams not only as a function of the applied perturbation but also of the variability of the raw material.

This topic should be investigated more in-depth to determine the role of water and interactions with plant tissues during storage.

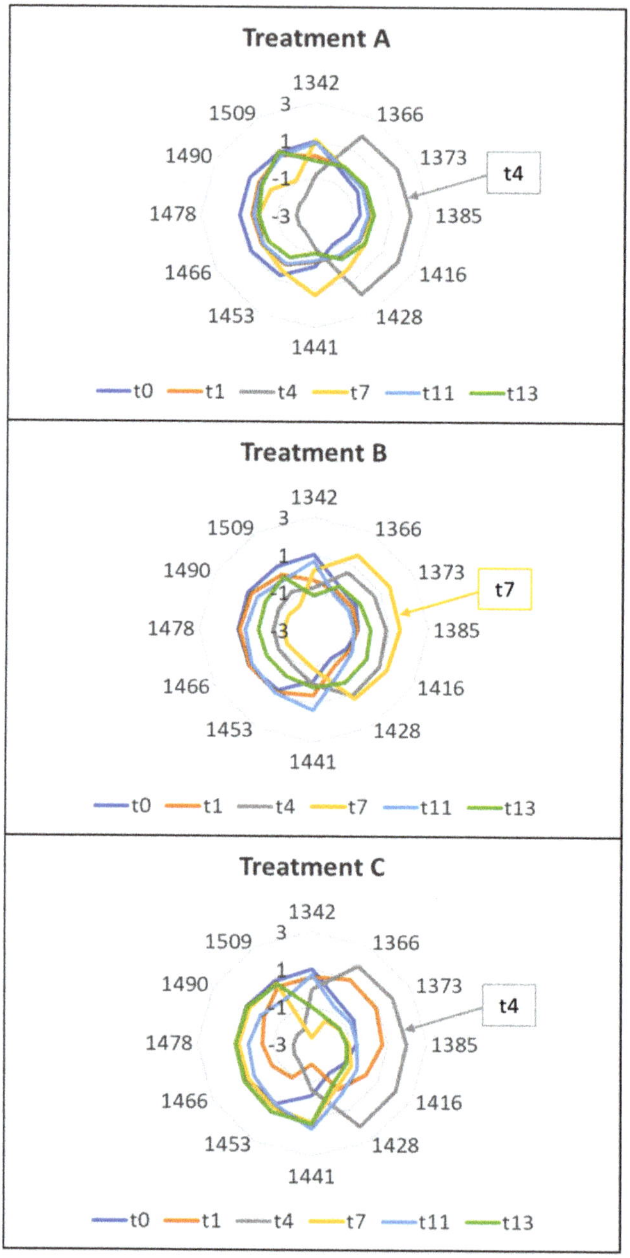

Figure 10. Aquagrams of the rocket samples belonging to the three treatments during the storage: Trial 2.

3. Materials and Methods

Two experimentations were carried out at the Research Centre for Engineering and Agro-Food Processing of the Council for Agricultural Research and Economics (CREA IT, Milan, Italy). Freshly harvested rocket leaves (*Eruca sativa* Mill.) were purchased from a local grower in Milan (Italy). The first test was carried out in spring on the first cut rocket (Trial 1), while for the second experiment second cut autumn rocket (Trial 2) was used. The fresh salad was immediately transported to the CREA-IT lab and inspected for impurity and visual defects, discarding damaged and dehydrated leaves. The product underwent washing in mildly chlorinated water (1% sodium hypochlorite solution) for 1 min, followed by rinsing in cold water, and centrifugation to remove the remaining water. Rocket leaves (ca. 60 g) were packed in polypropylene film bags, and each bag was sealed under atmospheric and modified headspace conditions. The following gas mixtures were used: treatment A, atmospheric air (21% O_2, 78% N_2); treatment B, 30% O_2, 70% N_2; treatment C, 10% CO_2, 5% O_2, 85% N_2. Three bags were prepared for each evaluation day for each treatment. All samples were stored at 4 ± 1 °C for 13 days and subjected to NIR, E-nose, and electrolyte leakage analyses at scheduled sampling points: 0, 1, 4, 7, 11, and 13 days for NIR and electrolyte leakage analyses; 1, 4, 7, 11, and 13 days for E-nose analyses.

3.1. E-Nose Analyses

The E-nose measurements were performed in triplicate on 3 bags for each treatment through a pierceable Silicon/Teflon disk, using a commercial portable electronic nose (PEN3, Win Muster Airsense Analytic Inc., Schwerim, Germany). The instrument is made up of a sampling apparatus, a detector unit containing the sensor array, and pattern-recognition software (Win Muster v.16) for data recording. The sensor array is composed of 10 metal oxide semiconductor (MOS) type chemical sensors: W1C (aromatic compounds), W5S (broad range), W3C (aromatic compounds), W6S (hydrogen), W5C (alkanes, aromatic compounds, less polar compounds), W1S (broad range, methane), W1W (terpenes, organic sulfur compounds, limonene, pyrazine), W2S (alcohols, broad range), W2W (aromatic compounds, organic sulfur compounds), and W3S (methane aliphatic, reacts on high concentrations > 100 mg/kg). The sensor response is given by the ratio between the conductivity response of the sensors to both the sample gas (G) and the carrier gas (G_0) over time (G/G_0). The E-nose analyses were performed following the conditions reported by Vanoli et al. [49]. For each measurement, the conductivity G/G_0 of the 10 sensors at the time corresponding to the normalized maximum of all signals was taken as the vector of the sensors' signal. The average of the measurements of each replicate was used for statistical analysis. Data were subjected to one-way analysis of variance (ANOVA) for means comparison using Statgraphics ver. 5.1 (Manugistic Inc, Rockville, MD, USA) software package. The means were separated using a Tukey's HSD test, and their statistical significance was determined at 5% ($p < 0.05$) level. The E-nose data were also analyzed by principal component analysis (PCA) with the Unscrambler software package (v 9.7, Camo, Inondhcim, Norway).

3.2. Electrolyte Leakage Test

The index of leaf damage (I_{LD}) was measured by an electrolyte leakage test. The analysis was performed in triplicate on 3 bags for each treatment. A method modified from Kim et al. [33] was used for ion leakage evaluation. Rocket leaf blades were cut into 1 cm^2 pieces, washed in distilled water, and blotted dry with paper towels. Two grams of the cut samples were placed in a falcon tube containing 25 mL of Milli-Q water and shaken for 1 h in a horizontal shaker at 100 strokes/minute. The initial conductivity (IC) of the solution was measured with a digital conductivity meter (Accumet AR20, Fisher Scientific, Waltham, MA, USA), and the tubes were frozen at −20 °C for one week. Frozen samples were then held at room temperature for 24 h, shaken for 1 h, and final conductivity (FC) was measured. The index of leaf damage was calculated as follows: $I_{LD} = (IC/FC) * 100$. Differences among averages were calculated by one-way ANOVA (Statgraphics 5.1 statistic software) and a least significant difference (LSD) post-hoc test. All the averages whose difference exceeds the LSD value are statistically significant ($p < 0.05$).

3.3. NIR Spectroscopy

Near-infrared spectra were collected in reflectance mode using the MicroNIR OnSite-W (VIAVI Solutions Italia S.r.l., Monza, Italy) portable spectrometer. Spectra were acquired in the spectral range between 900 and 1600 nm (50 scans; 125 reading points) on 3 bags for each treatment, on both sides of the bags. Ten replicates for each side were collected, for a total of 60 spectra for each treatment. Spectra of PET packaging (#10) were also collected, and the average spectrum was subtracted from each sample spectrum. Before the analysis, the instrument underwent calibration for the black, on the air, and for the white, on the supplied standard tile.

3.4. Chemometrics and Aquaphotomics

Chemometric analysis of the NIR data was performed using the Unscrambler software package (v 9.7, Camo, Inondhcim, Norway).

An explorative PCA was applied on spectra pre-processed using the Moving Average smoothing (gap size 15 points) and the first derivative Norris Gap transformation (gap size 21 points) in the range of the first overtone of water (1300–1600 nm).

Predictive NIR models for the I_{LD} index were computed by partial least square (PLS) regression on spectra pretreated with the Standard Normal Variate (SNV) and the second derivative Savitzky–Golay transformation (gap size 11 points).

Spectra were also pretreated according to Tsenkova et al. [24]: the second derivative Savitzky–Golay filter (second-order polynomial fit and 21 points) and Multiplicative Scatter Correction were applied to absorbance spectra to remove potential scatter effects. The transformed spectra were then normalized by applying the following formula:

$$(A\lambda - \mu\lambda)/\sigma\lambda \quad (1)$$

where $A\lambda$ is the transformed absorbance, $\mu\lambda$ is the mean value of all spectra and $\sigma\lambda$ is the standard deviation of all spectra at wavelength λ. The normalized spectra were then properly averaged using MS Excel®.

Twelve wavelengths that showed the maximum or minimum values in the normalized spectrum and the most impacting PCA or PLS loadings were chosen. The aquagrams were then built up using the selected wavelengths.

4. Conclusions

E-nose and I_{LD} results agreed in identifying the B atmosphere as the best for maintaining the freshness of RTE rocket salad in both experiments.

According to E-nose results, the A and B atmospheres confirmed the plausible positive and active role of oxygen concentration in maintaining the freshness of ready-to-eat rocket and minimizing the occurrence of anaerobic fermentations. Treatment C with low oxygen concentration seemed to lead to a switch to anaerobic respiration with a release of alcohols.

Similarly, the index of leaf damage suggested that in the C atmosphere composition, the cell membrane underwent more degradation and damage than in the other treatments.

NIR spectroscopy was useful in observing samples distribution according to the storage time, mainly based on wavelengths corresponding to the absorbance of the water solvation shells. The aquagram proved to be a promising tool for detecting changes in the water structure during storage in atmospheres with different gaseous compositions. For Trial 1 the spider-charts gave rise to different WASPs for each sampling time and treatment, suggesting that treatment B was the best at preserving the freshness of rocket salad, according to the E-nose and I_{LD} results. For Trial 2, aquagrams could not provide a clear interpretation of the changes that occurred inside the bags. However, it was possible to identify a greater variability in the WASPs in the C treatment during the shelf-life, suggesting greater changes in the water structure compared to the A and B atmospheres.

Although the data are very preliminary, the good agreement between the NIR spectra and the I_{LD} data makes NIR spectroscopy a promising technique for non-destructively evaluating the damage status of the plant membrane of the RTE rocket salad during the shelf-life.

NIR coupled with Aquaphotomics should be investigated more in-depth to determine the role of water and interactions with plant tissues during shelf-life in order to confirm these preliminary results.

Some other destructive parameters, such as consistency, fluorescence, ripening index, are under evaluation to confirm these results obtained, using mainly rapid and non-destructive techniques.

Author Contributions: Conceptualization, T.M.P.C. and L.M.; methodology, L.M.; software, L.M. and M.B.; validation, L.M., G.B. and M.B.; formal analysis, T.M.P.C., L.M., G.B. and M.B.; investigation, L.M., G.B. and M.B.; resources, T.M.P.C.; data curation, L.M., G.B. and M.B.; writing—original draft preparation, L.M.; writing—review and editing, T.M.P.C., L.M., G.B. and M.B.; supervision, T.M.P.C.; project administration, T.M.P.C.; funding acquisition, T.M.P.C. All authors have read and agreed to the published version of the manuscript.

Funding: This study was funded from the Italian Ministry of Agriculture, Agridigit project, sub-project Agrofiliere (D.M. 36503/7305/2018, approved on 20 December 2018).

Institutional Review Board Statement: Not applicable.

Informed Consent Statement: Not applicable.

Data Availability Statement: The data presented in this study are not publicly available due to the privacy related to the Agridigit project.

Acknowledgments: The authors are grateful to Tsukino Shizuku Foundation and the Chairperson Tomoko MataHari Miula for their financial support for the publication.

Conflicts of Interest: The authors declare no conflict of interest.

Sample Availability: No samples are available from the authors.

References

1. Pereira, M.J.; Amaro, A.L.; Oliveira, A.; Pintado, M. Bioactive compounds in Ready-to-Eat Rocket leaves as affected by oxygen partial pressure and storage time: A Kinetic Modelling. *Postharvest Biol. Technol.* **2019**, *158*, 110985. [CrossRef]
2. Ghidelli, C.; Pérez-Gago, M.B. Recent advances in Modified Atmosphere Packaging and edible coatings to maintain quality of fresh-cut fruits and vegetables. *Crit. Rev. Food Sci. Nutr.* **2018**, *58*, 662–679. [CrossRef] [PubMed]
3. Cefola, M.; Pace, B. Application of oxalic acid to preserve the overall quality of rocket and baby spinach leaves during storage: Oxalic acid postharvest treatment. *J. Food Process. Preserv.* **2015**, *39*, 2523–2532. [CrossRef]
4. Siomos, A.S.; Koukounaras, A. Quality and postharvest physiology of rocket leaves. *Fresh Prod.* **2007**, *1*, 59–65.
5. Lamy, E.; Schröder, J.; Paulus, S.; Brenk, P.; Stahl, T.; Mersch-Sundermann, V. Antigenotoxic properties of *Eruca sativa* (rocket plant), erucin and erysolin in human hepatoma (HepG2) cells towards benzo(a)pyrene and their mode of action. *Food Chem. Toxicol.* **2008**, *46*, 2415–2421. [CrossRef] [PubMed]
6. Wang, C.Y. Leafy, floral and succulent vegetables. In *Postharvest Physiology and Pathology of Vegetables*, 2nd ed.; Bartz, J.A., Brecht, J.K., Eds.; Marcel Dekker, Inc.: New York, NY, USA, 2003; pp. 599–623.
7. Kumar, S.; Sharma, S.; Kumar, V.; Sharma, R.; Minhas, A.; Boddu, R. Chapter 20—Cruciferous vegetables: A mine of phytonutrients for functional and nutraceutical enrichment. In *Current Advances for Development of Functional Foods Modulating Inflammation and Oxidative Stress*; Hernández-Ledesma, B., Martínez-Villaluenga, C., Eds.; Academic Press: Cambridge, MA, USA, 2022; pp. 401–426. [CrossRef]
8. Torales, A.C.; Gutiérrez, D.R.; Rodríguez, S.d.C. Influence of passive and active modified atmosphere packaging on yellowing and chlorophyll degrading enzymes activity in fresh-cut rocket leaves. *Food Packag. Shelf Life* **2020**, *26*, 100569. [CrossRef]
9. Waghmare, R.B.; Mahajan, P.V.; Annapure, U.S. Modelling the effect of time and temperature on respiration rate of selected fresh-cut produce. *Postharvest Biol. Technol.* **2013**, *80*, 25–30. [CrossRef]
10. La Zazzera, M.; Amodio, M.L.; Colelli, G. Designing a Modified Atmosphere Packaging (MAP) for fresh-cut artichokes. *Adv. Hortic. Sci.* **2015**, *29*, 24–29. [CrossRef]
11. La Zazzera, M.; Rinaldi, R.; Amodio, M.L.; Colelli, G. Influence of high CO2 atmosphere composition on fresh-cut artichoke quality attributes. *Acta Hortic.* **2012**, *934*, 633–640. [CrossRef]
12. Castro-Ibáñez, I.; Gil, M.I.; Allende, A. Ready-to-eat vegetables: Current problems and potential solutions to reduce microbial risk in the production chain. *LWT Food Sci. Technol.* **2017**, *85*, 284–292. [CrossRef]

13. Rico, D.; Martín-Diana, A.B.; Barat, J.M.; Barry-Ryan, C. Extending and measuring the quality of fresh-cut fruit and vegetables: A review. *Trends Food Sci. Technol.* **2007**, *18*, 373–386. [CrossRef]
14. Buccheri, M.; Cantwell, M. Damage to intact fruit affects quality of slices from ripened tomatoes. *LWT Food Sci. Technol.* **2014**, *59*, 327–334. [CrossRef]
15. Kou, L.; Luo, Y.; Park, E.; Turner, E.R.; Barczak, A.; Jurick, W.M. Temperature abuse timing affects the rate of quality deterioration of commercially packaged ready-to-eat baby spinach. Part I: Sensory analysis and selected quality attributes. *Postharvest Biol. Technol.* **2014**, *91*, 96–103. [CrossRef]
16. Hu, W.; Jiang, A.; Tian, M.; Liu, C.; Wang, Y. Effect of ethanol treatment on physiological and quality attributes of fresh-cut eggplant: Physiological and quality attributes of fresh-cut eggplant. *J. Sci. Food Agric.* **2010**, *90*, 1323–1326. [CrossRef] [PubMed]
17. Luca, A.; Kjær, A.; Edelenbos, M. Volatile organic compounds as markers of quality changes during the storage of wild rocket. *Food Chem.* **2017**, *232*, 579–586. [CrossRef] [PubMed]
18. Gardner, J.W.; Bartlett, P.N. A brief history of electronic noses. *Sens. Actuators B Chem.* **1994**, *18*, 210–211. [CrossRef]
19. Baldwin, E.A.; Bai, J.; Plotto, A.; Dea, S. Electronic noses and tongues: Applications for the food and pharmaceutical industries. *Sensors* **2011**, *11*, 4744–4766. [CrossRef]
20. Nielsen, T.; Bergström, B.; Borch, E. The origin of off-odours in packaged rucola (*Eruca sativa*). *Food Chem.* **2008**, *110*, 96–105. [CrossRef]
21. Yahya, H.N.; Lignou, S.; Wagstaff, C.; Bell, L. Changes in bacterial loads, gas composition, volatile organic compounds, and glucosinolates of fresh bagged Ready-To-Eat rocket under different shelf life treatment scenarios. *Postharvest Biol. Technol.* **2019**, *148*, 107–119. [CrossRef]
22. Tsenkova, R. Aquaphotomics: Dynamic spectroscopy of aqueous and biological systems describes peculiarities of water. *J. Near Infrared Spectrosc.* **2009**, *17*, 303–313. [CrossRef]
23. Tsenkova, R. Aquaphotomics: Water in the biological and aqueous world scrutinised with invisible light. *Spectrosc. Eur.* **2010**, *22*, 6–10.
24. Tsenkova, R.; Munćan, J.; Pollner, B.; Kovacs, Z. Essentials of aquaphotomics and its chemometrics approaches. *Front. Chem.* **2018**, *6*, 363. [CrossRef] [PubMed]
25. Marinoni, L.; Bianchi, G.; Cattaneo, T.M.P. The Aquaphotomics and E-nose approaches to evaluate the shelf-life of ready-to-eat rocket salad. In Proceedings of the 20th International Conference on Near Infrared Spectroscopy, Beijing, China, 18–21 October 2021; pp. 304–305.
26. Mastrandrea, L.; Amodio, M.L.; Pati, S.; Colelli, G. Effect of modified atmosphere packaging and temperature abuse on flavor related volatile compounds of rocket leaves (*Diplotaxis tenuifolia* L.). *J. Food Sci. Technol.* **2017**, *54*, 2433–2442. [CrossRef] [PubMed]
27. Hansen, M.E.; Sørensen, H.; Cantwell, M. Changes in acetaldehyde, ethanol and amino acid concentrations in broccoli florets during air and controlled atmosphere storage. *Postharvest Biol. Technol.* **2001**, *22*, 227–237. [CrossRef]
28. Luca, A.; Mahajan, P.V.; Edelenbos, M. Changes in volatile organic compounds from wild rocket (*Diplotaxis tenuifolia* L.) during modified atmosphere storage. *Postharvest Biol. Technol.* **2016**, *114*, 1–9. [CrossRef]
29. Allende, A.; Luo, Y.; McEvoy, J.L.; Artés, F.; Wang, C.Y. Microbial and quality changes in minimally processed baby spinach leaves stored under super atmospheric oxygen and modified atmosphere conditions. *Postharvest Biol. Technol.* **2004**, *33*, 51–59. [CrossRef]
30. Tudela, J.A.; Marín, A.; Martínez-Sánchez, A.; Luna, M.C.; Gil, M.I. Preharvest and postharvest factors related to off-odours of fresh-cut iceberg lettuce. *Postharvest Biol. Technol.* **2013**, *86*, 463–471. [CrossRef]
31. Rux, G.; Caleb, O.J.; Geyer, M.; Mahajan, P.V. Impact of water rinsing and perforation-mediated MAP on the quality and off-odour development for rucola. *Food Packag. Shelf Life* **2017**, *11*, 21–30. [CrossRef]
32. López-Gálvez, G.; Peiser, G.; Nie, X.; Cantwell, M. Quality changes in packaged salad products during storage. *Z. Lebensm. Unters. Forsch. A* **1997**, *205*, 64–72. [CrossRef]
33. Kim, J.G.; Luo, Y.; Tao, Y.; Saftner, R.A.; Gross, K.C. Effect of initial oxygen concentration and film oxygen transmission rate on the quality of fresh-cut romaine lettuce. *J. Sci. Food Agric.* **2005**, *85*, 1622–1630. [CrossRef]
34. Mastrandrea, L.; Amodio, M.L.; de Chiara, M.L.V.; Pati, S.; Colelli, G. Effect of temperature abuse and improper atmosphere packaging on volatile profile and quality of rocket leaves. *Food Packag. Shelf Life* **2017**, *14*, 59–65. [CrossRef]
35. Bjorkman, M.; Klingen, I.; Birch, A.N.E.; Bones, A.M.; Bruce, T.J.A.; Johansen, T.J. Phytochemicals of Brassicaceae in plant protection and human health—Influences of climate, environment and agronomic practice. *Phytochemistry* **2011**, *72*, 538–556. [CrossRef] [PubMed]
36. Wiedenhoeft, M.H.; Barton, B.A. Management and environment effects on brassica forage quality. *Agron. J.* **1994**, *86*, 227–232. [CrossRef]
37. Bianco, V.V. Rocket, an ancient underutilized vegetable crop and its potential. In *Rocket Genetic Resource Network*; Padulosi, S., Ed.; International Plant Genetic Resources Institute: Rome, Italy, 1995; pp. 35–57.
38. Hall, M.K.D.; Jobling, J.J.; Rogers, G.S. Factors affecting growth of perennial wall rocket and annual garden rocket. *Int. J. Veg. Sci.* **2012**, *18*, 393–411. [CrossRef]
39. Alcántara, C.; Pujadas, A.; Saavedra, M. Management of cruciferous cover crops by mowing for soil and water conservation in southern Spain. *Agric. Water Manag.* **2011**, *98*, 1071–1080. [CrossRef]

40. Ustin, S.L.; Jacquemoud, S. How the optical properties of leaves modify the absorption and scattering of energy and enhance leaf functionality. In *Remote Sensing of Plant Biodiversity*; Cavender-Bares, J., Gamon, J.A., Townsend, P.A., Eds.; Springer International Publishing: Cham, Switzerland, 2020; pp. 349–384. [CrossRef]
41. Tucker, C.J.; Garratt, M.W. Leaf optical system modeled as a stochastic process. *Appl. Opt.* **1977**, *16*, 635–642. [CrossRef]
42. Maier, S.W.; Lüdeker, W.; Günther, K.P. SLOP: A revised version of the stochastic model for leaf optical properties. *Remote Sens. Environ.* **1999**, *68*, 273–280. [CrossRef]
43. Edelenbos, M.; Løkke, M.M.; Seefeldt, H.F. Seasonal variation in color and texture of packaged wild rocket (*Diplotaxis tenuifolia* L.). *Food Packag. Shelf Life* **2017**, *14*, 46–51. [CrossRef]
44. Bonasia, A.; Lazzizera, C.; Elia, A.; Conversa, G. Nutritional, biophysical and physiological characteristics of wild rocket genotypes as affected by soilless cultivation system, salinity level of nutrient solution and growing period. *Front. Plant Sci.* **2017**, *8*, 300. [CrossRef]
45. Afzal, A.; Duiker, S.W.; Watson, J.E. Leaf Thickness to Predict Plant Water Status. *Biosyst. Eng.* **2017**, *156*, 148–156. [CrossRef]
46. Aday, M.S. Application of electrolyzed water for improving postharvest quality of mushroom. *LWT Food Sci. Technol.* **2016**, *68*, 44–51. [CrossRef]
47. Muncan, J.; Matovic, V.; Nikolic, S.; Askovic, J.; Tsenkova, R. Aquaphotomics approach for monitoring different steps of purification process in water treatment systems. *Talanta* **2020**, *206*, 120253. [CrossRef] [PubMed]
48. Næs, T.; Isaksson, T.; Fearn, T.; Davies, T. *A User-Friendly Guide to Multivariate Calibration and Classification*, 2nd ed.; IM Publications Open: Chichester, UK, 2017. [CrossRef]
49. Vanoli, M.; Grassi, M.; Buccheri, M.; Rizzolo, A. Influence of Edible Coating on Postharvest Physiology Ana Quality of Honeydew Melon Fruit (*Cucumis melo* L. *inodorus*). *Adv. Hortic. Sci.* **2015**, *29*, 65–74. [CrossRef]

molecules

Article

Aquaphotomics Research of Cold Stress in Soybean Cultivars with Different Stress Tolerance Ability: Early Detection of Cold Stress Response

Jelena Muncan [1], Balasooriya Mudiyanselage Siriwijaya Jinendra [2], Shinichiro Kuroki [3] and Roumiana Tsenkova [1,*]

[1] Aquaphotomics Research Department, Graduate School of Agricultural Science, Kobe University, Kobe 657-8501, Japan; jmuncan@people.kobe-u.ac.jp
[2] Department of Agricultural Engineering, Faculty of Agriculture, University of Ruhuna, Mapalana 81100, Sri Lanka; jinendra@agri.ruh.ac.lk
[3] Laboratory for Information Engineering of Bioproduction, Graduate School of Agricultural Science, Kobe University, Kobe 657-8501, Japan; skuroki@dragon.kobe-u.ac.jp
* Correspondence: rtsen@kobe-u.ac.jp; Tel.: +81-78-308-5911

Abstract: The development of non-destructive methods for early detection of cold stress of plants and the identification of cold-tolerant cultivars is highly needed in crop breeding programs. Current methods are either destructive, time-consuming or imprecise. In this study, soybean leaves' spectra were acquired in the near infrared (NIR) range (588–1025 nm) from five cultivars genetically engineered to have different levels of cold stress tolerance. The spectra were acquired at the optimal growing temperature 27 °C and when the temperature was decreased to 22 °C. In this paper, we report the results of the aquaphotomics analysis performed with the objective of understanding the role of the water molecular system in the early cold stress response of all cultivars. The raw spectra and the results of Principal Component Analysis, Soft Independent Modeling of Class Analogies and aquagrams showed consistent evidence of huge differences in the NIR spectral profiles of all cultivars under normal and mild cold stress conditions. The SIMCA discrimination between the plants before and after stress was achieved with 100% accuracy. The interpretation of spectral patterns before and after cold stress revealed major changes in the water molecular structure of the soybean leaves, altered carbohydrate and oxidative metabolism. Specific water molecular structures in the leaves of soybean cultivars were found to be highly sensitive to the temperature, showing their crucial role in the cold stress response. The results also indicated the existence of differences in the cold stress response of different cultivars, which will be a topic of further research.

Keywords: cold stress; stress tolerance; soybean; water; near infrared spectroscopy; aquaphotomics; water molecular species

Citation: Muncan, J.; Jinendra, B.M.S.; Kuroki, S.; Tsenkova, R. Aquaphotomics Research of Cold Stress in Soybean Cultivars with Different Stress Tolerance Ability: Early Detection of Cold Stress Response. *Molecules* **2022**, *27*, 744. https://doi.org/10.3390/molecules27030744

Academic Editor: Stefano Materazzi

Received: 5 January 2022
Accepted: 19 January 2022
Published: 24 January 2022

1. Introduction

Soybean (*Glycine max* (L.) Merr.) is one of the most important crops in the legume family with significant economic importance. It is a highly valued food in human and animal diet [1,2] and has important medicinal and industrial applications [2,3]. Soybean plants are susceptible to cold stress: cold halts the growth or results in injuries during all stages of development [4–9]. Despite these constraints, soybean has continued its expansion into cool climatic areas of the world [10,11]. In such areas, plants often undergo several degrees of low-temperature stress, and occasional cold stress injuries lead to decreased crop productivity and significant economic losses [12].

Soybean quality and production are dramatically affected by various abiotic stresses and a thorough understanding of the plant stress response is important for developing and breeding soybean with improved stress tolerance ability. Plants respond to all abiotic stresses with a series of morphological, physiological, cellular, biochemical and molecular changes [13]. Their purpose is the adaptation to the existing stress conditions and counteracting stress effects [14]. Cold stress, defined as the temperature in a range low enough to suppress growth without ceasing cellular functions, is known to induce several abnormalities at various levels of cellular organization [15]: (1) altered fluidity and damage of the membranes [16]; (2) the decrease in the uptake of nutrients and water, leading to cell desiccation and starvation [17]; (3) the conformational changes of proteins and nucleic acids [9]; (4) the decline in the rate of metabolic processes, reframing of gene expression [18] and reduced cellular respiration [19]; (5) accumulation of osmolytes and cryoprotectants [20] and (6) generation of reactive oxygen species [9,19,21].

The ability to measure plant stress responses in vivo is becoming increasingly important and methods are sought for rapid assessment of the stress response. Therefore, the development of non-destructive, rapid methodologies for early detection of plant response to cold stress during its growth, on the spot, is of high importance for both development of new varieties and as feedback in the agricultural industry.

Short-wavelength near-infrared (NIR) spectroscopy is a promising technique for fast and non-destructive analysis of biological materials. This region, called the "optical window", is the most useful region in the NIR for analyzing biological samples since it allows deeper penetration and non-destructive measurements. The acquired NIR spectra allow simultaneous analysis of many biomolecules in vivo. The absorption of molecules in the NIR region is due to the combinations and overtones of vibrations such as stretching and bending of CH, –OH and –NH functional groups, which engage in hydrogen bonding [22]. These functional groups are the primary structural components of major plant compounds—water, proteins, oils and starch [23–25]. Compared to the water content, the rest of the plant compounds are present in small quantities, resulting in their low signal in the NIR region—their absorbance bands are often overpowered by water absorption. However, water, with its strong capacity for hydrogen bonding, is very sensitive to any compositional or environmental changes that a biosystem experiences, which in turn produces differences in its spectrum, making it a source of information about the system as a whole and its current environmental conditions [26]. This property of water—that in an interaction with light it behaves like a mirror, revealing the structure (and function) of the system as a whole—is the basis of the aquaphotomics method and scientific discipline [26]. It extends the possibilities of traditional spectroscopy and offers a novel tool for studying biological systems [27].

Many forms of biotic stress, such as viruses [28], and abiotic stress, such as cold, drought, or salinity [29], affect water behavior on a cellular as well as on the whole plant level, which provides the rationale to apply aquaphotomics to study the stress response. The overall performance of a plant towards cold stress is a complex molecular phenomenon [30] strongly linked to the water response at the molecular structure level. The usefulness of aquaphotomics NIR spectroscopy was already demonstrated for non-destructive detection of early response to biotic stress in virus-inoculated soybean plants 2 weeks prior to the appearance of visual symptoms [28]. That work was the first to report evidence of a considerable impact from a virus infection on the hydrogen bonding network of water molecules in the infected soybean leaves and to suggest that reorganization of water at the molecular level is a part of a plant's response to stress conditions. The subsequent research on abiotic stress, specifically, desiccation stress and differences in response between resurrection plants (extremely desiccation-tolerant) and non-resurrection plants, has also provided significant new insights into the importance of the molecular structure of water for the preservation of plant tissues and survival in stressful conditions [31].

This paper reports the results obtained using a portable, non-destructive NIR instrument for detection of cold stress response in leaves of different soybean cultivars genetically modified to have different tolerances to cold stress. Using an aquaphotomics approach to NIR spectral analysis, we specifically aimed at achieving the following objectives: (1) obtaining the NIR spectral signature of cold stress in soybean cultivars' leaves that can serve as a tool for early stress detection, and (2) better understanding the physiological role of water molecular species in a cold stress response.

2. Results

2.1. Raw Absorbance Spectra of Stressed and Non-Stressed Soybean Plants

The mean leaf absorbance spectra (LogT^{-1}, where T is leaf transflectance) for soybean cultivar varieties grown continually for three weeks at 27 °C (from now on, referred to as "normal" or "no stress" conditions) and those grown for two weeks at 27 °C and then for one week at 22 °C (from now on, referred to as "cold stress" conditions) are plotted in Figure 1. The main feature of these spectra is a large absorbance peak in the visible region between 650 and 660 nm. This spectral feature is related to the light absorption by chlorophylls in the soybean leaves, which occurs in the visible part of the spectrum; the largest amount of energy is absorbed by chlorophyll *a* around 660 nm [32–34]. In the near-infrared domain (700–1050 nm), except for the differences in baseline, such strong spectral features are not visible.

The mean absorbance spectra of soybean leaves before the imposed temperature stress showed a small difference in the baseline offset between the cultivars, with the highest baseline spectral profile belonging to the most susceptible cultivar E (cyan solid line, Figure 1a, inset) and the lowest to the least susceptible cultivar A (black solid line, Figure 1a, inset). However, when the temperature was decreased to 22 °C, the mean absorbance spectra of soybean leaves showed decreased absorbance over the entire region. Comparison of the spectra averaged for all the plants grown at 27 °C and for all of the plants exposed to a 5 °C decrease in temperature (Figure 1b), revealed that decreased absorbance in the entire range is, on average, a common spectral behavior of all cultivars.

From the different spectra calculated for each cultivar, by subtracting the average spectrum of the plants grown in stressed conditions from the average spectrum of the plants grown in normal conditions (Figure 1c), we also observed that this decrease is the least intensive in the most cold-tolerant cultivar A and the most intensive in the cold susceptible cultivar E. Interestingly, only cultivar A displayed the unique feature of an actual subtle increase in absorbance, in the area 870 to 890 nm (approximately around 872 nm), which is usually attributed to the band of carbohydrates [35].

The near infrared part of the spectra when enlarged (~700–1050 nm, insets in Figure 1a–c) shows a strong baseline offset caused by light scattering (which increases the effective pathlength) or other physical differences in thickness or anatomy of the leaves. Despite this, subtle nuances in the shape of the spectral lines suggest that spectral differences also arise from the structural changes in the components of the leaves, which is especially noticeable in difference spectra in Figure 1c at the indicated wavelengths 782, 815, 872, 944 and 998 nm. In the analyzed range, both the second and thrid vibrational frequency overtones of the water OH stretching vibrations are located: second overtone around 970 nm and the third around 738 nm [36–38]; also around 836 nm is the third overtone of the combination band [39]. Since in the normal conditions the relative water content of soybean leaves is around 90% [40], it can be assumed that changes in the spectra of leaves in this region would predominantly originate from the water absorbance bands. Water is a strong absorber of NIR light and the spectra of samples with high water contents (>80%) are strongly dominated by the signature from water [41].

The changes in baseline might occur due to several reasons. First, the thickness of the leaves, which gives rise to different optical pathlengths is closely related to the water content of the leaves, as it was reported not only for soybean, but other plants as well [42]. There are reports connecting the cold stress in soybean with a decrease in the relative water content in leaves but at temperatures lower than employed in this research [43]. Furthermore, a horizontal shift in part of the 950–970 nm region was reported to be related to changes in plant leaf water status during water stress [44,45].

In order to analyze all the spectral changes in more depth, in the following analysis, the baseline shift and slope were removed using adequate preprocessing techniques.

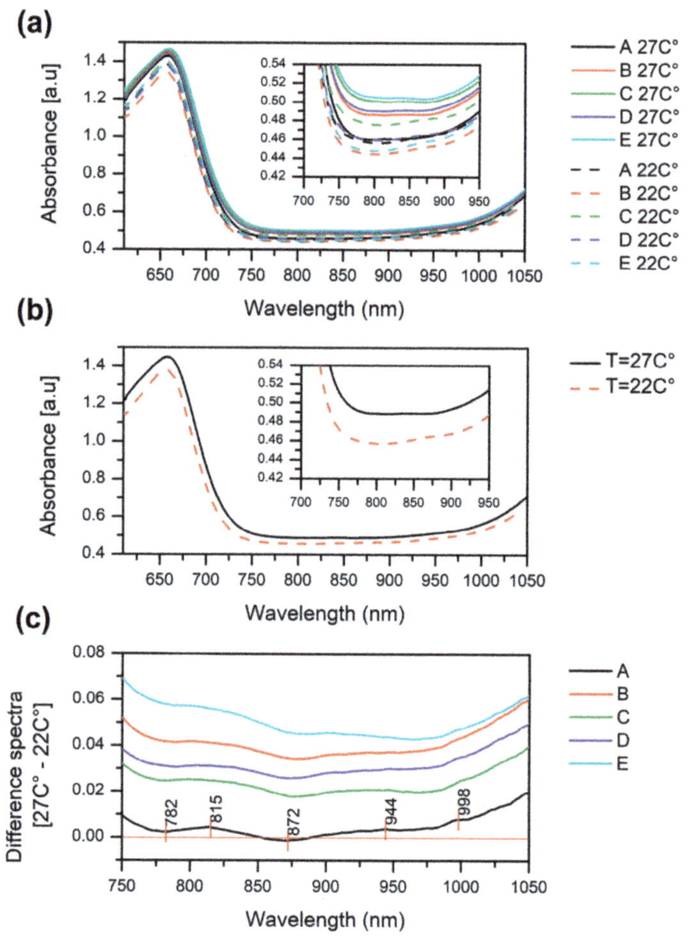

Figure 1. (**a**) Raw absorbance spectra of non-stressed (solid lines) and stressed (dashed lines) soybean plants' leaves in the vis-NIR region. Averaged for each cultivar separately—in normal growing conditions (27 °C) and in the mild cold stress conditions (22 °C); (**b**) averaged spectra for all cultivars together—in the absence of stress and in the cold stress conditions; (**c**) the difference spectra calculated as the averaged spectrum for each cultivar at 22 °C was subtracted from the average spectrum of the same cultivar at 27 °C.

2.2. Principal Component Analysis (PCA)—Exploratory Analysis of Cold Stress Effects on Spectra of Soybean Cultivars' Leaves

In order to better examine the changes in leaves due to the imposed stress and enhance the absorption effects in the spectra, further analysis was performed on the truncated region 780–1000 nm, excluding the part attributed to pigments that may dominate the analysis.

The results of PCA, presented as scores and loadings plots in Figure 2 helped in the detection of patterns in the spectral behavior of examined leaves. The scores plot for the first three principal components (which together described 97% of the variance in the spectra) showed sharp separation in two large clusters along the direction of PC1 (Figure 2a). On closer inspection, it was revealed that the PC1 component (which explained 81.3% of total variance) separated the group of non-stressed plants located in the negative part of PC1 from the group of plants exposed to cold stress located in the positive part. The loadings of principal components showed the importance of variables (wavelengths) for the computation of each of the PCs. The loading of PC1, which was the most important for separation of the plants in no-stress and stress conditions, showed several important features: positive peaks at 815, 926, 944 nm (specific for the plants during cold stress conditions) and negative peaks at 873 and 985 nm (specific for the plants in the absence of cold stress) (Figure 2a). The bands 926, 944 and 985 nm, being located in the second overtone of water, can be attributed to absorbance of different water molecular species. Specifically, 926 nm can be attributed to the bands of proton hydrates [46,47] or water hydration shell [48], 944 nm to free water molecules [49,50], while 985 nm to hydrogen-bonded water [51]. The band at 926 nm can alternately be assigned to lipids; around 930 nm in biological samples there is usually a characteristic small lipid peak [52–54] to the lipid–water mixture [55], though we cannot exclude the water–lipid interaction spectral feature. Bands at 815 nm and 873 nm may be attributed to carbohydrates, although in different forms, soluble carbohydrates and starch, respectively. The more detailed assignments will be provided later in the Discussion.

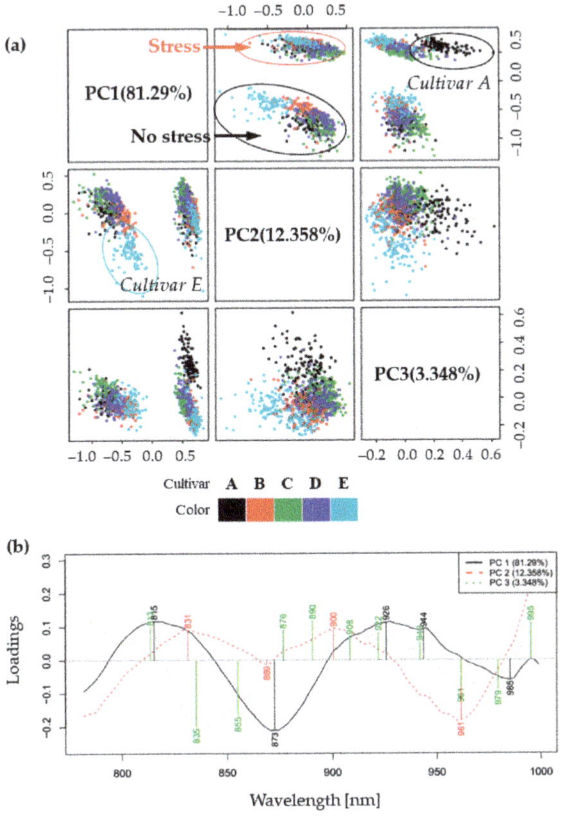

Figure 2. Principal component analysis results: (**a**) Score plots for the first three components revealed separation of plants according to the growing conditions. Two large groups of scores in the PC1-PC2 space correspond to the spectra of plants in the optimal growing conditions and during cold stress. In the score plots PC1-PC3 and PC2-PC3, differences were observed between cultivar A and cultivar E, respectively, compared to the other cultivars; (**b**) loadings of the first three principal components describe 97% variation in the spectra. The loading of the PC1 describes variations in the spectra of plants' leaves as a result of changes in the temperature of the growing environment, while the PC2 and PC3 loading show spectral characteristics that distinguish cultivar E and cultivar A, respectively, compared to the other cultivars.

Next, in the PC1-PC2 scores plot, it can be seen that PC2 separates cold-susceptible cultivar E in the non-stressed conditions—its scores are located in the negative part of PC2, in contrast to all others. The loading vector of PC2 shows positive peaks at 831 and 900 nm, while in the negative part there is a large, broad peak around 869 nm and a smaller one at 961 nm. Further, in the PC1-PC3 scores plot, PC3 separates cold-tolerant cultivar A during stress conditions from all other cultivars—scores of this cultivar are located in the positive part of PC3. The loading vector of PC3 shows positive peaks at 813, 876, 890, 908, 922, 942 and 995 nm and negative at 835, 855, 961 and 979 nm.

In summary, PCA analysis showed sharp separation between the spectra of plant leaves from the investigated soybean cultivars when they were grown at optimal temperature and after the temperature decrease. Further, the information from lower-order PC components showed the existence of differences between cultivars, particularly separating the weakest cultivar E during normal conditions, while the strongest cultivar A showed a marked difference during stress conditions.

2.3. *Soft Independent Modeling of Class Analogies for Detection of Plants' Response to Cold Stress—Discrimination of Non-Stressed and Stressed Plants*

Soft independent modeling of class analogies (SIMCA) was first applied with the purpose of supervised classification of plant leaves' spectra according to the conditions at which they were grown, i.e., no stress and cold stress, in order to develop a model for cold stress detection.

The classification accuracy for the test set was 100%, while the interclass distance (Mahalanobis distance) was 4.53, which shows reliable, strong separation between the classes [56,57] (Figure 3a). Interestingly, on Cooman's plot (Figure 3a) in the class of cold stress, a separation was detected within the class-cultivar A (the most cold-tolerant) in which it appeared separated from the others, further supporting the results of the PCA analysis in that there is a difference in the reaction of this cultivar to cold stress when compared to the rest of the cultivars.

To further explore this finding, SIMCA analysis was repeated in the same way as before, but after the spectra of cultivar A were excluded from the dataset. The classification accuracy in this case was also 100%, while the interclass distance increased to 6.67 (Figure 3b). In this case, the class seemed well-defined without any cultivars standing out. The increase in interclass distance indicates that the exclusion of cultivar A actually influences better separation of the classes of normal and cold stress conditions, as if the difference in cultivar A before and after cold stress is not so big. It is interesting to note that, in both analyses, plants in the normal conditions, in general, showed more variations within the class (scattering of scores can be observed in Figure 3a,b), in contrast to the cold stress class scores.

The discriminating powers of both SIMCA analyses were investigated for the wavelengths in the NIR spectra with the highest contribution for the distinction between classes (not stressed vs. stressed plants) (Figure 3c). The most significant wavelengths (highest discriminating power) in the case of the first SIMCA analysis, performed on the whole dataset, were observed at 799–03, 827, 868–874, 880, 900, 908, 918–922, 928, 934, 943–946, 959, 973, 985 and 995–996 nm. When the spectra of cultivar A were excluded, the discriminating power lacked a peak at 827 nm, showing this absorbance band is specifically important for separation of other cultivars and A cultivar; it lacks the discriminating power when B, C, D and E cultivar are being compared. The peak at 868–880 nm also changed, adding much more weight to the band at 880 nm and making it the most influential variable for discrimination of cultivars B, C, D and E.

2.4. *Aquagrams*

Because this part of the NIR spectra contains numerous overlapping bands it was deemed necessary to examine in more detail the nature of absorbance bands and how their assignments and interpretation can be related to what was already observed during the analysis. Therefore, the first step of the analysis was to calculate aquagrams in order to present the differences in the stress response of all cultivars together as spectral patterns to find the general features of the cold stress response in soybean (Figure 4).

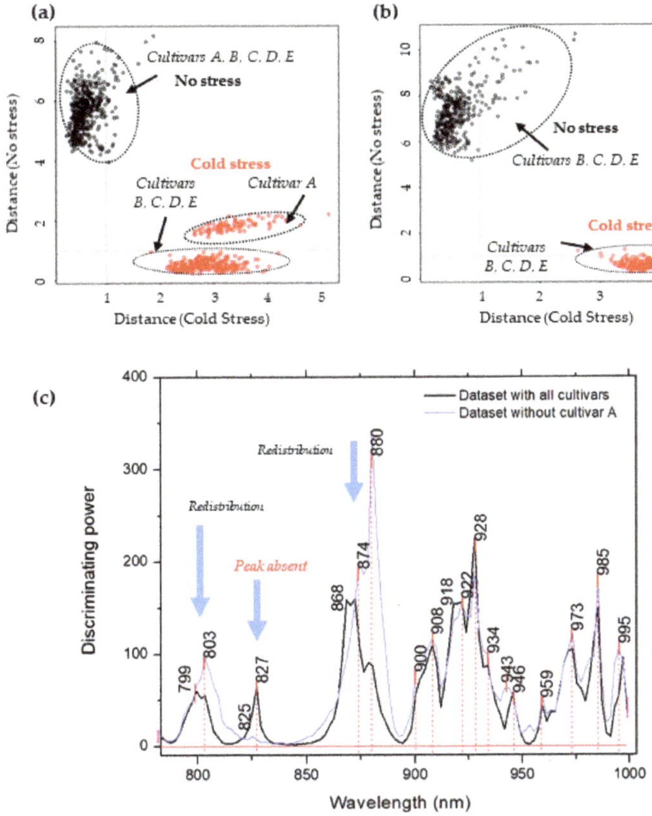

Figure 3. (**a**) SIMCA analysis results when modeling was performed using the dataset with all cultivars (A, B, C, D and E). Cooman's plot of plants grown in normal conditions (27 °C) (black) and plants exposed to mild cold stress for one week (22 °C) (red) shows excellent separation between plants and reveals distinctive stress response in cultivar A; (**b**) SIMCA analysis results when modeling was performed after the spectra of cultivar A were excluded from the analysis. Cooman's plot of plants grown in normal conditions (black) and plants exposed to mild cold stress for one week (red) shows strong, reliable separation of classes without distinction of cultivars within the class; (**c**) discriminating powers of SIMCA analyses. Comparison of discriminating powers shows that in both cases almost the same wavelengths contributed to the successful separation of classes of plants grown at normal temperature and in cold stress conditions. The exception is a peak at 827 nm, which is missing in the discriminatory power of SIMCA performed on the dataset without cultivar A.

The aquagram was calculated over the entire spectral region to indicate the regions of importance for separation between the cultivars grown in normal and temperature stress conditions, from the aspect of main leaf tissue chromophores.

The aquagram indicated six regions that show a marked difference in leaves after the cold stress, which can be interpreted as follows:

1. Region 772–799 nm: part of the third overtone of water stretching vibrations encompassing bands of hydrogen-bonded or ice-like water [36,58,59] found to be highly

correlated to the sample temperature [59,60]. The temperature stress resulted in a marked decrease in absorbance.

2. Region 800–830 nm: absorbance region that we tentatively assigned to CH of carbohydrates or hydrocarbons, not excluding their cumulative effect on the water molecular structure. The literature sources report the following absorbance bands and their interpretation in this range: 810 nm—related to oxidative metabolism in various cell types and cell proliferation [3,7–11], 815 nm—related to oxidation and the state of chloroplasts [61], 813 nm—absorbance band of aliphatic hydrocarbons [58,62], such as ethylene—a plant hormone with a role in the regulation of oxidative stress [63], shown to be produced during temperature stress in soybean leading to the oxidative injury [64]. The region also contains absorbance bands that may be attributed to water; specifically, 827–830 nm can be an absorbance band of small protonated clusters [46,51,59,65,66], while 814–816 nm a protein–water interaction (unpublished data) or carbohydrate–water interaction ([67], unpublished data). The temperature stress resulted in a marked increase in absorbance in this region.
3. Region 830–840 nm: Absorbing region of both carbohydrates and water, with water being a stronger absorber [35]. Centered at 836 nm is the second overtone of the combination band of water [39]. According to numerous sources, the 835–841 nm can be attributed to water highly influenced by temperature [59,60,68–71]. Several absorbance bands of small proton hydrates are identified within this region: at 837 nm-(+H(H_2O), +H$(H_2O)_2$), +H$(H_2O)_4$, +H$(H_2O)_6$ [46,51,59,65,66] and at 841–841.5 nm-(+H(H_2O), +H$(H_2O)_2$), +H$(H_2O)_4$, (H+·$(H_2O)_5$) +H$(H_2O)_6$ [46,51,59,65,66]. The absorbance at wavelength 840 nm was found to be related to the sample pathlength [60].
4. Region 841–900 nm: In this region both water and carbohydrates absorb, but at 870–890 nm is a strong absorbance region of carbohydrates [35,72], in particular the band 878 nm can be attributed to starch [72], major component of the leaves, and one of the key molecules mediating plant responses to abiotic stress, reported to decrease in response to abiotic stress independently of plant species [73]. The absorbance in this region shows a decrease in response to imposed temperature stress.
5. Region 900–959 nm: second overtone of water, the region that can be attributed to various water molecular species that are not involved in hydrogen bonding, i.e., less hydrogen-bonded water. The literature sources show rich information on particular absorbance bands corresponding to the specific water molecular conformations, which can all be connected to their respective locations in the first overtone region (1350–1439 nm), encompassing C1 to C6 Water Matrix Coordinates—WAMACs, that is, water solvation shells, proton hydrates, water vapor, trapped water, free water molecules and the hydration band [26,74,75]. The aquagram shows increased absorbance in this region after temperature stress, which is consistent with our previous findings of biotic stress [28].
6. Region 960–1000 nm: Second overtone of water, the region that can be attributed to various water molecular species that participate in hydrogen bonding, i.e., hydrogen-bonded water. Similar to the previous region, this one can be related to the WAMACs C7 to C11 in the first overtone of water, that is: water dimers, water solvation shells, physi-adsorbed water or bulk water, and water molecules with 2, 3 and 4 hydrogen bonds [26,74]. The aquagram shows decreased absorbance in this region after temperature stress (with the exception of a very small increase at 995 nm) in agreement with what was also observed in region 1, from the 3rd overtone of the same absorbance bands.

The aquagrams show that the absorbance spectral pattern of soybean leaves after the imposed low-temperature stress is vastly different compared to the optimal growing temperature (represented by zero line on aquagram). The difference can be related to the known and reported stress responses in soybean: changes in the water status and water molecular structure reorganization, changes in oxidative metabolism, possibly related to the ethylene hormone and the state of the chloroplasts, increased moisture (gas phase) in the leaves and their thickness and decrease in starch content. However, most importantly, the absorbance bands of water that literature sources indicate as highly influenced by temperature, were found to be the strong signature of the plant leaves' spectral changes as a reaction to temperature stress, showing direct relationship with the influence of the environment on the water metabolism. The aquagram, Figure 4, testifies about the change in the interaction of light energy and leaf tissues in soybean as a consequence of temperature stress and can serve as a quick visualizing tool for the occurrence of a stress response.

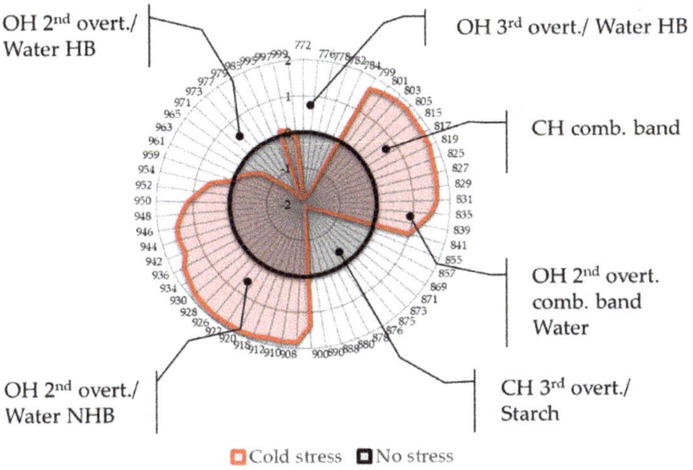

Figure 4. Aquagrams showing differences in the average spectral pattern of all cultivars calculated over the whole spectral range to present general effects of the cold stress response. The main features of the stress response are found in the 2nd overtone of water region, 2nd overtone of water combination band and 2 regions that can be attributed to 3rd overtone and combination bands of CH compounds. (HB—hydrogen bonded, NHB—non-hydrogen bonded).

Lastly, retaining only the absorbance bands that showed high importance in the previous analyses, a simple aquagram is made using 12 absorbance bands as radial axes (Figure 5).

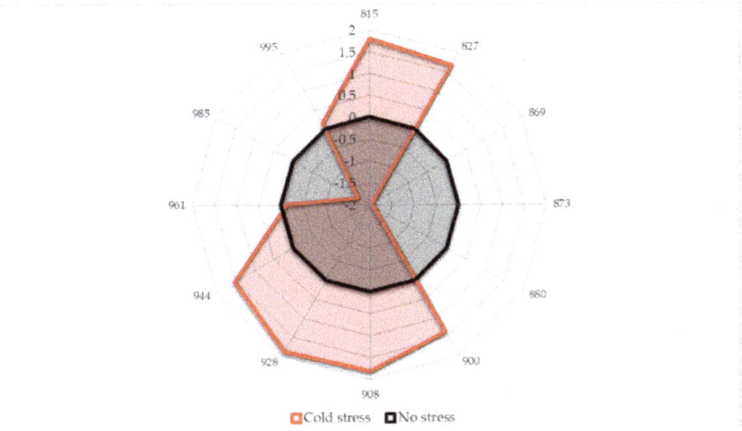

Figure 5. Aquagrams showing differences in the average spectral pattern of all soybean cultivars in the conditions of no stress and during cold stress.

The absorbance bands where increased absorbance of soybean leaves occurs in response to cold stress are located at 815, 827, 900, 908, 928 and 944 nm. This absorbance pattern speaks of increased solute accumulation (815, 827 nm [58,59,76–80]), increased interaction of water and these solutes (900, 908 and 928 nm [26,46,48,75,81]) and increased amount of free water molecules (944 nm [26,49,50]). All three phenomena are well-known to occur in plants subjected to stress. While at this point it is not possible to clearly identify what particular solutes are involved, it does not diminish the diagnostic value of the aquagram to clearly show if the plants are under stress or not. Using only 12 wavelengths to form a diagnostic marker also creates a good basis for the development of simply designed and low-cost portable sensors for applications in the field.

3. Discussion

In this paper, we used aquaphotomics based on a near infrared spectroscopy method for the evaluation of soybean plants in situ during imposed low-level temperature stress. The research was directed toward two goals: (1) early temperature stress detection in soybean based on the NIR spectral signature of cultivars' leaves, and (2) better understanding the molecular structure of water in leaves and how it is related to the overall stress response.

All our results, starting from the raw spectra analysis, over PCA exploration, SIMCA discrimination and visual representation using aquagrams, consistently showed strong evidence that a decrease of only 5 °C from the optimal growing temperature produced a response in plant tissues that was captured in the spectra. This decrease could be considered very mild cold stress, indicating that our method captured an early response to the changes in the environment of plants. Previous studies on living systems revealed that even such a small temperature decrease or increase is enough to induce antioxidant activities [82], which means that the method employed in this work is sensitive enough to capture the plants' stress response early, before the damage of the tissues. It is interesting to notice that detection of cold stress and discrimination analysis produced much poorer results when the whole vis-NIR region was used in the analysis (data not shown), indicating superior power of NIR spectroscopy because of the mild water absorbance used here as a source of information.

In the raw spectra the change in environmental temperature brought a downward shift of the baseline, caused by both physical and chemical changes in the leaves. Even in this initial step of analysis, the differences in cold stress response between the cultivars started to appear. The least cold-tolerant cultivar E showed the most intense change in the spectral profile, while the most cold-tolerant cultivar A, the smallest change, being most stable to the environmental perturbation.

The PCA analysis performed on preprocessed data, from which the effects of physical differences were removed, showed that temperature change is the cause of the largest variation in the spectral data, separating into two distinct groups scores of plants grown at optimal temperature, from the scores of the same plants after the temperature stress. In addition, lower-order PCA components showed distinctive characteristics of cold-susceptible cultivar E, whose scores were separated from the rest of the cultivars even in the conditions of optimal growing temperature, while the characteristics of cold-tolerant cultivar A became more distinguished after the exposure to lower temperatures. These findings indicated that the NIR spectra contain information not only about the stress response but also shed light on the specifics of cultivars and their individual stress responses.

SIMCA analysis further confirmed the results of PCA analysis, allowing persuasive discrimination of classes of plants grown at normal temperature and after they were exposed to cold stress. The value of interclass distance was large enough to confirm distinctive spectral features that characterize the plants before and after the cold stress. The accuracy of discrimination between the plants' growth at optimal temperature and after the temperature decreased for only 5 °C testifies to the high sensitivity of NIR spectroscopy and the power of utilizing the spectral pattern as a multidimensional biomarker for capturing the systematic stress response. Here, in this analysis, cultivar A was also distinguished compared to others when the stress occurred, once more indicating fewer variations in the less susceptible plant to be its specific stress response. The difference in discriminating power of SIMCA analyses performed with and without cultivar A in the dataset showed a particular absorbance band located at 827 nm to be the feature that is highly specific for the most cold-tolerant cultivar in relation to others.

By presenting the spectral profiles in aquagrams, the general, average reaction of all cultivars showed visually clear distinction of plants' leaves before and after cold stress. The observed spectral differences were large in six wavelength regions indicated in the aquagram, each of which was related to the main absorbers in leaf tissues and their involvement in the stress response and the wavelength assignment was supported by the current scientific literature. Throughout the analysis, we could witness the consistently repeating several absorbance bands, all of which belong to the indicated six regions found to be related mainly either to absorbance of water or carbohydrates. In summary, the findings based on the aquagram profile show that the early cold stress response is characterized by a decrease in the absorbance of hydrogen-bonded water and starch and increase in weakly hydrogen-bonded water, free water and moisture. It is interesting to notice that water absorbance bands of trapped water and strongly bound water, which are reported as a water spectral pattern related to dehydration and damage of biological tissues [27,74,83], were not observed during this study, indicating that at this stage of cold stress, the leaves did not suffer injuries.

Further on, the changes in absorbance profile were connected to changes in starch metabolism, oxidative metabolism and possibly other indicators of plant stress, such as plant hormones and state of chloroplasts. Starch metabolism has recently emerged as a key determinant of plant fitness under adverse conditions and is well-documented in various plant species but still with fragmentary knowledge about the roles in the stress response [73]. There are indications of its involvement in sugar metabolism enzymes, with differences between soybean genotypes, particularly with respect to starch characteristics in chloroplast ultrastructure [84]. The equal importance of the role of water and starch in the spectral pattern of cold stress in soybean places a new spotlight on the water functionality in the stress response. In particular, the interesting finding of the study is that specific water species, which literature sources describe as highly related to the sample temperature, were found as an important part of the stress response. The studies have reported that plants have the ability to, for example, cool their leaves below that of the temperature of the environment [85]. The temperatures of plants show that even with a 10 °C difference compared to the air temperature, physiological measurements correlated highly with a plant water stress index [86,87]. Plants have the ability to be cooled by transpiration, and in reverse when the stomata are closed, the plant temperature increases. The existing thermal imaging studies have shown the significant effects of cold and water stress on thermal infrared spectra of different plants [88]. Similarly, infrared thermography had been utilized for screening Arabidopsis plants with altered stomatal responses to drought based on the leaf temperature because their leaves appeared colder compared to the wild type [89].

In our research, the result that soybean plants in response to cold stress decrease the absorbance of hydrogen-bonded water and increase the absorbance of weakly hydrogen-bonded water (which is also evident from the changes in the baseline offset) show that plants work against cold environment by "internal heating", i.e., reorganizing the water molecular structure to be as if the temperature is higher. The observation that the magnitude of changes was highest in cold-susceptible cultivar E while lowest in cold-tolerant cultivar A suggests the possibility that the water in leaves of a cold-tolerant cultivar is already in the more favorable state, which opens up a new line of research direction aimed at examining the relationship between genetic modification and the end-result of a specific water molecular structure in the leaves of cold-tolerant plants.

The existing findings, in addition to the observation of this research, strongly support the possibility that water, not only its content but its structure, has an important role in the regulation of the plant's internal temperature, and certain water species that are temperature sensitive serve as signaling molecules, possibly initiating a cascade of events in the stress defense system.

As we witnessed in the results of the present research, the genomic base of the soybean cultivars may also dictate how sensitive the water molecular matrix of the leaves is to the perturbation coming from the environment. However, this is a research topic of future physiological, genetic and aquaphotomics studies. Hopefully, the integrated studies of these various omics disciplines may uncover the specifics of the mechanism underlying the different responses among cultivars and result in new strategies to breed soybean for future climates.

4. Materials and Methods

4.1. Plant Materials

Seeds of five different soybean (*Glycine max*) cultivars that have different degrees of cold stress tolerance, Kitamusume (A), Toyoharuka (B), Toyokomachi (C), Toyomusume (D), Hokkaihadaka (E), with cultivar A being the most cold-tolerant and E being the most cold-sensitive, were obtained from the Tokachi Agricultural Experiment Station (TAES), Hokkaido, Japan. The cold stress tolerance level was based on the Tokachi Agricultural Experiment Station grading based on the field performance. The cold tolerance of the studied cultivars, their cold tolerant index (CTI), was assigned based on the multiple field experiments. There are several research studies that have investigated the cold tolerance ability and field performance of the soybean cultivars studied in this work, and other cultivars as well, which can be used as a source of more information about the genotypic differences [10,11,90–93].

4.2. Experimental Protocol—Experimental Conditions for Cold Stress Investigation

Two hundred plants, 40 plants per cultivar, were grown in plastic pots at 27 °C, 14 h light/10 h dark (day/night) supply (22,000 Lux) for two weeks. After two weeks, 20 plants from each cultivar were moved to 22 °C phytothron ("cold stress" conditions) and the rest were kept continuously at 27 °C for up to three weeks ("normal" conditions—no stress). The temperature of 27 °C was chosen because it is usually encountered in real field conditions, while the mild cold stress temperature of 22 °C, i.e., decrease of only 5 °C, was chosen because it is still within the optimum temperature window for soybean growth (between 20 and 30 °C, [94]). If further reduced, prolonged exposure to low temperatures (15–10 °C) may induce cultivar cold acclimation attributes [95], which was not an objective of this study.

4.3. NIR Spectroscopy Measurements

Measurements were carried out non-destructively on single leaves using a handheld type NIR spectrometer FQA-NIR Gun (Shizuoka Shibuya Seiki, Hamamatsu, Japan). Five transflectance spectra (588 nm up to 1025 nm at 2 nm steps) from the first trifoliate leaves of each plant were acquired using a custom designed reflectance probe as previously described (Figure 6) [28]. Briefly, the modified probe allowed constant measuring conditions for all leaves by preventing the environmental light interference, and a hinge-type bottom plate of the modified probe provided a constant white background for all the measurements. The sampled leaf was kept immobile, and spectral acquisition was performed within few seconds, thus minimally interfering with the leaf functionality.

The acquired leaf reflectance spectra (R) were converted to absorbance spectra ($A = \log R^{-1}$). For 5 cultivars with 40 biological replicates per cultivar and 5 acquired spectra from the first trifoliate of each biological replicate, a dataset of 1000 absorbance spectra for the analysis was obtained (500 for the plants grown in normal, and 500 for the plants grown in stressed conditions).

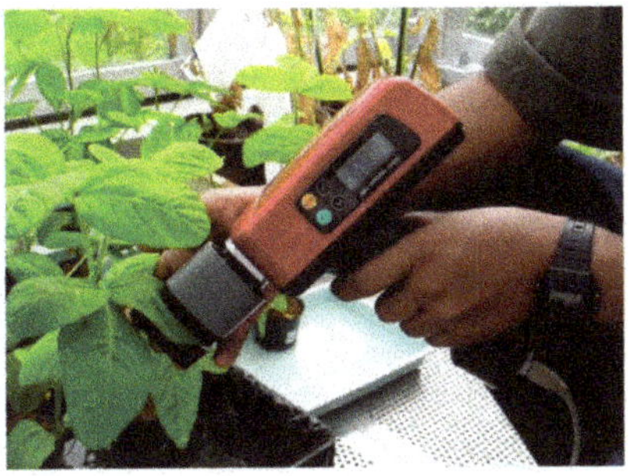

Figure 6. Acquiring soybean leaf spectra by handheld NIR spectrometer with a custom designed probe.

4.4. Data Processing and Analysis

Principal component analysis (PCA) [96] of the whole spectral dataset in the spectral range 780–1000 nm was performed after detrend and standard normal variate transformation [97] preprocessing to remove the baseline effects and improve separation of the overlapping bands [98]. PCA was used on the whole dataset—firstly, for the general inspection and removal of outliers based on the values of the Mahalanobis distance [99]. Secondly, the aim of performing PCA was to examine the information present in the dataset and to detect possible existing patterns in data and relationships with variables. PCA transforms the original data into new, orthogonal, variables called principal components (PCs) where only the first few contain most of the useful information. The loadings of PCA indicate the importance of wavelengths for computation of each PC.

Soft independent modeling of class analogies (SIMCA) [100] was applied to build a supervised classification model for discrimination of plants in normal and stressed conditions. A SIMCA model was tested on an independent test set containing 50% of the original dataset, formed by selecting every other spectra (odd numbered spectra were used for calibration, even numbered for validation). The test set used for validation was left completely out during the modeling based on the calibration set.

An aquagram was used to visualize the changes in the water molecular matrix in the leaves of all cultivars together in response to cold stress. Aquagrams were calculated using the method for classic aquagrams [99], according to the following equation:

$$A'_\lambda = \frac{A_\lambda - \mu_\lambda}{\sigma_\lambda} \quad (1)$$

In the equation, A'_λ is a normalized absorbance, which is displayed on the aquagram, and A_λ is the absorbance after detrend [98] and standard normal variate transformation (SNV) [97] performed on spectral data acquired in the normal conditions and cold stress conditions separately. The value μ_λ is the mean, while σ_λ is the standard deviation of all the preprocessed spectra together after separately performed transformations. First, the aquagrams were presented using as the wavelengths λ all the wavelengths from the whole spectral range. This way of representing differences allowed for better identification of major absorbers in the leaves and how they changed in response to stress. Finally, as is usual practice in the aquaphotomics analysis protocol, only the most influential absorbance bands were retained based on the frequency of their occurrence throughout the analysis [98], and the simple aquagram was made using only 12 absorbance bands as radial axes.

The two transformations—detrending and standard normal variate transformations—were performed prior to the aquagram calculation to cancel the differences in baseline effects and were performed separately on data acquired during normal and during stress conditions because the raw spectra showed differences in the baseline effects depending on the conditions.

The transformation of spectral data, data analysis and visualizations were performed using the aquap2 package [101] in R Project statistical software [102]. Spectral subtraction and peak detections in second derivative spectra and difference spectra were performed using OriginPro® version 8.5 (OriginLab Corporation, Northampton, MA, USA). Aquagram calculations were performed using Microsoft Excel 2016 (Microsoft Corp., Redmond, WA, USA).

5. Conclusions

This study was conducted using near infrared spectroscopy and aquaphotomics as a novel method for non-destructive detection of the cold stress response.

The research showed that the method was sensitive enough to detect the response of the soybean plants even in very mild cold stress conditions and to discriminate with 100% accuracy the plants grown at optimal growing temperature and plants after they were exposed to the cold stress.

The information in spectra that allowed the successful detection of cold stress response was largely based on the water absorbance bands, testifying to the water structure playing an important part in the primary stress response in soybean plants' leaves. Additionally, the role of carbohydrates and their interaction with water was found to be strongly associated with the cold stress response.

Our results cast new light on the importance of water in plants' adaptive response to temperature change and its role in the cold tolerance ability of different soybean cultivars contributing to a better understanding of this phenomenon, while at the same time providing a novel principle for the development of rapid, non-destructive methods for cold stress detection that can be performed in the field.

Author Contributions: Conceptualization, B.M.S.J., S.K. and R.T.; methodology, B.M.S.J., S.K. and R.T; software, J.M.; validation, J.M. and R.T.; formal analysis, J.M.; investigation, B.M.S.J., S.K. and J.M; resources, R.T.; data curation, B.M.S.J. and R.T.; writing—original draft preparation, B.M.S.J. and J.M.; writing—review and editing, J.M.; visualization, J.M.; supervision, R.T.; project administration, S.K. and R.T.; funding acquisition, R.T. All authors have read and agreed to the published version of the manuscript.

Funding: This research received no external funding.

Institutional Review Board Statement: Not applicable.

Informed Consent Statement: Not applicable.

Data Availability Statement: The data presented in this study are available on request from the corresponding author.

Acknowledgments: The author J.M. gratefully acknowledges the Japanese Society for Promotion of Science (P17406) for the financial support for postdoctoral fellowship during which the majority of the analysis and writing of this paper has been performed. The authors wish to thank Naoki Mori, Yukio Tosa, Hiromichi Ito and Sugimoto Toshio for providing the space for plant growth and other forms of support to accomplish this work. The authors are also grateful to the Tokachi Agricultural research station, as without their help this research would never have been materialized.

Conflicts of Interest: The authors declare no conflict of interest.

References

1. Liu, K.S. Chemistry and nutritional value of soybean. In *Soybean: Chemistry, Technology, and Utilization*; Chapman & Hall: New York, NY, USA, 1997; p. 532. ISBN 9780834212992.
2. Thao, N.P.; Tran, L.-S.P. Potentials toward genetic engineering of drought-tolerant soybean. *Crit. Rev. Biotechnol.* **2012**, *32*, 349–362. [CrossRef] [PubMed]
3. Wu, Z.; Schenk-Hamlin, D.; Zhan, W.; Ragsdale, D.W.; Heimpel, G.E. The Soybean Aphid in China: A Historical Review. *Ann. Entomol. Soc. Am.* **2009**, *97*, 209–218. [CrossRef]
4. Schor, A.; Fossati, A.; Soldat, A.; Stamp, P. Cold tolerance in soybean (*Glycine max* L. Merr.) in relation to flowering habit, pod set and compensation for lost reproductive organs. *Eur. J. Agron.* **1993**, *2*, 173–178. [CrossRef]

5. Ohnishi, S.; Miyoshi, T.; Shirai, S. Low temperature stress at different flower developmental stages affects pollen development, pollination, and pod set in soybean. *Environ. Exp. Bot.* **2010**, *69*, 56–62. [CrossRef]
6. Yamaguchi, N.; Ohnishi, S.; Miyoshi, T. Screening for Chilling-Tolerant Soybeans at the Flowering Stage Using a Seed Yield- and Maturity-Based Evaluation Method. *Crop Sci.* **2018**, *58*, 312. [CrossRef]
7. Rys, M.; Szaleniec, M.; Skoczowski, A.; Stawoska, I.; Janeczko, A. FT-Raman spectroscopy as a tool in evaluation the response of plants to drought stress. *Open Chem.* **2015**, *13*, 1091–1100. [CrossRef]
8. Cheesbrough, T.M. Decreased growth temperature increases soybean stearoyl-acyl carrier protein desaturase activity. *Plant Physiol.* **1990**, *93*, 555–559. [CrossRef]
9. Nouri, M.-Z.; Toorchi, M.; Komatsu, S. Proteomics Approach for Identifying Abiotic Stress Responsive Proteins in Soybean. In *Soybean-Molecular Aspects of Breeding*; In Tech Open Limited: London, UK, 2011.
10. Funatsuki, H.; Kawaguchi, K.; Matsuba, S.; Sato, Y.; Ishimoto, M. Mapping of QTL associated with chilling tolerance during reproductive growth in soybean. *Theor. Appl. Genet.* **2005**, *111*, 851–861. [CrossRef]
11. Funatsuki, H.; Ohnishi, S. Recent Advances in Physiological and Genetic Studies on Chilling Tolerance in Soybean. *Japan Agric. Res. Q. JARQ* **2009**, *43*, 95–101. [CrossRef]
12. Kurosaki, H.; Yumoto, S. Effects of Low Temperature and Shading during Flowering on the Yield Components in Soybeans. *Plant Prod. Sci.* **2003**, *6*, 17–23. [CrossRef]
13. Sanghera, G.S.; Wani, S.H.; Hussain, W.; Singh, N.B. Engineering Cold Stress Tolerance in Crop Plants. *Curr. Genomics* **2011**, *12*, 30–43. [CrossRef] [PubMed]
14. Rodziewicz, P.; Swarcewicz, B.; Chmielewska, K.; Wojakowska, A.; Stobiecki, M. Influence of abiotic stresses on plant proteome and metabolome changes. *Acta Physiol. Plant.* **2014**, *36*, 1–19. [CrossRef]
15. Balestrasse, K.B.; Tomaro, M.L.; Batlle, A.; Noriega, G.O. The role of 5-aminolevulinic acid in the response to cold stress in soybean plants. *Phytochemistry* **2010**, *71*, 2038–2045. [CrossRef] [PubMed]
16. Xing, W.; Rajashekar, C. Glycine betaine involvement in freezing tolerance and water stress in Arabidopsis thaliana. *Environ. Exp. Bot.* **2001**, *46*, 21–28. [CrossRef]
17. Miura, K.; Tada, Y. Regulation of water, salinity, and cold stress responses by salicylic acid. *Front. Plant Sci.* **2014**, *5*, 4. [CrossRef]
18. Chinnusamy, V.; Zhu, J.; Zhu, J.-K. Cold stress regulation of gene expression in plants. *Trends Plant Sci.* **2007**, *12*, 444–451. [CrossRef]
19. Lee, T.-M.; Lur, H.-S.; Chu, C. Role of abscisic acid in chilling tolerance of rice (*Oryza sativa* L.) seedlings. *Plant Sci.* **1997**, *126*, 1–10. [CrossRef]
20. Bhandari, K.; Nayyar, H. Low Temperature Stress in Plants: An Overview of Roles of Cryoprotectants in Defense. In *Physiological Mechanisms and Adaptation Strategies in Plants Under Changing Environment*; Springer: New York, NY, USA, 2014; pp. 193–265.
21. Abdel Latef, A.A.H.; Chaoxing, H. Arbuscular mycorrhizal influence on growth, photosynthetic pigments, osmotic adjustment and oxidative stress in tomato plants subjected to low temperature stress. *Acta Physiol. Plant.* **2011**, *33*, 1217–1225. [CrossRef]
22. Sakudo, A.; Suganuma, Y.; Kobayashi, T.; Onodera, T.; Ikuta, K. Near-infrared spectroscopy: Promising diagnostic tool for viral infections. *Biochem. Biophys. Res. Commun.* **2006**, *341*, 279–284. [CrossRef]
23. van der Meer, F.; De Jong, S.; Bakker, W. Imaging Spectrometry: Basic Analytical Techniques. In *Imaging Spectrometry: Basic Principles and Prospective Applications (Remote Sensing and Digital Image Processing, 4)*; Kluwer Academic: Dordrecht, The Netherlands, 2002; pp. 17–62.
24. Jinendra, B. Near Infrared Spectroscopy and Aquaphotomics: Novel Tool for Biotic and Abiotic Stress Diagnosis of Soybean. Ph.D. Thesis, Kobe University, Kobe, Japan, 2011.
25. Lee, H.; Kim, M.S.; Song, Y.-R.; Oh, C.-S.; Lim, H.-S.; Lee, W.-H.; Kang, J.-S.; Cho, B.-K. Non-destructive evaluation of bacteria-infected watermelon seeds using visible/near-infrared hyperspectral imaging. *J. Sci. Food Agric.* **2017**, *97*, 1084–1092. [CrossRef]
26. Tsenkova, R. Aquaphotomics: Dynamic spectroscopy of aqueous and biological systems describes peculiarities of water. *J. Near Infrared Spectrosc.* **2009**, *17*, 303–313. [CrossRef]
27. Muncan, J.; Tsenkova, R. Aquaphotomics-From Innovative Knowledge to Integrative Platform in Science and Technology. *Molecules* **2019**, *24*, 2742. [CrossRef] [PubMed]
28. Jinendra, B.; Tamaki, K.; Kuroki, S.; Vassileva, M.; Yoshida, S.; Tsenkova, R. Near infrared spectroscopy and aquaphotomics: Novel approach for rapid in vivo diagnosis of virus infected soybean. *Biochem. Biophys. Res. Commun.* **2010**, *397*, 685–690. [CrossRef] [PubMed]
29. Beck, E.H.; Fettig, S.; Knake, C.; Hartig, K.; Bhattarai, T. Specific and unspecific responses of plants to cold and drought stress. *J. Biosci.* **2007**, *32*, 501–510. [CrossRef] [PubMed]
30. Levitt, J. *Responses of Plants to Environmental Stress, Volume 1: Chilling, Freezing, and High Temperature Stresses*; Academic Press: New York, NY, USA, 1980.
31. Kuroki, S.; Tsenkova, R.; Moyankova, D.P.; Muncan, J.; Morita, H.; Atanassova, S.; Djilianov, D. Water molecular structure underpins extreme desiccation tolerance of the resurrection plant Haberlea rhodopensis. *Sci. Rep.* **2019**, *9*, 3049. [CrossRef] [PubMed]
32. Olascoaga, B. Leaf Optical Properties and Dynamics of Photosynthetic Activity. Ph.D. Thesis, Faculty of Agriculture and Forestry of the University of Helsinki, Helsinki, Finland, 2018.

33. Sims, D.A.; Gamon, J.A. Relationships between leaf pigment content and spectral reflectance across a wide range of species, leaf structures and developmental stages. *Remote Sens. Environ.* **2002**, *81*, 337–354. [CrossRef]
34. Kaspary, T.E.; Lamego, F.P.; Cutti, L.; Aguiar, A.C.M.; Bellé, C. Determination of photosynthetic pigments in fleabane biotypes susceptible and resistant to the Herbicide Glyphosate. *Planta Daninha* **2014**, *32*, 417–426. [CrossRef]
35. McGlone, V.A.; Kawano, S. Firmness, dry-matter and soluble-solids assessment of postharvest kiwifruit by NIR spectroscopy. *Postharvest Biol. Technol.* **1998**, *13*, 131–141. [CrossRef]
36. Golic, M.; Walsh, K.; Lawson, P. Short-wavelength near-infrared spectra of sucrose, glucose, and fructose with respect to sugar concentration and temperature. *Appl. Spectrosc.* **2003**, *57*, 139–145. [CrossRef]
37. Abe, H.; Kusama, T.; Kawano, S.; Iwamoto, M. Analysis of hydrogen bond state of water by band decomposition of near infrared absorption spectrum. *Bunko Kenkyu* **1995**, *44*, 247–253. [CrossRef]
38. Osborne, B.; Fearn, T.; Hindle, P. *Practical NIR Spectroscopy with Applications in Food and Beverage Analysis-UCL Discovery*, 2nd ed.; Longman Scientific and Technical: Essex, UK, 1993.
39. Chaplin, M. Water Structure and Science. Available online: http://www1.lsbu.ac.uk/water/water_vibrational_spectrum.html (accessed on 29 January 2019).
40. Hossain, M.M.; Liu, X.; Qi, X.; Lam, H.-M.; Zhang, J. Differences between soybean genotypes in physiological response to sequential soil drying and rewetting. *Crop J.* **2014**, *2*, 366–380. [CrossRef]
41. Büning-Pfaue, H. Analysis of water in food by near infrared spectroscopy. *Food Chem.* **2003**, *82*, 107–115. [CrossRef]
42. Afzal, A.; Duiker, S.W.; Watson, J.E. Leaf thickness to predict plant water status. *Biosyst. Eng.* **2017**, *156*, 148–156. [CrossRef]
43. Yildiztugay, E.; Ozfidan-Konakci, C.; Kucukoduk, M. Improvement of cold stress resistance via free radical scavenging ability and promoted water status and photosynthetic capacity of gallic acid in soybean leaves. *J. Soil Sci. Plant Nutr.* **2017**, *17*, 366–384. [CrossRef]
44. Peñuelas, J.; Filella, I. Visible and near-infrared reflectance techniques for diagnosing plant physiological status. *Trends Plant Sci.* **1998**, *3*, 151–156. [CrossRef]
45. Kumar, L.; Schmidt, K.; Dury, S.; Skidmore, A. Imaging spectroscopy and vegetation science. In *Imaging Spectrometry: Basic Principles and Prospective Applications*; Van der Meer, S.M., De Jong, S.M., Eds.; Kluwer Academic: Dordrecht, The Netherlands, 2001; pp. 111–155.
46. Headrick, J.M.; Diken, E.G.; Walters, R.S.; Hammer, N.I.; Christie, R.A.; Cui, J.; Myshakin, E.M.; Duncan, M.A.; Johnson, M.A.; Jordan, K.D. Spectral signatures of hydrated proton vibrations in water clusters. *Science* **2005**, *308*, 1765–1769. [CrossRef]
47. Shin, J.-W.W.; Hammer, N.I.; Diken, E.G.; Johnson, M.A.; Walters, R.S.; Jaeger, T.D.; Duncan, M.A.; Christie, R.A.; Jordan, K.D. Infrared signature of structures associated with the H+(H 2O)n (n = 6 to 27) clusters. *Science* **2004**, *304*, 1137–1140. [CrossRef]
48. Robertson, W.H.; Diken, E.G.; Price, E.A.; Shin, J.-W.; Johnson, M.A. Spectroscopic determination of the OH^- solvation shell in the $OH^- \cdot (H_2O)_n$ clusters. *Science* **2003**, *299*, 1367–1372. [CrossRef]
49. Suzuki, T. Hydrogen-bond studies of thin film water using near-infrared spectroscopy in the 970 nm spectral region. *Appl. Surf. Sci.* **2002**, *187*, 261–265. [CrossRef]
50. Ozaki, Y. Applications in Chemistry. In *Near-Infrared Spectroscopy. Principles, Instruments, Applications*; Siesler, H.W., Ozaki, Y., Kawata, S., Heise, H., Eds.; Wiley-VCH Verlag GmbH: Weinheim, Germany, 2002; pp. 179–213. ISBN 3527301658.
51. Mizuse, K.; Fujii, A. Tuning of the Internal Energy and Isomer Distribution in Small Protonated Water Clusters $H^+(H_2O)4$–8: An Application of the Inert Gas Messenger Technique. *J. Phys. Chem. A* **2012**, *116*, 4868–4877. [CrossRef]
52. Zuzak, K.J.; Naik, S.C.; Alexandrakis, G.; Hawkins, D.; Behbehani, K.; Livingston, E. Intraoperative bile duct visualization using near-infrared hyperspectral video imaging. *Am. J. Surg.* **2008**, *195*, 491–497. [CrossRef]
53. Wilson, R.H.; Nadeau, K.P.; Jaworski, F.B.; Tromberg, B.J.; Durkin, A.J. Review of short-wave infrared spectroscopy and imaging methods for biological tissue characterization. *J. Biomed. Opt.* **2015**, *20*, 030901. [CrossRef]
54. Kukreti, S.; Cerussi, A.E.; Tromberg, B.J.; Gratton, E. Intrinsic tumor biomarkers revealed by novel double-differential spectroscopic analysis of near-infrared spectra. *J. Biomed. Opt.* **2007**, *12*, 020509. [CrossRef]
55. Zuzak, K.J.; Naik, S.C.; Alexandrakis, G.; Hawkins, D.; Behbehani, K.; Livingston, E.H. Characterization of a Near-Infrared Laparoscopic Hyperspectral Imaging System for Minimally Invasive Surgery. *Anal. Chem.* **2007**, *79*, 4709–4715. [CrossRef]
56. Blomquist, G.; Johansson, E.; Söderström, B.; Wold, S. Data analysis of pyrolysis—Chromatograms by means of simca pattern recognition. *J. Anal. Appl. Pyrolysis* **1979**, *1*, 53–65. [CrossRef]
57. Brereton, R.G. *Multivariate Pattern Recognition in Chemometrics: Illustrated by Case Studies*; Elsevier Science Publishers: Amsterdam, The Netherlands, 1992; ISBN 9780080868363.
58. Workman, J.J.; Weyer, L. *Practical Guide and Spectral Atlas for Interpretive Near-Infrared Spectroscopy*, 2nd ed.; CRC Press Taylor & Francis Group: Boca Raton, FL, USA, 2012; ISBN 978-1-4398-7526-1.
59. Kovacs, Z.; Muncan, J.; Ohmido, N.; Bazar, G.; Tsenkova, R. Water Spectral Patterns Reveals Similarities and Differences in Rice Germination and Induced Degenerated Callus Development. *Plants* **2021**, *10*, 1832. [CrossRef]
60. Miyamoto, K.; Kitano, Y. Non-Destructive Determination of Sugar Content in Satsuma Mandarin Fruit by near Infrared Transmittance Spectroscopy. *J. Near Infrared Spectrosc.* **1995**, *3*, 227–237. [CrossRef]
61. Klughammer, C.; Schreiber, U. Analysis of Light-Induced Absorbance Changes in the Near-Infrared Spectral Region I. Characterization of Various Components in Isolated Chloroplasts. *Z. Naturforsch. C J. Biosci.* **1991**, *46*, 233–244. [CrossRef]

62. Williams, P.; Antoniszyn, J.; Manley, M. *Near Infrared Technology: Getting the Best out of Light*; AFRICAN SUN MeDIA: Stellenbosch, South Africa, 2019; ISBN 978-1-928480-30-3.
63. Ishibashi, Y.; Koda, Y.; Zheng, S.H.; Yuasa, T.; Iwaya-Inoue, M. Regulation of soybean seed germination through ethylene production in response to reactive oxygen species. *Ann. Bot.* **2013**, *111*, 95–102. [CrossRef]
64. Djanaguiraman, M.; Prasad, P.V.V.; Al-Khatib, K. Ethylene perception inhibitor 1-MCP decreases oxidative damage of leaves through enhanced antioxidant defense mechanisms in soybean plants grown under high temperature stress. *Environ. Exp. Bot.* **2011**, *71*, 215–223. [CrossRef]
65. Ojamäe, L.; Shavitt, I.; Singer, S.J. Potential energy surfaces and vibrational spectra of H5O2+ and larger hydrated proton complexes. *Int. J. Quantum Chem.* **1995**, *56*, 657–668. [CrossRef]
66. Rhine, P.; Williams, D.; Hale, M.; Querry, M.R. Infrared Optical Constants of Aqueous Solutions of Electrolytes. Acids and Bases. *J. Phys. Chem.* **1974**, *78*, 1405–1410. [CrossRef]
67. Tsenkova, R.; Muncan, J. *Aquaphotomics for Bio-diagnostics in Dairy-Applications of Near-Infrared Spectroscopy*; Springer Nature Singapore Pte Ltd.: Singapore, 2021; ISBN 978-981-16-7113-5.
68. Chauchard, F.; Roger, J.M.; Bellon-Maurel, V. Correction of the Temperature Effect on near Infrared Calibration—Application to Soluble Solid Content Prediction. *J. Near Infrared Spectrosc.* **2004**, *12*, 199–205. [CrossRef]
69. Kawano, S.; Abe, H.; Iwamoto, M. Development of a Calibration Equation with Temperature Compensation for Determining the Brix Value in Intact Peaches. *J. Near Infrared Spectrosc.* **1995**, *3*, 211–218. [CrossRef]
70. Langford, V.S.; McKinley, A.J.; Quickenden, T.I. Temperature dependence of the visible-near-infrared absorption spectrum of liquid water. *J. Phys. Chem. A* **2001**, *105*, 8916–8921. [CrossRef]
71. Bell, J.T.; Krohn, N.A. The near-infrared spectra of water and heavy water at temperatures between 25 and 39. deg. *J. Phys. Chem.* **1970**, *74*, 4006. [CrossRef]
72. Williams, P.; Norris, K.H. *Near Infrared Technology in the Agricultural and Food Industries*; American Association of Cereal Chemists: St Paul, MN, USA, 1987.
73. Thalmann, M.; Santelia, D. Starch as a determinant of plant fitness under abiotic stress. *New Phytol.* **2017**, *214*, 943–951. [CrossRef]
74. Malegori, C.; Muncan, J.; Mustorgi, E.; Tsenkova, R.; Oliveri, P. Analysing the water spectral pattern by near-infrared spectroscopy and chemometrics as a dynamic multidimensional biomarker in preservation: Rice germ storage monitoring. *Spectrochim. Acta Part A Mol. Biomol. Spectrosc.* **2022**, *265*, 120396. [CrossRef]
75. Kojić, D.; Tsenkova, R.; Tomobe, K.; Yasuoka, K.; Yasui, M. Water confined in the local field of ions. *ChemPhysChem* **2014**, *15*, 4077–4086. [CrossRef]
76. Ge, Z.; Cavlnato, A.G.; Callls, J.B. Noninvasive Spectroscopy for Monitoring Cell Density in a Fermentation Process. *Anal. Chem.* **1994**, *66*, 808–890. [CrossRef]
77. Wang, Y.; Huang, Y.Y.; Wang, Y.; Lyu, P.; Hamblin, M.R. Red (660 nm) or near-infrared (810 nm) photobiomodulation stimulates, while blue (415 nm), green (540 nm) light inhibits proliferation in human adipose-derived stem cells. *Sci. Rep.* **2017**, *7*, 1–10. [CrossRef] [PubMed]
78. Karu, T.I.; Afanasyeva, N.I.; Kolyakov, S.F.; Pyatibrat, L.V.; Welser, L. Changes in Absorbance of Monolayer of Living Cells Induced by Laser Radiation at 633, 670 and 820 nm. *IEEE J. Sel. Top. Quantum Electron.* **2001**, *7*, 982–988. [CrossRef]
79. Amaroli, A.; Ferrando, S.; Benedicenti, S. Photobiomodulation Affects Key Cellular Pathways of all Life-Forms: Considerations on Old and New Laser Light Targets and the Calcium Issue. *Photochem. Photobiol.* **2019**, *95*, 455–459. [CrossRef]
80. Bhattacharya, M.; Dutta, A. Computational modeling of the photon transport, tissue heating, and cytochrome C oxidase absorption during transcranial near-infrared stimulation. *Brain Sci.* **2019**, *9*, 179. [CrossRef]
81. Xantheas, S.S. Theoretical Study of Hydroxide Ion-Water Clusters. *J. Am. Chem. Soc.* **1995**, *117*, 10373–10380. [CrossRef]
82. Roth, M.S.; Deheyn, D.D. Effects of cold stress and heat stress on coral fluorescence in reef-building corals. *Sci. Rep.* **2013**, *3*, 1421. [CrossRef]
83. Muncan, J.; Aouadi, B.; Tsenkova, R. New perspectives in plant and plant-based food quality determination: Aquaphotomics. In *Plant-Based Bioactives, Functional Foods, Beverages and Medicines: Processing, Analysis and Health Benefit*; Goyal, M.R., Kovacs, Z., Nath, A., Suleria, H., Eds.; Apple Academic Press, Taylor and Francis: Palm Bay, FL, USA, 2020.
84. Du, Y.; Zhao, Q.; Chen, L.; Yao, X.; Zhang, W.; Zhang, B.; Xie, F. Effect of drought stress on sugar metabolism in leaves and roots of soybean seedlings. *Plant Physiol. Biochem.* **2020**, *146*, 1–12. [CrossRef]
85. Herritt, M.T.; Fritschi, F.B. Characterization of Photosynthetic Phenotypes and Chloroplast Ultrastructural Changes of Soybean (*Glycine max*) in Response to Elevated Air Temperatures. *Front. Plant Sci.* **2020**, *11*, 153. [CrossRef]
86. Humplík, J.F.; Lazár, D.; Husičková, A.; Spíchal, L. Automated phenotyping of plant shoots using imaging methods for analysis of plant stress responses-A review. *Plant Methods* **2015**, *11*, 1–10. [CrossRef]
87. Idso, S.B.; Reginato, R.J.; Radin, J.W. Leaf diffusion resistance and photosynthesis in cotton as related to a foliage temperature based plant water stress index. *Agric. Meteorol.* **1982**, *27*, 27–34. [CrossRef]
88. Buitrago, M.F.; Groen, T.A.; Hecker, C.A.; Skidmore, A.K. Changes in thermal infrared spectra of plants caused by temperature and water stress. *ISPRS J. Photogramm. Remote Sens.* **2016**, *111*, 22–31. [CrossRef]
89. Merlot, S.; Mustilli, A.C.; Genty, B.; North, H.; Lefebvre, V.; Sotta, B.; Vavasseur, A.; Giraudat, J. Use of infrared thermal imaging to isolate Arabidopsis mutants defective in stomatal regulation. *Plant J.* **2002**, *30*, 601–609. [CrossRef] [PubMed]

90. Funatsuki, H.; Matsuba, S.; Kawaguchi, K.; Murakami, T.; Sato, Y. Methods for evaluation of soybean chilling tolerance at the reproductive stage under artificial climatic conditions. *Plant Breed.* **2004**, *123*, 558–563. [CrossRef]
91. Funatsuki, H.; Kurosaki, H.; Murakami, T.; Matsuba, S.; Kawaguchi, K.; Yumoto, S.; Sato, Y. Deficiency of a cytosolic ascorbate peroxidase associated with chilling tolerance in soybean. *Theor. Appl. Genet.* **2003**, *106*, 494–502. [CrossRef] [PubMed]
92. Yamaguchi, N.; Yamazaki, H.; Ohnishi, S.; Suzuki, C.; Hagihara, S.; Miyoshi, T.; Senda, M. Method for selection of soybeans tolerant to seed cracking under chilling temperatures. *Breed. Sci.* **2014**, *64*, 103–108. [CrossRef] [PubMed]
93. Kasai, A.; Ohnishi, S.; Yamazaki, H.; Funatsuki, H.; Kurauchi, T.; Matsumoto, T.; Yumoto, S.; Senda, M. Molecular Mechanism of Seed Coat Discoloration Induced by Low Temperature in Yellow Soybean. *Plant Cell Physiol.* **2009**, *50*, 1090–1098. [CrossRef] [PubMed]
94. Wang, Z.; Reddy, V.R.; Quebedeaux, B. Growth and photosynthetic responses of soybean to short-term cold temperature. *Environ. Exp. Bot.* **1997**, *37*, 13–24. [CrossRef]
95. Robison, J.; Arora, N.; Yamasaki, Y.; Saito, M.; Boone, J.; Blacklock, B.; Randall, S. *Glycine max* and *Glycine soja* are capable of cold acclimation. *J. Agron. Crop Sci.* **2017**, *203*, 553–561. [CrossRef]
96. Cowe, I.A.; McNicol, J.W. The Use of Principal Components in the Analysis of Near-Infrared Spectra. *Appl. Spectrosc.* **1985**, *39*, 257–266. [CrossRef]
97. Dhanoa, M.S.; Barnes, R.J.; Lister, S.J. Standard Normal Variate Transformation and De-trending of Near-Infrared Diffuse Reflectance Spectra. *Appl. Spectrosc.* **1989**, *43*, 772–777.
98. Tsenkova, R.; Munćan, J.; Pollner, B.; Kovacs, Z. Essentials of Aquaphotomics and Its Chemometrics Approaches. *Front. Chem.* **2018**, *6*, 363. [CrossRef]
99. Wold, S.; Sjostrom, M. SIMCA: A Method for Analyzing Chemical Data in Terms of Similarity and Analogy. In *Chemometrics: Theory and Application*; Kowalski, B.R., Ed.; American Chemical Society: San Francisco, CA, USA, 1977; pp. 243–282.
100. Wold, S.; Albano, C.; Dunn, W.J.; Edlund, U.; Esbensen, K.; Geladi, P.; Hellberg, S.; Johansson, E.; Lindberg, W.; Sjöström, M. Multivariate Data Analysis in Chemistry. In *Chemometrics*; Springer: Dordrecht, The Netherlands, 1984; pp. 17–95.
101. Pollner, B.; Kovacs, Z. R-Package aquap2-Multivariate Data Analysis Tools for R including Aquaphotomics Methods 2016. Available online: https://www.aquaphotomics.com/aquap2/ (accessed on 20 December 2021).
102. R Development Core Team R: A Language and Environment for Statistical Computing 2017. Available online: https://www.r-project.org/ (accessed on 20 December 2021).

molecules

MDPI

Review

Water as a Link between Membrane and Colloidal Theories for Cells

E. Anibal Disalvo *, A. Sebastian Rosa, Jimena P. Cejas and María de los A. Frias

Applied Biophysics and Food Research Center (Centro de Investigaciones en Biofisica Aplicada y Alimentos, CIBAAL, Laboratory of Biointerphases and Biomimetic Systems, National University of Santiago del Estero and CONICET), RN 9-Km 1125, Santiago del Estero 4206, Argentina
* Correspondence: disalvoanibal@yahoo.com.ar

Abstract: This review is an attempt to incorporate water as a structural and thermodynamic component of biomembranes. With this purpose, the consideration of the membrane interphase as a bidimensional hydrated polar head group solution, coupled to the hydrocarbon region allows for the reconciliation of two theories on cells in dispute today: one considering the membrane as an essential part in terms of compartmentalization, and another in which lipid membranes are not necessary and cells can be treated as a colloidal system. The criterium followed is to describe the membrane state as an open, non-autonomous and responsive system using the approach of Thermodynamic of Irreversible Processes. The concept of an open/non-autonomous membrane system allows for the visualization of the interrelationship between metabolic events and membrane polymorphic changes. Therefore, the Association Induction Hypothesis (AIH) and lipid properties interplay should consider hydration in terms of free energy modulated by water activity and surface (lateral) pressure. Water in restricted regions at the lipid interphase has thermodynamic properties that explain the role of H-bonding networks in the propagation of events between membrane and cytoplasm that appears to be relevant in the context of crowded systems.

Keywords: lipid hydration; water interphases; crowded systems; restricted environments; H bonding propagation

Citation: Disalvo, E.A.; Rosa, A.S.; Cejas, J.P.; Frias, M.d.l.A. Water as a Link between Membrane and Colloidal Theories for Cells. *Molecules* **2022**, *27*, 4994. https://doi.org/10.3390/molecules27154994

Academic Editors: Roumiana Tsenkova and Jelena Muncan

Received: 7 July 2022
Accepted: 1 August 2022
Published: 5 August 2022

Publisher's Note: MDPI stays neutral with regard to jurisdictional claims in published maps and institutional affiliations.

1. Introduction

> *The air-water interface of a drop of water has its specific heat and hence its entropy potential, i.e., an entropy potential independent of the bulk. A perturbation of such an interface is conserved. This inevitably leads—due to the conservation of momentum and the laws of thermodynamics—to propagation phenomena.*
>
> *(Einstein, 1901)*

According to cell membrane theory, membranes form the boundary of living cells and regulate transport in and out of the cell by providing a dynamic barrier between the cellular constituents and the extracellular environment. Within this paradigm, the basic structure of the biological membrane is the lipid bilayer. The interactions between the constituent lipid molecules are at expense of water which plays a major role in the membrane properties such as stability, permeation and related functions [1].

The membrane theory has received most of the attention from physiologists and biophysicists due to the acceptance of the Fluid Mosaic Membrane (FMM) model formulated originally by Singer and Nicholson [2] and modified by others [3,4].

All of them take the lipids as the responsible for forming a semipermeable membrane encapsulating the cytoplasm which is justified from an evolution point of view with the argument that one of the first steps in life is the formation of closed supramolecular structures confining a reactive electrolytic media [5,6].

Opposed to this view, the Association Induction Hypothesis (AIH) describes a cell as a colloidal coacervate of gel proteins in water in which the protoplasm responds to metabolic events through changes in protein conformation [7,8].

While the cell membrane theories mostly ignore water as part of the structure and the thermodynamic (functional) properties derived from it, the AIH put emphasis on water ignoring membranes and lipids. However, both theories contain relevant concepts to understand cell physiology, which are in certain aspects, complementary to a unified cell theory considering its functionality as the final goal.

For this purpose, the unique properties of water linked to membranes appear to be a way by which the two proposals may converge. This requires a deeper knowledge of water structure and hydration in biological membranes. Specifically, its role in surface phenomena in different lipid assemblies and in contact with crowded systems. For this purpose, a new view of the membrane in which the interphase region is taken as an open bidimensional solution of lipid head groups is discussed.

With this aim, this article deals with the following concepts:

- A brief review of the membrane and coacervate theories

  The membrane theory.
  The coacervate theory

- The membrane interphase model.
- The membrane as an open system. Thermodynamic consequences.
- Membrane hydration and membrane state.
- The surface domains. Excluded volume concept.
- Critical water activity and the cut-off surface pressure

  Critical states: packing and cut off pressure.
  Cut off and critical water activity.

- Hydration and phase transition.
- The limits of the membrane in crowded systems and signal propagation.
- Unifying membrane approach with water colloid systems.
- The thermodynamic response: membrane state/hydration state/state- function relationship.

  Responsive structures and H bond networks.

- Concluding remarks: Membrane hydration and membrane state. An alternative way to membrane response.

2. A Brief Review of the Membrane and Coacervate Theories

2.1. The Membrane Theory

The classical paradigms supporting the actual membrane models are resumed below.

The lipid bilayer is the backbone of the membrane in which proteins can be inserted. In some conditions, non-lamellar aggregates can be formed as transient structures depending on the lipid composition [1].

The lipid bilayer conformation is a selective permeability barrier in which water and non-polar solutes can cross driven by a concentration gradient. Permeability is evaluated as a partition-diffusion process in which the lamellar conformation is not altered. Under this paradigm, solutes dissolve in the membrane and water copermeates. On the other hand, ions and most polar solutes cannot permeate the lipid membrane, and therefore, it occurs due to the presence of specialized proteinaceous carriers or channels coupled to metabolism (active transport). The cell is filled with ordinary water with small solutes including K^+ in solution. To compensate for the passive leaks, ion pumps located at the membrane continuously operate, a process that is considered energetically impossible [8].

Under this view, ions and other biocompounds such as aminoacids are excluded from membrane bulk due to their low solubility in the hydrocarbon region [9]. However, experimental evidences have shown that water can be found as pockets in the membrane structure favoring the permeation of some polar aminoacids [10,11]. Thus, the classical concept of permeability in which the bilayer is considered as a hydrocarbon slab where the dielectric constant is 2 has strong limitations.

Based on the concept of the lipid assemble as a phase, the bilayer suffers structural changes induced by temperature and water content by which permeability, area per lipid, and thickness are drastically modified. The phase transition is mainly ascribed to the fusion process of the hydrocarbon region in fully hydrated membranes.

The current models focus on the presence of different lipid lateral arrangements in the membrane plane (domains) due to the heterogeneity in composition. Some lipids in their pure form can stabilize in water forming non-lamellar structures such as phosphatidylethanolamines (PE) and glyceryl monooleate (GMO) [12,13]. Therefore, it has been speculated that when those lipids are present in the membrane, non-bilayer structures may be formed and therefore explain changes in permeability to ions and polar solutes. In these conditions, some lipids may act as ionophores [14]. However, the phenomena seem to be an all or none process, in which selectivity, specificity for ions, and gradual modulation are not described. In all cases, little or no role of the water surface state of the membrane has been considered.

The proposal of membrane theory relies on rules mainly deduced for bulk phases large enough to neglect interfacial phenomena. Under this view, permeation occurs driven by a chemical potential difference of the permeant between the bulk phases on both sides of the membrane. Thus, permeability is interpreted in terms of the Henry law (partition of a single solute between bulk water and the hydrocarbon region without water). In addition, diffusion is considered to be governed by Fick's law, meaning that the diffusion coefficient is constant during the process.

The solubility-diffusion theory was questioned introducing the role of the polar head group arrangements in a three-layer theory that incorporates the area dependence as a primary modulating parameter [15]. This theory implicitly considers the presence of water in the bilayer structure.

For convenience, bilayers (liposomes, vesicles) and monolayers (extended on the air-water surface) have been extensively used as experimental model systems in a nearly independent way. Monolayers' behavior was mostly analyzed considering that lipids behave as a van der Waals gas spread on the water surface [16,17]. The water/lipid interaction is not taken into account and, consequently, the membrane is described as a closed system in thermodynamic equilibrium with the adjacencies. On the other hand, bilayers are modeled as fully hydrated lipids in which lateral pressure cannot be controlled [17,18].

From the phenomenological point of view, an extensive discussion has led to some consensus on the conditions in which monolayers may be considered equivalent to a bilayer of the same lipid species. The bilayer equivalent pressure is accepted to be at around $\Pi = 30$ mN/m at which the phospholipase A_2 activity is similar in both systems [19–21]. Estimation of the bilayer equivalent pressure is purely theoretical because bilayer lateral pressure is not experimentally measurable. Another frequently cited point is the bilayer equivalent molecular area, which for DPPC bilayers is ~64 Å^2, which is coincident with that determined in monolayers at a saturation point [22,23].

2.2. *The Coacervate Theory*

The coacervate theory was first proposed by the Russian biochemist A.I. Oparin in 1936 [24]. According to it, the origin of life was preceded by the formation of mixed colloidal units called 'coacervates'. These are particles composed of two or more colloids which might be proteins, lipids, or nucleic acids.

Under the view of this theory, the cell is described as a colloid with distribution coefficients and adsorption coefficients as prime physical-chemical parameters allowing a negative-entropy driven bioenergetics based on coherence [25].

Ling developed a complete colloid model for the living cell, the so-called 'association-induction-hypothesis' (AIH), which is claimed to be able to explain the coherent behavior of cells without the need to invoke the presence of the membrane [26].

In short, the membrane theory favors the idea that a cell is a solution of proteins while the coacervate view considers the cell as proteins dissolving water.

In this review, the consideration of water in the membrane extending the interphase to the cell interior gives the possibility to reconcile both views in terms of considering the cell as a crowded system [27].

3. The Membrane Interphase Model

The point that the bilayer/monolayer system cannot be appropriately treated with laws defined for bulk macroscopic systems derives from the need to consider new paradigms introducing concepts of surface physical chemistry [28]. This new view is based on Einstein's words in the heading of this article. Moreover, other physical chemists, namely Guggenheim, Defay and Prigogine among others have called attention to the particular phenomena of interphase, but they have not been explicitly incorporated into the classical membrane literature.

The common factor behind the redefinitions of membrane properties within the new paradigm of physical chemistry of surfaces is that water is not considered as part of the membrane structure. Therefore, to include it, it is necessary to examine experimental evidence concerning water in membranes and therefore to choose the right thermodynamic approach in relation to surfaces.

There are, at least, three ways to describe the surface phenomena (Figure 1). The first, defined by Gibbs, considers the interface as an ideal plane separating two milieus of different physical-chemical properties (Figure 1A). This definition, when applied to the membrane, takes into account the hydrocarbon core framed by the polar regions being of similar properties than bulk water. In lipid membranes, the interface corresponds to the plane running along the glycerol backbone in which carbonyl groups can be oriented either towards the membrane or to the aqueous phase. This definition gives importance to the separation of the non-polar region from the polar one, without giving relevance to the physical-chemical properties of the head polar group region. Within this approach, the capacitance and the thickness of the bilayer have been calculated. Although the thickness of the bilayer does not fit a pure hydrocarbon slab, which suggests a more complex structure in terms of dielectrics; most biophysical studies use this interface idea [29].

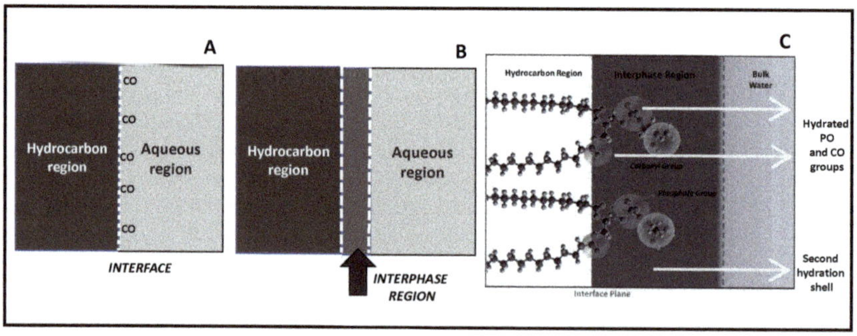

Figure 1. Different schematical descriptions of the interface: (**A**) The Gibbs model, (**B**) The Guggenheim model and (**C**) The membrane interphase model.

In another definition, provided by Guggenheim, two phases of quite different polarities are separated not by a plane but by a finite region (called the interphase) whose properties differ from the bulk phase which is in contact (Figure 1B). This region has quite different properties in comparison with the two pure bulk phases in contact. It is, to some extent, considered as a mixture of the two components although the exact ratios are not easy to assess.

The Guggenheim model is particularly appropriate to adapt to a lipid membrane if the contribution of the head group region is taken into account (Figure 1C). In connection with this definition, the thermodynamics of a monolayer was described by Defay-Prigogine (and extended by Damoradam and Disalvo) as a bidimensional solution of polar head groups embedded in water [30–32]. This visualization of the interphase makes that monolayers' and bilayers' behavior can be compared considering the physical chemistry of this region as an aqueous polar solutions, something that in the current biological literature is absent [33].

The principal feature of the interphase is that it is conformed by an aqueous solution of hydrated head groups that can be treated as ions in the solution. Thus, the physical chemistry of that region can be reasonably evaluated in terms of surface solution components (head groups, ions, and water) in a bidimensional arrangement.

A direct consequence of this lipid membrane model is that water becomes a crucial component of the membrane structure that defines its thermodynamic state.

In terms of structure, it gives a more realistic picture since the microscopic water organization around the different membrane groups can be related with the macroscopic response. The dynamics of these structures give place to fluctuations between water populations with different energy and entropy contributions.

4. The Membrane as an Open System: Thermodynamic Consequences

The introduction of water as a membrane component changes the definition of a membrane system from a closed to an open one. In consequence, the time-invariant state is not an equilibrium in a closed system in which the maximum entropy or minimum energy is reached when all forces are zero. In contrast, in an open system, the entropy is maintained constant in a time-invariant state (steady-state) in which non null forces are canceled out. In this state, the membrane exchanges water with the adjacent milieu at given surface pressure. An unbalance either of surface pressure or water exchange produces a transient state that the system tries to compensate for.

The approach of Defay-Prigogine in which the interphase is an ionic solution (Figure 1C) is particularly adequate to describe this process and illustrative to extend the role of water in the membrane in accordance with the coupled processes between solute and water named above. According to these authors, when a solute is injected in the subphase of a monolayer, it can diffuse from the bulk aqueous solution to the interphase driven by a concentration gradient. In this process, the water activity at the interphase decreases which produces a coupled flux of water into the interphase. This can explain the increase in surface pressure produced by the insertion of bioeffector in the monolayers at a constant area, and extended to bilayers also when the decrease in membrane density is considered [32,34]. It must be taken into account that this increase in surface pressure is indeed a decrease in the surface tension of the interphase, a point that will be analyzed in detail later.

Consequently, several of the above paradigms concerning permeability and dielectric properties must be revised. Permeability is described by the interrelation of a partition process of the permeant between water and membrane bulk, which is taken as a pure hydrocarbon phase without water, and its diffusion in a homogeneous phase. This is supposed to be valid for single water permeation driven by a permeant solute gradient of concentration across the membrane. A more realistic picture was offered when Thermodynamics of Irreversible Processes (TIP) was applied to explain the permeation of nonelectrolytes. It was concluded that solute diffusion promotes a water flux and that osmosis induces also solute permeation. These conclusions were sustained for the process across the membrane, but no consideration of the changes in water content in the membrane itself was made [35]. This point is discussed in the next session.

5. Membrane Hydration and Membrane State

The introduction of the interphase as a binary aqueous solution as part of the membrane structure and the notion of an open system regarding water imposes a different thermodynamic approach to understanding membrane processes.

The thermodynamics of the membrane as an open system is given by the entropy production (dS/dt) that can be written in terms of the sum of forces (X_i) and fluxes (J_i) operating on the system defined in two dimensions as in Equation (1):

$$\frac{dS}{dt} = \sum J_i X_i \tag{1}$$

Thus,

$$\frac{dS}{dt} = \frac{\Pi dA}{dt} + \frac{\Delta\,\mu\, dn_W}{dt} = J_a\Pi + J_w\Delta\mu = 0 \tag{2}$$

where Π is suface pressure; $\frac{dA}{dt} = J_a$ is the change in area (A); $\Delta\,\mu$ is the gradient of chemical potential of water and $\frac{dn_W}{dt} = J_w$ is the water flux.

For the sake of simplicity, the system is taken at constant temperature and in the absence of electric fields and chemical reactions (this can be extended but it is beyond the aim of this work).

When the system is in the steady state, the entropy production is constant and thus dS/dt = 0.

Then,

$$J_a\Pi = J_W\,\Delta\mu \tag{3}$$

As the surface pressure (π) can be expressed by the difference between the surface tension of pure water (γ^0) and surface tension of water with lipids (γ)

$$\pi = \left(\gamma^0 - \gamma\right) \tag{4}$$

$$\text{Considering that} \quad \Delta\mu = \Gamma_W RT\ln a_W \tag{5}$$

with Γ_W equal to surface water concentration and a_W equal to water activity,

It results in

$$\gamma = \gamma^0 - \Gamma_W RT\ln a_W \tag{6}$$

In this condition, each value of water activity would correspond to a value of surface tension. In other words, water activity fixes the surface tension, and vice versa, surface pressure (surface tension) would give place to a given water activity.

This analysis denotes the importance of water in the determination of the thermodynamic properties of monolayers and bilayers, mainly its propensity to react in the presence of solute in the bulk phase. According to Equation (6), any process that affects water activity will affect surface tension and hence denoted as a surface pressure increase. Therefore, at a given water activity the membrane surface free energy state is fixed, and thus its propensity to respond to solutes in the bulk adjacencies [22,36].

The point here is to define the properties of water in lipids in terms of its free energy (i.e., surface tension)

6. The Surface Domains: Excluded Volume Concept

Cellular membranes are laterally heterogeneous systems that are probably involved in function. The composition of membrane rafts as the archetypical lipid-driven plasma membrane domains has been extensively discussed. The complexity and flexibility of lipid-mediated membrane organization could be functionalized by cells. The different lateral compositional heterogeneity is a ubiquitous feature of cellular membranes on various length scales, conforming molecular assemblies. The nature of the micrometric domains in terms of specific physicochemical properties is a matter of discussion [4,37].

The water content and its organization as H bond networks is concomitant to the composition of lipids and its topology, such as rafts or domains. The mechanical properties to these water regions surrounding the lipid domains acts as a plasticizer along its compressibility modulus [38].

Thus, the friction between lipids and water at this point implies changes in water properties (structure, density, and polarity among others) [33,39] and hence propensity to H bond rearrangements.

These arrangements are affected by the surface pressure (i.e. the area available for the lipids) and therefore its excess free energy of the regions exposed to bulk water changes consequently. Therefore, the propensity of the membrane to "react" to bioeffectors (i.e., biologically relevant compounds in the bulk adjacency) is modulated by water activity and the corresponding surface tension of those regions (Equation (6)).

Different lipid packing states in biomembranes that form coexisting domains (i.e., relatively ordered and disordered domains such as lipids in the liquid condensed or the liquid expanded state) are assumed to have functional characteristics [40]. However, it must be considered that each packing state implies different water levels and arrangements giving place to regions in which water surface tension is different, i.e., the excess of surface free energy. Thus, they act as an energy reservoir that would explain the responsiveness of lipid membrane to bioeffectors present in the adjacent media (aminoacids, peptides, enzymes, etc.). The changes in surface tension, as stated in Equation (6), are modulated by the influence of lipids on water structure and this is manifested in conditions in which lipids form a coherent array (at c.a. 5–10 mN/m) ending at the collapse pressure (c.a. 45 mN/m) depending on the lipid [41]. Thus, a correlation between lipid packing and water activity is inherent to functional activity.

To make explicit the role of surface activity in terms of water activity it is necessary to extend some features of hydration of membranes in analogy to studies made on protein hydration. This is particularly important if the aim is to explain the properties of a membrane in the context of crowded systems [27].

Biological membranes can assume a number of different lipid packing states that may correspond to domains in live cell membranes [42].

Packing is referred to in different structural membrane studies but the thermodynamic properties inherent to it are not rigorously explained. These two aspects are related to surface tension and excluded volume concept as will be explained below.

Excluded volume is a term that represents the unavailable volume of solvent for a solute in a solution. In a simple description, solute dissolves in a salt solution in the water beyond that the hydration shell of the ions. It is also applied to concentrated solutions of macromolecules in which water as a solvent is drastically reduced. This view has been particularly used to refer to the cell as a crowded system [43].

The mutual impenetrability of solute molecules into the hydration shell of the ions and the steric repulsion between ions themselves plays a fundamental role in intermolecular interactions. The activity of a solute depends on the volume that is available for each molecular specie. The steric freedom (entropy) is a function of the size and shape of the solute.

In terms of the bidimensional solution defined as the interphase, the impenetrability in a lipid membrane is given by the polar head group surrounded by the hardcore of hydration molecules (Figure 2) [44].

The hardcore region (blue region) only changes in drastic conditions of dehydration or by the presence of certain compounds that may replace water such as sugars such as trehalose [45–47].

Tightly bound water determines the excluded volume of the interphase region contributing to the permeability barrier [48]. In this view, water layers are of a similar magnitude to the hydrocarbon region itself and constitute a repulsion barrier for many permeant solutes and for membrane adhesion [49–52].

Assuming that the lipid hardcore of hydration is constant, expansion/contraction processes change the water available for solutes in a lipid membrane beyond this hardcore. Thus, the membrane state at a given surface pressure is determined by the relationship of the amount of loosely bound water in relation to the hardcore which is influenced by the presence of the lipids.

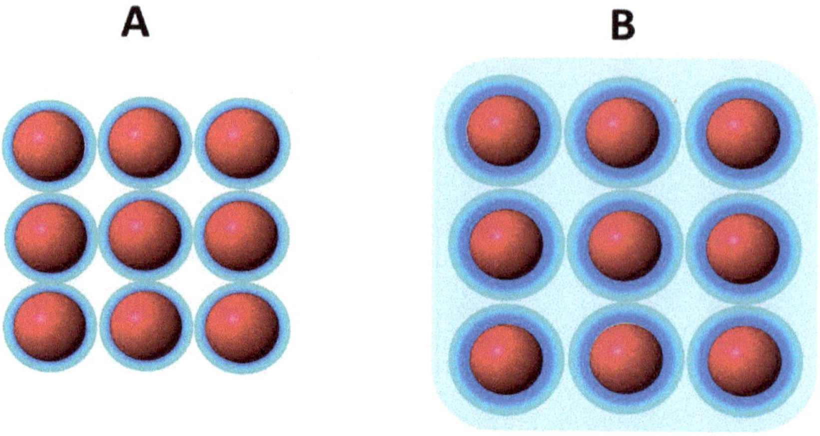

Figure 2. Schematic representation of the excluded volume in the head group region (red spheres) of a lipid membrane. (**A**). Blue region: hardcore first hydration shell. (**B**). Light blue region: water available as solvent (confined water) although of different properties than bulk water.

In this regard, the thermodynamic response of an interphase (i.e., the change in surface tension) to bioeffectors is related to water organized around the lipids beyond the first hardcore hydration shell. This type of water between lipids beyond the first hydration shell sustains the original model of Defay-Prigogine in which the interphase is a bidimensional solution of hydrated head groups immersed in water [28,32].

7. Critical Water Activity and the Cut off Surface Pressure

7.1. Critical States: Packing and Cut off Pressure

Recalling that the surface tension of water varies according to the dimension and quality of its environment, it is not difficult to comprehend that the physical chemistry of water confined between lipids (the light blue region in Figure 2) with its hydration hardcore (dark blue) can determine the membrane thermodynamic response.

The typical curves in Figure 3A denote the response of a monolayer at a given initial surface pressure to a bioeffector added to the subphase. The plot of the magnitude of the response ($\pi_f - \pi_i$) as a function of the initial surface pressure (π_i) indicates that there is a cut off surface pressure above which no membrane response is observed. This behavior is usually related to the packing of the lipids at the interphase. In a simplistic interpretation, there is no area available to the bioeffector to penetrate the monolayer.

However, the insertion process is not driven by the area but by free energy changes. Therefore, other properties concerning the interphase must be relevant.

Packing is frequently taken as the equivalent of the ordered state. However, packing is referred to lipid molecules i.e., the special arrangement in terms of distance. Such ordering is ascribed to lipids immersed in water since properties are assumed to be measured in fully hydrated membranes. The packing increased by compression enhances the hydrophobic interactions of the monolayer or bilayer promoting a decrease in water order. Therefore, the two concepts must be compatibilized with each other.

Packing is a geometric criterium and order-disorder is a thermodynamic one. However, the geometrical criterium to some extent can be translated into thermodynamic terms if the energy contribution is considered in terms of the excluded volume as described above.

7.2. Cut off and Critical Water Activity

The surface pressure can be expressed in terms of water activity (a^i_w according to equation $\pi = -C\,\Gamma_w\,RT \ln (a^i_w)$, where Γ_w is the water concentration at the interface and

C is function of the frictional coefficient lipid-lipid, lipid water and water lipid [33]. Thus, the cut-off pressure reflects a critical water activity.

At the cut-off pressure, water activity beyond the hardcore is zero and no water domains are formed. Thus, no effect of bioeffectors is found. This is produced at the critical water activity (Figure 3D) above which water domains are formed (Figure 2B) and the excess free energy triggers the bioeffector perturbation [32]. The water domains are characterized by a surface tension fixed by the water activity according to Equation (6).

For a given water activity at the membrane, the perturbation ($\Delta\Pi$) depends on the type of bioeffector, and of lipids and it may have different consequences. Among them, drastic changes in the dielectric permittivity of the membrane maintaining the bilayer conformation allow permeation of polar and ionic solutes, a process that cannot be explained by the classical non-polar slab of the bilayer in classical models [28,53]. Another consequence is the induction of non bilayered structure abandoning the bilayer conformation [54].

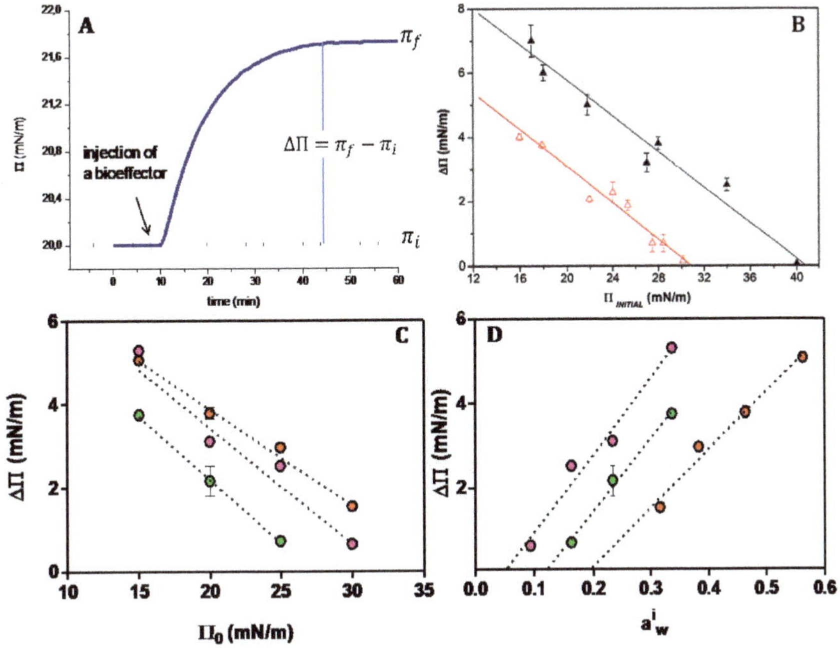

Figure 3. Perturbation of a responsive membrane to the different bioffectors. (**A**) Typical changes of the monolayer surface pressure upon the addition of a bioeffector. (**B**) Difference of the final and initial surface pressure for different initial surface pressures induced by a soluble protease as a bioffector on DMPC (Δ) and DMPE (Δ) monolayers (taken from Ref. [55]). (**C**) Difference of the final and initial surface pressure for different initial surface pressures induced by chlorogenic acid on DPPC (•), Di 16:0 ether PC (•), DMPC (•) (taken from Ref. [56]). (**D**) Difference of the final and initial surface pressure as a function of the initial water activity in the monolayer calculated according to $\pi = -C\,\Gamma_w\,RT \ln (a^i_w)$ for DPPC (•), Di 16:0 ether PC (•), DMPC (•) (See text).

Compression produces the collapse of the lipid monolayer at high pressures. In this stage, lipids are packed to a limit in which the hard core first hydration layers are in contact (Figure 2A). This is the minimum excluded volume (blue spheres) which implies a volume non available for solutes. In a $\Delta\Pi/\Pi$ curve as in Figure 3B,C, this value is reflected by the critical cut-off, i.e., the pressure at which no response is observed. The response is observed when the initial surface pressure is below the cut off, which is somewhat below the collapse pressure. In consequence, the water activity at the cut-off is higher than that at the collapse (Table 1).

Table 1. Comparison of surface pressure and the corresponding water activities at the collapse and cut off pressures [55,56].

Type of Lipid	Bioeffector	$\pi_{saturation} \pm$ sd (mN/m)	$\pi_{cut\ off} \pm$ sd (mN/m)	a_w (Saturation)	a_w (Cut Off)
DPhPC	Aqueous protease	48.0 ± 0.7	39.6 ± 0.4	0.308	0.378
DOPC	Aqueous protease	47.2 ± 0.9	41.4 ± 0.3	0.314	0.362
DMPC	Aqueous protease	47.8 ± 0.8	41.5 ± 0.5	0.309	0.361
DPPC	Aqueous protease	46.6 ± 0.6	39.5 ± 0.9	0.034	0.057
DMPE	Aqueous protease	45.0 ± 0.5	30.6 ± 0.1	0.038	0.108
Di(ether) PC	Aqueous protease	48.0 ± 0.7	31.9 ± 0.3	0.307	0.457
Di(ether) PE	Aqueous protease	44.5 ± 0.5	29.4 ± 0.6	0.040	0.118
DMPC	CGA	47.8 ±0.8	36.9 ± 0.3	0.160	0.243
DPPC	CGA	61.4 ± 1.3	27.2 ± 0.3	0.011	0.134
16:0 dieter PC	CGA	58.5 ± 1.1	32.4 ± 0.1	0.013	0.092

This means that the excluded volume sensitive for membrane response is larger than the hardcore water inferred from the collapse pressure. This implies that the geometrical space created is much lower than the molecule volume of the bioeffector. Therefore, the insertion of the biocompounds can be more suitably explained in terms of energetic considerations.

8. Hydration and Phase Transition

The increase in surface pressure produced by a bioeffector is a measure of the decrease in surface tension. This means that the initial surface tension, which reflects a particular free energy state of the membrane, is reduced and this can only be produced if initial water arrangements have certain level of potential energy. These arrangements should be reflected in the thermodynamic properties of the membrane.

Being the membrane composed of two slabs of a strongly different physical chemical nature, the main phase transition should be an emergent of the system.

Heat causes a global thermal transition due to the interplay of molecular interactions between the nonpolar and polar regions with water playing a fundamental role.

Considering the presence of water, the total enthalpic change in the transition can be written as

$$\Delta H = \Delta H_f + \Delta H_l \quad (7)$$

where ΔH_f is the enthalpy of fusion of the hydrocarbon chains and ΔH_l is the energy involved in the ionic network in the aqueous excluded region. In turn,

$$\Delta H_l = E_r + \Delta H_h \quad (8)$$

where E_r energy of fusion of the ionic (polar groups) lattice and ΔH_h the enthalpy of hydration of the head groups.

ΔH_f and E_r are endothermic processes and ΔH_h is an exothermic one. Thus, how endothermic ΔH is, would depend, to a great extent, on the hydration of the polar groups [57].

Thus, the lipid propensity for membrane responsiveness involves water rearrangements reflected in the ΔH values.

9. The Limits of the Membrane in Crowded Systems and Signal Propagation

The limits confining the interphase are not sharp. Water may penetrate the first 4C atoms, and the presence of the polar groups may affect layers of water in the bulk solution. In terms of Molecular Dynamics (MD) this may have an extension of around

12 Å [58]. This implies water facing different kinds of molecular residues and thus with different free energy content with different capabilities to exchange.

There is a great content of ambiguity in the definition of the cell limits and cell membranes: boundaries become in barriers and these in membranes, which finally are resumed in bilayers giving to them the same hierarchy.

This confusing nomenclature is due, in our view, to macroscopic observations disregarding the definition of interphases as a region separating two well-characterized (continuous) regions.

A great deal of care has been taken to establish the limit between the hydrocarbon core and the aqueous phase since Luzzati et al. [59] interpreted the X-ray diagram of lipid suspensions, considering the former proposal of the lipoidal nature of the cellular boundary by Overton [60].

Over the years, many assumptions have been made in order to calculate area per lipid from measurements of interbilayer distance and membrane thickness [23,49,61,62]. The membrane thickness also includes the polar head groups. Needless to say, in these calculations a simplification is dragged, e.g., the density of water (molar volume) is constant and similar to the bulk [63].

Further, with the aid of molecular dynamics and new scattering methodologies, the limit between water and the hydrocarbon region has become diffuse. Water can extend into the first 4–5 C atoms below the carbonyl groups and from the plane of the phosphates and the different polar residues attached to it, toward the external water. Consequently, the neat differentiation of water near the groups and the bulk is gradually diluted [49,58,64]. In spite of these uncertainties, the phase properties of the membrane have been mostly interpreted in terms of the properties of the non-polar region. However, the only region that can be considered properly as a hydrocarbon phase is that at the terminal -CH_3 residue in the center of the bilayer. That is why most of the interpretations lay on the idea that the phase transition is due to the fusion of the hydrocarbon chains that are affected by water, but no consideration of the thermal properties of the water region itself is made [65]. However, in the phase transition water structure also changes and this change is implicit in dynamic process [57].

The behavior of water beyond the hardcore (blue light region in Figure 2B) at the phase transition is shown in Figure 4.

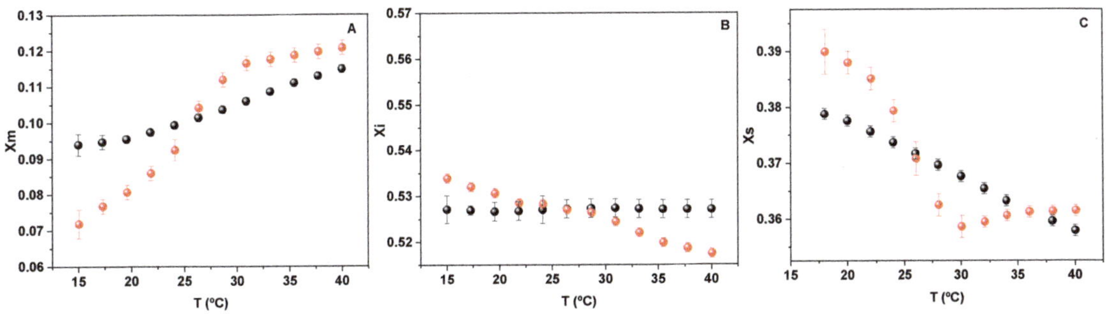

Figure 4. Molar fraction of water monomer (**A**) water bound with less than four H bonds (**B**) and tetracoordinated water molecules (**C**) as a function of temperature. Black symbols correspond to pure water, red symbols correspond to water in the presence of lipids.

The data in Figure 4 clearly indicates that the thermodynamic properties of water between lipids are different in comparison to bulk water, since a clear break is observed in the presence of lipids that is absent in pure water. The main observation is that the molar fraction of water monomers increases (part A) parallel to the water tetramer decrease (part C), indicating an order-disorder transition. In both cases, a break is observed at the phase transition followed by the phospholipid groups (red dots) that is not present in pure water (black dots). Thus, the transition in water associated with the membrane reflects the membrane state.

If a living cell is represented by a water solution of proteins and ions enclosed by the membrane as a bilayer, the general criterium is to take water inside having no major differences from normal liquid water bathing the cells. In contrast, from the colloidal point of view, cytoplasmic water is stabilized, essentially continuously, by interactions with proteins, forming an extensive, ordered lattice in which the water molecules have reduced translational and orientational freedom and ordered microscopic arrangements compared with free water [64]. However, the so-called "bound" water invoked by the Ling's AIH can not only be ascribed to the presence of macromolecules in the microscopic heterogeneity of the cytoplasm (due to the influence of cell organelles) but also to the presence of lipid aggregates such as a membrane [65–67]. These concepts may be incorporated into membrane theories without entering into conflict with Ling's theory.

It is precisely the dynamics of lipid-water and water-lipid association that make it possible to think in a dynamic, coherent coacervate responding to and driven by cell metabolism. Moreover, the propensity of lipids to stabilize in different topological and conformational arrays beside lamellas seems to be driven by lyotropic transitions, i.e., water activity variations at a constant temperature [68,69].

The view of including water as a component of membrane structure inquires the concept of bilayer as a permeability barrier. In addition, it introduces water as a participant in the lipid conformational changes.

Despite this, it is quite reasonable that lipids in that context can suffer lyotropic phase transitions maintaining the bilayer conformation and/or polymorphic changes abandoning the lamellar conformation, in such a way that the bilayer, as usually pictured, is not a continuous barrier [13,70].

Lipids interact between them by short-range (weak) forces that make them considered a soft material. However, lipids have specific sites of hydration (phosphate-PO_2^- and carbonyl-CO groups) and acyl chains that impose a particular ordering of water molecules. Moreover, the correlation of polar-polar and chain-chain interactions are modulated by water content giving place to cooperative phenomena as described elsewhere [57,71–73].

In this regard, following the TIP approach [28,33] it is important to point out that water content may be modulated by osmosis, and this should not be considered as a process to produce a flux across the membrane (such as in the classical membrane theory) but as one in which water is extruded from the membrane itself. That is to say, it may cause lyotropic transitions. Even in the case that the bilayer is preserved, permeability is a much more complex process than that described by partition and diffusion in the classical membrane theory. This is so because the partition is not uniform along the membrane thickness, and diffusion is not given by a constant coefficient as described by Fick's law [32]. In contrast, it varies along the process due to the relaxation of the water structure. Different water activities can give place to changes in the lipid conformation different from bilayers in extreme cases of dehydration [28].

10. Unifying Membrane Approach with Water Colloid Systems

If the membrane is taken, thermodynamically speaking, as an open system, it is thought that exchanges of matter with the surroundings are allowed. The classical idea of close systems is that membrane material is constant. The exchange of water through the membrane barrier (transient or non-stationary water) is explained without altering its composition and even maintaining constant its density (packing) along the process. However, density can change maintaining the lipid constant, at surface pressures well below the collapse, because the water content is modified. This is more noticeable when water is dragged by a permeant. Water dissolves in kinks affecting the density of the lipid matrix [41,57,72] and its dielectric properties due to solute penetration [53,74]. In this sense, both, open and non-autonomous systems are interrelated concepts.

In a non-autonomous system, the limit of the aqueous layer is not determined by the membrane itself but by the media which is in contact with. Thus, if the membrane faces a colloid aqueous one, such as cytoplasm, it will have different states than if the media is pure bulk water.

In terms of compartmentalization, continuous semipermeable membranes are not required as the FMM model does. Compartmentalization can be taken as a kinetic process and not necessarily as a physical barrier. Different kinetics of solute penetration were found at different cholesterol ratios in lipid monolayers and constant areas and at different surface pressures, all of them related to changes in water activity in the interphase [22,41,75].

It is possible that the presence of lipids with the propensity to stabilize in non-bilayer ensembles strongly affects the kinetics of permeation. The proposal that the dependence of the conformation of the lipids with the state of the internal cytosol is an extension of the concept of an open (non-autonomous) system, since it considers a structural change in the lipid arrangement much more drastic than the lipid density changes in bilayers. This would deserve further analysis within the frame of Thermodynamics of Irreversible Processes (TIP) [33].

11. The Thermodynamic Response: Membrane State/Hydration State/State-Function Relationship

As said, the concept of the open/non autonomous phase can be framed in terms of Gibbs free energy. J.W. Gibbs was a visionary. It is not known if he was conscious of that, but the extension of the physical thermodynamics to chemical systems is one of the most relevant theoretically based experimental formalisms on which science is based today [76,77].

The free energy decrease can be enthalpically or entropically driven. If water is the messenger in order to make coherent the biochemical processes in cells including lipids, the two aspects are fundamental. First, the energy exchange is driven by the energy of hydrogen bond networks (water-water, water-lipid interactions) and by the entropy change due to the unique properties of the structure of water itself. An example of this is the water exchange between monomers and tetramers shown in Figure 4.

The important observation that the periodicity of glycolytic oscillations and that the attendant coupled oscillations in water relaxation are slowed down by deuterium oxide (heavy water) makes it reasonable that this is a consequence of the stronger energy of the D-bonds in comparison to the H-bonds [54]. Thus, this increase in stability enhances hydrophobic interactions and dampens oscillations.

Therefore, unstable or metastable systems have the root in the H bond strength of water with itself and with the walls in a restricted environment [64,77–79]. Therefore, more details in relation to hydrogen bonding energy in different spatial configurations are needed.

Responsive Structures and H Bond Networks

The presence of a cellular component governs the emergent properties that would affect the cellular interior dynamically. This implies that water organization mainly by hydrogen bonding should be higher, in terms of extension and stability, than bulk water. If this is so it should be reflected in dielectric relaxation and NMR results [53,78]. However, no more than 10% of cell water is supposed to be highly structured. The possibility of highly organized water was thought to be confirmed when the polywater was apparently discovered but was promptly demonstrated as a failure [80,81]. In addition, if the highly structured water exists the strength of H bonds would damp oscillations as occurs in D_2O as denoted above [54].

However, the new perspective of introducing water as a structural/functional component in cytoplasm and membranes can be reasonably accepted if interphase phenomena are considered to play a key role [82]. This is more logical when the cell interior is thought of as a crowded system, in comparison to a broth of protein ionic solution. In this regard, volume chemistry should be replaced by surface chemistry [27,83,84].

Lipids are part of the complex and crowded system and may determine kinetic and relaxation phenomena that are not restricted to permeation across the membrane. The relaxation implies the reorganization of water arrangements and therefore, changes in polarization, density, and compressibility. These are noticeable properties of water derived from hydrogen bonding network with noticeable plasticity [38].

The relaxation of water in the vicinity of lipid head polar groups measured with fluorescence probes in cellular aggregates of lipids is a strong indication that responsive behavior is due to water at the *interphase* which may be coupled to the cytosol [85–87]. The physical coupling can be a combination of properties emerging from water arrangements by H-bonds. As observed by FTIR, water bands are modified by the presence of lipids in different states (gel or liquid crystalline). These bands change at the phase transition mirroring the phase transition in the lipid phase [57]. The changes in bands are a consequence of the evolution of water populations from tetrahedral array (4H bonds) along 3, 2, 1, and 0H -bonded species [64]. The transition in the water populations "resonates" with the lipid state, and probably with the interior cell structure and central metabolism as well [88,89].

The strong cohesion in the cytoplasm can be extended not only between proteins and water but also between lipids and water. This statement fits with the association claimed in the association-induction hypothesis.

The living state is defined as a *cooperative* state indicating that each state is well defined and discrete and that there are neighbor-to-neighbor interactions among the individual elements. These features have been found in lipid molecules in the processes of adsorption of aminoacids and proteins to lipid membranes [90].

The cooperativity gives place to propagation. Polarized multilayers of water are not only in proteins but also in lipids and its propagation from and to the interphase is a property of the H bonds. According to AIH theory, fixed charges and associated counter-ions are separated by up to three dielectrically saturated water layers. This is comparable to the thickness of water layers in the membrane interphase polarized by charges such as phosphate and carbonyl groups, constituting the excluded volume which contributes to the repulsion forces and the responsiveness of the membrane (see Figures 2 and 3) [28,32,50,58]. The complete restriction of reorientation applies to the first hydration layer of these groups. However, the shells beyond it and in between the acyl chains can be modulated by surface pressure, mechanical constriction imposed by the water activity [65,91]. Membrane expansion-contraction may be induced by intrinsic processes of the cell driven by metabolic activity or by mechanical stress imposed by the external environmental conditions (osmotic swelling and shrinkage) [92].

The dynamic behavior of water at a constant temperature can be of electrical nature, more precisely derived from the dielectric properties implied in the polarization measured with fluorescent probes.

The dielectric permittivity is, in turn, much higher in ice than in liquid water explained by the higher degree of association of water molecules in a periodic array of tetrahedral coordination (4H-bond population predominates).

The dielectric permittivity is due to the orientation in an electric field of the dipoles. The common picture is that the reorientation implies the breaking of hydrogen bonds. However, a complete rotation of the dipole can be achieved by displacement of the H along with the H bond that remains unbroken. The water dipolar relaxation (rotational dynamics) is represented schematically below (Figure 5).

The inversion in the direction of the water molecular dipole (arrows) can be conducted without rotation of the molecule (i.e., without breaking H bonds), but with a displacement of the protons along with the linear H bond. The extent of the propagation will be limited by the density of states of 4, 3, 2, and 1-coordinated molecules by H-bonds giving a multiplicity of polarization states. Thus, polarization at the interphase and the propagation to the cell interior can be due to H displacement as in the Grothuss mechanism.

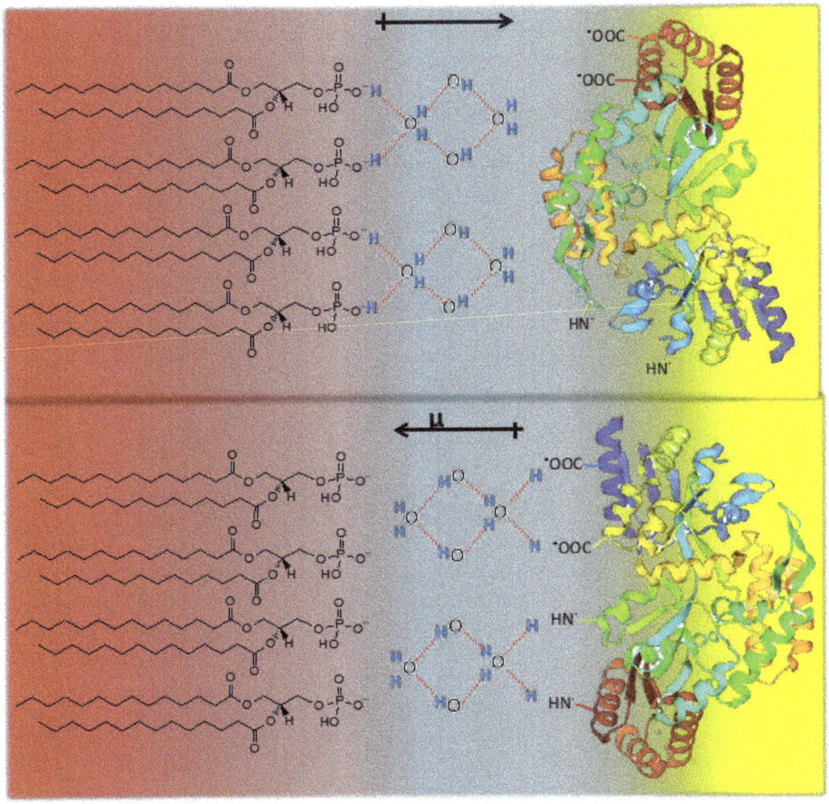

Figure 5. Inversion of dipole direction by displacement of protons without molecular rotation. Protein conformation may change inducing a water polarization by proton displacement that propagates to the membrane interphase and vice versa.

Moreover, if water populations change as a consequence of changes in lipid phase states or internal cell processes, a complex (and fast) response of polarization can result. The lack of water would alter this propagation essential for the living state [88,89].

Thus, "dynamic interphase hydration" can be controlling the probability of lyotropic mesomorphic transitions, allowing lipid self-assemblies and metabolically reactive structures in the cell to be coupled.

12. Concluding Remarks: Membrane Hydration and Membrane State. An Alternative Way to Membrane Response

The consideration of the interphase as a bidimensional hydrated polar head group solution coupled to the hydrocarbon region whose polarity varies according to its water content deserves a new thermodynamic interpretation.

In this regard, the consideration of the excluded volume in the free energy of the lipid interphase is useful to have a picture of the membrane in crowded and confined systems.

Thus, the description and characterization of crowding- and confinement-induced effects in living organisms, which have been focused on considering proteins in the cell cytoplasm, can be extended by the inclusion of the membrane itself as a crowded system and in connection with the cell interior.

The presence of water in the first 4C atoms and around the polar groups affects the water properties and implies water with different free energy content in comparison to pure bulk water, and hence with different capabilities to react.

Excluded volume can be modified by different chemical and physical conditions, such as surface pressure, osmosis, mechanical forces, and membrane components (e.g., unsaturated lipids and cholesterol) that may alter the lipid water ratio. This is the basic criterium to describe the membrane state as an open, non-autonomous and responsive system as it has been discussed [28,33].

The concept of an open/non-autonomous membrane system is visualized in the interrelationship between metabolic events and membrane polymorphic changes.

Therefore, the AIH and lipid properties interplay should consider hydration in terms of free energy modulated by water activity and surface (lateral) pressure.

This review is an attempt to incorporate the membrane as a structural component following the AIH and coacervate proposal.

In a recent review, the breakdown of current paradigms in the bilayer knowledge has been analyzed considering water as a fundamental structural and thermodynamic component of membrane systems [28,33]. This proposal can be extended to lipids organized in non-bilayer structures.

This criterium may also contribute to linking the role of lipids with Ling's cell theory, giving the water a central role from the thermodynamic viewpoint.

Thus, the challenging step forward is to take water organization at the limits of the membrane as a structural, dynamic, and functional element in living cells that may penetrate lipid membranes [32,90]. In this view, the new physical-chemical tool includes Thermodynamic of Irreversible Process formalisms and their dissipative and non-dissipative components to comprehend complex systems, such as cells and cell structures [28,87,92].

Author Contributions: A.S.R. and J.P.C. designed and carried out the experiments and statistical analysi; E.A.D. conceptualization; E.A.D. and M.d.l.A.F. wrote and revised the paper; M.d.l.A.F. supervised the study. All authors have read and agreed to the published version of the manuscript.

Funding: This work was supported by funds from CONICET and ANPCyT.

Institutional Review Board Statement: Not applicable.

Informed Consent Statement: Not applicable.

Data Availability Statement: Not applicable.

Conflicts of Interest: The authors declare that they have no known competing financial interest or personal relationship that could have appeared to influence the work reported in this paper.

References

1. Luckey, M. *Membrane Structural Biology: With Biochemical and Biophysical Foundations*; Cambridge University Press: Cambridge, UK, 2014.
2. Nicolson, G.L. The Fluid—Mosaic Model of Membrane Structure: Still relevant to understanding the structure, function and dynamics of biological membranes after more than 40 years. *Biochim. Biophys. Acta (BBA)-Biomembr.* **2014**, *1838*, 1451–1466. [CrossRef] [PubMed]
3. Israelachvili, J.N. Refinement of the fluid-mosaic model of membrane structure. *Biochim. Biophys. Acta* **1977**, *469*, 221–225. [CrossRef]
4. Goñi, F.M. The basic structure and dynamics of cell membranes: An update of the Singer–Nicolson model. *Biochim. Biophys. Acta (BBA)-Biomembr.* **2014**, *1838*, 1467–1476. [CrossRef] [PubMed]
5. Luisi, P.L. *The Emergence of Life: From Chemical Origins to Synthetic Biology*; Cambridge University Press: Cambridge, UK, 2016.
6. Deamer, D. The role of lipid membranes in life's origin. *Life* **2017**, *7*, 5. [CrossRef]
7. Chaplin, M. Do we underestimate the importance of water in cell biology? *Nat. Rev. Mol. Cell Biol.* **2006**, *7*, 861. [CrossRef]
8. Ling, G.N. The physical state of water in living cell and model systems. *Ann. N. Y. Acad. Sci.* **1993**, *125*, 401–417. [CrossRef]
9. Wimley, W.C.; White, S.H. Membrane partitioning: Distinguishing bilayer effects from the hydrophobic effect. *Biochemistry* **1993**, *32*, 6307–6312. [CrossRef]
10. MacCallum, J.L.; Bennett, W.D.; Tieleman, D.P. Distribution of amino acids in a lipid bilayer from computer simulations. *Biophys. J.* **2008**, *94*, 3393–3404. [CrossRef]

11. Bouchet, A.; Lairion, F.; Disalvo, E.A. Role of guanidinium group in the insertion of l-arginine in DMPE and DMPC lipid interphases. *Biochim. Biophys. Acta* **2010**, *1798*, 616–623. [CrossRef]
12. Seddon, J.M. Structure of the inverted hexagonal (HII) phase, and non-lamellar phase transitions of lipids. *Biochim. Biophys. Acta-Rev. Biomembr.* **1990**, *1031*, 1–69. [CrossRef]
13. Caffrey, M. A comprehensive review of the lipid cubic phase or in meso method for crystallizing membrane and soluble proteins and complexes. *Acta Crystallogr. Sect. F Struct. Biol. Commun.* **2015**, *71*, 3–18. [CrossRef] [PubMed]
14. Raja, M.; Spelbrink, R.E.; de Kruijff, B.; Killian, J.A. Phosphatidic acid plays a special role in stabilizing and folding of the tetrameric potassium channel KcsA. *FEBS Lett.* **2007**, *581*, 5715–5722. [CrossRef] [PubMed]
15. Nagle, J.F.; Mathai, J.C.; Zeidel, M.L.; Tristram-Nagle, S. Theory of passive permeability through lipid bilayers. *J. Gen. Physiol.* **2008**, *131*, 77–85. [CrossRef]
16. Duncan, S.L.; Larson, R.G. Comparing experimental and simulated pressure-area isotherms for DPPC. *Biophys. J.* **2008**, *94*, 2965–2986. [CrossRef] [PubMed]
17. Marsh, D. Lateral pressure in membranes. *Biochim. Biophys. Acta-Rev. Biomembr.* **1996**, *1286*, 183–223. [CrossRef]
18. Shinitzky, M.; Barenholz, Y. Fluidity parameters of lipid regions determined by fluorescence polarization. *Biochim. Biophys. Acta* **1978**, *515*, 367–394. [CrossRef]
19. MacDonald, R.; Simon, S. Lipid monolayer states and their relationships to bilayers. *Proc. Natl. Acad. Sci. USA* **1987**, *84*, 4089–4093. [CrossRef]
20. Blume, A. A comparative study of the phase transitions of phospholipid bilayers and monolayers. *Biochim. Biophys. Acta (BBA)-Biomembr.* **1979**, *557*, 32–44. [CrossRef]
21. Pattus, F.; Slotboom, A.; de Haas, G. Regulation of phospholipase A2 activity by the lipid-water interface: A monolayer approach. *Biochemistry* **1979**, *18*, 2691–2697. [CrossRef]
22. Disalvo, E.A.; Lairion, F.; Martini, F.; Tymczyszyn, E.; Frías, M.; Almaleck, H.; Gordillo, G.J. Structural and functional properties of hydration and confined water in membrane interfaces. *Biochim. Biophys. Acta* **2008**, *1778*, 2655–2670. [CrossRef]
23. Nagle, J.F.; Tristram-Nagle, S. Structure of lipid bilayers. *Biochim. Biophys. Acta-Rev. Biomembr.* **2000**, *1469*, 159–195. [CrossRef]
24. Lazcano, A.; Alexandr, I. Oparin and the origin of life: A historical reassessment of the heterotrophic theory. *J. Mol. Evol.* **2016**, *83*, 214–222. [CrossRef] [PubMed]
25. Schrodinger, E. *What Is Life*; Cambridge University Press: Cambridge, UK, 1944.
26. Ling, G.N. *Physical Theory of the Living State*; Blaisdell: Waltham, MA, USA, 1962.
27. Zhou, H.-X.; Rivas, G.; Minton, A.P. Macromolecular crowding and confinement: Biochemical, biophysical, and potential physiological consequences. *Annu. Rev. Biophys.* **2008**, *37*, 375–397. [CrossRef] [PubMed]
28. Frías, M.; Disalvo, E. Breakdown of classical paradigms in relation to membrane structure and functions. *Biochim. Biophys. Acta (BBA)-Biomembr.* **2020**, *1863*, 183512. [CrossRef]
29. McIntosh, T.; Simon, S.; Dilger, J. Location of the water-hydrocarbon interface in lipid bilayers. *Water Transp. Biol. Membr.* **1989**, *1*, 1–15.
30. Defay, R.; Prigogine, I.; Bellemans, A. *Surface Tension and Adsorption*; Wiley: New York, NY, USA, 1966.
31. Damodaran, S. Water activity at interfaces and its role in regulation of interfacial enzymes: A hypothesis. *Colloids Surf. B Biointerfaces* **1998**, *11*, 231–237. [CrossRef]
32. Disalvo, E.A.; Hollmann, A.; Semorile, L.; Martini, M.F. Evaluation of the Defay-Prigogine model for the membrane interphase in relation to biological response in membrane-protein interactions. *Biochim. Biophys. Acta* **2013**, *1828*, 1834–1839. [CrossRef]
33. Pinto, O.; Disalvo, E. A new model for lipid monolayer and bilayers based on thermodynamics of irreversible processes. *PLoS ONE* **2019**, *14*, e0212269. [CrossRef]
34. Viera, L.; Senisterra, G.; Disalvo, E. Changes in the optical properties of liposome dispersions in relation to the interlamellar distance and solute interaction. *Chem. Phys. Lipids* **1996**, *81*, 45–54. [CrossRef]
35. van Zoelen, E.; Blok, M.; Stafleu, G.; Lancée-Hermkens, A.; de Jesus, C.H.; de Gier, J. A molecular basis for an irreversible thermodynamic description on non-electrolyte permeation through lipid bilayers. *Biochim. Biophys. Acta (BBA)-Biomembr.* **1978**, *511*, 320–334. [CrossRef]
36. Wennerström, H.; Sparr, E. Thermodynamics of membrane lipid hydration. *Pure Appl. Chem.* **2003**, *75*, 905–912. [CrossRef]
37. Levental, I.; Veatch, S.L. The continuing mystery of lipid rafts. *J. Mol. Biol.* **2016**, *428*, 4749–4764. [CrossRef] [PubMed]
38. Pfeiffer, H. Hydration forces between lipid bilayers: A theoretical overview and a look on methods exploring dehydration. *Subcell. Biochem.* **2015**, *71*, 69–104. [PubMed]
39. Swenson, J.; Kargl, F.; Berntsen, P.; Svanberg, C. Solvent and lipid dynamics of hydrated lipid bilayers by incoherent quasielastic neutron scattering. *J. Chem. Phys.* **2008**, *129*, 07B616. [CrossRef]
40. Srivastava, A.; Malik, S.; Karmakar, S.; Debnath, A. Dynamic coupling of a hydration layer to a fluid phospholipid membrane: Intermittency and multiple time-scale relaxations. *Phys. Chem. Chem. Phys.* **2020**, *22*, 21158–21168. [CrossRef] [PubMed]
41. Disalvo, E.A.; Pinto, O.A.; Martini, M.F.; Bouchet, A.M.; Hollmann, A.; Frías, M.A. Functional role of water in membranes updated: A tribute to Trauble. *Biochim. Biophys. Acta* **2015**, *1848*, 1552–1562. [CrossRef]
42. Heimburg, T. *Thermal Biophysics of Membranes*; John Wiley & Sons: Berlin, Germany, 2008.
43. Rivas, G.; Ferrone, F.; Herzfeld, J. *Life in a Crowded World: Workshop on the Biological Implications of Macromolecular Crowding*; John Wiley & Sons, Ltd.: Chichester, UK, 2004.

44. Miyazaki, K.; Schweizer, K.; Thirumalai, D.; Tuinier, R.; Zaccarelli, E. The Asakura–Oosawa theory: Entropic forces in physics, biology, and soft matter. *J. Chem. Phys.* **2022**, *156*, 080401. [CrossRef]
45. Andersen, H.D.; Wang, C.; Arleth, L.; Peters, G.H.; Westh, P. Reconciliation of opposing views on membrane–sugar interactions. *Proc. Natl. Acad. Sci. USA* **2011**, *108*, 1874–1878. [CrossRef]
46. Luzardo, M.C.; Amalfa, F.; Nunez, A.M.; Diaz, S.; de Lopez, A.C.B.; Disalvo, E.A. Effect of trehalose and sucrose on the hydration and dipole potential of lipid bilayers. *Biophys. J.* **2000**, *78*, 2452–2458. [CrossRef]
47. Lairion, F.; Disalvo, E.A. Effect of trehalose on the contributions to the dipole potential of lipid monolayers. *Chem. Phys. Lipids* **2007**, *150*, 117–124. [CrossRef]
48. Disalvo, E.; de Gier, J. Contribution of aqueous interphases to the permeability barrier of lipid bilayers for non-electrolytes. *Chem. Phys. Lipids* **1983**, *32*, 39–47. [CrossRef]
49. White, S.H.; Jacobs, R.E.; King, G.I. Partial specific volumes of lipid and water in mixtures of egg lecithin and water. *Biophys. J.* **1987**, *52*, 663. [CrossRef]
50. Marčelja, S.; Radić, N. Repulsion of interfaces due to boundary water. *Chem. Phys. Lett.* **1976**, *42*, 129–130. [CrossRef]
51. LeNeveu, D.-M.; Rand, R. Measurement and modification of forces between lecithin bilayers. *Biophys. J.* **1977**, *18*, 209–230. [CrossRef]
52. Simon, S.; Fink, C.; Kenworthy, A.; McIntosh, T. The hydration pressure between lipid bilayers. Comparison of measurements using x-ray diffraction and calorimetry. *Biophys. J.* **1991**, *59*, 538–546. [CrossRef]
53. Sun, W.Q. Dielectric relaxation of water and water-plasticized biomolecules in relation to cellular water organization, cytoplasmic viscosity, and desiccation tolerance in recalcitrant seed tissues. *Plant Physiol.* **2000**, *124*, 1203–1216. [CrossRef] [PubMed]
54. Bagatolli, L.A.; Stock, R.P. Lipids, membranes, colloids and cells: A long view. *Biochim. Biophys. Acta (BBA)-Biomembr.* **2021**, *1863*, 183684. [CrossRef] [PubMed]
55. Martini, M.; Disalvo, E. Influence of electrostatic charges and non-electrostatic components on the adsorption of an aspartyl protease to lipid interfaces. *Colloids Surf. B Biointerfaces* **2001**, *22*, 219–226. [CrossRef]
56. Cejas, J.; Rosa, A.; Nazareno, M.; Disalvo, E.; Frías, M. Interaction of chlorogenic acid with model lipid membranes and its influence on antiradical activity. *Biochim. Biophys. Acta (BBA)-Biomembr.* **2021**, *1863*, 183484. [CrossRef]
57. Rosa, A.S.; Disalvo, E.A.; Frías, M.A. Water behaviour at the phase transition of phospholipid matrixes assesed by FTIR. *J. Phys. Chem. B* **2020**, *124*, 6236–6244. [CrossRef]
58. Calero, C.; Franzese, G. Membranes with different hydration levels: The interface between bound and unbound hydration water. *J. Mol. Liq.* **2019**, *273*, 488–496. [CrossRef]
59. Luzzati, V.; Tardieu, A.; Taupin, D. A pattern-recognition approach to the phase problem: Application to the X-ray diffraction study of biological membranes and model systems. *J. Mol. Biol.* **1972**, *64*, 269–286. [CrossRef]
60. Overton, C.E. On the general osmotic properties of the cell, their probably origin and their significance for physiology. *Vierteljahr. Nat. Ges Zur.* **1899**, *44*, 88–135.
61. Tristram-Nagle, S. Use of X-ray and neutron scattering methods with volume measurements to determine lipid bilayer structure and number of water molecules/lipid. *Subcell. Biochem.* **2015**, *71*, 17–43.
62. Nickels, J.D.; Katsaras, J. Water and Lipid Bilayers. In *Membrane Hydration: The Role of Water in the Structure and Function of Biological Membranes*; Springer: Cham, Switzerland, 2015; pp. 45–67.
63. Disalvo, E.A. *Membrane Hydration: The Role of Water in the Structure and Function of Biological Membranes*; Springer: Cham, Switzerland, 2015.
64. Alarcón, L.M.; Frías, M.d.; Morini, M.A.; Sierra, M.B.; Appignanesi, G.A.; Disalvo, E.A. Water populations in restricted environments of lipid membrane interphases. *Eur. Phys. J. E* **2016**, *39*, 94. [CrossRef]
65. Heerklotz, H.; Epand, R.M. The enthalpy of acyl chain packing and the apparent water-accessible apolar surface area of phospholipids. *Biophys. J.* **2001**, *80*, 271–279. [CrossRef]
66. Wiggins, P. Life depends upon two kinds of water. *PLoS ONE* **2008**, *3*, e1406. [CrossRef] [PubMed]
67. Chattopadhyay, M.; Krok, E.; Orlikowska, H.; Schwille, P.; Franquelim, H.G.; Piatkowski, L. Hydration Layer of Only a Few Molecules Controls Lipid Mobility in Biomimetic Membranes. *J. Am. Chem. Soc.* **2021**, *143*, 14551–14562. [CrossRef]
68. Epand, R.M.; Leon, B.T. Hexagonal phase forming propensity detected in phospholipid bilayers with fluorescent probes. *Biochemistry* **1992**, *31*, 1550–1554. [CrossRef]
69. Han, X.; Gross, R. Nonmonotonic alterations in the fluorescence anisotropy of polar head group labeled fluorophores during the lamellar to hexagonal phase transition of phospholipids. *Biophys. J.* **1992**, *63*, 309–316. [CrossRef]
70. Seddon, J.; Templer, R. Polymorphism of lipid-water systems. In *Handbook of Biological Physics*; Elsevier: Amsterdam, The Netherlands, 1995; Volume 1, pp. 97–160.
71. Rosa, A.S.; Cejas, J.P.; Disalvo, E.A.; Frías, M.A. Correlation between the hydration of acyl chains and phosphate groups in lipid bilayers: Effect of phase state, head group, chain length, double bonds and carbonyl groups. *Biochim. Biophys. Acta (BBA)-Biomembr.* **2019**, *1861*, 1197–1203. [CrossRef] [PubMed]
72. Disalvo, E.; Bouchet, A.; Frías, M. Connected and isolated CH2 populations in acyl chains and its relation to pockets of confined water in lipid membranes as observed by FTIR spectrometry. *Biochim. Biophys. Acta (BBA)-Biomembr.* **2013**, *1828*, 1683–1689. [CrossRef] [PubMed]

73. Pérez, H.A.; Cejas, J.; Rosa, A.S.; Giménez, R.E.; Disalvo, E.A.; Frías, M.A. Modulation of Interfacial Hydration by Carbonyl Groups in Lipid Membranes. *Langmuir* **2020**, *36*, 2644–2653. [CrossRef] [PubMed]
74. Van Zoelen, E.; de Jesus, C.H.; de Jonge, E.; Mulder, M.; Blok, M.; de Gier, J. Non-electrolyte permeability as a tool for studying membrane fluidity. *Biochim. Biophys. Acta (BBA)-Biomembr.* **1978**, *511*, 335–347. [CrossRef]
75. Pérez, H.A.; Disalvo, A.; de los Ángeles Frías, M. Effect of cholesterol on the surface polarity and hydration of lipid interphases as measured by Laurdan fluorescence: New insights. *Colloids Surf. B Biointerfaces* **2019**, *178*, 346–351. [CrossRef] [PubMed]
76. Davies, J.T. *Interfacial Phenomena*; Elsevier: Amsterdam, The Netherlands, 2012.
77. Whittaker, J.; Delle Site, L. Investigation of the hydration shell of a membrane in an open system molecular dynamics simulation. *Phys. Rev. Res.* **2019**, *1*, 033099. [CrossRef]
78. Volke, F.; Eisenblätter, S.; Galle, J.; Klose, G. Dynamic properties of water at phosphatidylcholine lipid-bilayer surfaces as seen by deuterium and pulsed field gradient proton NMR. *Chem. Phys. Lipids* **1994**, *70*, 121–131. [CrossRef]
79. Walter, J.; Hope, A. Nuclear magnetic resonance and the state of water in cells. *Prog. Biophys. Mol. Biol.* **1971**, *23*, 1–20. [CrossRef]
80. Derjaguin, B. Polywater reviewed. *Nature* **1983**, *301*, 9–10. [CrossRef]
81. de Paz, M.; Pozzo, A.; Vallauri, M. Mass-spectrometric evidence against "Polywater". *Chem. Phys. Lett.* **1970**, *7*, 23–24. [CrossRef]
82. Snead, W.T.; Gladfelter, A.S. The control centers of biomolecular phase separation: How membrane surfaces, PTMs, and active processes regulate condensation. *Mol. Cell* **2019**, *76*, 295–305. [CrossRef] [PubMed]
83. Długosz, M.; Trylska, J. Diffusion in crowded biological environments: Applications of Brownian dynamics. *BMC Biophys.* **2011**, *4*, 3. [CrossRef] [PubMed]
84. Dix, J.A.; Verkman, A. Crowding effects on diffusion in solutions and cells. *Annu. Rev. Biophys.* **2008**, *37*, 247–263. [CrossRef] [PubMed]
85. Bagatolli, L. LAURDAN fluorescence properties in membranes: A journey from the fluorometer to the microscope. In *Fluorescent Methods to Study Biological Membranes*; Springer: Berlin/Heidelberg, Germany, 2012; pp. 3–35.
86. Dutta, C.; Mammetkuliyev, M.; Benderskii, A.V. Re-orientation of water molecules in response to surface charge at surfactant interfaces. *J. Chem. Phys.* **2019**, *151*, 034703. [CrossRef] [PubMed]
87. Bagatolli, L.A.; Stock, R.P.; Olsen, L.F. Coupled response of membrane hydration with oscillating metabolism in live cells: An alternative way to modulate structural aspects of biological membranes? *Biomolecules* **2019**, *9*, 687. [CrossRef]
88. Clegg, J.; Szwarnowski, S.; McClean, V.; Sheppard, R.; Grant, E. Interrelationships between water and cell metabolism in Artemia cysts X. Microwave dielectric studies. *Biochim. Biophys. Acta-Mol. Cell Res.* **1982**, *721*, 458–468. [CrossRef]
89. Clegg, J.S. Hydration-dependent metabolic transitions and the state of cellular water in Artemia cysts. In *Dry Biological Systems, Proceedings of the 1977 American Institute of Biological Sciences Symposium, East Lansing, MI, USA, 21–26 August 1977*; Academic Press: Cambridge, MA, USA, 1978; pp. 117–153.
90. Disalvo, E.; Lairion, F.; Martini, F.; Almaleck, H.; Diaz, S.; Gordillo, G. Water in biological membranes at interfaces: Does it play a functional role? *An. Asoc. Quím. Argent.* **2004**, *92*, 1–22.
91. Soderlund, T.; Alakoskela, J.M.; Pakkanen, A.L.; Kinnunen, P.K. Comparison of the effects of surface tension and osmotic pressure on the interfacial hydration of a fluid phospholipid bilayer. *Biophys. J.* **2003**, *85*, 2333–2341. [CrossRef]
92. Heimburg, T. Linear nonequilibrium thermodynamics of reversible periodic processes and chemical oscillations. *Phys. Chem. Chem. Phys.* **2017**, *19*, 17331–17341. [CrossRef]

molecules

Article

Increase in the Intracellular Bulk Water Content in the Early Phase of Cell Death of Keratinocytes, Corneoptosis, as Revealed by 65 GHz Near-Field CMOS Dielectric Sensor

Keiichiro Shiraga [1,2,3,*], Yuichi Ogawa [1], Shojiro Kikuchi [4], Masayuki Amagai [2,5] and Takeshi Matsui [2,6]

1 Graduate School of Agriculture, Kyoto University, Kyoto 606-8502, Japan; ogawa.yuichi.4u@kyoto-u.ac.jp
2 RIKEN Center for Integrative Medical Sciences, Yokohama 230-0045, Japan; amagai@keio.jp (M.A.); matsuitks@stf.teu.ac.jp (T.M.)
3 PRESTO, Japan Science and Technology Agency, Kawaguchi 332-0012, Japan
4 Institute for Advanced Medical Sciences, Hyogo College of Medicine, Nishinomiya 663-8501, Japan; skikuchi@hyo-med.ac.jp
5 Department of Dermatology, Keio University School of Medicine, Tokyo 160-8582, Japan
6 School of Bioscience and Biotechnology, Tokyo University of Technology, Tokyo 192-0982, Japan
* Correspondence: shiraga.keiichiro.3a@kyoto-u.ac.jp

Abstract: While bulk water and hydration water coexist in cells to support the expression of biological macromolecules, how the dynamics of water molecules, which have long been only a minor role in molecular biology research, relate to changes in cellular states such as cell death has hardly been explored so far due to the lack of evaluation techniques. In this study, we developed a high-precision measurement system that can discriminate bulk water content changes of ±0.02% (0.2 mg/cm^3) with single-cell-level spatial resolution based on a near-field CMOS dielectric sensor operating at 65 GHz. We applied this system to evaluate the temporal changes in the bulk water content during the cell death process of keratinocytes, called corneoptosis, using isolated SG1 (first layer of stratum granulosum) cells in vitro. A significant irreversible increase in the bulk water content was observed approximately 1 h before membrane disruption during corneoptosis, which starts with cytoplasmic high Ca^{2+} signal. These findings suggest that the calcium flux may have a role in triggering the increase in the bulk water content in SG1 cells. Thus, our near-field CMOS dielectric sensor provides a valuable tool to dissect the involvement of water molecules in the various events that occur in the cell.

Keywords: bulk water content; near-field CMOS dielectric sensor; fluorescence imaging; corneoptosis; SG1 cell

Citation: Shiraga, K.; Ogawa, Y.; Kikuchi, S.; Amagai, M.; Matsui, T. Increase in the Intracellular Bulk Water Content in the Early Phase of Cell Death of Keratinocytes, Corneoptosis, as Revealed by 65 GHz Near-Field CMOS Dielectric Sensor. *Molecules* **2022**, *27*, 2886. https://doi.org/10.3390/molecules27092886

Academic Editor: Stefano Materazzi

Received: 25 February 2022
Accepted: 28 April 2022
Published: 30 April 2022

1. Introduction

Since the birth of primitive life in the ocean about 3.5 billion years ago, life has evolved on the basis of water. It is known that chemical reactions in living organisms would not be possible without water, which forms the medium that accounts for most of the weight of mammalian cells [1]. One of the most important roles of water molecules is the hydration of biological macromolecules, as their conformation is stabilized by the presence of surrounding hydration water [2]. Hence, the hydration environment in the cell is considered to be a mirror of the cell activity [3–5], and some theoretical studies have predicted that most of the water in a cell crowded with many biomolecules exists as dynamically restrained hydration water [6,7]. However, in the past 15 years, sporadic studies have experimentally evaluated water dynamics in cells, revealing that the majority of intracellular water molecules exhibit bulk-like orientation and translational motions, with only a fraction of hydration water [8–14]. This result suggests that both bulk water and hydration water interacting with biomolecules are involved in some way in intracellular activities, and therefore, the equilibrium between bulk and hydration water may play an important biological role in cellular functions.

Research to assess the amount of bulk and hydration water in cells originated in nuclear magnetic relaxation and neutron scattering experiments in the 2000s [8–11]. However, these techniques require deuterium substitution or tissue freezing to highlight intracellular water dynamics, and have not been able to observe intracellular water in its true physiological state. Later, using terahertz spectroscopy [15–17], it was shown that about a quarter of intracellular water in cultured human-derived cells under physiological conditions exists as hydration water, but its uncertainty (more than ±5%) would not be small enough to observe slight changes in the hydration state accompanied by changes in cell conditions [17]. In addition, the wavelength of terahertz waves (300 μm at 1 THz) is sufficiently large for the size of a cell and so it is difficult to obtain spatial resolution at the level of a single cell with far-field spectroscopy, and thus, the water dynamics that can be obtained are limited to the spatial average of a cell monolayer. Therefore, in order to clarify how intracellular water is involved in cellular functions, an improved technique to evaluate the bulk or hydration water content in cells with high precision at single-cell-level spatial resolution is required.

In recent years, we have found that the complex dielectric constant, $\tilde{\varepsilon} = \varepsilon' - i\varepsilon''$, in the millimeter-wave region (30–300 GHz) can be used to quantitatively evaluate the bulk water content without interference from macromolecules and hydration water (including confined water), because the contribution of dipolar relaxation of bulk water is far more dominant in this region [18–21]. We developed a dielectric sensor with embedded LC resonators oscillating at ~65 GHz, whose resonance conditions change to reflect the complex dielectric constant of the sample, and analyzed the change in the bulk water content based on the change in resonance frequency, thereby reducing the uncertainty of the evaluated bulk water content by an order of magnitude compared to conventional spectroscopic measurements [20]. The sensor consists of a two-dimensional array of resonators that sense the dielectric responses of the near-field, and the information of all elements can be read out in a CMOS circuit, so that the complex dielectric constant in the 65 GHz region (wavelength of 4.6 mm) can be recognized with a spatial resolution of about 50 μm at video rate [22]. Therefore, this new dielectric sensor can be expected to be an elemental technology for highly precise real-time evaluation of the bulk water content changes occurring in a single cell, which will help elucidate the role of intracellular water.

In this study, we aim to evaluate the relationship between changes in cell state and in the intracellular bulk water content using the near-field CMOS dielectric sensor operating at 65 GHz, using cell death as an example, which involves enormous and irreversible changes in cell physiology. Since changes in the position and morphology of cells may have a significant effect on the measurement results when using near-field sensors, we focus on corneoptosis, which is a process by which non-migratory SG1 cells (keratinocytes located in the superficial layer of stratum granulosum of the skin epidermis) die under high [Ca^{2+}] and acidic conditions to transform into nonviable anuclear corneocytes that perform barrier functions in the epidermis [23,24]. In this study, we develop an experimental system that can characterize the bulk water content with ultimate precision using the 65 GHz near-field CMOS dielectric sensor, and present changes in the bulk water content during corneoptosis of SG1 cells isolated from mouse epidermis, in parallel with time-lapse fluorescence imaging.

2. Materials and Methods

2.1. Near-Field CMOS Dielectric Sensor Operating at 65 GHz

The CMOS dielectric sensor used in this study was a custom-made product, manufactured by Sharp Corporation, with a measurement area of 3 × 4 mm on a 50 × 65 mm sensor chip, in which LC resonators operating at around 65 GHz are arrayed in 24 rows, with even- and odd-numbered rows vertically shifted by forming a zigzag arrangement within each row, as illustrated in Figure 1a [20]. Each LC resonator is coupled to a voltage-controlled oscillator (VCO) and embedded in a frequency synthesizer loop, and its oscillation frequency is detected by a 32-bit frequency counter after down-conversion to ~100 MHz output frequency by divide-by-3 injection-locked frequency divider and divide-by-200 divider [22]. This LC resonator, defined by the capacitance C_0 and inductance L_0, is implemented in a top metal layer, on which a passivation layer (capacitance: C_1) of several μm thickness is formed. When the measurement sample with $C_2 - iG_2 \propto \varepsilon_2' - i\varepsilon_2''$ is applied on it, the resonant frequency f of this LC resonator is given by [20,22]:

$$f = \left[2\pi \sqrt{L_0 \left\{ C_0 + C_1 \frac{C_1 C_2 + {C_2}^2 + {G_2}^2}{(C_1 + C_2)^2 + {G_2}^2} \right\}} \right]^{-1} \tag{1}$$

Equation (1) indicates that each LC resonator acts as a sensing element that measures the complex dielectric constant of the sample through the resonant frequency f. The C_0 and L_0 of the resonators are strictly locked in a self-sustained manner according to the VCO, and even with a gating time of 200 μs, the variation in the resonant frequency is limited within ±0.17 MHz (under ideal circumstances), which is extremely small compared to the center frequency (~65 GHz) [22]. Given that the impact of dipolar relaxation on the complex dielectric constant (ε_2' and ε_2'') in the 65 GHz region is sufficiently larger for bulk water than for macromolecules or hydration water [18–21], each resonator element serves as a highly sensitive dielectric sensor that can characterize the bulk water content by distinguishing small changes in the complex dielectric constant in the 65 GHz region, and the two-dimensional spatial distribution of the bulk water content can be also evaluated in real time by reading out a total of 1488 arrayed elements in the CMOS circuit. However, the detection sensitivity of this dielectric sensor is not spatially uniform; the dielectric properties of the sample near the gap of the LC resonator are most sensitive to the resonance frequency in the planar direction, and the detection sensitivity decays exponentially with depth [22]. As a result, each LC resonator works as a near-field sensor reflecting the complex dielectric constant at around 65 GHz in a region limited to ~50 μm in diameter and ~10 μm depth, which is determined by the resonator structure and the thickness of the passivation layer, thus enabling the precise evaluation of the bulk water content with single-cell-level spatial resolution as long as the cell is located in the sensitive area of the LC resonator.

2.2. Experimental Setup of Fluorescence Imaging

To assess the morphology of the cells by acquiring the fluorescence images in parallel with the dielectric sensor measurements, we set up a custom-made Tokai Hit imaging chamber on the manual translation stage of a Nikon upright microscope (Eclipse Ni-U). Inside the chamber was kept at 37 °C with humidified air containing 5% CO_2 supplied from a controller STGX (Tokai Hit, Fujimiya, Japan), and the dielectric sensor chip was mounted on the substrate in the chamber. A stainless steel well with a diameter of 16 mm and a depth of 5 mm is fixed around the measurement area of the dielectric sensor as a liquid reservoir. A 20× water immersion lens (CFI Fluor 20× W, Nikon, Tokyo, Japan) is approached through an opening in the chamber canopy until it is immersed in the liquid filling the well, allowing acquisition of the fluorescence image of the dielectric sensor chip surface in the upright position.

2.3. Preparation of SG1/SG2 Cell Suspension

By injecting exfoliative toxin-A into the dorsal skin of 4-month-old $EGFP^{SG1}$ knock-in mice (male), epidermal sheets (approximately 5 × 15 mm) containing SG2 cells (keratinocytes in the 2nd layer of stratum granulosum) and SC cells (keratinized dead cells; corneocytes) as well as SG1 cells were detached [23], and all cells were separated from the sheets in trypsin solution containing Hoechst 33342 and CellMask Orange Plasma (Thermo Fisher Scientific Inc., Waltham, MA, USA) at final concentrations of 10 μg/mL and 15 μg/mL, respectively. After that, the extracellular [Ca^{2+}] was reduced to less than ca. 1 nM by adding 1 mM ethylene glycol tetraacetic acid, and then SG1/SG2 cell suspensions were prepared by adding MCDB 153 medium at pH 7.2 containing 3 μM DRAQ7 (Biostatus

Ltd., Shepshed, UK) after centrifuge. As shown in the confocal images in Figure 1b, SG1 cells isolated by this procedure express EGFP in the entire cytoplasm except for numerous intracellular granules, whereas SG2 cells are EGFP-negative. In the skin epidermis, SG1 cells are known to have a flattened Kelvin's tetrakaidecahedron-like shape [25], but during the isolation process, the expansion rate differs between the apical and basolateral side of the cells, resulting in a polygonal saucer-like morphology. While SG1 cells can be cultured in a viable state, SG2 cells are dead in the final cell suspension, presumably because the cell membrane is directly damaged for a longer period of time than SG1 cells during trypsin treatment.

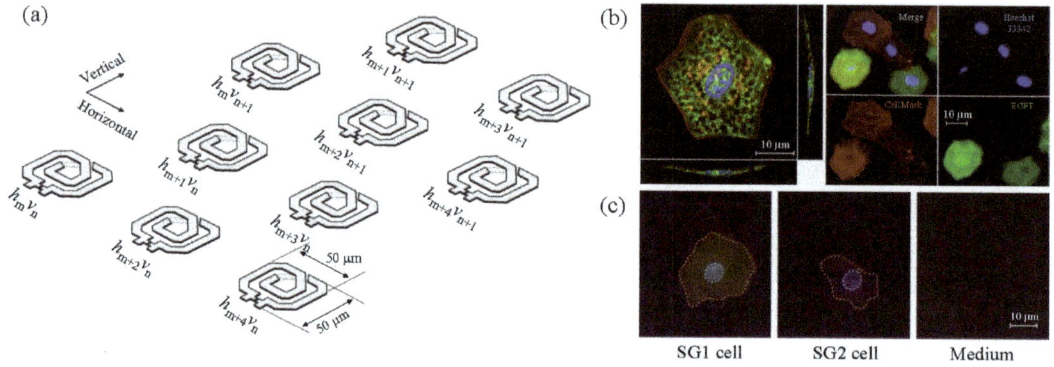

Figure 1. (**a**) Illustration of the LC resonator array. Each resonator element is numbered by $h_m v_n$ (m-th in horizontal and n-th in vertical direction; $0 \leqq m \leqq 62$, $0 \leqq n \leqq 24$), and even- and odd-numbered columns in the same row are vertically shifted in a zigzag arrangement. (**b**) Left: Confocal fluorescence images of isolated SG1 cells (EGFP; green) stained with Hoechst 33342 (blue) and CellMask (orange). Note that the scale of the cross-section planes is compressed to 50% compared to that of the top view. Right: Tiled fluorescent labeling of SG1/SG2 cells stained with Hoechst 33342 and CellMask. EGFP expression allows SG1 cells (EGFP-positive) to be fluorescently distinguished from SG2 cells (EGFP-negative). (**c**) Upright fluorescence microscopy images of measured SG1 (EGFP-positive; green) and SG2 (EGFP-negative) cells that meet the "single cell on a single element" condition at $t = 0$ h. Both cells are stained with Hoechst 33342 (blue), CellMask (orange), and DRAQ7 (magenta). The contours of the resonator structures, cells, and nuclei recognized by these fluorescent dyes are manually traced with white, orange, and cyan lines.

2.4. *Simultaneous Evaluation of SG1 Cell Death by Dielectric Sensor and Microscopy*

We applied 600 μL of the SG1/SG2 cell suspension onto the measurement area of the dielectric sensor placed at the focal point of the upright microscope and waited for about 10 min until the cells were completely settled. After that, by observing the entire measurement area (3 × 4 mm) while manually moving the translation stage of the microscope, we identified 13 resonator elements that had only one cell on the sensitive area, i.e., elements that satisfied the "single cell on a single element" condition. By discriminating SG1 cells from SG2 based on the EGFP expression, we found that 7 of the 13 cells were SG1 cells and the remaining 6 were SG2 cells. After fixing the manual stage in the field of view where one SG1 cell and one SG2 cell (Figure 1c), each of which fulfilled the "single cell on a single element" condition, could be observed simultaneously, corneoptosis of SG1 cells was induced by gently replacing the medium in the wells with MCDB 153 medium at pH 6.1 supplemented with 1 mM $CaCl_2$ and 3 μM DRAQ7 at final concentration. After the entire surface of the sensor was observed within 10 min to ensure that no change in the position of the cells had occurred due to the replacement of the medium, simultaneous data acquisition of the dielectric sensor and upright fluorescence microscope was performed at 10-minute intervals with the initial measurement, $t = 0$ h, until the 16th hour in total.

Since the dielectric sensor scans all 1488 elements in the CMOS circuit in a few seconds, the resonant frequencies of all the elements with seven SG1 cells and six SG2 cells were acquired almost simultaneously. With the fluorescence microscope, on the other hand, the fluorescence of one SG1 and one SG2 cell each was only observed, because it performed fixed-point observation in the same field of view.

3. Results and Discussion

3.1. Establishment of a High-Precision Evaluation for Resonant Frequency Changes

Figure 2a shows the time-dependent change in the resonant frequency f of a randomly selected element with no cells in the sensitive area (hereafter referred to as the "primary element"), which observes only the dielectric responses of the culture medium. The resonant frequency f fluctuated non-monotonically during the 16 h of continuous measurement, with a maximum change of 0.0161 GHz (16.1 MHz). However, since stability of the center frequency of the resonator in this dielectric sensor is typically controlled within ±1 MHz in our experimental setup [20], this 16.1 MHz variation is considered to reflect fluctuations in the dielectric properties of the medium rather than fluctuations in the resonator itself, such as C_0 and L_0. The dielectric response of bulk water, which makes up most of the medium, has a pronounced temperature dependence in the 65 GHz region [26], and the resonant frequency f of the dielectric sensor downshifts by about 26 MHz for every 1 °C increase in bulk water temperature [20]. Therefore, a change in the resonance frequency of 16.1 MHz corresponds to about 0.6 °C in terms of temperature, but this level of temperature fluctuation is conventionally tolerated in general cell culture, and besides, it is not technically easy to keep the temperature more strictly constant over 10 h. However, since the LC resonators in the dielectric sensor used in this study are arrayed at 50 μm intervals, the temperature between two adjacent resonators is expected to be extremely close, and by calculating their difference, the effect of temperature fluctuation on the resonant frequency can be compensated over a long period of time. In fact, as shown in Figure 2a, the f of the resonator element vertically adjacent to the primary element ("reference element") shows a quite similar time variation, keeping a constant difference of ~4 MHz regardless of time, which originates from differences in the device constants such as the resonator (C_0, L_0) and the passivation layer (C_1) for each element. Therefore, in order to take into account this effect, the frequency shift Δf at time t for an individual LC resonator is defined as [20,22]:

$$\Delta f(t) = f_0 - f(t) \quad (2)$$

where f_0 is the resonance frequency when there is no sample on the resonator. Since the frequency shift Δf represents the change in f of the same element with and without the sample, it can effectively cancel the effect of the device constant. The calculated frequency shifts Δf of the primary and the adjacent reference elements in Figure 2b show that they were in good agreement, indicating that the difference in the resonant frequency f by 4 MHz seen in Figure 2a is indeed due to the difference in the device constants (C_0, L_0 and C_1) between the elements, and there is little difference in the dielectric properties (=temperature) of the sample sensed by the two adjacent elements. Here, we define the difference between the frequency shift $\Delta f_{\mathrm{ref}}(t)$ of the reference element and the frequency shift $\Delta f(t)$ of the primary element,

$$\delta[\Delta f(t)] = \Delta f_{\mathrm{ref}}(t) - \Delta f(t) \quad (3)$$

as the difference frequency shift. As shown in Figure 2c, the $\delta[\Delta f(t)]$ calculated from Figure 2b was maintained at 0.02 ± 0.24 MHz for 16 h, allowing precise observation of the change in resonance frequency over time. Using Equations (1)–(3), it is calculated that the variation in the resonance frequency of ±0.24 MHz is comparable with changes of 0.002 in the real part (ε_2') and 0.004 in the imaginary part (ε_2'') of the dielectric constant [20], which are far smaller than the dielectric constant of pure water at 65 GHz (14.9 for the real and 23.7 for the imaginary part at 37 °C). Assuming that the dielectric constant change is solely due to the change in the bulk water content, the frequency shift of ±0.24 MHz corresponds to a ±0.02% (i.e., ~0.2 mg/cm^3 according to the water density of ~1.0 g/cm^3) change in the bulk water content using the analysis algorithm established in our previous study [20]. Therefore, this technique can identify changes in the bulk water content as a significant difference if it is 0.02% or more.

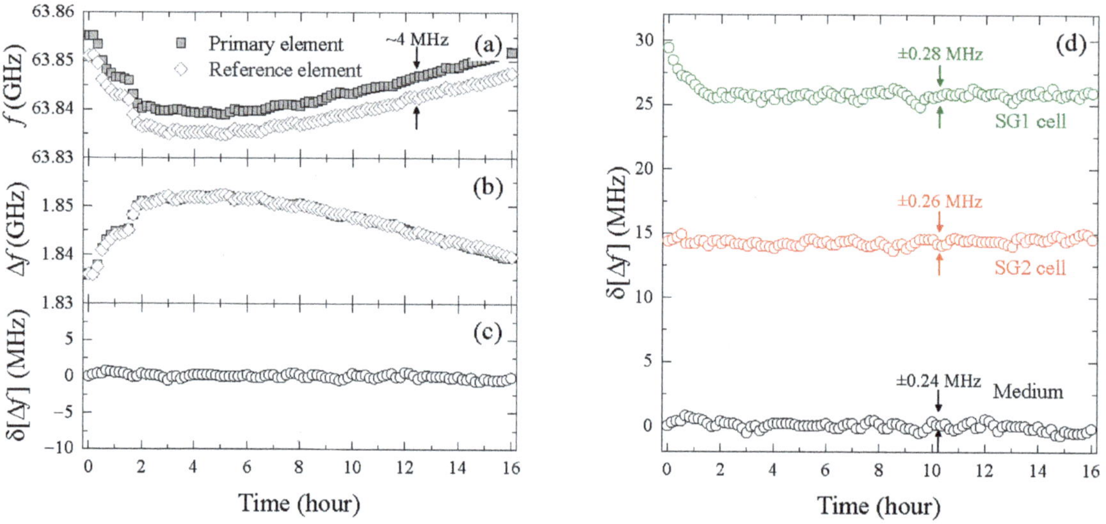

Figure 2. (**a**) Oscillation frequency $f(t)$ and (**b**) frequency shift $\Delta f(t)$ of the primary resonator element with the liquid medium on top and its vertically adjacent resonator element (reference element). (**c**) Time-dependent difference frequency shift $\delta[\Delta f(t)]$ defined by Equation (3). (**d**) Difference frequency shift $\delta[\Delta f(t)]$ for the SG1 cell (green), the dead SG2 cell (red), and liquid medium (gray) observed simultaneously by fluorescence microscopy. Standard deviations over 3–16 h (SG1 cell) and 0–16 h (SG2 cell and medium) are given for reference.

3.2. Evaluation of Intracellular Bulk Water Content Changes during SG1 Cell Death

Next, the element in which the cell is included in the sensitive area is considered to be the primary element, and its adjacent element with no cells is used as the reference. The difference frequency shift $\delta[\Delta f(t)]$ in the live SG1 cell (at $t = 0$ h) and dead SG2 cells measured while observing with the upright fluorescence microscope, and the same result as in Figure 2c, named medium, are shown in Figure 2d. The medium showed almost zero $\delta[\Delta f(t)]$ throughout the entire measurement time, while that of the dead SG2 cells averaged about 15 MHz over time, with a similar time variation (±0.26 MHz). Based on Equation (3), this result indicates that $\Delta f(t)$ is smaller than the frequency shift $\Delta f_{\text{ref}}(t)$ of the reference element (liquid medium) by ~15 MHz. Given that the complex dielectric constant in the 65 GHz region decreases in both real and imaginary parts as the bulk water content in the sample decreases [20], which results in a decrease in the frequency shift Δf (or an increase in f), the larger time-averaged difference frequency shift $\delta\langle\Delta f(t)\rangle$ in the SG2 cell than in the medium indicates that the bulk water content in the SG2 cell is lower than in the liquid medium. This result is considered to be natural because water accounts for about 99% of the weight of the MCDB153 medium [27,28], while the water content is relatively low due to the presence of organelles and some of the water is hydrated to biomolecules in the cells [15–17]. As the dielectric sensor used in this study has a spatially non-uniform sensitivity distribution [22], at this point, we are not able to determine the absolute value of the bulk water content in the cell due to the presence of extracellular water, but it is possible to observe the time-dependent change in the bulk water content above 0.02%.

Figure 2d shows that the difference frequency shift $\delta[\Delta f(t)]$ in the SG1 cell decreases monotonically until the second hour after induction of corneoptosis at $t = 0$ h and then converges to a constant value at ~26 MHz, in contrast to the constant $\delta[\Delta f(t)]$ of the dead SG2 cell and liquid medium during 16 h of the continuous measurement (the larger $\delta\langle\Delta f(t)\rangle$ than that of the SG2 cell is because the observed SG1 cell occupies a larger part of the sensitive area of the resonator element). By fitting this result with a single exponential function, it was found that $\delta[\Delta f(t)]$ of the SG1 cell decreased by 3.64 MHz with a time constant $\tau = 0.55$ h, which means that it takes 0.55 h for $\delta[\Delta f(t)]$ to reach 63.2% (=$1-e^{-1}$) of equilibrium. In light of the above, the significant decrease in $\delta[\Delta f(t)]$ during $0 \leqq t \leqq 2$ h indicates that the dielectric sensor reflects some phenomenon related to the initial process of corneoptosis by the SG1 cell.

To confirm whether the monotonic decrease in $\delta[\Delta f(t)]$ immediately after the corneoptosis induction is also observed in different cells, the measured $\delta[\Delta f(t)]$ of the SG1 cells ($n = 7$) that met the condition of "single cell on a single element", as secured by fluorescence microscopy, were collected. In order to evaluate their response to time, ignoring the effect of cell position on the sensitive area of the resonator element, the normalized $\delta[\Delta f(t)]$ adjusted to take values between 0 and 1 was derived, and then fitted with the exponential function, as shown in Figure 3a. Considering that SG1 cells isolated from mouse epidermis were used in this study, the time constant τ, which varied from 0.38 to 2.48 h, reflects the heterogeneity among cells. However, the characteristic of the temporal change—$\delta[\Delta f(t)]$ monotonically decreasing immediately after cell death induction and then reaching a plateau—was common to all seven SG1 cells. The normalized $\delta[\Delta f(t)]$ of the $n = 7$ average of the SG1 cells, as well as the SG2 cells ($n = 6$) and liquid medium ($n = 9$), are summarized in Figure 3b,c. The dead SG2 cells and medium showed almost constant $\delta[\Delta f(t)]$ over the 16 h of measurement, but only that of the SG1 cells showed a significant exponential decrease, confirming the reproducibility of the results seen in Figure 2d. Based on this finding, in the following, we will deepen the interpretation of $\delta[\Delta f(t)]$ by limiting it to the SG1 cell shown in Figure 2d, and compare it with biological findings obtained by fluorescence labeling.

If we assume that the decrease in $\delta[\Delta f(t)]$ of the SG1 cell by 3.64 MHz, found in Figure 2d, is solely due to the change in the dielectric properties at around 65 GHz, this result can be interpreted as an increase in the intracellular bulk water content in the early stage of corneoptosis in SG1 cells (according to Equations (1)–(3), $\delta[\Delta f(t)]$ decreases as the bulk water content increases, and becomes $\delta[\Delta f(t)] = 0$ MHz when it is the same as the liquid medium). However, each resonator element works as a near-field sensor that is sensitive only to a spatially limited area, and therefore, the dielectric properties of the sample sensed by the resonator change as the relative position of the cell to the resonator element or the thickness of the cell changes. Hence, in order to understand the origin of the $\delta[\Delta f(t)]$ observed in Figure 2d, it is essential to observe the changes in cell position and morphology based on microscopy. Figure 4a shows the temporal changes in the upright fluorescence microscope images taken in parallel with the dielectric sensor measurement. The SG1 cells express endogenous EGFP (green) with additional staining by CellMask (red) for the plasma membrane, and membrane-permeable Hoechst 33342 (blue) and membrane-impermeable DRAQ7 (orange) for the nucleus. Figure 4a shows that the isolated SG1 cell do not migrate in parallel or rotate within the measurement time. Furthermore, time-lapse imaging using confocal microscopy of a SG1 cell isolated from different mice on different days revealed that in vitro corneoptosis causes loss of Hoechst 33342 fluorescence but little change in depth and thickness, which is common to all observed cells ($n = 7$); a cross-sectional image of one of them is shown in Figure 4b. These observations suggest that SG1 cells are not migratory and that their three-dimensional morphology is largely preserved throughout corneoptosis, at least in the in vitro environment. Therefore, we can exclude the possibility that changes in the position or morphology of SG1 cells affect the change in $\delta[\Delta f(t)]$, and hence, the decrease in $\delta[\Delta f(t)]$ seen in Figure 2d can be attributed to an increased bulk water content in the cell. Calculated in the same manner as above, a decrease in $\delta[\Delta f(t)]$ of 3.64 MHz corresponds to an increase in the bulk water content of 0.3% (~3 mg/cm^3) [20]. Nevertheless, as SG1 cells have a convexly curved shape (Figure 1b) and the liquid medium outside the cells also occupies the sensitive area of the dielectric sensor, the bulk water content in the SG1 cell is considered to increase by more than 0.3% in actuality.

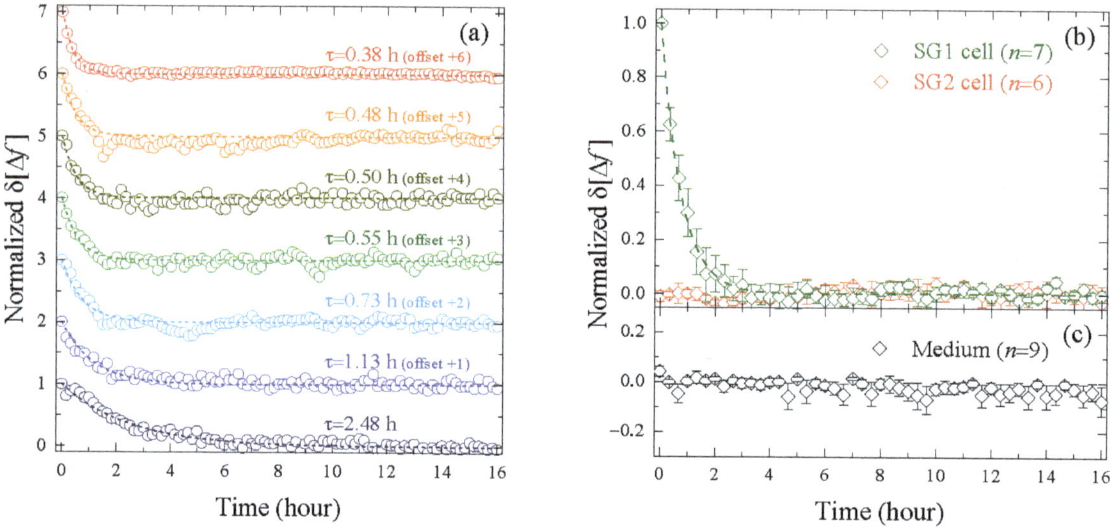

Figure 3. (**a**) Normalized $\delta[\Delta f(t)]$ of seven elements with a SG1 cell located in the sensitive area of the resonator (offsetting is applied to avoid data overlap). Each of the experimental results was fitted with the single exponential function with the time constant τ. The data with $\tau = 0.55$ h represent a normalized version of the results shown in Figure 2d. (**b**) Normalized $\delta[\Delta f(t)]$ averaged over the examined SG1 cells ($n = 7$) and SG2 cells ($n = 6$), and (**c**) liquid medium ($n = 9$). The error bars represent the standard error.

In living cells, cellular stability is accomplished by a number of homeostatic processes, and the cell volume (in other words, the intracellular water content) is maintained within a certain range. However, when cell death is induced, failure of these homeostatic processes results in volume changes specific to the cell death process [29,30]. For example, in apoptosis, monovalent cations, mainly sodium and potassium [31], are released from the cell, and the resulting osmotic shock causes rapid loss of water through aquaporins [32], leading to a tens of percent decrease in cell volume. On the other hand, in corneoptosis of SG1 cells, the nucleus and mitochondria, which are essential for cell survival, are lost, while the keratin network [33] and cornified envelope are developed in the cell [34] and the remaining cell body is taken over by the corneocyte. Thus, the three-dimensional morphology of SG1 cells maintains its mechanical strength even after cell death, and as a result, no discernible volume change is observed in corneoptosis in vitro, unlike other cell deaths. Nevertheless, it is intriguing to note that corneoptosis, as well as other cell deaths such as apoptosis (although the intracellular "bulk" water content was not directly assessed), share the same event of changes in intracellular water content, and it is worth noting what causes the one-step irreversible increase in the bulk water content seen in corneoptosis and what biological significance it has in the cell death process.

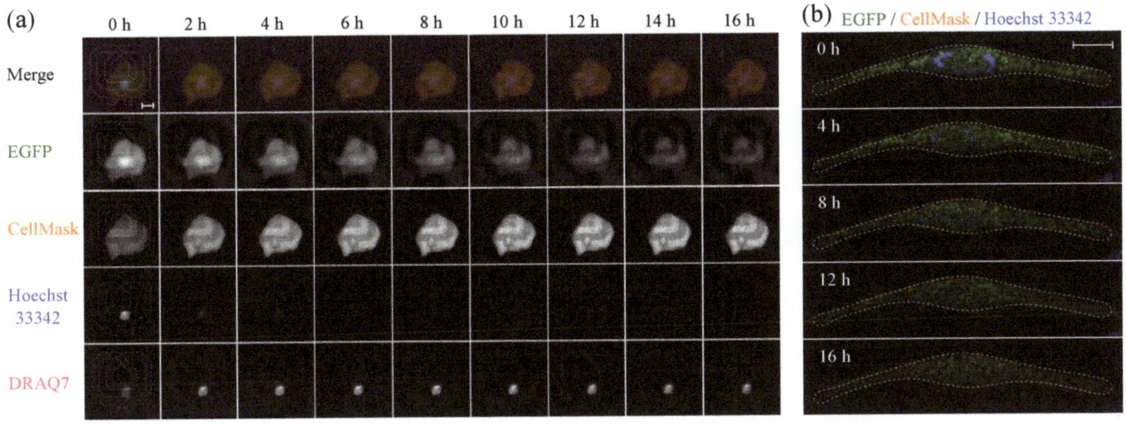

Figure 4. (**a**) Time-lapse fluorescence images of the SG1 cell (EGFP-positive) stained with CellMask (orange), Hoechst 33342 (blue), and DRAQ7 (magenta) under pH 6.1 and 1 mM [Ca^{2+}] conditions (scale bar, 10 μm). The resonator structure is manually traced with white dotted line at $t = 0$ h to show the relative position of the cell (nucleus) and the resonator. (**b**) Cross-sectional images of a SG1 cell isolated from different mice on different days at 4-hour intervals observed with a confocal microscope (scale bar, 10 μm). The cross-sectional outline at 0 h is superimposed to confirm that there are no three-dimensional morphology changes in the cell.

3.3. Comparison of Changes in Intracellular Water and Cell Membrane Permeability

To further understand the relationship between changes in the intracellular bulk water content and biological processes during corneoptosis, we will now quantitatively compare $\delta[\Delta f(t)]$ and fluorescence imaging in the same SG1 cell. In this experiment, nuclei of the cells were stained with membrane-permeable Hoechst 33342 and membrane-impermeable DRAQ7, and Figure 4a shows that the former showed strong fluorescence from $t = 0$ h, while the latter increased its intensity from 0 to 4 h followed by a gradual decrease. In order to interpret this temporal change, the fluorescence intensity of DRAQ7, $I_{\mathrm{DRAQ}}(t)$, normalized to a value between 0 and 1 is shown in Figure 5a. Consistent with a recent report [23], the rapid increase in $I_{\mathrm{DRAQ}}(t)$ seen immediately after induction of corneoptosis reflects the binding of DRAQ7 dye to intracellular DNA due to the increase in cell membrane permeability. However, once corneoptosis begins to set in, DNA degradation also progresses due to the activation of deoxyribonuclease, and after the increase in membrane permeability subsides, the effect of DNA degradation becomes apparent as a slow and monotonous decrease in $I_{\mathrm{DRAQ}}(t)$. In order to make a quantitative comparison with the change in $\delta[\Delta f(t)]$ seen in Figure 2d, the normalized $I_{\mathrm{DRAQ}}(t)$ was fitted with the following biexponential function:

$$I_{\mathrm{DRAQ}}(t) = \Delta I_{\mathrm{p}}(1 - \exp[-t/\tau_{\mathrm{p}}]) + \Delta I_{\mathrm{d}} \exp[-t/\tau_{\mathrm{d}}] \quad (4)$$

where the first term on the right-hand side corresponds to the increase in DRAQ7 intensity due to the increased cell membrane permeability, and the second term corresponds to the gradual intensity decrease due to DNA degradation, with ΔI and τ representing the amplitude and time constant of each process, respectively. Based on the best-fitting parameters, the time evolution of cell membrane permeability and DNA degradation is reproduced in the inset of Figure 5a.

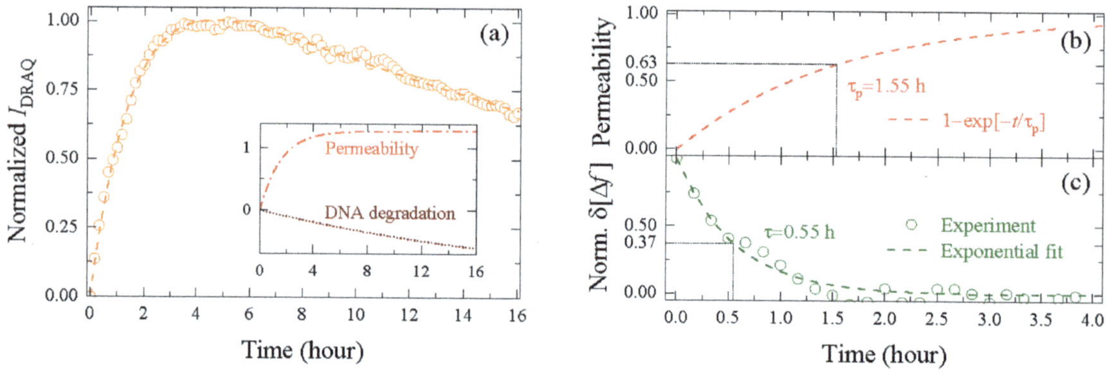

Figure 5. (**a**) Normalized fluorescence intensity of DRAQ7, $I_{\mathrm{DRAQ}}(t)$, and its best-fitting biexponential functions (dashed lines). The inset shows the time variation of the membrane permeability and DNA degradation components of the biexponential function given by Equation (4). (**b**) Membrane permeability defined by $1-\exp\left[-t/\tau_{\mathrm{p}}\right]$, and (**c**) normalized $\delta[\Delta f(t)]$ and its exponential fit of the same SG1 cell.

The observed membrane permeabilization is not limited to corneoptosis of SG1 cells, but is also observed in other cell deaths [29], and hence, the increased intensity of membrane-impermeable dye is widely used as a probe of cell death accompanied by plasma membrane disruption. Since the permeability of DRAQ7 with a molecular weight of about 400 Da allows smaller water molecules to pass through the cell membrane in and out of the cell, the increase in the bulk water content in the cell may be related to increased membrane permeability. Aiming to evaluate this effect, we compared the membrane permeability, $1-\exp\left[-t/\tau_{\mathrm{p}}\right]$, and the normalized frequency shift, $\delta[\Delta f(t)]$, of the same SG1 cell in Figure 5b,c. The results show that the time constant of $\delta[\Delta f(t)]$ ($\tau = 0.55$ h) is separated from $\tau_{\mathrm{p}} = 1.55$ h by as much as one hour, even though the same cell was observed simultaneously by the dielectric sensor and fluorescence microscope. Matsui et al. recently reported that τ_{p} was in good agreement with the time constant for the leakage of the fluorescent dye Rhod4-AM out of the cell [23], indicating that τ_{p} is a direct index of the rate of cell membrane disruption because the time required for DRAQ7 molecules to bind to DNA and show fluorescence after penetrating the cell membrane is sufficiently small compared to τ_{p}. Therefore, the fact that the time constant of $\delta[\Delta f(t)]$ was one hour shorter than τ_{p} suggests that the bulk water content increased in the cell before the permeability of the cell membrane increased. In addition, the fact that $\delta[\Delta f(t)]$ reaches a plateau after $t = 2$ h indicates that the intracellular bulk water content is almost unaffected by membrane permeabilization and DNA degradation.

Previously, it was shown that when isolated SG1 cells were exposed to acidic medium containing 1 mM [Ca^{2+}], instantaneous calcium flux into SG1 cells was observed within 5 min, which possibly activates enzymes such as transglutaminase, deoxyribonuclease, and aspartic protease in the cells, resulting in the progression of death into anuclear cells with the cornified envelope [23]. In general, when an enzyme specifically binds to a substrate, a portion of the hydration water immobilized in its active site is displaced [35,36], increasing the number of water molecules that behave in a bulk-like manner [37]. Although it is possible in principle to consider that the increase in the intracellular bulk water content observed in this study is due to such a release of hydration water, the bulk water content increased by enzyme-substrate binding cannot be more than 0.1% (~1 mg/cm^3) at most since the number of hydration molecules occupying the active site of the enzyme is small, nor can it explain the irreversible change in $\delta[\Delta f(t)]$. On the other hand, it has been shown that calcium plays an important regulatory role in the function of aquaporins, which are involved in the rapid volume loss (water outflow) that occurs during apoptosis [38,39].

This makes a possible scenario that elevated cytoplasmic [Ca^{2+}] activates aquaporins at the same time that corneoptosis is initiated, causing a water influx into the cell. The irreversible increase in the bulk water content may alter a vital entropy sink for biochemical reactions in the cell [40], resulting in changes in protein folding, self-assembly of membranes, and expression of macromolecular functions [2].

4. Conclusions

While physicochemical studies have revealed that water is closely associated to the functional expression of biological macromolecules, little is known about the involvement of water in the actual cell crowded with numerous molecules. In this study, we aimed to understand this issue in a paradoxical way by observing temporal changes of the intracellular bulk water content during SG1 cell death (corneoptosis) into anuclear corneocytes. Using a near-field CMOS dielectric sensor capable of measuring the complex dielectric constant in the 65 GHz region with high sensitivity, we developed a measurement system that can observe changes in the bulk water content of ± 0.2 mg/cm^3. We then found that the bulk water content significantly increases by more than 3 mg/cm^3 in an isolated SG1 cell in the early stage of corneoptosis, which is triggered by an increase in cytoplasmic [Ca^{2+}]. Simultaneous observation of the membrane-impermeable DRAQ7 fluorescence intensity revealed that the time constant τ for the increase in the intracellular bulk water content was found to be about one hour shorter than that for the change in DRAQ7 intensity, indicating that changes in water dynamics in SG1 cells precede membrane permeabilization in corneoptosis. Since such temporal changes in the bulk water content were not observed in dead SG2 cells, it is possible that although living SG1 cells have a mechanism to actively maintain low bulk water content, the induction of cell death by corneoptosis may upset the equilibrium of water dynamics maintained in the cell, probably due to cytoplasmic calcium-induced activation of aquaporin, which in turn promotes changes in the state of macromolecules and hence the progression of cell death.

Although it is not possible to speculate further at this time due to the lack of available experimental evidence, if this state-of-the-art near-field CMOS dielectric sensor, which is still capable of acquiring data with high time resolution at video rates, can be further developed to improve measurement precision and spatial resolution, and if it can be integrated with surface modification technologies to reduce cellular migration, it is expected that further studies using a wide range of cells and bacteria will elucidate, in a real-time and non-invasive manner, the involvement of bulk water in various cell activities, not just cell death.

Author Contributions: Conceptualization, K.S., Y.O., S.K. and T.M.; methodology, K.S. and T.M.; software, K.S.; validation, K.S.; formal analysis, K.S.; investigation, K.S.; resources, Y.O. and T.M.; data curation, K.S.; writing—original draft preparation, K.S.; writing—review and editing, M.A. and T.M.; visualization, K.S.; supervision, M.A. and T.M.; project administration, Y.O. and T.M.; funding acquisition, Y.O., S.K. and T.M. All authors have read and agreed to the published version of the manuscript.

Funding: This work was financially supported by the RIKEN Special Postdoctoral Researcher Program; by RIKEN Incentive Research Projects; by JST Industry Academia Collaborative R&D; by JST PRESTO grant number JPMJPR2008; by Grant-in-Aid Scientific Research (B) grant number JP22H03; and by AMED grant numbers 19gm1010001, 18gm1010001, 19ek0410058, and 18ek0410028.

Institutional Review Board Statement: Animal experiments were approved by the Institutional Animal Care and Use Committee of the RIKEN Yokohama Branch (2019-008(2)), in accordance with institutional policies, and conducted in the laboratory.

Informed Consent Statement: Not applicable.

Data Availability Statement: The data presented in this study are available on request from the corresponding author.

Acknowledgments: We acknowledge Rika Yokoo and Mako Urabe (RIKEN Center for Integrative Medical Sciences) for assistance in the experiments. We would also like to thank Yasuhiro Nishimura, Masako Ino (Nikon Solutions, Co., Ltd., Tokyo, Japan), and Nanako Kadono-Maekubo (Chifure Corporation, Kawagoe, Japan) for their help in acquiring confocal images of SG1 cells, and Tomoko Inose (Kyoto University) for her assistance in image analysis.

Conflicts of Interest: The authors declare no conflict of interest.

Sample Availability: Not available.

References

1. Ball, P. Water as an Active Constituent in Cell Biology. *Chem. Rev.* **2008**, *108*, 74–108. [CrossRef] [PubMed]
2. Chaplin, M. Do We Underestimate the Importance of Water in Cell Biology? *Nat. Rev. Mol. Cell Biol.* **2006**, *7*, 861–866. [CrossRef] [PubMed]
3. Wiggins, P. High and Low Density Water and Resting, Active and Transformed Cells. *Cell Biol. Int.* **1996**, *20*, 429–435. [CrossRef] [PubMed]
4. Häussinger, D. The Role of Cellular Hydration in the Regulation of Cell Function. *Biochem. J.* **1996**, *313*, 697–710. [CrossRef] [PubMed]
5. Davidson, R.M.; Lauritzen, A.; Seneff, S. Biological Water Dynamics and Entropy: A Biophysical Origin of Cancer and Other Diseases. *Entropy* **2013**, *15*, 3822–3876. [CrossRef]
6. Fullerton, G.D.; Cameron, I.L. Water Compartments in Cells. In *Methods in Enzymology*; Academic Press Inc.: Cambridge, MA, USA, 2007; Volume 428, pp. 1–28, ISBN 9780123739216.
7. Mentré, P. Water in the Orchestration of the Cell Machinery. Some Misunderstandings: A Short Review. *J. Biol. Phys.* **2012**, *38*, 13–26. [CrossRef]
8. Ford, R.C.; Ruffle, S.V.; Ramirez-Cuesta, A.J.; Michalarias, I.; Beta, I.; Miller, A.; Li, J. Inelastic Incoherent Neutron Scattering Measurements of Intact Cells and Tissues and Detection of Interfacial Water. *J. Am. Chem. Soc.* **2004**, *126*, 4682–4688. [CrossRef]
9. Tehei, M.; Franzetti, B.; Wood, K.; Gabel, F.; Fabiani, E.; Jasnin, M.; Zamponi, M.; Oesterhelt, D.; Zaccai, G.; Ginzburg, M.; et al. Neutron Scattering Reveals Extremely Slow Cell Water in a Dead Sea Organism. *Proc. Natl. Acad. Sci. USA* **2007**, *104*, 766–771. [CrossRef]
10. Stadler, A.M.; Embs, J.P.; Digel, I.; Artmann, G.M.; Unruh, T.; Büldt, G.; Zaccai, G. Cytoplasmic Water and Hydration Layer Dynamics in Human Red Blood Cells. *J. Am. Chem. Soc.* **2008**, *130*, 16852–16853. [CrossRef]
11. Persson, E.; Halle, B. Cell Water Dynamics on Multiple Time Scales. *Proc. Natl. Acad. Sci. USA* **2008**, *105*, 6266–6271. [CrossRef]
12. Sebastiani, F.; Orecchini, A.; Paciaroni, A.; Jasnin, M.; Zaccai, G.; Moulin, M.; Haertlein, M.; de Francesco, A.; Petrillo, C.; Sacchetti, F. Collective THz Dynamics in Living Escherichia Coli Cells. *Chem. Phys.* **2013**, *424*, 84–88. [CrossRef]
13. Martins, M.L.; Dinitzen, A.B.; Mamontov, E.; Rudić, S.; Pereira, J.E.M.; Hartmann-Petersen, R.; Herwig, K.W.; Bordallo, H.N. Water Dynamics in MCF-7 Breast Cancer Cells: A Neutron Scattering Descriptive Study. *Sci. Rep.* **2019**, *9*, 8704. [CrossRef] [PubMed]
14. Martins, M.L.; Bordallo, H.N.; Arrese-Igor, S.; Alegría, A.; Colmenero de Leon, J. Effect of Paclitaxel in the Water Dynamics of MCF-7 Breast Cancer Cells Revealed by Dielectric Spectroscopy. *ACS Omega* **2020**, *5*, 18602–18607. [CrossRef] [PubMed]
15. Shiraga, K.; Ogawa, Y.; Suzuki, T.; Kondo, N.; Irisawa, A.; Imamura, M. Determination of the Complex Dielectric Constant of an Epithelial Cell Monolayer in the Terahertz Region. *Appl. Phys. Lett.* **2013**, *102*, 053702. [CrossRef]
16. Shiraga, K.; Ogawa, Y.; Suzuki, T.; Kondo, N.; Irisawa, A.; Imamura, M. Characterization of Dielectric Responses of Human Cancer Cells in the Terahertz Region. *J. Infrared Millim. Terahertz Waves* **2014**, *35*, 493–502. [CrossRef]
17. Shiraga, K.; Suzuki, T.; Kondo, N.; Tanaka, K.; Ogawa, Y. Hydration State inside HeLa Cell Monolayer Investigated with Terahertz Spectroscopy. *Appl. Phys. Lett.* **2015**, *106*, 253701. [CrossRef]
18. Shiraga, K.; Ogawa, Y.; Kondo, N. Hydrogen Bond Network of Water around Protein Investigated with Terahertz and Infrared Spectroscopy. *Biophys. J.* **2016**, *111*, 2629–2641. [CrossRef]
19. Shiraga, K.; Tanaka, K.; Arikawa, T.; Saito, S.; Ogawa, Y. Reconsideration of the Relaxational and Vibrational Line Shapes of Liquid Water Based on Ultrabroadband Dielectric Spectroscopy. *Phys. Chem. Chem. Phys.* **2018**, *20*, 26200–26209. [CrossRef]
20. Shiraga, K.; Urabe, M.; Matsui, T.; Kikuchi, S.; Ogawa, Y. Highly Precise Characterization of the Hydration State upon Thermal Denaturation of Human Serum Albumin Using a 65 GHz Dielectric Sensor. *Phys. Chem. Chem. Phys.* **2020**, *22*, 19468–19479. [CrossRef]
21. Shiraga, K.; Fujii, Y.; Koreeda, A.; Tanaka, K.; Arikawa, T.; Ogawa, Y. Dynamical Collectivity and Nuclear Quantum Effects on the Intermolecular Stretching Mode of Liquid Water. *J. Phys. Chem. B* **2021**, *125*, 1632–1639. [CrossRef]
22. Mitsunaka, T.; Sato, D.; Ashida, N.; Saito, A.; Iizuka, K.; Suzuki, T.; Ogawa, Y.; Fujishima, M. CMOS Biosensor IC Focusing on Dielectric Relaxations of Biological Water With 120 and 60 GHz Oscillator Arrays. *IEEE J. Solid-State Circuits* **2016**, *51*, 2534–2544. [CrossRef]
23. Matsui, T.; Kadono-Maekubo, N.; Suzuki, Y.; Furuichi, Y.; Shiraga, K.; Sasaki, H.; Ishida, A.; Takahashi, S.; Okada, T.; Toyooka, K.; et al. A Unique Mode of Keratinocyte Death Requires Intracellular Acidification. *Proc. Natl. Acad. Sci. USA* **2021**, *118*, e2020722118. [CrossRef] [PubMed]

24. Moore, J.L.; Greco, V. Functional Cell Death, Corneoptosis, Requires Temporally Controlled Intracellular Acidification. *Proc. Natl. Acad. Sci. USA* **2021**, *118*, e2106633118. [CrossRef] [PubMed]
25. Yokouchi, M.; Atsugi, T.; van Logtestijn, M.; Tanaka, R.J.; Kajimura, M.; Suematsu, M.; Furuse, M.; Amagai, M.; Kubo, A. Epidermal Cell Turnover across Tight Junctions Based on Kelvin's Tetrakaidecahedron Cell Shape. *eLIFE* **2016**, *5*, e19593. [CrossRef] [PubMed]
26. Buchner, R.; Barthel, J.; Stauber, J. The Dielectric Relaxation of Water between 0 °C and 35 °C. *Chem. Phys. Lett.* **1999**, *306*, 57–63. [CrossRef]
27. Tsao, M.C.; Walthall, B.J.; Ham, R.G. Clonal Growth of Normal Human Epidermal Keratinocytes in a Defined Medium. *J. Cell. Physiol.* **1982**, *110*, 219–229. [CrossRef]
28. Boyce, S.T.; Ham, R.G. Calcium-Regulated Differentiation of Normal Human Epidermal Keratinocytes in Chemically Defined Clonal Culture and Serum-Free Serial Culture. *J. Investig. Dermatol.* **1983**, *81*, S33–S40. [CrossRef]
29. Galluzzi, L.; Vitale, I.; Aaronson, S.A.; Abrams, J.M.; Adam, D.; Agostinis, P.; Alnemri, E.S.; Altucci, L.; Amelio, I.; Andrews, D.W.; et al. Molecular Mechanisms of Cell Death: Recommendations of the Nomenclature Committee on Cell Death 2018. *Cell Death Differ.* **2018**, *25*, 486–541. [CrossRef]
30. Bortner, C.D.; Cidlowski, J.A. Ions, the Movement of Water and the Apoptotic Volume Decrease. *Front. Cell Dev. Biol.* **2020**, *8*, 611211. [CrossRef]
31. McCarthy, J.V.; Cotter, T.G. Cell Shrinkage and Apoptosis: A Role for Potassium and Sodium Ion Efflux. *Cell Death Differ.* **1997**, *4*, 756–770. [CrossRef]
32. Day, R.E.; Kitchen, P.; Owen, D.S.; Bland, C.; Marshall, L.; Conner, A.C.; Bill, R.M.; Conner, M.T. Human Aquaporins: Regulators of Transcellular Water Flow. *Biochim. Biophys. Acta (BBA)-Gen. Subj.* **2014**, *1840*, 1492–1506. [CrossRef] [PubMed]
33. Bragulla, H.H.; Homberger, D.G. Structure and Functions of Keratin Proteins in Simple, Stratified, Keratinized and Cornified Epithelia. *J. Anat.* **2009**, *214*, 516–559. [CrossRef] [PubMed]
34. Candi, E.; Schmidt, R.; Melino, G. The Cornified Envelope: A Model of Cell Death in the Skin. *Nat. Rev. Mol. Cell Biol.* **2005**, *6*, 328–340. [CrossRef] [PubMed]
35. Ben-Naim, A. Molecular Recognition—Viewed through the Eyes of the Solvent. *Biophys. Chem.* **2002**, *101–102*, 309–319. [CrossRef]
36. Li, Z.; Lazaridis, T. The Effect of Water Displacement on Binding Thermodynamics: Concanavalin A. *J. Phys. Chem. B* **2005**, *109*, 662–670. [CrossRef]
37. Grossman, M.; Born, B.; Heyden, M.; Tworowski, D.; Fields, G.B.; Sagi, I.; Havenith, M. Correlated Structural Kinetics and Retarded Solvent Dynamics at the Metalloprotease Active Site. *Nat. Struct. Mol. Biol.* **2011**, *18*, 1102–1108. [CrossRef]
38. Sidhaye, V.K.; Guler, A.D.; Schweitzer, K.S.; D'Alessio, F.; Caterina, M.J.; King, L.S. Transient Receptor Potential Vanilloid 4 Regulates Aquaporin-5 Abundance under Hypotonic Conditions. *Proc. Natl. Acad. Sci. USA* **2006**, *103*, 4747–4752. [CrossRef]
39. Conner, M.T.; Conner, A.C.; Bland, C.E.; Taylor, L.H.J.; Brown, J.E.P.; Parri, H.R.; Bill, R.M. Rapid Aquaporin Translocation Regulates Cellular Water Flow. *J. Biol. Chem.* **2012**, *287*, 11516–11525. [CrossRef]
40. Zaccai, G. Molecular Dynamics in Cells: A Neutron View. *Biochim. Biophys. Acta (BBA)-Gen. Subj.* **2020**, *1864*, 129475. [CrossRef]

molecules

MDPI

Article

Bovine Respiratory Syncytial Virus (BRSV) Infection Detected in Exhaled Breath Condensate of Dairy Calves by Near-Infrared Aquaphotomics

Mariana Santos-Rivera [1], Amelia R. Woolums [2], Merrilee Thoresen [2], Florencia Meyer [1] and Carrie K. Vance [1,*]

1 Department of Biochemistry, Molecular Biology, Entomology, and Plant Pathology, Mississippi State University, Starkville, MS 39762, USA; jms2033@msstate.edu (M.S.-R.); fsm28@msstate.edu (F.M.)

2 College of Veterinary Medicine, Pathobiology & Population Medicine, Mississippi State University, Starkville, MS 39762, USA; aw1873@msstate.edu (A.R.W.); mt1657@msstate.edu (M.T.)

* Correspondence: ckv7@msstate.edu

Abstract: Bovine respiratory syncytial virus (BRSV) is a major contributor to respiratory disease in cattle worldwide. Traditionally, BRSV infection is detected based on non-specific clinical signs, followed by reverse transcriptase-polymerase chain reaction (RT-PCR), the results of which can take days to obtain. Near-infrared aquaphotomics evaluation based on biochemical information from biofluids has the potential to support the rapid identification of BRSV infection in the field. This study evaluated NIR spectra (n = 240) of exhaled breath condensate (EBC) from dairy calves (n = 5) undergoing a controlled infection with BRSV. Changes in the organization of the aqueous phase of EBC during the baseline (pre-infection) and infected (post-infection and clinically abnormal) stages were found in the WAMACS (water matrix coordinates) C1, C5, C9, and C11, likely associated with volatile and non-volatile compounds in EBC. The discrimination of these chemical profiles by PCA-LDA models differentiated samples collected during the baseline and infected stages with an accuracy, sensitivity, and specificity >93% in both the calibration and validation. Thus, biochemical changes occurring during BRSV infection can be detected and evaluated with NIR-aquaphotomics in EBC. These findings form the foundation for developing an innovative, non-invasive, and in-field diagnostic tool to identify BRSV infection in cattle.

Keywords: absorbance; biofluid; cattle; chemometrics; discrimination; NIRS; transmittance; virus

Citation: Santos-Rivera, M.; Woolums, A.R.; Thoresen, M.; Meyer, F.; Vance, C.K. Bovine Respiratory Syncytial Virus (BRSV) Infection Detected in Exhaled Breath Condensate of Dairy Calves by Near-Infrared Aquaphotomics. *Molecules* **2022**, *27*, 549. https://doi.org/10.3390/molecules27020549

Academic Editors: Roumiana Tsenkova and Jelena Muncan

Received: 15 December 2021
Accepted: 13 January 2022
Published: 16 January 2022

1. Introduction

Bovine respiratory syncytial virus (BRSV) is an enveloped, non-segmented, negative-stranded RNA virus that belongs to the order *Mononegavirales*. It is a member of the *pneumovirus* genus within the *Pneumovirinae* subfamily of the *Paramyxoviridae* family [1,2]. The BRSV virion is made up of a lipid envelope generated from the host plasma membrane; it contains three virally encoded transmembrane surface glycoproteins that are arranged independently on the surface as spikes. These glycoproteins are the large glycoprotein G, the fusion protein F, and the small hydrophobic protein SH [1,2]. BRSV is very contagious and spreads through respiratory aerosols and via animal-to-animal contact [3]. During the incubation period (2–5 days), BRSV replicates primarily in ciliated respiratory epithelial cells and type II pneumocytes. After incubation, BRSV infection can be asymptomatic, or clinical signs such as fever (39.4–42.2 °C) and cough with a seromucoid nasal and ocular discharge can be present [2]. Clinical signs are typically mild; however, immunological suppression and mucosal damage in the respiratory tract might lead to subsequent bacterial infection, leading to BRDC (bovine respiratory disease complex) [1,4]. BRDC is the most costly disease affecting young calves worldwide [5–7]. As a result, it is critical to design new ways to prevent the spread of the primary causes of infection by this complex, which requires fast and non-invasive diagnostic tools to detect early cases of BRSV infection in the herd.

Field diagnosis of BRDC and BRSV infection is conventionally based on visual-clinical diagnosis (VCD) of the appearance and behavior of cattle, which is not specific for detecting and treating the causal agent [8–10]. Specialized techniques to detect BRSV infection have been developed and may include lung lavage, tracheal washes, and nasal swabs collected from live cattle or post-mortem samples for virus isolation and recognition of cytopathic effects in cell cultures [1,3]. Serological tests such as immunofluorescent antibody (IF) and enzyme-linked immunosorbent (ELISA) assays are also used to detect viral infection, exhibiting 47% and 60% sensitivity for BRSV, respectively. By comparison, analysis using reverse transcription-polymerase chain reaction (RT-PCR), which is currently considered the gold standard for BRSV diagnosis, has 99% sensitivity and specificity [1,3,11]. More recently, analytical techniques such as nuclear magnetic resonance (NMR) and gas chromatography based mass spectrometry (GC-MS) have been used in blood plasma, blood serum, nasal secretions, and exhaled breath condensate to identify biomarkers related to BRDC to create new diagnostic tools that facilitate appropriate treatment [12–17].

Near-infrared spectroscopy (NIRS) is a type of vibrational spectroscopy that measures absorption resulting from the interaction of NIR light (700–2500 nm) with functional groups of organic matter [18,19]. The application of NIRS to biological systems has often been confounded by the strong overtone signal of the water matrix, which acts to not only solvate biomolecules through hydrogen bonding but also has a complex and dynamic microstructure [18]. Aquaphotomics is a recent discipline in which the water spectrum arises from the interactions of water with specific biological components, while also focusing on how the biological composition influences the formation of water coordination spheres, clusters, and ions, which have distinct absorbance bands described by the water matrix coordinates (WAMACS) [20–23]. Thus, aquaphotomics is being increasingly applied to detect changes in water-based systems and is particularly applicable to biological fluid matrices in which a suite of biochemical changes occurs in response to shifts in organismal homeostasis [24,25].

Exhaled breath condensate (EBC) can be collected non-invasively and has been used to monitor respiratory disease in humans and animals [26–29]. EBC contains metabolites or substances such as adenosine, ammonia, cytokines (small proteins ~5–25 kDa), hydrogen peroxide, isoprostanes (free radical lipid peroxidation of arachidonate), leukotriene B4, nitrogen oxides (NO_2^- and NO_3^-), and peptides demonstrated to be helpful in evaluating oxidative stress and inflammatory response in the respiratory system [26,30], and which have been detected by GC-MS [14,16,31–33]. We propose that with these known indicators of inflammation evident in EBC, NIRS-based aquaphotomics coupled with chemometrics may provide a mode of rapid analysis of respiratory disease that can be conducted in the field. In this research, dairy calves were challenged with BRSV, and the EBC samples that were collected before and after infection were assessed by NIRS-aquaphotomics to create disease profiles and prediction equations, with a specific inquiry into the early stages of disease progression.

2. Materials and Methods

2.1. Animals and Controlled Challenge

BRSV strain GA-1, P5 was propagated in Madin-Darby bovine kidney cell lines grown in Dulbecco's minimal essential medium with 10% fetal bovine serum and 2 mM of Gibco™ GlutaMAX™ Supplement. On day 7 post-inoculation of cells, the cell culture supernatant containing −5.20 $TCID_{50}$ units of BRSV per mL was collected. Then, 5 mL of the supernatant was administered via a nebulizer (DeVilbiss Pulmo-Neb) through a custom-made face mask to each of five non-vaccinated three-month-old Holstein steers weighing approximately 130 kg and housed in outdoor pens isolated from other cattle at Mississippi State University (Animal Care and Use Committee IACUC-19-037) [17]. Clinical signs (VCD) of respiratory infection, including rectal temperature, heart rate, respiratory rate, assessment of nasal and ocular discharge, presence of cough, breathing pattern, and character of lung sounds, were evaluated before and after infection (Figure 1) [17,34].

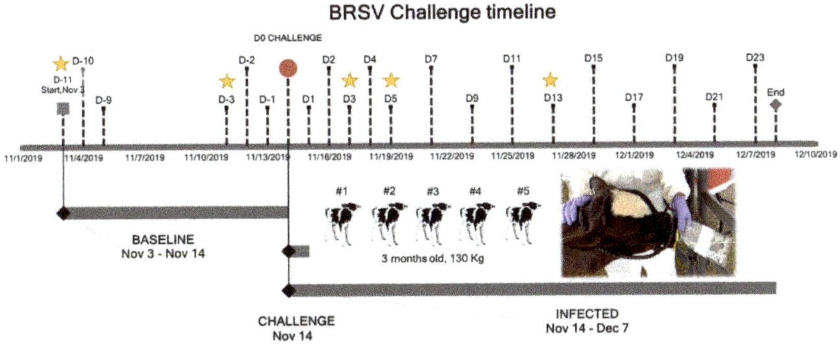

Figure 1. Timeline for the BRSV controlled challenge carried out in five dairy calves. The stars point out the days of the EBC collection.

2.2. Exhaled Breath Condensate (EBC) Collection

Samples were collected before and after the controlled challenge (D0). For the collection of EBC ($n = 24$), a sterile Nasco Whirl-PaK® sample bag with puncture-proof tabs (cat# B01489) was placed over one of the calf's nostrils for 15 min, ensuring that the breath was blown into the collection bag (Figure 1). The bag with the aerosolized particles was stored at −80 °C for 24 h, then thawed at room temperature (21 °C) to allow the condensation of the particles forming liquid droplets. The droplets (approximately 500 µL total volume) were stored in sterile Eppendorf tubes at −80 °C until NIRS analysis. To avoid discomfort in the dairy calves, these samples were collected only five times on the following days: D-11, D-3, D3, D5, and D13.

2.3. Spectral Signature Acquisition

Transmittance NIR spectra ($n = 240$) were collected from 300 µL of EBC using a portable ASD FieldSpec®3 spectrophotometer and Indico®Pro software (Malvern Panalytical, ASD Analytical Spectral Devices Inc. Boulder, CO. USA) as previously described by the authors [32]. Ten spectral signatures were collected independently per sample. Each NIR spectrum was taken across the wavelength range 350–2500 nm (interval = 1.4 nm for the region 350–1000 nm and 2 nm for the region 1000–2500 nm; 50 scans; 34 ms integration). Spectral signatures from sterile distilled water were collected as the reference solution required for the aquaphotomics analysis [34].

2.4. Data Analysis

Based on the clinical signs (VCD) evaluated before and after the BRSV challenge, the samples were classified as having been collected during the baseline, Asymptomatic, infected, or Recovered stages relative to challenge. To avoid interference of the asymptomatic phase or the recovery process in the interpretation of the aquaphotomics profiles, only an equal number of samples designated as baseline (pre-infection) and infected (post-infection and clinically abnormal) were used in the aquaphotomics evaluation and the statistical and multivariate analyses (MVA) [34]. The absorbance of EBC and the reference solution was transformed with the mathematical pre-treatments of SNV (Standard Normal Variate) with de-trending (polynomial order: 2), baseline Offset & Linear baseline Correction, and a 2nd derivative (polynomial order: 2, Gap Size: 25, Segment Size: 19, Savitzky-Golay smoothing points: 25) (Unscrambler® X v.11, Aspen Technology Inc, MA, USA).

2.5. Aquaphotomics Approach

Aquaphotomics was applied to determine the molecular organization of the aqueous phase of EBC as a method to identify the biochemical changes caused by the infection. PCA (principal component analysis) was performed on the mean-centered matrix of the aquaphotomics region (1300–1600 nm) using full random cross-validation and the algorithm SVD (singular value decomposition) as a first step in revealing trends in the spectra with the goal of exploring the data, identifying dominant peaks in the loadings, and looking for outliers (Hotelling's T^2 influence plot) [23]. Previously described WAMACS were used to create barcodes and aquagrams using a spectral database containing samples from all the calves ($n = 200$) [20,21,23,34]. Using Microsoft Excel 365®, the absorbance was normalized by subtracting the mean transformed absorbance of distilled sterile water as the reference solution from the mean transformed absorbance of each group (baseline or infected) and then dividing the results by the standard deviation (SD) of each category [21,23]. For the barcodes, WABS (water absorbance bands) within the WAMACS were identified by plotting the normalized absorbance to identify the direction of the peaks before detecting the WABS in each point of absorbance of the 12 WAMACS. These identified points were colored in the barcode according to each category to compare chemical shifts [34]. For the aquagram, the identified WABS for the baseline were selected as the points to be plotted in a radar chart to obtain the WASPS (water absorbance spectral patterns), which indicate the trends in the organization of the water molecules of the evaluated samples [21,23].

2.6. Chemometrics

The chemometric analysis was performed on the first overtone region of the near-infrared transformed absorbance between 1300 and 1600 nm. Balanced databases ($n = 200$) were generated to control the disproportion and diversity of the total number of samples collected [34]. These databases were used to create five datasets by stratified random sampling and analyzed in a leave-one-animal-out approach to develop five PCA-LDA (linear discriminant analysis) models using the Mahalanobis method [35,36]. To produce the calibration and internal validation sets (128/32), spectra from four calves were partitioned into an 80/20 percent distribution; spectra from the fifth calf were utilized as the external validation set ($n = 40$) (Unscrambler® X v.11.0, Aspen Technology Inc, Bedford, MA, USA). Within each model, nine predictions were tested using PCs (principal components), explaining from 95% to 99.9% of the variation of the databases using the top-down approach for PC selection methodology [34,37]. A total of 45 predictions were evaluated; however, only the results from the ones with the best performance are shown in the results section. Quality parameters, including the percentage of accuracy, sensitivity, and specificity, were carried out to establish the technique's ability to classify true positive and true negative samples [34,38]. ANOVA, and a pairwise mean comparison using Tukey-Kramer HSD (honestly significant difference) test with alpha = 0.05 were used to assess significance between models (JMP® 14.0, SAS Institute Inc., Cary, NC, USA); in addition, a pairwise mean comparison using Student's t-test with alpha = 0.05 was used to evaluate differences between categories (baseline vs. infected).

3. Results

3.1. Aquaphotomics Findings

The aquaphotomic analysis for NIR spectral signatures collected for breath condensate from dairy calves infected with BRSV revealed a consistent and expected spectral water pattern in the wavelength range between 1300 and 1600 nm (Figure 2a). This region corresponds to the first overtone of the functional groups O-H, C-H, and N-H forming molecules containing water (H_2O), alcohols (ROH), phenols (ArOH), simple amides ($CONH_2$), amides (CONHR), monoamides (RNH_2), methylene (CH_2), and methyl radicals (CH_3) [18], which are, in this case, likely related to the high content of water and the volatile and non-volatile compounds in the EBC [30]. The pattern in the transformed absorbance (Figure 2b) was also expected due to the application of a second derivative and Savitzky-Golay smoothing in the pre-treatment [39]. Chemical similarities were observed in the trends of the PCA scores plot (Figure 2c), where both categories overlap. The dominant peaks identified in the positive and negative directions of the PCA loadings (PC-1 = 1347, 1396, 1454, 1528 nm; PC-2 = 1396, 1418, 1539 nm; PC-3 = 1338, 1380, 1431, 1524, 1576 nm) explained the aforementioned patterns, with the first three PCs accounting for 97% of the variation in the spectral database (Figure 2d). There were no outliers in the Hotelling's T^2 influence plot (not shown). These findings highlight the need to use both, aquaphotomics and chemometrics-based MVA to reveal discriminating biochemical profiles of BRSV infection in EBC.

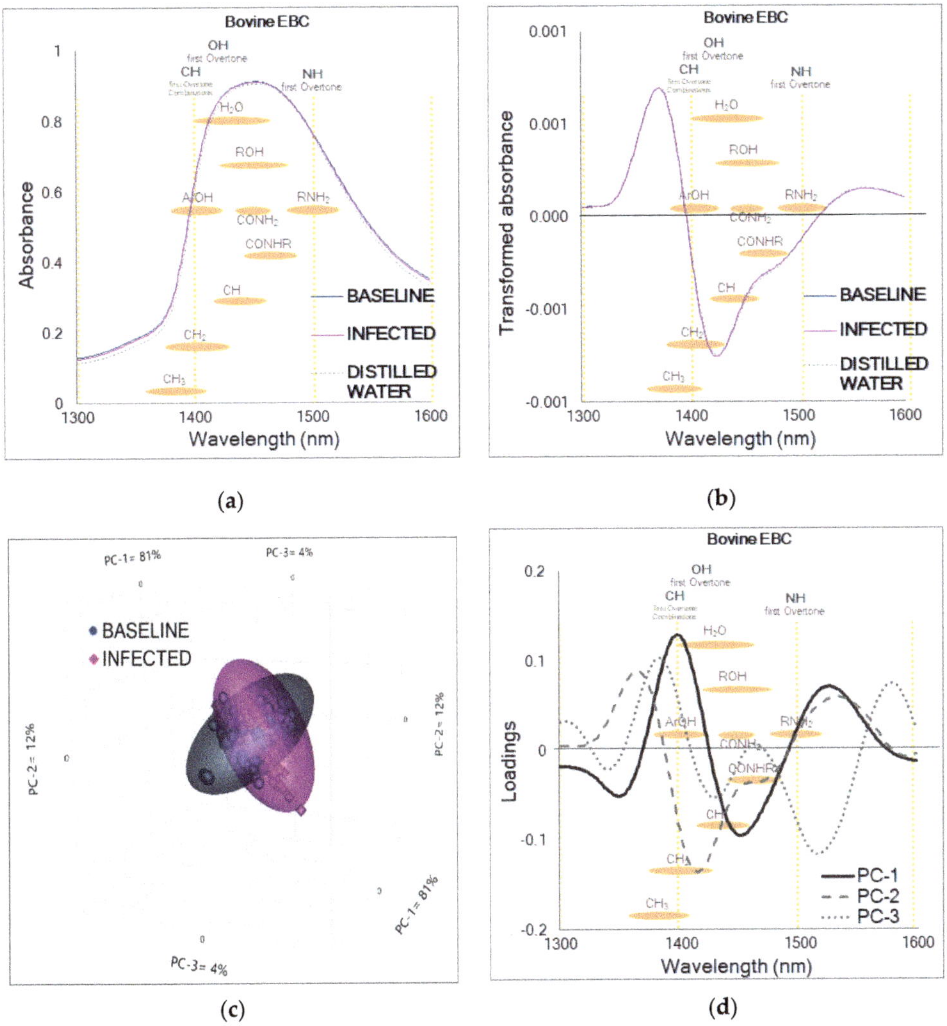

Figure 2. NIR absorbance from bovine EBC collected before and after BRSV infection. (**a**) Raw or unprocessed NIR absorbance from baseline (n = 100) and infected (n = 100) stages relative to infection, showing the characteristic water spectral pattern. (**b**) Transformed or processed absorbance from baseline (n = 100) and infected (n = 100) stages displaying two prominent features at 1376 and 1424 nm. (**c**) PCA scores plot for samples of the baseline and infected stages from all the calves (n = 5) challenged in this study (n = 200). (**d**) PCA loadings showing the dominant peaks influencing the positive and negative trends in the scores plot: PC-1 = 81%, PC-2 = 12%, PC-3 = 4%.

The normalized absorbance of EBC collected in the pre-infection baseline stage and the infected stage when calves had clinical signs of disease revealed different patterns for both categories, indicating differences in the chemical composition of EBC from healthy and sick dairy calves (Figure 3a). Interestingly, at 1574 nm, a prominent feature in the normalized absorbance from the infected stage was unveiled; this wavelength corresponds to the first overtone of N-H stretching vibration and is not included in the current described WAMACS.

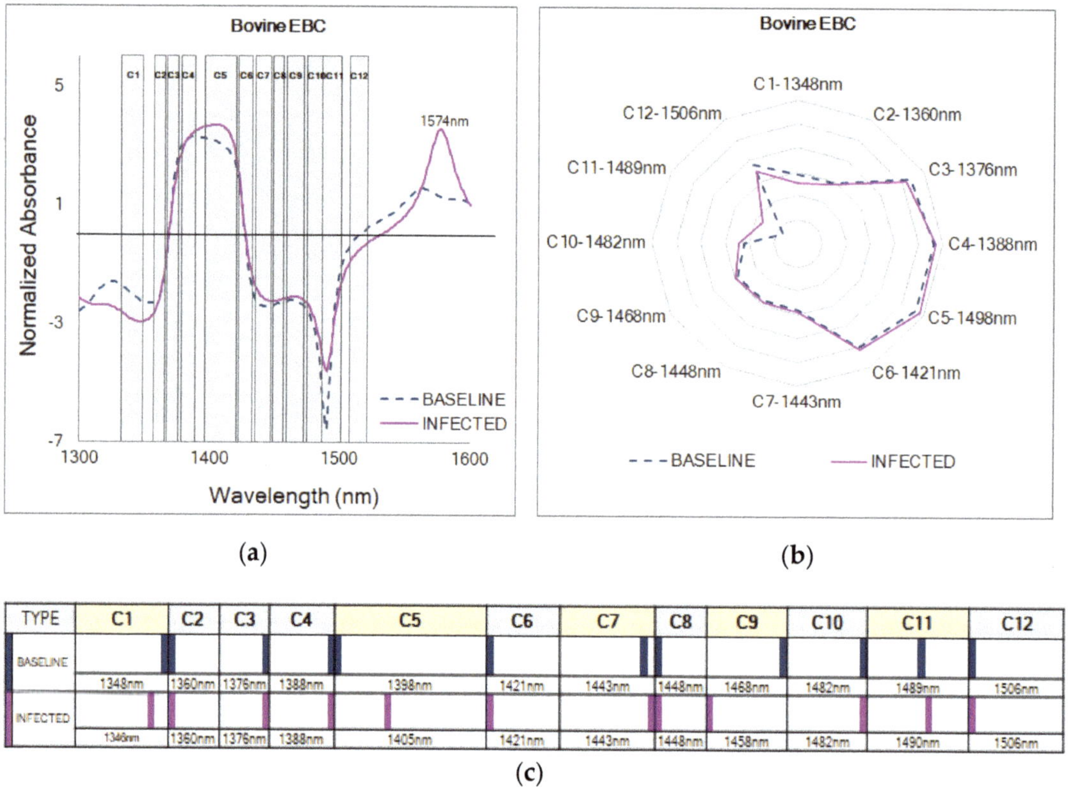

Figure 3. Aquaphotomics of EBC from dairy calves infected with BRSV. (**a**) Normalized absorbance for samples from the baseline (n = 100) and infected (n = 100) stages from all the calves (n = 5) challenged in this study. (**b**) Aquagram created with the key WABS from the baseline stage. (**c**) WAMACS barcode showing chemical shifts.

The WASPS in the aquagram (Figure 3b) indicate that water molecules in EBC from both categories were highly organized in the WAMACS C3, C4, C5, and C6 and less organized in the coordinates C7 to C12, which are related to water dimers (S_1) and water clusters with two, three, and four hydrogen bonds (S_2, S_3, and S_4) [21,23]. In this case, baseline samples showed the highest absorbance at C4, and samples from the infected stage showed the highest absorbance at C5. At C4 (1380–1388 nm), a change in the formation of complex three-dimensional molecular spheres or hydration shells around solute molecules can be implied, mainly concerning the lipid (total lipids, phospholipids, cholesterol, triglycerides, eicosanoids, free fatty acids) and cytoplasmic (glucose, ammonia, lactate; pyruvic, succinic, and oxaloacetic acids) metabolites known to increase in EBC during chronic pulmonary disease [21,40–44]. At C5 (1398–1418 nm), two types of changes in the water matrix of EBC can be inferred, the first one related to water molecules confined in a local field of ions and the second related to water molecules with free hydroxide ion (OH-) [21,23]. Moreover, higher absorbances at C3 (1370–1376 nm) suggest that molecules were structured in water symmetrical and asymmetrical stretching vibrations ($\nu_1 + \nu_3$) related to variations in the EBC solute composition during the baseline or infected stage [21,23]. In addition, at C6 (1421–1430 nm), changes in the HOH bending frequency are suggested to occur [21,23].

The barcode (Figure 3c) shows shifts between EBC samples collected in both the baseline and infected stages in five of the 12 known WAMACS in the coordinates C1, C5, C7, C9, and C11 likely related to changes in the ratios of volatile and non-volatile compounds. In the normalized absorbance from EBC collected during the infected stage, NIR spectral peaks were right-shifted in C5 (1398–1418 nm), C7 (1432–1444 nm), and C11 (1482–1495 nm), more specifically to 1405, 1443, and 1490 nm, in comparison with initial peaks at 1398, 1443, and 1489 nm found in spectra of the baseline samples, suggesting a shift towards free water (C5), water dimers (C7), and water clusters with four hydrogen bonds (C11) [21,23]. At C1 (1336–1348 nm) and C9 (1458–1468 nm), NIR spectral peaks were left-shifted in samples from the infected stage at 1346 and 1458 nm in comparison to 1348 and 1489 nm during baseline, thus indicating a shift towards molecules structured in water asymmetrical stretching vibrations (ν_3) and water clusters with two hydrogen bonds (S_2) [21,23].

3.2. Discriminant Analysis Results

The results from the PCA-LDA models for classifying NIR-transformed absorbance (1300–1600 nm) of EBC collected from calves before and after the BRSV infection can be found in Table 1. On average, 7 ± 2 PCs explaining 99.6 ± 0.4% of the variation of the database were selected to perform the analyses. In this case, no significant differences ($p < 0.05$) were detected for the values of correctly predicted categories between the models (1–5) or between stages (baseline and infected) when applying the ANOVA or the Student's t-tests. When evaluating the quality parameters from all the models simultaneously, significant differences ($p < 0.05$) were detected for the calibration values in comparison to the internal validation and the external validation. During the calibration, percentages of accuracy, sensitivity, and specificity of 97 ± 6, 98 ± 4, and 96 ± 9%, respectively, were achieved, indicating that 2 ± 4% of the transformed absorbance from samples of the infected stage were classified as false negatives, and 4 ± 9% of the transformed absorbance from samples of the baseline stage were classified as false positives. In the internal validation, the percentages 96 ± 8, 99 ± 3, and 93 ± 17% were obtained for the accuracy, sensitivity, and specificity, respectively. Hence, 1 ± 3% of the transformed absorbance from samples of the infected stage were classified as false negatives, and 7 ± 17% of the transformed absorbance from samples of the baseline stage were classified as false positives. Additionally, the external validation set containing the spectra from the calf excluded during the calibration was classified with percentages of 74 ± 21, 71 ± 27, and 76 ± 23%, for the accuracy, sensitivity, and specificity, correspondingly. Here, 29 ± 27% of the transformed absorbance were classified as false negatives, and 26 ± 23% were false positives to the viral infection. All the calibration PCA-LDA plots showed similar tendencies where two well-defined groups were found; in Figure 4, Model 4, omitting Calf 4, is shown as a representative of the five performed models. These results suggest that the biochemical differences found in the aquaphotomics evaluation due to changes in EBC composition during the infection can be discriminated using chemometrics-based MVA methods with quality parameters higher than the traditional clinical signs (VCD) and serological methods to detect this infection.

Table 1. PCA-LDA for transformed absorbance (1300–1600 nm) classification and quality parameters for bovine EBC collected before and after the BRSV challenge.

Model	# Selected PCs	% Explained Variance	Category and Quality	% PCA-LDA Mahalanobis		
				Cal 80%	Val 20%	External Validation
1 (Calf 1 out)	8	99.8	baseline	64/64	16/16	7/20
			infected	64/64	16/16	9/20
			% Accuracy	100	100	40
			% Sensitivity	100	100	45
			% Specificity	100	100	35
2 (Calf 2 out)	9	99.9	baseline	64/64	16/16	16/20
			infected	64/64	16/16	20/20
			% Accuracy	100	100	90
			% Sensitivity	100	100	100
			% Specificity	100	100	80
3 (Calf 3 out)	7	99.6	baseline	64/64	16/16	18/20
			infected	64/64	15/16	10/20
			% Accuracy	100	97	70
			% Sensitivity	100	94	50
			% Specificity	100	100	90
4 (Calf 4 out)	5	98.9	baseline	54/64	10/16	17/20
			infected	59/64	16/16	20/20
			% Accuracy	86	81	93
			% Sensitivity	92	100	100
			% Specificity	80	63	85
5 (Calf 5 out)	8	99.9	baseline	63/64	16/16	18/20
			infected	64/64	16/16	12/20
			% Accuracy	99	100	75
			% Sensitivity	100	100	60
			% Specificity	98	100	90
Mean ± SD	7 ± 2	99.6 ± 0.4	% Accuracy	97 ± 6 (a)	96 ± 8 (a,b)	74 ± 21 (b)
			% Sensitivity	98 ± 4 (a)	99 ± 3 (a)	71 ± 27 (b)
			% Specificity	96 ± 9 (a)	93 ± 17 (a)	76 ± 23 (a)

Values with different letters were significantly different ($p < 0.05$) between the calibration (Cal 80%), the internal validation (Val 20%), and the external validation. No significant differences were detected in the prediction values between models after applying ANOVA and Tukey-Kramer HSD (honestly significant difference).

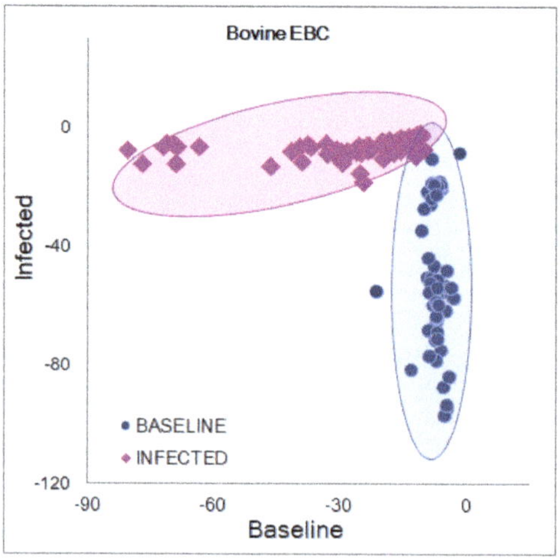

Figure 4. PCA-LDA plot for the calibration of Model 4 developed with the transformed absorbance (1300–1600 nm) from EBC collected before and after the BRSV challenge.

4. Discussion

The exhaled breath condensate (EBC) comprises >99.9% condensed water vapor and <0.1% aerosols [29,30]. While the condensing water absorbs water-soluble volatile compounds, respiratory droplets containing non-volatile molecules compose a minor fraction of the condensate [29,30]. The use of EBC as a biofluid to evaluate and detect respiratory diseases in small and large animals has gained special relevance in veterinary medicine [28,29]. The chemical composition of EBC from healthy and sick calves has been previously reported [28–30]. In healthy animals, hydrogen peroxide (H_2O_2), which is a volatile molecule in EBC, is well-known for its involvement in airway homeostasis [45,46]. During respiratory disease, H_2O_2 in EBC is considered a biomarker of inflammation and oxidative stress caused by the release of reactive oxygen species (ROS) and nitrogen species (RNS) from inflammatory leukocytes (neutrophils, eosinophils), monocytes (macrophages), and airway epithelial cells [30,47]. EBC from Holstein calves with bronchopneumonia ($n = 15$) also demonstrated higher levels of H_2O_2 in comparison to healthy neonatal calves ($n = 15$) [33]. Similarly, significant increases ($p < 0.05$) in H_2O_2 were detected in EBC collected from Holstein calves with mild ($n = 20$) and aggravated ($n = 20$) respiratory disease ($n = 20$) [32]. The increase in H_2O_2 causes bronchoconstriction and coughing when the mucous membranes of the trachea and bronchi become irritated as a result of their heightened sensitivity [32,48]. Here, the right shifts in the C5 and C7 WAMACS and WASPs from the aquaphotomics analysis are in alignment with increases in H_2O_2 found in infected individuals.

The eicosanoid leukotriene B_4 (LTB_4) is a pro-inflammatory mediator produced by neutrophils, eosinophils, macrophages, and epithelial cells that have been stimulated [28,49]. Leukotriene B_4 ($C_{20}H_{32}O_4$) is a known non-volatile component of bovine EBC and is considered a biomarker of inflammation during respiratory disease [28–30,49,50]. Increased levels of LTB_4 in EBC were detected in two out of four calves infected with BRSV in comparison with baseline values [49], similar to calves with *Pasteurella multocida* serovar *D*, which also led to an increase in LTB_4 after infection [49,50]. The observed changes in the aquaphotomics parameters, a left shift of C1 and C9, for inducing localized water structure would be consistent with increases in LTB_4, and other lipid-based compounds known to increase in response to infection. Urea (CH_4N_2O) and ammonia (NH_3) are other constituents of bovine EBC [26,51,52], and during homeostasis, the concentration of these compounds is related to food intake and ventilation [52]. However, the EBC from calves with induced bacterial pneumonia ($n = 20$) showed an increase in urea and ammonia, which was attributed to a change in the permeability of the lung-capillary barrier [52]. Other volatile organic compounds, such as acetaldehyde (C_2H_4O) and decanal ($C_{10}H_{20}O$), have also been reported in the EBC from steers ($n = 3$) diagnosed with BRDC by clinical signs (VCD), while heptane (C_7H_{16}), octanal ($C_8H_{16}O$), 2,3-butadione (C_6H_{10}), hexanoic acid ($C_6H_{12}O_2$), and phenol (C_6H_6O) were associated with healthy animals ($n = 3$) [14]. More volatile compounds, as well as some chemical elements, have been detected at significant levels in bovine EBC using an electronic nose, finding potential biomarkers for animals with respiratory disease [31] that can be associated with the aquaphotomics profile found in the present study. The compounds 1,2-dimethylcyclohexylamine ($C_8H_{17}N$), aliphatic acids C_2–C_5, ammonia (NH_3), cyclohexylamine ($C_6H_{13}N$), ethandal, methylamine (CH_3NH_2), methylglyoxal ($C_3H_4O_2$), and pyridine-carbaldehyde (C_6H_5NO) were detected in calves with respiratory disease in comparison to healthy calves that only exhaled alkyl-, cyclic amines [31]. Chemical elements evaluated in the EBC from 18 sick Holstein calves with bronchopneumonia showed a significant decrease ($p < 0.05$) in Se and Zn, and an increase in Al, Co, Mn, Mo, Na, P, Pb, and Sn in comparison to the EBC from 12 healthy subjects [16].

Biofluid spectroscopy is a novel clinical research technology that provides a straightforward approach to gathering diagnostic information from easily obtained samples [19,53–55]. The NIR spectra of biofluids provide a plethora of information and may be viewed as a biochemical fingerprint of the sample state [56–58]. This is the first report on the use of NIRS to successfully evaluate and discriminate BRSV infection from EBC for disease diagnosis in animals. The decrease in the values for the external validation in the PCA-LDA are likely related to each individual calf's immune response contributing to different biochemical changes for the classification of the samples. The chemical profile found in the aquaphotomics evaluation, and chemometric-based MVA analyses of NIR spectra are likely the result of the absorbance of the functional groups O-H, C-H, and N-H forming the molecules structuring the volatile and non-volatile compounds described for EBC from healthy and sick calves with respiratory disease.

5. Conclusions

NIR-aquaphotomics profiles were established for EBC collected from dairy calves challenged with BRSV based on the clinical signs following infection and the associated biochemical changes occurring with cell signaling and immune response activation. The aquaphotomics evaluation revealed changes in the organization of the aqueous phase of EBC acquired during the baseline and infected stages in the WAMACS C1, C5, C9, and C11 likely to be associated with both, the volatile and non-volatile compounds conforming this biofluid. Furthermore, the discrimination of the chemical profiles by PCA-LDA models distinguished EBC from pre-infected and infected calves with an accuracy, sensitivity, and specificity >93% in the calibration and validation. Here, the potential of NIRS in combination with aquaphotomics and chemometrics-based MVA to profile and discriminate this viral infection in unprocessed samples was demonstrated, providing evidence that the method could be used to develop an innovative, rapid, and non-invasive tool to support more effective diagnosis strategies for this problematic disease.

Author Contributions: M.S.-R. was involved in the research conceptualization, funding acquisition, and resources, supervised the sample collection, carried out the NIRS experiments, data collection, data curation, formal data analysis and validation of results, manuscript visualization, design, and writing. A.R.W. was involved in the research conceptualization, funding acquisition, supervision of animal experiments, and data collection. M.T. prepared the virus, collected samples, and organized clinical data. F.M. participated in research conceptualization, experimental design, funding acquisition, and resources. C.K.V. was in charge of the research conceptualization, experimental design, funding acquisition, supervision, resources, and manuscript editing. All authors contributed to the final review and editing of the manuscript and have given their approval for submission. All authors have read and agreed to the published version of the manuscript.

Funding: This project was supported by the Mississippi Agricultural and Forestry Experiment Station, the National Institute of Food and Agriculture, the U.S. Department of Agriculture, Hatch project under accession number W3173, and the U.S. Department of Agriculture, Agricultural Research Service, Biophotonics project 6066-31000-015-00D.

Institutional Review Board Statement: This study was conducted following MSU-IACUC guidelines and regulations (IACUC-19-037).

Informed Consent Statement: Not applicable.

Data Availability Statement: Data are available upon request from Carrie K. Vance (ckv7@msstate.edu).

Acknowledgments: Special thanks to Ellianna Blair, Amanda Free, Hannah Bostick, Matt Harjes, Victoria Jefferson, and Matt Scott (DVM) for their assistance with the sample collection.

Conflicts of Interest: The authors declare no conflict of interest. The funding sources played no role in the study design, data collection, data analysis and interpretation, manuscript writing, or manuscript submission for publication.

Sample Availability: EBC Samples are available upon request from Carrie K. Vance (ckv7@msstate.edu).

References

1. Larsen, L.E. Bovine Respiratory Syncytial Virus (BRSV): A review. *Acta Vet. Scand.* **2000**, *41*, 1–24. [CrossRef]
2. Valarcher, J.-F.; Taylor, G. Bovine respiratory syncytial virus infection. *Vet. Res.* **2007**, *38*, 153–180. [CrossRef] [PubMed]
3. Brodersen, B.W. Bovine respiratory syncytial virus. *Vet. Clin. N. Am. Food Anim. Pract.* **2010**, *26*, 323–333. [CrossRef] [PubMed]

4. Bell, R.L.; Turkington, H.L.; Cosby, S.L. The bacterial and viral agents of BRDC: Immune evasion and vaccine developments. *Vaccines* **2021**, *9*, 337. [CrossRef] [PubMed]
5. Snowder, G.D.; Van Vleck, L.D.; Cundiff, L.V.; Bennett, G.L. Bovine respiratory disease in feedlot cattle: Environmental, genetic, and economic factors. *J. Anim. Sci.* **2006**, *84*, 1999–2008. [CrossRef]
6. Kurćubić, V.; Đoković, R.; Ilić, Z.; Petrović, M. Etiopathogenesis and economic significance of bovine respiratory disease complex (BRDC). *Acta Agric. Serbica* **2018**, *23*, 85–100. [CrossRef]
7. Peel, D.S. The Effect of Market Forces on Bovine Respiratory Disease. *Vet. Clin. N. Am. Food Anim. Pract.* **2020**, *36*, 497–508. [CrossRef]
8. Fulton, R.W.; Confer, A.W. Laboratory test descriptions for bovine respiratory disease diagnosis and their strengths and weaknesses: Gold standards for diagnosis, do they exist? *Can. Vet. J.* **2012**, *53*, 754–761. [PubMed]
9. White, B.J.; Goehl, D.R.; Amrine, D.E.; Booker, C.; Wildman, B.; Perrett, T. Bayesian evaluation of clinical diagnostic test characteristics of visual observations and remote monitoring to diagnose bovine respiratory disease in beef calves. *Prev. Vet. Med.* **2016**, *126*, 74–80. [CrossRef]
10. Timsit, E.; Dendukuri, N.; Schiller, I.; Buczinski, S. Diagnostic accuracy of clinical illness for bovine respiratory disease (BRD) diagnosis in beef cattle placed in feedlots: A systematic literature review and hierarchical Bayesian latent-class meta-analysis. *Prev. Vet. Med.* **2016**, *135*, 67–73. [CrossRef] [PubMed]
11. Nefedchenko, A.V.; Glotov, A.G.; Koteneva, S.V.; Glotova, T.I. Developing and Testing a Real-Time Polymerase Chain Reaction to Identify and Quantify Bovine Respiratory Syncytial Viruses. *Mol. Genet. Microbiol. Virol.* **2020**, *35*, 168–173. [CrossRef]
12. Blakebrough-Hall, C.; Dona, A.; D'occhio, M.J.; McMeniman, J.; González, L.A. Diagnosis of Bovine Respiratory Disease in feedlot cattle using blood 1H NMR metabolomics. *Sci. Rep.* **2020**, *10*, 115. [CrossRef] [PubMed]
13. Maurer, D.L.; Koziel, J.A.; Engelken, T.J.; Cooper, V.L.; Funk, J.L. Detection of volatile compounds emitted from nasal secretions and serum: Towards non-invasive identification of diseased cattle biomarkers. *Separations* **2018**, *5*, 18. [CrossRef]
14. Spinhirne, J.P.; Koziel, J.A.; Chirase, N.K. Sampling and analysis of volatile organic compounds in bovine breath by solid-phase microextraction and gas chromatography-mass spectrometry. *J. Chromatogr. A* **2004**, *1025*, 63–69. [CrossRef]
15. Kuchmenko, T.; Shuba, A.; Umarkhanov, R.; Chernitskiy, A. Portable Electronic Nose for Analyzing the Smell of Nasal Secretions in Calves: Toward Noninvasive Diagnosis of Infectious Bronchopneumonia. *Vet. Sci.* **2021**, *8*, 74. [CrossRef] [PubMed]
16. Safonov, V.A.; Kuchmenko, T.A.; Chernitskiy, A. Chemical elements in exhaled breath condensate of calves with infectious bronchopneumonia. In Proceedings of the 45th FEBS Congress, Molecules of Life: Toward New Horizons, Ljubljana, Slovenia, 3–8 July 2021.
17. Santos-Rivera, M.; Fitzkee, N.C.; Hill, R.A.; Baird, R.E.; Blair, E.; Thoresen, M.; Woolums, A.R.; Meyer, F.; Vance, C. Nuclear Magnetic Resonance-based Metabolomics of Blood Plasma from Dairy Calves Infected with the Main Causal Agents of Bovine Respiratory Disease (BRD). *Sci. Rep.* **2022**, 1–31. [CrossRef]
18. Williams, P.; Antoniszyn, J.; Manley, M. *Near Infrared Technology. Getting the Best out of Light;* 1st ed.; AFRICAN SUN Media: Stellenbosch, South Africa, 2019; ISBN 978-1-928480-30-3.
19. Beć, K.B.; Grabska, J.; Huck, C.W. Near-infrared spectroscopy in bio-applications. *Molecules* **2020**, *25*, 2948. [CrossRef]
20. Tsenkova, R. Introduction aquaphotomics: Dynamic spectroscopy of aqueous and biological systems describes peculiarities of water. *J. Near Infrared Spectrosc.* **2009**, *17*, 303–314. [CrossRef]
21. Muncan, J.; Tsenkova, R. Aquaphotomics-From Innovative Knowledge to Integrative Platform in Science and Technology. *Molecules* **2019**, *24*, 2742. [CrossRef]
22. Tsenkova, R. AquaPhotomics: Water Absorbance Pattern as a Biological Marker. *NIR News* **2006**, *17*, 13–23. [CrossRef]
23. Tsenkova, R.; Munćan, J.; Pollner, B.; Kovacs, Z. Essentials of Aquaphotomics and Its Chemometrics Approaches. *Front. Chem.* **2018**, *6*, 363. [CrossRef]
24. Tsenkova, R. Aquaphotomics: Acquiring Spectra of Various Biological Fluids of the Same Organism Reveals the Importance of Water Matrix Absorbance Coordinates and the Aquaphotome for Understanding Biological Phenomena. *NIR News* **2008**, *19*, 13–15. [CrossRef]
25. Tsenkova, R. AquaPhotomics: Water Absorbance Pattern as a Biological Marker for Disease Diagnosis and Disease Understanding. *NIR News* **2007**, *18*, 14–16. [CrossRef]
26. Kazani, S.; Israel, E. Utility of exhaled breath condensates across respiratory diseases. *Am. J. Respir. Crit. Care Med.* **2012**, *185*, 791–792. [CrossRef] [PubMed]
27. Houspie, L.; De Coster, S.; Keyaerts, E.; Narongsack, P.; De Roy, R.; Talboom, I.; Sisk, M.; Maes, P.; Verbeeck, J.; Van Ranst, M. Exhaled breath condensate sampling is not a new method for detection of respiratory viruses. *Virol. J.* **2011**, *8*, 98. [CrossRef] [PubMed]
28. Zollinger, E.; Clauss, M.; Steinmetz, H.W.; Hatt, J.M. Collection of exhaled breath and exhaled breath condensate in veterinary medicine. A review. *Vet. Q.* **2006**, *28*, 105–117. [CrossRef]
29. Reinhold, P.; Knobloch, H. Exhaled breath condensate: Lessons learned from veterinary medicine. *J. Breath Res.* **2010**, *4*. [CrossRef] [PubMed]
30. Horváth, I.; Hunt, J.; Barnes, P.J.; Alving, K.; Antczak, A.; Baraldi, E.; Becher, G.; van Beurden, W.J.C.; Corradi, M.; Dekhuijzen, R.; et al. Exhaled breath condensate: Methodological recommendations and unresolved questions. *Eur. Respir. J.* **2005**, *26*, 523–548. [CrossRef]

31. Kuchmenko, T.A.; Umarkhanov, R.U.; Shuba, A.A.; Dorovskaya, E.S.; Chernitskiy, A.E. Analysis of the volatile compounds' condensate exhaled air "electronic nose" based on piezoelectric sensor to assess the status of calves. *IOP Conf. Ser. Earth Environ. Sci.* **2021**, *640*, 072028. [CrossRef]
32. Chernitskiy, A.E.; Safonov, V.A. Early detection of bovine respiratory disease in calves by induced cough. *IOP Conf. Ser. Earth Environ. Sci.* **2021**, *677*, 042047. [CrossRef]
33. Chernitskiy, A.; Safonov, V.A. Exhaled hydrogen peroxide as a potential marker of lower airway inflammation in neonatal calves. In Proceedings of the 45th FEBS Congress, Molecules of Life: Toward New Horizons, Ljubljana, Slovenia, 3–8 July 2021; pp. 102–103.
34. Santos-Rivera, M.; Woolums, A.; Thoresen, M.; Blair, E.; Jefferson, V.; Meyer, F.; Vance, C.K. Profiling Mannheimia haemolytica infection in dairy calves using near infrared spectroscopy (NIRS) and multivariate analysis (MVA). *Sci. Rep.* **2021**, *11*, 1392. [CrossRef]
35. Garrido-Varo, A.; Garcia-Olmo, J.; Fearn, T. A note on Mahalanobis and related distance measures in WinISI and The Unscrambler. *J. Near Infrared Spectrosc.* **2019**, *27*, 253–258. [CrossRef]
36. Fearn, T. Mahalanobis and Euclidean Distances. *NIR News* **2010**, *21*, 12–14. [CrossRef]
37. Messick, N.J.; Kalivas, J.H.; Lang, P.M. Selecting factors for partial least squares. *Microchem. J.* **1997**, *55*, 200–207. [CrossRef]
38. Lalkhen, A.G.; McCluskey, A. Clinical tests: Sensitivity and specificity. *Contin. Educ. Anaesth. Crit. Care Pain* **2008**, *8*, 221–223. [CrossRef]
39. Rinnan, Å.; van den Berg, F.; Engelsen, S.B. Review of the most common pre-processing techniques for near-infrared spectra. *TrAC-Trends Anal. Chem.* **2009**, *28*, 1201–1222. [CrossRef]
40. Robertson, W.H.; Diken, E.G.; Price, E.A.; Shin, J.W.; Johnson, M.A. Spectroscopic determination of the OH^- solvation shell in the $OH^-\cdot(H_2O)_n$ clusters. *Science* **2003**, *299*, 1367–1372. [CrossRef]
41. Bázár, G.; Kovacs, Z.; Tanaka, M.; Furukawa, A.; Nagai, A.; Osawa, M.; Itakura, Y.; Sugiyama, H.; Tsenkova, R. Water revealed as molecular mirror when measuring low concentrations of sugar with near infrared light. *Anal. Chim. Acta* **2015**, *896*, 52–62. [CrossRef]
42. Beganović, A.; Beć, K.B.; Grabska, J.; Stanzl, M.T.; Brunner, M.E.; Huck, C.W. Vibrational coupling to hydration shell—Mechanism to performance enhancement of qualitative analysis in NIR spectroscopy of carbohydrates in aqueous environment. *Spectrochim. Acta-Part A Mol. Biomol. Spectrosc.* **2020**, *237*, 118359. [CrossRef]
43. Makarevich, A.E.; Ivashkevich, D.L. Dynamics of Intermediate Substrates of Carbohydrates Metabolism in Exhaled Breath Condensate During Copd Development. *Chest* **2006**, *130*, 170S. [CrossRef]
44. Makarevich, A.E. Lipid and carbohydrate metabolites changes in exhaled breath condensate and blood in acute exacerbation of chronic bronchitis and chronic obstructive. *Практикуючий Лікар* **2018**, *7*, 30–36.
45. Conner, G.E.; Salathe, M.; Forteza, R. Lactoperoxidase and hydrogen peroxide metabolism in the airway. *Am. J. Respir. Crit. Care Med.* **2002**, *166*, S57–S61. [CrossRef]
46. Knobloch, H.; Becher, G.; Decker, M.; Reinhold, P. Evaluation of H_2O_2 and pH in exhaled breath condensate samples: Methodical and physiological aspects. *Biomarkers* **2008**, *13*, 319–341. [CrossRef] [PubMed]
47. Horváth, I.; MacNee, W.; Kelly, F.J.; Dekhuijzen, P.N.R.; Phillips, M.; Döring, G.; Choi, A.M.K.; Yamaya, M.; Bach, F.H.; Willis, D.; et al. "Haemoxygenase-1 induction and exhaled markers of oxidative stress in lung diseases", summary of the ERS Research Seminar in Budapest, Hungary, September, 1999. *Eur. Respir. J.* **2001**, *18*, 420–430. [CrossRef] [PubMed]
48. Skulachev, V.P. The H_2O_2 sensors of lungs and blood vessels and their role in the antioxidant defense of the body. *Biokhimiya* **2001**, *66*, 1425–1429.
49. Reinhold, P.; Becher, G.; Rothe, M. Evaluation of the measurement of leukotriene B4 concentrations in exhaled condensate as a noninvasive method for assessing mediators of inflammation in the lungs of calves. *Am. J. Vet. Res.* **2000**, *61*, 742–749. [CrossRef]
50. Reinhold, P.; Langenberg, A.; Becher, G.; Rothe, M. Exhaled condensate—A medium obtained by a non-invasive method for the detection of inflammation mediators of the lung. *Berl. Munch. Tierarztl. Wochenschr.* **1999**, *112*, 254–259.
51. Reinhold, P.; Langenberg, A.; Foedisch, G.; Jena, M.R. The influence of variables of ventilation on the concentration of urea and ammonia in the exhaled breath condensate Member's Comments. *Eur Respir J.* **2004**, *24*, 2486.
52. Reinhold, P.; Langenberg, A.; Seifert, J.; Rothe, M.; Jena, G.B. Ammonia and urea in the exhaled breath condensate (EBC) and in corresponding blood samples Member's Comments. *Eur Respir J.* **2002**, *20*, 3034.
53. Theakstone, A.G.; Rinaldi, C.; Butler, H.J.; Cameron, J.M.; Confield, L.R.; Rutherford, S.H.; Sala, A.; Sangamnerkar, S.; Baker, M.J. Fourier-transform infrared spectroscopy of biofluids: A practical approach. *Transl. Biophotonics* **2021**, *3*, e2020000255. [CrossRef]
54. Rutherford, S.H.; Nordon, A.; Hunt, N.T.; Baker, M.J. Biofluid Analysis and Classification using IR and 2D-IR Spectroscopy. *Chemom. Intell. Lab. Syst.* **2021**, *217*, 104408. [CrossRef]
55. Shaw, R.A.; Mantsch, H.H. Infrared Spectroscopy of Biological Fluids in Clinical and Diagnostic Analysis. In *Encyclopedia of Analytical Chemistry*; John and Wiley and Sons: Hoboken, NJ, USA, 2008. [CrossRef]
56. Ollesch, J.; Drees, S.L.; Heise, H.M.; Behrens, T.; Brüning, T.; Gerwert, K. FTIR spectroscopy of biofluids revisited: An automated approach to spectral biomarker identification. *Analyst* **2013**, *138*, 4092–4102. [CrossRef] [PubMed]

57. Fabian, H.; Lasch, P.; Naumann, D. Analysis of biofluids in aqueous environment based on mid-infrared spectroscopy. *J. Biomed. Opt.* **2005**, *10*, 031103. [CrossRef] [PubMed]
58. Baker, M.J.; Hussain, S.R.; Lovergne, L.; Untereiner, V.; Hughes, C.; Lukaszewski, R.A.; Thiéfin, G.; Sockalingum, G.D. Developing and understanding biofluid vibrational spectroscopy: A critical review. *Chem. Soc. Rev.* **2016**, *45*, 1803–1818. [CrossRef]

molecules

Article

Changes in Water Properties in Human Tissue after Double Filtration Plasmapheresis—A Case Study

Felix Scholkmann [1,*] and Roumiana Tsenkova [2]

[1] Biomedical Optics Research Laboratory, Department of Neonatology, University Hospital Zurich, University of Zurich, 8091 Zurich, Switzerland

[2] Aquaphotomics Research Department, Graduate School of Agricultural Science, Kobe University, Kobe 657-8501, Japan; rtsen@kobe-u.ac.jp

* Correspondence: felix.scholkmann@usz.ch; Tel.: +41-44-255-93-26

Abstract: Double-filtration plasmapheresis (DFPP) is a blood cleaning technique that enables the removal of unwanted substances from the blood. In our case study, we performed near-infrared (NIR) spectroscopy measurements on the human hand tissue before and after a specific DFPP treatment (INUSpheresis with a TKM58 filter), along with NIR measurements of the substances extracted via DFPP (eluate). The spectral data were analyzed using the aquaphotomics approach. The analysis showed that the water properties in the tissue change after DFPP treatment, i.e., an increase in small water clusters, free water molecules and a decrease in hydroxylated water as well as superoxide in hydration shells was noted. The opposite effect was observed in the eluates of both DFPP treatments. Our study is the first that documents changes in water spectral properties after DFPP treatments in human tissue. The changes in tissue water demonstrated by our case study suggest that the positive physiological effects of DFPP in general, and of INUSpheresis with the TKM58 filter in particular, may be associated with improvements in water quality in blood and tissues.

Keywords: double-filtration plasmapheresis; INUSpheresis; near-infrared spectroscopy; aquaphotomics; water

Citation: Scholkmann, F.; Tsenkova, R. Changes in Water Properties in Human Tissue after Double Filtration Plasmapheresis—A Case Study. *Molecules* **2022**, *27*, 3947. https://doi.org/10.3390/molecules27123947

Academic Editor: Stefano Materazzi

Received: 18 May 2022
Accepted: 10 June 2022
Published: 20 June 2022

1. Introduction

Introduced in the early 1980s by Agishi et al. [1], double-filtration plasmapheresis (DFPP) allows the removal particles in blood plasma having sizes between the pore size of the first (plasma separator) and second filter membrane (plasma fractionator). This is realized by first separating the blood into plasma and blood cells (with the plasma separator) and then fractioning the separated plasma into large and small molecular weight components. Although the blood cells and plasma with small molecular weight components are transfused back to the patient, the large molecular weight components (eluate) are filtered out. DFPP is an effective, efficient and patient-friendly blood purification procedure.

The DFPP technique allows pathophysiological relevant molecules (e.g., circulating autoantigens, autoantibodies, circulating immune complexes, damaged proteins) and toxins (e.g., environmental toxins and toxins from microorganisms) to be removed from the blood of a subject. This blood cleaning procedure has been successfully used therapeutically in many diseases [2–4], including myasthenia gravis [5–12], chronic inflammatory demyelinating polyneuropathy [12], anti-glomerular basement membrane disease [13], hypoglycemia and hyperglycemia induced by insulin antibodies [14], pancreatitis induced by hypertriglyceridemia [15–17], Guillain–Barré syndrome [12,18–21], Crow–Fukase syndrome [12], rheumatoid arthritis [22–24], chronic hepatitis C [25,26], pemphigus [27,28], bullous pemphigoid [29,30], atopic dermatitis [31], dermatomyositis [12], polymyositis [12], membranous nephropathy [32], acute thallotoxicosis [33], antibody-associated vasculitis [34–36], antisynthetase syndrome [37], diffuse proliferative lupus nephritis [38], refractory chronic urticaria [39], systemic lupus erythematosus associated with autoimmune thyroid disease [40], rhesus D-incompatible pregnancy [41], anti-PP1Pk isoantibodies-incompatible pregnancy [42], adult onset Still's disease [43], multiple sclerosis [12,44–46], Eaton–Lambert syndrome [12], hemorrhagic fever [47], acquired thrombotic thrombocytopenic purpura [48], neuromyelitis optica [49,50], Graves' disease [51], antiphospholipid syndrome [52], age-related macular degeneration [53], diffuse cutaneous systemic sclerosis [54], co-infection infection with Hepatitis C and human immunodeficiency virus [55], acute atherothrombotic brain infarction [56], cryoglobulinemia [57], inflammatory polyneuropathy [58], chronic inflammatory demyelinating polyradiculoneuropathy [59], prevention of antibody-dependent xenograft rejection [60,61] and even cancer [62].

Although DFPP has been widely and routinely used in clinical practice in Asia, especially in Japan, for decades, its use is not yet widespread in the West. For a few years now, however, DFPP has been attracting increasing attention in Europe, largely due to the development of a specific type of DFPP, called INUSpheresis, by developers and scientists from Germany. For example, these researchers have recently shown that this type of DFPP has great therapeutic potential for the treatment of metabolic and non-metabolic peripheral neuropathy [63], borreliosis [64], Alzheimer's disease [65] and chronic post-COVID-19 syndrome ("long-COVID") [66].

In the case of the treatment of neuropathy patients [63], a significant reduction in total cholesterol, triglycerides, LDL-cholesterol, serum C-reactive protein (sCRP), tumor necrosis factor-α (TNF-α), eosinophilic cationic protein (ECP), fibrinogen and the chemokine RANTES (Regulated And Normal T cell Expressed and Secreted) could be achieved. Furthermore, a significant amount of environmental toxins (including heavy metals and pesticides) in the blood of neuropathy patients could be removed by applying this type of DFPP. Such an improvement in the lipid profile and in inflammatory markers was also evident in borreliosis patients treated with this type of DFPP [64], including a decrease in the inflammatory lipid lipoprotein-associated phospholipase A2 (Lp-PLA2). A clinical improvement in the patients was also evident. In case of Alzheimer's disease patients treated with this type of DFPP [65], a significant reduction in the concentration of RANTES, fibrinogen, sCRP, ECP, TNF-α, and α2-macroglobulin (a marker of neuronal injury and generally increased in Alzheimer's disease [67,68]) was evident. A significant amount of toxins (e.g., aluminum and organophosphorus pesticides) could be also removed from the blood of these patient with this procedure. In another recently published report, this specific type of DFPP was described to be able to remove neurotransmitter receptor antibodies against ß-adrenergic and muscarinic receptors (linked to myalgic encephalomyelitis/chronic fatigue syndrome, ME/CFS) present in the blood of patients with post-COVID-19 syndrome [66]. The treatment alleviated symptoms of CFS in these patients.

The blood composition of people treated with DPFF using the INUSpheresis technology with a specific filter (TKM58) has recently been shown to change significantly [69]. A decrease was found in the concentration of albumin, γ-globulins, triglycerides, total cholesterol, HDL-cholesterol, LDL-cholesterol, liporotein(a), ferritin, fibrinogen, IgG, IgM, IgA, total protein, INR, quick, platelets and an increase in erythrocytes, haematocrit and leukocytes. Furthermore, proteomics showed significant changes in the concentration of apolipoprotein-related proteins, parameters of the coagulation system, immunoglobulins, parameters of the complement system and other inflammation-related proteins.

Human blood consists about 55% of plasma which is composed of 91% of water, 7% of proteins (i.e., 57% albumin, 38% globulins, 4% fibrinogen and 1% prothrombin) and 2% of other solutes [70]. The composition of the human body is also characterized by a high water content. An adult human consists of about 40 L (men) and 30 L (women), respectively, of water [71,72]. This total body water can be subdivided into intracellular water (ICW) and extracellular water (ECW). Men have about 25 L of ICW and 15 L of ECW, women have 17 L of ICW and 11 L of ECW, and the ECW-to-ICW ratio (which can be determined by bioelectrical impendence analysis) increases with age [72].

Water in the tissue and blood exists in the form of free and bound water. Around dissolved ions or dipoles, the dipoles of the water molecules are oriented and form a hydration shell. The hydration shell of ions contains strongly bound water in the first hydration layer, and less bound water in the further layers. In case of proteins, water plays an essential role for folding, stability, and binding with other molecules [73]. Single water monomers interact with each other, forming water clusters of the form $(H_2O)_n$ which can be neutral, protonated, deprotonated or auto-ionized [74,75]. Water in the blood (plasma) and tissue is present in a variety of structures and states, which makes water so special in biological systems.

Since the physicochemical properties of water can change when passing through a filter or when the concentration of substances in the water change, we hypothesized that such changes in the water of the blood plasma would also have to occur with blood washing using DFPP. In order to verify this experimentally, we carried out corresponding measurements using near-infrared (NIR) spectroscopy before and after a specific DFPP treatment (INUSpheresis with the TKM58 filter) in one subject as a case study. It has not previously been investigated how DFPP affects the water in the tissue and what water properties the eluate has.

2. Material and Methods

2.1. Double-Filtration Plasmapheresis Treatments and Spectroscopic Measurements

DFPP INUSpheresis (with TKM58 filter) treatments were performed on a 39-year-old man (first author, FS) at a private clinic in Switzerland in February 2022 on two different days, one day apart. Each treatment lasted about 2.5 h. No official ethical approval was necessary to conduct the measurements and report the results since it is a case report (Kantonale Ethikkommission, Kanton Zürich) and measurements were conducted by and on the first author (FS). The DFPP treatment was performed as part of a routine medical treatment.

A portable and ultra-compact NIR spectrometer (MicroNIR 1700, Viavi, Milpitas, CA, USA) was used to measure the diffuse reflectance spectra of the hand palm of the left hand and of the eluate. Measurements were performed in the spectral range 950–1650 nm with a nominal spectral resolution of 6.25 nm, an integration time of 11.7 ms and an average of 1000 scans for each spectrum to ensure an optimal signal-to-noise ratio. 15 consecutive measurements were performed for each measurement. Measurements were conducted in the morning one day before the first DFPP treatment (day 1), in the morning on the day of the first DFPP treatment (day 2), 1 h after the first DFPP treatment (day 2), in the morning on the day of the second DFPP treatment (day 4), 1 h after the second treatment (day 4) and in the morning one day after the second DFPP treatment (day 5). For each measurement it was ensured that the hand had subjectively the same temperature and the NIR spectrometer had also always the same temperature (T = 31.5 °C). Furthermore, the eluate of the first and second DFPP treatment was also measured by placing the NIR spectrometer on the plastic bag with the eluate inside and also measuring the spectrum of the plastic bag as a reference. This measurement was performed at an instrument temperature of T = 35.4, 35.5 and 35.6 °C.

2.2. Data Analysis

First, the spectra of the hand tissue and eluate measurements were pre-processed applying the SNV (standard normal variate) algorithm for baseline correction. SNV normalization was performed on both datasets separately.

For the analysis of the hand tissue measurements, the difference spectra ($\mathbf{X}_{\mathrm{Diff}}$) were calculated for the first and second DFPP treatment according to

$$\mathbf{X}_{\text{Diff}}^{\text{1st DFPP}}(\text{A}_1) = \mathbf{X}(\text{after 1}^{\text{st}}\text{ DFPP (day 2)}) - \mathbf{X}(\text{before 1}^{\text{st}}\text{ DFPP (day 2)}) \quad (1)$$

$$\mathbf{X}_{\text{Diff}}^{\text{1st DFPP}}(\text{A}_2) = \mathbf{X}(\text{after 1}^{\text{st}}\text{ DFPP (day 2)}) - \mathbf{X}(\text{before 1}^{\text{st}}\text{ DFPP (day 1)}) \quad (2)$$

$$\mathbf{X}_{\text{Diff}}^{\text{2nd DFPP}}(\text{B}_1) = \mathbf{X}\left(\text{after 2}^{\text{nd}}\text{ DFPP (day 4)}\right) - \mathbf{X}\left(\text{before 2}^{\text{nd}}\text{ DFPP (day 4)}\right) \quad (3)$$

$$\mathbf{X}_{\text{Diff}}^{\text{2nd DFPP}}(\text{B}_2) = \mathbf{X}\left(\text{after 2}^{\text{nd}}\text{ DFPP (day 5)}\right) - \mathbf{X}\left(\text{before 2}^{\text{nd}}\text{ DFPP (day 4)}\right) \quad (4)$$

while the indices A_1 and A_2 (and B_1 and B_2, respectively) refer to the calculation of the difference spectra for the 1st DFPP (2nd DFPP, respectively) based on the data measured on the same day (A_1, B_1) and 24 h apart (A_2, B_2). With this approach, the spectroscopic measurement after the DFPP treatments were compared to two baselines (i.e., at the same day and before/after 24 h).

For the analysis of the eluate measurements, the spectrum of the empty plastic bag containing the eluate was removed from the spectrum of the eluate measured through the plastic bag. With this, the spectra of the eluate itself was obtained.

To analyze the water spectral changes, the aquaphotomics approach was used [76–81]. 12 spectral regions of particular interest in the region of the 1st overtone of water (C*i*, *i* = 1–12; Water Matrix Absorbance Coordinates, WAMACS) were analyzed in particular by calculating the absorbance of the difference spectra in these 12 spectral regions and visualizing the results on aquagrams to determine the specific water absorbance spectral pattern [76,77]. A listing of the WAMACS with the corresponding water properties can be found in Table 1 in Muncan et al. [79].

Data processing and visualizations were carried out in Matlab (R2017a, MathWorks, Inc., Natick, MA, USA) and R (2022.02.0).

3. Results

The spectroscopic analysis of the hand tissue before and after the DFPP treatments revealed clear differences in the spectral features in the first overtone spectral region of water, i.e., in the region of the 12 WAMACS (Figure 1). The corresponding aquagram (Figure 3a) shows the strongest increase in C6 (1421–1430 nm), corresponding to the water hydration band [79], the H–O–H bending mode, as well as the O-H stretch vibration mode, linked to the hydrogen bound strength of the water molecules [82]. The strongest decrease was found to be in C4 (1380–1388 nm), corresponding to water hydration shells ($OH\text{-}(H_2O)_{,1,4}$), hydrated superoxide water clusters ($O_2\text{-}(H_2O_4)$) and the H_2O symmetrical stretch vibration ($2\nu_1$) [79]. In general, there was a decrease in C2 (1360–1366 nm) to C4 (1380–1388 nm) (linked to weaker H-bounded water) and an increase in C5 (1392–1412 nm) to C11 (1492–1494 nm) (linked to free water molecules and small water clusters). Interestingly, this specific change in spectral properties was evident after the first as well as the second DFPP treatment, whereas the first treatment caused the most pronounced effect. After the first DFPP treatment, the number of small and large water clusters increased, whereas after the second DFPP treatment, only the number of small water clusters increased while the larger ones decreased slightly.

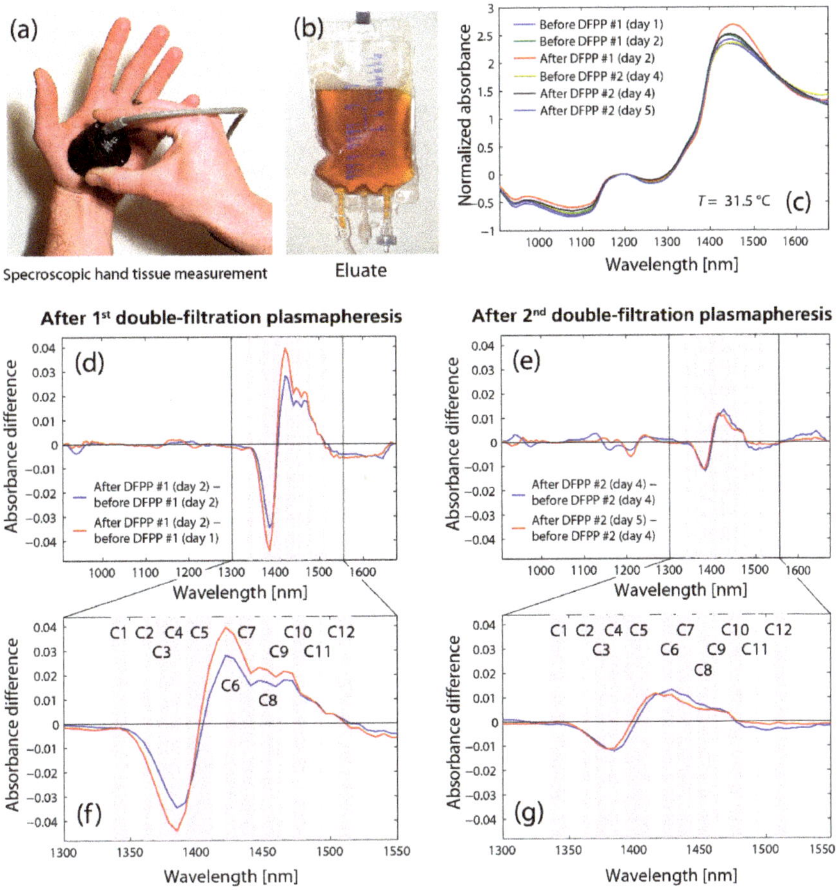

Figure 1. (**a**) Measurement performed on the palm of the left hand. (**b**) Bag with eluate extracted during the first DFPP treatment. The yellowish-brown color is striking, which is due to a high concentration of filtered substances. Normal blood plasma is clearer and more yellowish. (**c**) Raw spectra. (**d**) and (**e**) Difference spectra of the tissue measurements after the first ($\mathbf{X}_{\mathrm{Diff}}^{\mathrm{1st\ DFPP}}(\mathrm{A}_1)$, $\mathbf{X}_{\mathrm{Diff}}^{\mathrm{1st\ DFPP}}(\mathrm{A}_2)$) and second ($\mathbf{X}_{\mathrm{Diff}}^{\mathrm{1st\ DFPP}}(\mathrm{B}_1)$, $\mathbf{X}_{\mathrm{Diff}}^{\mathrm{1st\ DFPP}}(\mathrm{B}_2)$) DFPP treatment. (**f**,**g**) show zoomed-in regions with the 12 WAMACS. A listing of the WAMACS with the corresponding water properties can be found in Table 1 in Muncan et al. [79].

The spectroscopic analysis of the eluate obtained after the first and second DFPP treatment also revealed clear differences in the spectral features in the first overtone spectral region of water (Figure 2). The corresponding aquagram (Figure 3b) shows the strongest increase in absorbance at C2 (1360–1366 nm), corresponding to water salvation shells ($OH\text{-}(H_2O)_{1,2,4}$) and C3 (1370–1379 nm), corresponding to symmetrical and asymmetrical stretching vibration of water molecules ($\nu_1 + \nu_3$) [79]. The strongest decrease in absorbance was at C6 (1421–1430) associated with the water hydration band, as well as the H-O-H bending mode and O-H stretch vibration mode. Fascinatingly, the specific water absorbance spectral pattern of the eluate is thus complementary to that measured in the tissue.

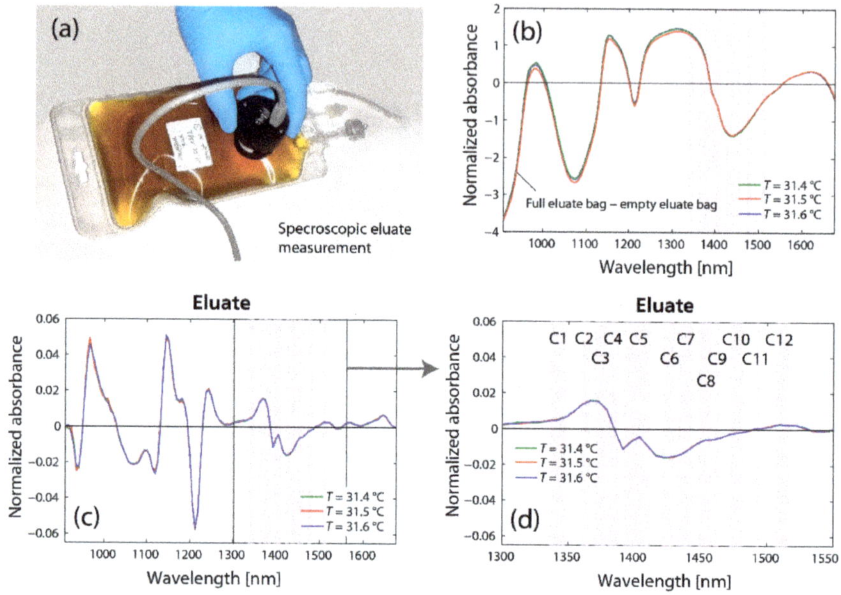

Figure 2. (**a**) Measurement of the eluate. (**b**) Raw spectra. (**c**) Difference spectra. (**d**) Zoomed-in part of (**c**) highlighting the region with the 12 WAMACS.

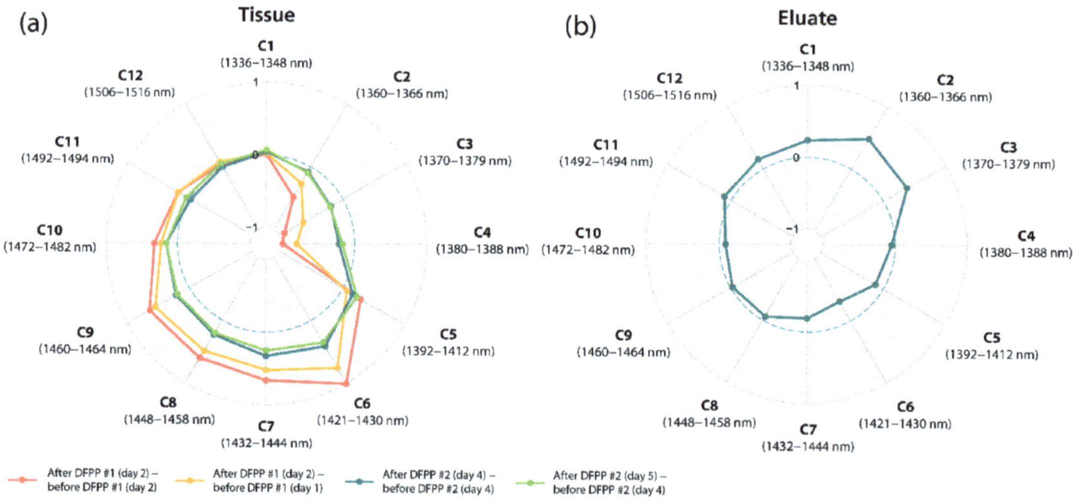

Figure 3. Aquagrams of the (**a**) tissue and (**b**) eluate spectra. The blue dashed circles refer to the zero baseline indicating no changes in the difference spectra. Note the complementary specific water absorbance spectral pattern of both aquagrams.

To complement the aquaphotomics-based NIR spectral analysis, the eluate obtained from both DFPP treatment was also analyzed for toxic ingredients (IGL Labor GmbH, Wittbek, Germany). The analysis revealed the presence of several toxins (Figure 4). The ten highest detected concentrations were from aflatoxin B1 (596.2 nmol/L), chromium-VI (591.0 nmol/L), lead (571.6 nmol/L), cadmium (558.1 nmol/L), arsenic (556.1 nmol/L), lindane (516.3 nmol/L), cobalt (509.5 nmol/L), polycyclic-aromatic-hydrocarbons (493.1 nmol/L), disulfoton (489.2 nmol/L) and aluminum (429.3 nmol/L). The concentration of toxins was generally significantly lower in the eluate from the second DFPP treatment compared to the first one. The concentration of some toxins increased after the second DFPP treatment (DDT, mercury, vinyl chloride), indicating that the first DFPP treatment most probably caused a diffusion gradient from the tissue to the blood, releasing these toxins from the tissue into the blood. The detoxification with DFPP is a multi-stage process whereby different compartments in the human organism are cleaned.

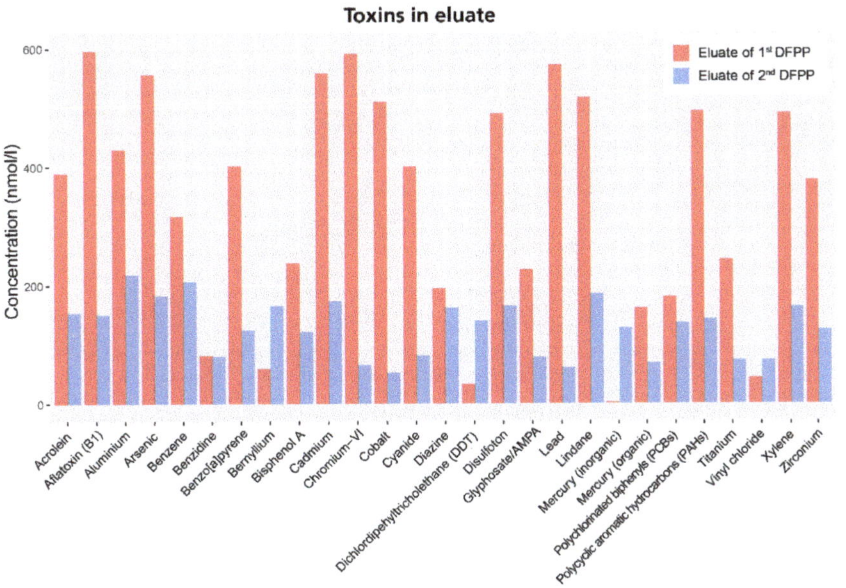

Figure 4. Concentration of toxins detected in the eluate of the first and second DFPP treatment. The first eluate showed a high amount of toxins whereas the amount was significantly reduced in the second eluate, highlighting the ability of DFPP to remove toxins from the blood/tissue.

4. Discussion and Conclusions

In this study, we have shown that the water properties in the tissue change after DFPP treatment (INUSpheresis with TKM58 filter). DFPP caused an increase in free water molecules, small water clusters and a decrease in hydroxylated water clusters, superoxides of water solvation shells and weaker H-bonded water. The opposite effect was observed in the eluates of both DFPP treatments.

In our opinion, these observations can be caused by two processes involved. First, the treatment filters out many molecules from the blood plasma to which water is bound in the form of hydration shells. This is the fraction of rather weakly H-bound water (which was reduced in the tissue after DFPP and was enriched in the eluates). Second, the process of filtration will cause water passing through the fine filter pores in a hydrophilic material to be structurally altered [83,84]. The formation of water clusters with stronger H-bonds is favored.

Our study is the first to date to investigate changes in tissue water after a DFPP treatment and also the first to perform a spectroscopic investigation of the eluates obtained by DFPP. In particular, it is also the first analysis of this kind concerning this specific type of DFPP, i.e., INUSpheresis with the TKM58 filter. We know of only one comparable study that investigated the dialysate after dialysis using NIR spectroscopy and the aquaphotomics approach [85]. This study showed that the absorption of 1398 nm and 1410 nm increased during dialysis. This finding is in line with our observation of an increase in this wavelength range after DFPP.

The changes in tissue water demonstrated by our case study suggest that the positive physiological effects of DFPP in general and of INUSpheresis with the TKM58 filter in particular, may be associated with improvements in water quality in blood and tissues related to the respective water molecular structures. Such an improvement in water quality could, for example, be associated later on with improved blood circulation and optimized metabolic processes. Our small study should serve as a stimulus to explore these possibilities through further, larger and more comprehensive studies.

It should be noted that our study is based on the measurements of a single person and two eluates. Generalizations of our results are only possible to a limited extent. As noted, our case study serves to stimulate further research on the interesting results and to show how an aquaphotomics-based analysis of NIRS data can be performed to investigate the effects of a DFPP.

Author Contributions: Conceptualization, F.S; methodology, F.S. and R.T.; formal analysis, F.S.; writing—original draft preparation, F.S.; writing—review and editing, R.T. and F.S.; visualization, F.S. All authors have read and agreed to the published version of the manuscript.

Funding: This research received no external funding.

Institutional Review Board Statement: Ethical review and approval were waived for this study since it is a case report and measurements were conducted by and on the first author (FS). The DFPP treatment was performed as part of a routine medical treatment.

Informed Consent Statement: Not applicable.

Data Availability Statement: The data will be made available by the corresponding author, upon reasonable request.

Acknowledgments: The authors are grateful to "Yunosato" Ltd., Japan for providing the NIRS spectrometer, to DTK Electronics LTD OOD, Sofia, Bulgaria for assisting the experiment and to the Tsuki no Shizuku Foundation. In addition, we thank Frank Oberle, Karin Bak and Jerry Pollack for discussions and for feedback on an earlier version of the manuscript.

Conflicts of Interest: The authors declare no conflict of interest.

Sample Availability: Samples of the compounds are not available from the authors.

References

1. Agishi, T.; Kaneko, I.; Hasuo, Y.; Hayasaka, Y.; Sanaka, T.; Ota, K.; Amemiya, H.; Sugino, N.; Abe, M.; Ono, T.; et al. Double Filtration Plasmapheresis. *ASAIO J.* **1980**, *26*, 406–411. [CrossRef]
2. Hirano, R.; Namazuda, K.; Hirata, N. Double filtration plasmapheresis: Review of current clinical applications. *Ther. Apher. Dial.* **2020**, *25*, 145–151. [CrossRef] [PubMed]
3. Lumlertgul, D.; Suteeka, Y.; Tumpong, S.; Bunnachak, D.; Boonkaew, S. Double Filtration Plasmapheresis in Different Diseases in Thailand. *Ther. Apher. Dial.* **2013**, *17*, 99–116. [CrossRef] [PubMed]
4. Mineshima, M.; Akiba, T. Double Filtration Plasmapheresis in Critical Care. *Ther. Apher. Dial.* **2002**, *6*, 180–183. [CrossRef]
5. Yeh, J.-H.; Chiu, H.-C. Comparison between double-filtration plasmapheresis and immunoadsorption plasmapheresis in the treatment of patients with myasthenia gravis. *J. Neurol.* **2000**, *247*, 510–513. [CrossRef]
6. Bennani, H.N.; Lagrange, E.; Noble, J.; Malvezzi, P.; Motte, L.; Chevallier, E.; Rostaing, L.; Jouve, T. Treatment of refractory myasthenia gravis by double-filtration plasmapheresis and rituximab: A case series of nine patients and literature review. *J. Clin. Apher.* **2020**, *36*, 348–363. [CrossRef]
7. Liu, J.-F.; Wang, W.-X.; Xue, J.; Zhao, C.-B.; You, H.-Z.; Lu, J.-H.; Gu, Y. Comparing the Autoantibody Levels and Clinical Efficacy of Double Filtration Plasmapheresis, Immunoadsorption, and Intravenous Immunoglobulin for the Treatment of Late-onset Myasthenia Gravis. *Ther. Apher. Dial.* **2010**, *14*, 153–160. [CrossRef]
8. Zhang, L.; Liu, J.; Wang, H.; Zhao, C.; Lu, J.; Xue, J.; Gu, Y.; Hao, C.; Lin, S.; Lv, C. Double filtration plasmapheresis benefits myasthenia gravis patients through an immunomodulatory action. *J. Clin. Neurosci.* **2014**, *21*, 1570–1574. [CrossRef]
9. Yeh, J.H.; Chiu, H.C. Double filtration plasmapheresis in myasthenia gravis—Analysis of clinical efficacy and prognostic parameters. *Acta Neurol. Scand.* **2009**, *100*, 305–309. [CrossRef]
10. Yeh, J.H.; Chen, W.H.; Chiu, H.C. Double filtration plasmapheresis in the treatment of myasthenic crisis—analysis of prognostic factors and efficacy. *Acta Neurol. Scand.* **2001**, *104*, 78–82. [CrossRef]

11. Liu, C.; Liu, P.; Ma, M.; Yang, H.; Qi, G. Efficacy and safety of double-filtration plasmapheresis treatment of myasthenia gravis. *Medicine* **2021**, *100*, e25622. [CrossRef] [PubMed]
12. Ito, Y.; Odaka, M.; Tabata, Y.; Soeda, K.; Hayashi, H.; Kobayashi, S.; Sato, T.; Yamane, S.; Isono, K. Clinical Experience of Double Filtration Plasmapheresis for Drug Refractory Neurological Diseases. *Biomater. Artif. Cells Immobil. Biotechnol.* **2009**, *19*, 27–35. [CrossRef] [PubMed]
13. Zhang, Y.-Y.; Tang, Z.; Chen, D.-M.; Gong, D.-H.; Ji, D.-X.; Liu, Z.-H. Comparison of double filtration plasmapheresis with immunoadsorption therapy in patients with anti-glomerular basement membrane nephritis. *BMC Nephrol.* **2014**, *15*, 128. [CrossRef] [PubMed]
14. Koyama, R.; Kato, M.; Yamashita, S.; Nakanishi, K.; Kuwahara, H.; Katori, H. Hypoglycemia and Hyperglycemia Due to Insulin Antibodies against Therapeutic Human Insulin: Treatment with Double Filtration Plasmapheresis and Prednisolone. *Am. J. Med. Sci.* **2005**, *329*, 259–264. [CrossRef]
15. Galán Carrillo, I.; Demelo-Rodriguez, P.; Rodríguez Ferrero, M.L.; Anaya, F. Double filtration plasmapheresis in the treatment of pancreatitis due to severe hypertriglyceridemia. *J. Clin. Lipidol.* **2015**, *9*, 698–702. [CrossRef]
16. Huang, S.-P.; Toh, D.-E.; Sue, Y.-M.; Chen, T.-H.; Cheng, S.-W.; Cheng, C.-Y. Double filtration plasmapheresis in treatment of acute pancreatitis associated with severe hypertriglyceridemia. *Medicine* **2018**, *97*, e12987. [CrossRef]
17. Lu, Z.; Chen, Y.; Wu, Y.; Lin, Y.; Yang, N.; Wang, X.; Guo, F. The role of double filtration plasmapheresis in hypertriglyceridemic pancreatitis: A propensity score matching analysis. *J. Clin. Apher.* **2020**, *35*, 388–397. [CrossRef]
18. Lyu, R.-K.; Chen, W.-H.; Hsieh, S.-T. Plasma Exchange Versus Double Filtration Plasmapheresis in the Treatment of Guillain-Barre Syndrome. *Ther. Apher. Dial.* **2002**, *6*, 163–166. [CrossRef]
19. Lin, J.-H.; Tu, K.-H.; Chang, C.-H.; Chen, Y.-C.; Tian, Y.-C.; Yu, C.-C.; Hung, C.-C.; Fang, J.-T.; Yang, C.-W.; Chang, M.-Y. Prognostic factors and complication rates for double-filtration plasmapheresis in patients with Guillain–Barré syndrome. *Transfus. Apher. Sci.* **2015**, *52*, 78–83. [CrossRef]
20. Cheng, B.-C.; Chang, W.-N.; Chen, J.-B.; Chee, E.C.-Y.; Huang, C.-R.; Lu, C.-H.; Chang, C.-J.; Hung, P.-L.; Chuang, Y.-C.; Lee, C.-T.; et al. Long-term prognosis for Guillain-Barré syndrome: Evaluation of prognostic factors and clinical experience of automated double filtration plasmapheresis. *J. Clin. Apher.* **2003**, *18*, 175–180. [CrossRef]
21. Chen, W.-H.; Yeh, J.-H.; Chiu, H.-C. Experience of double filtration plasmapheresis in the treatment of Guillain-Barré syndrome. *J. Clin. Apher.* **1999**, *14*, 126–129. [CrossRef]
22. Yu, X.; Ma, J.; Tian, J.; Jiang, S.; Xu, P.; Han, H.; Wang, L. A Controlled Study of Double Filtration Plasmapheresis in the Treatment of Active Rheumatoid Arthritis. *JCR J. Clin. Rheumatol.* **2007**, *13*, 193–198. [CrossRef] [PubMed]
23. Matsuda, Y.; Tsuda, H.; Takasaki, Y.; Hashimoto, H. Double Filtration Plasmapheresis for the Treatment of a Rheumatoid Arthritis Patient with Extremely High Level of C-reactive Protein. *Ther. Apher. Dial.* **2004**, *8*, 404–408. [CrossRef] [PubMed]
24. Liu, J.-D.; Zhang, C.; Li, W.-S.; Lun, L.-D. Double Filtration Plasmapheresis for the Treatment of Rheumatoid Arthritis: A Study of 21 Cases. *Artif. Organs* **2008**, *21*, 96–98. [CrossRef]
25. Fujiwara, K.; Kaneko, S.; Kakumu, S.; Sata, M.; Hige, S.; Tomita, E.; Mochida, S. Double filtration plasmapheresis and interferon combination therapy for chronic hepatitis C patients with genotype 1 and high viral load. *Hepatol. Res.* **2007**, *37*, 701–710. [CrossRef]
26. Kaneko, S.; Sata, M.; Ide, T.; Yamashita, T.; Hige, S.; Tomita, E.; Mochida, S.; Yamashita, Y.; Inui, Y.; Kim, S.R.; et al. Efficacy and safety of double filtration plasmapheresis in combination with interferon therapy for chronic hepatitis C. *Hepatol. Res.* **2010**, *40*, 1072–1081. [CrossRef]
27. Higashihara, T.; Kawase, M.; Kobayashi, M.; Hara, M.; Matsuzaki, H.; Uni, R.; Matsumura, M.; Etoh, T.; Takano, H. Evaluating the Efficacy of Double-Filtration Plasmapheresis in Treating Five Patients With Drug-Resistant Pemphigus. *Ther. Apher. Dial.* **2017**, *21*, 243–247. [CrossRef]
28. Liu, Y.; Zhang, B.; Ma, J.; Wang, H.; Fan, X.; Zheng, K.; Chen, L.; Li, X.; Qin, Y.; Li, L.; et al. Double-filtration plasmapheresis combined with immunosuppressive treatment for severe pemphigus: 10 years' experience of a single center in China. *J. Clin. Apher.* **2020**, *36*, 20–27. [CrossRef]
29. Hatano, Y.; Katagiri, K.; Arakawa, S.; Umeki, T.; Takayasu, S.; Fujiwara, S. Successful treatment by double-filtration plasmapheresis of a patient with bullous pemphigoid: Effects in vivo on transcripts of several genes for chemokines and cytokines in peripheral blood mononuclear cells. *Br. J. Dermatol.* **2003**, *148*, 573–579. [CrossRef]
30. Kitabata, Y.; Sakurane, M.; Orita, H.; Kamimura, M.; Siizaki, K.; Narukawa, N.; Kaketaka, A.; Abe, T.; Kobata, H.; Akizawa, T. Double Filtration Plasmapheresis for the Treatment of Bullous Pemphigoid: A Three Case Report. *Ther. Apher. Dial.* **2001**, *5*, 484–490. [CrossRef]
31. Kim, J.-Y.; Park, J.S.; Park, J.-C.; Kim, M.-E.; Nahm, D.-H. Double-Filtration Plasmapheresis for the Treatment of Patients With Recalcitrant Atopic Dermatitis. *Ther. Apher. Dial.* **2013**, *17*, 631–637. [CrossRef] [PubMed]
32. Podestà Manuel, A.; Gennarini, A.; Portalupi, V.; Rota, S.; Alessio Maria, G.; Remuzzi, G.; Ruggenenti, P. Accelerating the Depletion of Circulating Anti-Phospholipase A_2 Receptor Antibodies in Patients with Severe Membranous Nephropathy: Preliminary Findings with Double Filtration Plasmapheresis and Ofatumumab. *Nephron* **2020**, *144*, 30–35. [CrossRef] [PubMed]
33. Tian, Y.R.; Sun, L.L.; Wang, W.; Du, F.; Song, A.X.; Ni, C.Y.; Zhu, Q.; Wan, Q. A Case of Acute Thallotoxicosis Successfully Treated With Double-Filtration Plasmapheresis. *Clin. Neuropharmacol.* **2005**, *28*, 292–294. [CrossRef] [PubMed]

34. Gong, D.; Ji, D.; Xu, B.; Liu, Z. More Selective Removal of Myeloperoxidase-Anti-Neutrophil Cytoplasmic Antibody From the Circulation of Patients With Vasculitides Using a Novel Double-Filtration Plasmapheresis Therapy. *Ther. Apher. Dial.* **2013**, *17*, 93–98. [CrossRef] [PubMed]
35. Chen, Y.; Yang, L.; Li, K.; Liu, Z.; Gong, D.; Zhang, H.; Liu, Z.; Hu, W. Double Filtration Plasmapheresis in the Treatment of Antineutrophil Cytoplasmic Autoantibody Associated Vasculitis with Severe Renal Failure: A Preliminary Study of 15 Patients. *Ther. Apher. Dial.* **2016**, *20*, 183–188. [CrossRef] [PubMed]
36. Cheng, L.; Tang, Y.-Q.; Yi, J.; Ren, Q.; Yang, X.-Y.; Gou, S.-J.; Zhang, L.; Fu, P. Double Filtration Plasmapheresis in the Treatment of Anti-Neutrophil Cytoplasmic Antibody-Associated Vasculitis with Severe Kidney Dysfunction. *Blood Purif.* **2020**, *49*, 713–722. [CrossRef]
37. Bozkirli, D.E.E.; Kozanoglu, I.; Bozkirli, E.; Yucel, E. Antisynthetase syndrome with refractory lung involvement and myositis successfully treated with double filtration plasmapheresis. *J. Clin. Apher.* **2013**, *28*, 422–425. [CrossRef]
38. Li, M.; Wang, Y.; Qiu, Q.; Wei, R.; Gao, Y.; Zhang, L.; Wang, Y.; Zhang, X.; Chen, X. Therapeutic effect of double-filtration plasmapheresis combined with methylprednisolone to treat diffuse proliferative lupus nephritis. *J. Clin. Apher.* **2016**, *31*, 375–380. [CrossRef]
39. Jiang, X.; Lu, M.; Ying, Y.; Feng, J.; Ye, Y. A Case Report of Double-Filtration Plasmapheresis for the Resolution of Refractory Chronic Urticaria. *Ther. Apher. Dial.* **2008**, *12*, 505–508. [CrossRef]
40. Liu, L.-L.; Li, X.-L.; Wang, L.-N.; Yao, L.; Fan, Q.-L.; Li, Z.-L. Successful treatment of patients with systemic lupus erythematosus complicated with autoimmune thyroid disease using double-filtration plasmapheresis: A retrospective study. *J. Clin. Apher.* **2011**, *26*, 174–180. [CrossRef]
41. Kamei, K.; Yamaguchi, K.; Sato, M.; Ogura, M.; Ito, S.; Okada, T.; Wada, S.; Sago, H. Successful treatment of severe rhesus D-incompatible pregnancy with repeated double-filtration plasmapheresis. *J. Clin. Apher.* **2015**, *30*, 305–307. [CrossRef] [PubMed]
42. Taniguchi, F.; Horie, S.; Tsukihara, S.; Nagata, N.; Nishikawa, K.; Terakawa, N. Successful Management of a P-Incompatible Pregnancy Using Double Filtration Plasmapheresis. *Gynecol. Obstet. Investig.* **2003**, *56*, 117–120. [CrossRef] [PubMed]
43. Kato, T.; Kobayashi, T.; Nishino, H.; Hidaka, Y. Double-filtration plasmapheresis for resolution of corticosteroid resistant adult onset still's disease. *Clin. Rheumatol.* **2006**, *25*, 579–582. [CrossRef] [PubMed]
44. Ramunni, A.; De Robertis, F.; Brescia, P.; Saliani, M.T.; Amoruso, M.; Prontera, M.; Dimonte, E.; Trojano, M.; Coratelli, P. A Case Report of Double Filtration Plasmapheresis in an Acute Episode of Multiple Sclerosis. *Ther. Apher. Dial.* **2008**, *12*, 250–254. [CrossRef]
45. De Masi, R.; Orlando, S.; Accoto, S. Double Filtration Plasmapheresis Treatment of Refractory Multiple Sclerosis Relapsed on Fingolimod: A Case Report. *Appl. Sci.* **2020**, *10*, 7404. [CrossRef]
46. Matsuo, H. Plasmapheresis in acute phase of multiple sclerosis and neuromyelitis optica. *Nihon Rinsho. Jpn. J. Clin. Med.* **2014**, *72*, 1999–2002.
47. Meço, B.C.; Memikoğlu, O.; İlhan, O.; Ayyıldız, E.; Gunt, C.; Ünal, N.; Oral, M.; Tulunay, M. Double filtration plasmapheresis for a case of Crimean-Congo hemorrhagic fever. *Transfus. Apher. Sci.* **2013**, *48*, 331–334. [CrossRef]
48. Chauvel, F.; Reboul, P.; Cariou, S.; Aglae, C.; Renaud, S.; Trusson, R.; Garo, F.; Ahmadpoor, P.; Prelipcean, C.; Pambrun, E.; et al. Use of double filtration plasmapheresis for the treatment of acquired thrombocytopenic thrombotic purpura. *Ther. Apher. Dial.* **2020**, *24*, 709–717. [CrossRef]
49. Yoshida, H.; Ando, A.; Sho, K.; Akioka, M.; Kawai, E.; Arai, E.; Nishimura, T.; Shinde, A.; Masaki, H.; Takahashi, K.; et al. Anti-Aquaporin-4 Antibody-Positive Optic Neuritis Treated with Double-Filtration Plasmapheresis. *J. Ocul. Pharmacol. Ther.* **2010**, *26*, 381–385. [CrossRef]
50. Miyamoto, K.; Kusunoki, S. Intermittent Plasmapheresis Prevents Recurrence in Neuromyelitis Optica. *Ther. Apher. Dial.* **2009**, *13*, 505–508. [CrossRef]
51. Lew, W.H.; Chang, C.-J.; Lin, J.-D.; Cheng, C.-Y.; Chen, Y.-K.; Lee, T.-I. Successful preoperative treatment of a Graves' disease patient with agranulocytosis and hemophagocytosis using double filtration plasmapheresis. *J. Clin. Apher.* **2011**, *26*, 159–161. [CrossRef] [PubMed]
52. Otsubo, S.; Nitta, K.; Yumura, W.; Nihei, H.; Mori, N. Antiphospholipid Syndrome Treated with Prednisolone, Cyclophosphamide and Double-Filtration Plasmapheresis. *Intern. Med.* **2002**, *41*, 725–729. [CrossRef] [PubMed]
53. Yeh, J.-H.; Cheng, C.-K.; Chiu, H.-C. A Case Report of Double-Filtration Plasmapheresis for the Treatment of Age-related Macular Degeneration. *Ther. Apher. Dial.* **2008**, *12*, 500–504. [CrossRef] [PubMed]
54. Suga, K.; Yamashita, H.; Takahashi, Y.; Katagiri, D.; Hinoshita, F.; Kaneko, H. Therapeutic efficacy of combined glucocorticoid, intravenous cyclophosphamide, and double-filtration plasmapheresis for skin sclerosis in diffuse systemic sclerosis. *Medicine* **2020**, *99*, e19301. [CrossRef]
55. Mednikov, R.V.; Rabinovich, V.I.; Kizlo, S.N.; Belyakov, N.A.; Sokolov, A.A. Double Filtration Plasmapheresis in Treatment of Patients With Co-Infection of Hepatitis C and Human Immunodeficiency Virus. *Ther. Apher. Dial.* **2016**, *20*, 413–419. [CrossRef]
56. Hasegawa, Y.; Tagaya, M.; Fujimoto, S.; Hayashida, K.; Yamaguchi, T.; Minematsu, K. Extracorporeal double filtration plasmapheresis in acute atherothrombotic brain infarction caused by major artery occlusive lesion. *J. Clin. Apher.* **2003**, *18*, 167–174. [CrossRef]
57. Ramunni, A.; Brescia, P. Double Filtration Plasmapheresis: An Effective Treatment of Cryoglobulinemia. *HCV Infect. Cryoglobulinemia* **2012**, 337–341. [CrossRef]

58. Chiu, H.-C.; Chen, W.-H.; Yeh, J.-H. Double Filtration Plasmapheresis in the Treatment of Inflammatory Polyneuropathy. *Ther. Apher.* **1997**, *1*, 183–186. [CrossRef]
59. Kumazawa, K.; Yuasa, N.; Mitsuma, T.; Nagamatsu, M.; Sobue, G. Double filtration plasmapheresis (DFPP) in chronic inflammatory demyelinating polyradiculoneuropathy (CIDP). *Rinsho Shinkeigaku Clin. Neurol.* **1998**, *38*, 719–723.
60. Tagawa, Y.; Yuki, N.; Hirata, K. Ability to remove immunoglobulins and anti-ganglioside antibodies by plasma exchange, double-filtration plasmapheresis and immunoadsorption. *J. Neurol. Sci.* **1998**, *157*, 90–95. [CrossRef]
61. Vatazin, A.V.; Zulkarnaev, A.B. The impact of therapeutic plasma exchange and double filtration plasmapheresis on hemostasis in renal transplant recipients. *Ter. Arkhiv* **2018**, *90*, 22–27. [CrossRef] [PubMed]
62. Uchida, S.; Sakagami, K.; Miyazaki, M.; Shiozaki, S.; Fujiwara, T.; Haisa, M.; Saitou, S.; Orita, K. Efficacy of large-volume double filtration plasmapheresis as adjunctive therapy for cancers. *Jpn. J. Artif. Organs* **1990**, *19*, 933–936.
63. Straube, R.; Müller, G.; Voit-Bak, K.; Tselmin, S.; Julius, U.; Schatz, U.; Rietzsch, H.; Reichmann, H.; Chrousos, G.P.; Schürmann, A.; et al. Metabolic and Non-Metabolic Peripheral Neuropathy: Is there a Place for Therapeutic Apheresis? *Horm. Metab. Res.* **2019**, *51*, 779–784. [CrossRef] [PubMed]
64. Straube, R.; Voit-Bak, K.; Gor, A.; Steinmeier, T.; Chrousos, G.P.; Boehm, B.O.; Birkenfeld, A.L.; Barbir, M.; Balanzew, W.; Bornstein, S.R. Lipid Profiles in Lyme Borreliosis: A Potential Role for Apheresis? *Horm. Metab. Res.* **2019**, *51*, 326–329. [CrossRef] [PubMed]
65. Bornstein, S.R.; Voit-Bak, K.; Rosenthal, P.; Tselmin, S.; Julius, U.; Schatz, U.; Boehm, B.O.; Thuret, S.; Kempermann, G.; Reichmann, H.; et al. Extracorporeal apheresis therapy for Alzheimer disease—Targeting lipids, stress, and inflammation. *Mol. Psychiatry* **2019**, *25*, 275–282. [CrossRef]
66. Bornstein, S.R.; Voit-Bak, K.; Donate, T.; Rodionov, R.N.; Gainetdinov, R.R.; Tselmin, S.; Kanczkowski, W.; Müller, G.M.; Achleitner, M.; Wang, J.; et al. Chronic post-COVID-19 syndrome and chronic fatigue syndrome: Is there a role for extracorporeal apheresis? *Mol. Psychiatry* **2021**, *27*, 34–37. [CrossRef]
67. Shi, L.; Buckley, N.J.; Bos, I.; Engelborghs, S.; Sleegers, K.; Frisoni, G.B.; Wallin, A.; Lléo, A.; Popp, J.; Martinez-Lage, P.; et al. Plasma Proteomic Biomarkers Relating to Alzheimer's Disease: A Meta-Analysis Based on Our Own Studies. *Front. Aging Neurosci.* **2021**, *13*. [CrossRef]
68. Varma, V.R.; Varma, S.; An, Y.; Hohman, T.J.; Seddighi, S.; Casanova, R.; Beri, A.; Dammer, E.B.; Seyfried, N.T.; Pletnikova, O.; et al. Alpha-2 macroglobulin in Alzheimer's disease: A marker of neuronal injury through the RCAN1 pathway. *Mol. Psychiatry* **2016**, *22*, 13–23. [CrossRef]
69. Yin, X.; Takov, K.; Straube, R.; Voit-Bak, K.; Graessler, J.; Julius, U.; Tselmin, S.; Rodionov, R.; Barbir, M.; Walls, M.; et al. Precision Medicine Approach for Cardiometabolic Risk Factors in Therapeutic Apheresis. *Horm. Metab. Res. Horm. Und. Stoffwechs. Horm. Et. Metab.* **2022**, *54*, 238–249. [CrossRef]
70. Patton, K.T.; Thibodeau, G.A. *The Human Body in Health & Disease*, 7th ed.; Mosby: Maryland Heights, MI, USA, 2018.
71. Bossingham, M.J.; Carnell, N.S.; Campbell, W.W. Water balance, hydration status, and fat-free mass hydration in younger and older adults. *Am. J. Clin. Nutr.* **2005**, *81*, 1342–1350. [CrossRef]
72. Ohashi, Y.; Joki, N.; Yamazaki, K.; Kawamura, T.; Tai, R.; Oguchi, H.; Yuasa, R.; Sakai, K. Changes in the fluid volume balance between intra- and extracellular water in a sample of Japanese adults aged 15–88 yr old: A cross-sectional study. *Am. J. Physiol. Ren. Physiol.* **2018**, *314*, F614–F622. [CrossRef] [PubMed]
73. Levy, Y.; Onuchic, J.N. Water Mediation in Protein Folding and Molecular Recognition. *Annu. Rev. Biophys. Biomol. Struct.* **2006**, *35*, 389–415. [CrossRef] [PubMed]
74. Ludwig, R. Protonated Water Clusters: The Third Dimension. *ChemPhysChem* **2004**, *5*, 1495–1497. [CrossRef] [PubMed]
75. De Silva, N.; Adreance, M.A.; Gordon, M.S. Application of a semi-empirical dispersion correction for modeling water clusters. *J. Comput. Chem.* **2018**, *40*, 310–315. [CrossRef]
76. Tsenkova, R. Aquaphotomics: Dynamic Spectroscopy of Aqueous and Biological Systems Describes Peculiarities of Water. *J. Near Infrared Spectrosc.* **2009**, *17*, 303–313. [CrossRef]
77. Tsenkova, R. Aquaphotomics: Water in the biological and aqueous world scrutinised with invisible light. *Spectrosc. Eur.* **2010**, *22*, 6–10.
78. Tsenkova, R.; Munćan, J.; Pollner, B.; Kovacs, Z. Essentials of Aquaphotomics and Its Chemometrics Approaches. *Front. Chem.* **2018**, *6*, 363. [CrossRef]
79. Muncan, J.; Tsenkova, R. Aquaphotomics—From Innovative Knowledge to Integrative Platform in Science and Technology. *Molecules* **2019**, *24*, 2742. [CrossRef]
80. Tsenkova, R.; Kovacs, Z.; Kubota, Y. Aquaphotomics: Near Infrared Spectroscopy and Water States in Biological Systems. *Membr. Hydration* **2015**, *71*, 189–211. [CrossRef]
81. de Kraats, V.; Everine, B.; Munćan, J.; Tsenkova, R.N. Aquaphotomics—Origin, concept, applications and future perspective. *Substantia* **2021**, *3*, 13–28.
82. Seki, T.; Chiang, K.-Y.; Yu, C.-C.; Yu, X.; Okuno, M.; Hunger, J.; Nagata, Y.; Bonn, M. The Bending Mode of Water: A Powerful Probe for Hydrogen Bond Structure of Aqueous Systems. *J. Phys. Chem. Lett.* **2020**, *11*, 8459–8469. [CrossRef] [PubMed]
83. Zheng, J.M.; Chin, W.C.; Khijniak, E.; Khijniak, E., Jr.; Pollack, G.H. Surfaces and interfacial water: Evidence that hydrophilic surfaces have long-range impact. *Adv. Colloid Interface Sci.* **2006**, *127*, 19–27. [CrossRef] [PubMed]

84. Hwang, S.G.; Hong, J.K.; Sharma, A.; Pollack, G.H.; Bahng, G. Exclusion zone and heterogeneous water structure at ambient temperature. *PLoS ONE* **2018**, *13*, e0195057. [CrossRef] [PubMed]
85. Muncan, J.M.I.; Matovic, V.; Sakota Rosic, J.; Matija, L. The prospects of aquaphotomics in biomedical science and engineering. In Proceedings of the 2nd International Aquaphotomics Symposium, Kobe, Japan, 26–29 November 2016.

MDPI
St. Alban-Anlage 66
4052 Basel
Switzerland
Tel. +41 61 683 77 34
Fax +41 61 302 89 18
www.mdpi.com

Molecules Editorial Office
E-mail: molecules@mdpi.com
www.mdpi.com/journal/molecules

www.ingramcontent.com/pod-product-compliance
Lightning Source LLC
LaVergne TN
LVHW070240100526
838202LV00015B/2159
* 9 7 8 3 0 3 6 5 7 1 1 8 8 *